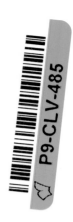

Food IS Medicine

EDIBLE PLANT FOODS,
FRUITS, AND SPICES
FROM A TO Z:
EVIDENCE FOR THEIR
HEALING PROPERTIES

....

VOLUME TWO

Brian R. Clement, PhD, NMD, LN

....

HIPPOCRATES PUBLICATIONS
SUMMERTOWN, TENNESSEE

© 2013 Brian R. Clement

Cover and interior design: Scattaregia Design

Hippocrates Publications
an imprint of Book Publishing Company
PO Box 99
Summertown, TN 38483
888-260-8458
bookpubco.com

ISBN: 978-1-57067-300-9

19 18 17 16 15 14 13   1 2 3 4 5 6 7 8 9

Library of Congress Cataloging-in-Publication Data is available upon request

Book Publishing Company is a member of Green Press Initiative. We chose to print this title on paper with 100% postconsumer recycled content, processed without chlorine, which saved the following natural resources:

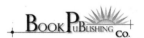

- 64 trees
- 1,990 pounds of solid waste
- 29,730 gallons of water
- 5,481 pounds of greenhouse gases
- 28 million BTU of energy

For more information on Green Press Initiative, visit www.greenpressinitiative.org. Environmental impact estimates were made using the Environmental Defense Fund Paper Calculator. For more information visit www.papercalculator.org.

Table of Contents

Introduction

by Brian R. Clement, Ph.D., NMD, LNC.

MEDICAL SCIENCE, with all of its many technological advancements, lost its way during most of the twentieth century in terms of finding the natural biological path to maintaining and enhancing human health. Western academic communities, with their mostly cerebral and arrogant approach to nature, distanced themselves from the roots of nutrition responsible for their very existence.

The time is ripe for a return to a fundamental foundation of biology so that we might not only employ what we have fabricated from nature, but also vigorously study and apply the genius found within it. As evidenced by the huge amount of documentation that you will find in the following pages, this process now seems well under way.

Within this book, volume two of the *Food IS Medicine* series, the focus is on scientific medical studies that evaluate the health benefits of specific edible plants—vegetables, fruits, and spices—and their nutrient factors. It was only in the mid-twentieth century that Western medical and nutritional science first stumbled upon this potential for nature to address all of the ills of human health, an awareness that had already been possessed by tribal cultures and ancient wisdom traditions since well before the time of Hippocrates and the other great Greek philosophers.

Now, after endless hours and billions of dollars spent internationally, a new and profound nutritional science has emerged that reaffirms many of the trial and error findings of ancient knowledge. Terms like "phytochemo," referring to the anticancer effect that certain food-based chemistries possess, have begun to replace terms familiar to the pharmaceutical industry. Even at this early stage of discovery, we have developed a wide catalogue of supported evidential science that is revolutionizing research into maladies, recovery, and aging.

My organization, the Hippocrates Health Institute, pioneered a renaissance in this new world view of nutrition and health more than half a century ago. Today, with validation of our approach being provided by thousands of peer-reviewed medical science studies, we are better able to understand the multitude of dimensions that interplay to bring about disease prevention, healing, and longevity.

This volume, *Edible Plant Foods, Fruits, and Spices from A to Z*, features thirty-nine of the most studied foods and spices and provides a compendium of discoveries about the health benefits of each. The medical science studies covered in this book, several thousand in all, come from reputable researchers and academic institutions worldwide and were published in mainstream peer-reviewed science journals.

Some of the foods have been studied most extensively by scientists within the cultures where those particular foods have long been a staple in both diets and medical traditions. For example, Japanese medical researchers have undertaken many of the studies on algae and sea vegetables, used as a food source for centuries in Japan. Research institutes in India have performed a large percentage of the studies on the health benefits of curcumin, a phytochemical abundant in the spice turmeric, which has a rich history of dietary and medical use in that culture dating back thousands of years.

From the studies on foods and spices detailed in this book, several patterns emerge that are worth identifying and bringing to your attention. Many lists of so-called superfoods that purportedly empower health already circulate in the mainstream media. Most of these lists carry little or no scientific weight and often simply reflect the list maker's wishful thinking and dietary agenda.

The following list of the top ten superfoods, however, is based purely on the weight of study evidence showing the variety of ailments these foods can potentially prevent or treat. The same is true for the top ten cancer fighting foods list. Think of these two lists as a handy reference point to guide you in making healthful food choices.

Top 10 Super Foods
(Based on Numbers of Conditions Prevented or Treated)

Algae : 44 conditions
Garlic: 32 conditions
Curcumin (in turmeric): 29 conditions
Resveratrol (in grapes and berries): 23 conditions
Onions: 20 conditions
Apples: 19 conditions
Blueberries: 19 conditions
Pomegranates: 16 conditions
Cranberries: 17 conditions
Strawberries: 15 conditions

Top 10 Cancer Fighting Foods
(Based on Cancer Types Prevented or Treated)

Garlic: 15 types

Curcumin (in turmeric): 14 types

Cranberries: 13 types

Broccoli: 11 types

Mushrooms: 11 types

Resveratrol (in grapes and berries): 10 types

Spinach: 9 types

Berries (in general): 8 types

Oranges: 7 types

Tomatoes: 9 types

When we combine the results from the two lists above, garlic and curcumin emerge as the top two superfoods in the arsenal of natural prevention and treatment therapies. They are the dynamic duo and have proven their value to human health both in science and in practice.

With this volume of the *Food IS Medicine* series in hand, no longer do you have to rely on abstract and shaky methods when treating either yourself or others. Getting back to simple proven techniques that rely on pure nutrition should be the future for all forms of legitimate medicine.

Join this potent revolution in quantum biology that will hopefully once and for all silence the fragile and historically tainted processes often called modern science.

Algae (see also Sea Vegetables)

ONCE DISMISSED BY MAINSTREAM MEDICINE as just "pond scum," blue-green algae, a single-cell organism also known as cyanobacteria, ranks as one of the oldest life-forms on the planet and one that has achieved new respectability as a source of healing agents. Fossilized remains of cyanobacteria have been found that date back to nearly three billion years ago. The types examined here can be found in both seawater and freshwater environments.

Spirulina is one of the therapeutic types of blue-green alga, with two species—*Arthrospira platensis* and *Arthrospira maxima*—now being used as dietary supplements. The Aztecs and other Mesoamerican cultures harvested spirulina from lakes and then dried it to create cakes eaten as a nutritious food. It has a long history of use in the African nation Chad, where it was harvested from ponds and lakes. It is rich in protein, containing up to 77 percent protein by dry weight, and contains all of the essential amino acids, making it a source of complete protein. It also has the B vitamins thiamin, riboflavin, niacinamide, pyridoxine, and folic acid and vitamins A, C, D, and E.

Chlorella is a single-celled green algae that contains the photosynthetic pigments chlorophyll a and chlorophyll b. It too is a complete protein. The composition of dried chlorella is nearly half protein and 10 percent vitamins and minerals, with the remainder being fats and carbohydrates. Like blue-green algae, chlorella acts as a detoxifier when absorbed by the human body and has been scientifically proven to reduce cholesterol and high blood pressure and enhance immune system function, among many other health benefits.

Aging

Dietary supplementation with blueberries, spinach, or spirulina reduces ischemic brain damage. Wang Y, Chang CF, Chou J, Chen HL, Deng X, Harvey BK, Cadet JL, Bickford PC. Exp Neurol. 2005 May;193(1):75-84. **Key Finding:** "Free radicals are involved in neurodegenerative disorders, such as **ischemia** and **aging**. We have previously demonstrated that treatment with diets enriched with blueberry, spinach, or spirulina have been shown to reduce neurodegenerative changes in aged animals. The purpose of this study was to determine if these diets have neuroprotective effects in focal ischemic brain in Sprague-Dawley rats. Animals treated with blueberry, spinach, or spirulina had significantly lower caspase-3 activity in the ischemic hemisphere. In conclusion, our data suggest that chronic treatment with blueberry, spinach, or spirulina reduces ischemia/reperfusion-induced apoptosis and cerebral infarction."

Diets enriched in foods with high **antioxidant** *activity reverse age-induced decreases in cerebellar beta-adrenergic function and increases in proinflammatory cytokines.* Gemma C. Mesches MH, Sepesi B, Choo K, Holmes DB, Bickford PC. J Neurosci. 2002 Jul 15;22(14):6114-20. **Key Finding:** "Antioxidants and diets supplemented with foods high in oxygen radical absorbance capacity (ORAC) reverse **age-**related decreases in cerebellar beta-adrenergic receptor function. Aged male Fischer 344 rats were given apple (5 mg dry weight), spirulina (5 mg) or cucumber (5 mg) daily for 14 days. Electrophysiologic techniques revealed a significant decrease in beta-adrenergic receptor function in aged control rats. Spirulina reversed this effect. Apple had an intermediate effect, and cucumber (low ORAC) had no effect, indicating that the reversal of beta-adrenergic receptor function decreases might be related to the ORAC dose."

Allergic Rhinitis

The effects of spirulina on **allergic rhinitis.** Cingi C, Conk-Dalay M, Cakli H, Bal C. Eur Arch Otorhinolaryngol. 2008 Oct;265(10):1219-23. **Key Finding:** "Spirulina consumption significantly improved the symptoms and physical findings compared with placebo including nasal discharge, sneezing, nasal congestion and itching. Spirulina is clinically effective on allergic rhinitis."

Effects of a Spirulina-based dietary supplement on cytokine production from **allergic rhinitis** *patients.* Mao TK, Van de Water J, Gershwin ME, J Med Food. 2005 Spring;8(1):27-30. **Key Finding:** "Although Spirulina seemed to be ineffective at modulating the secretion of Th1 cytokines (IFN-gamma and IL-2), we discovered that Spirulina, administered at 2,000 mg/day, significantly reduced IL-4 levels by 32% from PHA-stimulated cells. These results indicate that Spirulina can modulate the Th profile in patients with allergic rhinitis."

Experimental study of spirulina platensis in treating **allergic rhinitis** *in rats.* Chen LL, Zhang SF, Huang DN, Tan JQ, He SH. Zhong Nan Da Xue bao Yi Xue Ban (Chinese),2005 Feb;30(1):96-8. **Key Finding:** "Spirulina platensis can prevent and treat allergic rhinitis in rats, which implies the possibility of using it for AR patients in the future."

Alzheimer's

Oral phycocyanobilin may diminish the pathogenicity of activated brain microglia in **neuro-degenerative disorders**. McCarty MF, Barroso-Aranda J, Contreras F. Med Hypotheses. 2009 Jul 1. (Epub ahead of print). **Key Finding:** "There is considerable evidence that activated microglia play a central role in the pathogenesis of many prominent neurodegenerative disorders, including **Parkinson's** and **Alzheimer's** diseases. Phycocyanobilin, a chromophone derived from biliverdin that constitutes up to 1% of the dry weight of Spirulina, has been shown to be a potent inhibitor of NADPH oxidase. Phycocyanobilin supplements may have considerable potential for preventing or slowing the progression of a range of neurodegenerative disorders."

Neuroprotection by Spirulina platensis protean extract and phycocyanin against iron-induced toxicity in SH-SY5Y neuroblastoma cells. Bermejo-Bescos P, Piñero-Estrada E, Villar del Fresno AM. Toxicol In Vitro. 2008 Sep;22(6):1496-502. **Key Finding:** "These results suggested that S. platensis protean extract is a powerful antioxidant through a mechanism related to antioxidant activity, capable of interfering with radical-mediated cell death. S. platensis may be useful in diseases known to be aggravated by reactive oxygen species and in the development of novel treatments for neurodegenerative disorders as long as iron has been implicated in the neuropathology of several neurodegenerative disorders such as **Alzheimer's** and **Parkinson diseases**."

Blueberry- and spirulina-enriched diets enhance striatal dopamine recovery and induce a rapid, transient microglia activation after injury of the rat nigrostriatal dopamine system. Stromberg I, Gemma C, Vila J, Bickford PC. Exp Neurol. 2005 Dec;196(2):298-307. **Key Finding:** "Neuroinflammation plays a critical role in loss of dopamine neurons during brain injury and in **neurodegenerative diseases**. Diets enriched in foods with antioxidant and anti-inflammatory actions may modulate this neuroinflammation. Enhanced striatal dopamine recovery appeared in animals treated with diet enrich in antioxidants and anti-inflammatory phytochemicals (blueberry and spirulina) and coincided with an early, transient increase in OX-6-positive microglia."

Antibacterial

Antibacterial activity of volatile component and various extracts of Spirulina platensis. Ozdemir G, Karabay NU, Dalay MC, Pazarbasi B. Phytother Res. 2004 Sep;18(9):754-7.

Key Finding: "The methanol, dichloromethane, petroleum ether, ethyl acetate extracts and volatile components of Spirulina platensis were tested in vitro for their antimicrobial activity. GC-MS analysis of the volatile components of S. platensis resulted in the identification of 15 compounds which constituted 96.45% of the total compounds. The volatile components of S. platensis consisted of heptadecane (39.70%) and tetradecane (34.61%) as major components."

Anti-Inflammatories

Stimulation of cytokine production in human peripheral blood mononuclear cells by an aqueous Chlorella extract. Ewart HS, Bloch O, Girouard GS, Kralovec J, Barrow CJ, Ben-Yehudah G, Suarez ER, Rapoport MJ. Planta Med. 2007 Jul;73(8):762-8. **Key Finding:** "We conclude that an aqueous extract of Chlorella pyrenoidosa stimulation of human peripheral blood mononuclear cells induces a T-helper-1 patterned cytokine response and a strong **anti-inflammatory** regulatory cytokine response, observations that await confirmation in vivo."

Clinical potential of Spirulina as a source of phycocyanobilin. McCarty MF. J Med Food. 2007 Dec;10(4):566-70. **Key Finding:** "Phycocyanobilin from Spirulina supplementation may have versatile potential in prevention and therapy – particularly in light of rodent studies demonstrating that orally administered Spirulina or phycocyanin can exert a wide range of **anti-inflammatory** effects. A heaping tablespoon (about 15 g) of Spirulina can be expected to provide about 100 mg of PCB. By extrapolating from rodent studies, it can be concluded that an intake of 2 heaping tablespoons daily would be likely to have important antioxidant activity in humans. An intake of this magnitude can be clinically feasible is Spirulina is incorporated into 'smoothies' featuring such ingredients as soy milk, fruit juices, and whole fruits."

C-Phycocyanin, a selective cyclooxygenase-2 inhibitor, induces apoptosis in lipopolysaccharide-stimulated RAW 264.7 macrophages. Reddy MC, Subhashini J, Mahipal SV, Bhat VB, Srinivas Reddy P, Kiranmai G, Madyastha KM, Reddanna P. Biochem Biophys Res Commun. 2003 May 2;304(2):385-92. **Key Finding:** "C-Phycocyanin (C-PC) is one of the major biliproteins of Spirulina platensis with antioxidant and radical scavenging properties. It is also known to exhibit anti-**inflammatory** and anti-**cancer** properties. Previously, we have shown that C-PC selectively inhibits cyclooxygenase-2 (COX-2), an inducible isoform that is up regulated during inflammation and cancer. The present study is undertaken to test the effect of C-PC on LPS stimulated RAW 264.7 mouse macrophage cell line. These studies have shown a dose dependent reduction in the growth and multiplication of macrophage cell line by C-PC."

Antioxidation

Six-week supplementation with Chlorella has favorable impact on **antioxidant** *status in Korean male smokers.* Lee SH, Kang HJ, Lee HJ, Kang MH, Park YK. Nutrition. 2009 Aug 4. (Epub ahead of print). **Key Finding:** "Chlorella supplementation resulted in the conservation of plasma antioxidant nutrient status and improvement in erythrocyte antioxidant enzyme activities in subjects. Therefore, our results are supportive of an antioxidant role for Chlorella and indicate that Chlorella is an important whole-food supplement that should be included as a key component of a healthy diet."

Evaluation of antioxidant profile and activity of amalaki (Emblica officinalis), spirulina and wheat grass. Shukla V, Vashistha M, Singh SN. Ind J Clin Biochem. 2009 Jan;24(1):70-75. **Key Finding:** "Total antioxidant activity of aqueous extract of amalki, spirulina and wheat grass at 1mg/ml concentration were 7.78, 1.33 and 0.278 mmol/l respectively. Alcoholic extract of wheat grass showed 50% inhibition in FeCI2- ascorbic acid induced lipid peroxidation of rat liver homogenates in vitro. Both aqueous and alcoholic extracts of amalaki inhibited activity of rat liver glutathione S-transferase in vitro in dose dependent manner. The aqueous extracts of both amalki and spirulina also showed protection against t-BOOH induced cytotoxicity and production of ROS in cultured C6 glial cells."_

Hepatoprotection of chlorella against carbon tetrachloride-induced oxidative damage in rats. Peng HY, Chu YC, Chen SJ, Chou ST. In Vivo. 2009 Sep-Oct;23(5):747-54. **Key Finding:** "Chlorella may be useful as a hepatoprotective agent against chemical-induced **liver damage** in vivo."

Antioxidant *effect of the marine algae Chlorella vulgaris against naphthalene-induced oxidative stress in the albino rats.* Vijayavel K, Anbuselvam C, Balasubramanian MP. Mol Cell Biochem. 2007 Sep;303(1-2):39-44. **Key Finding:** "The present results suggest that Chlorella vulgaris extract exerts its chemo-preventive effect by modulating the antioxidants status and lipid peroxidation during naphthalene intoxication."

Antioxidant *and antiproliferative activities of Spirulina and Chlorella water extracts.* Wu LC, Ho JA, Shieh MC, Lu IW. J Agric Food Chem. 2005 May 18;53(10):4207-12. **Key Finding:** "Liver fibrosis is a chronic liver disease that will further develop to cirrhosis if severe damage continues to form. A potential treatment for liver fibrosis is to inhibit activated hepatic stellate cell (HSC) proliferation and, subsequently, to induce HSC apoptosis. In this study, the aqueous extract of spirulina was chosen as the source of antioxidant to investigate the inhibitory effect on the proliferation of HSC. The growth inhibitory effects of aqueous spirulina and chlorella extract on human **liver cancer** cells, HepG2, were also studied. Results indicated that the total phenol content of spirulina was almost five times greater than that of chlorella. The antioxidant activity of spirulina was higher than chlorella. The aqueous extracts of these two algae both showed antiproliferative effects on HSC and HepG2, but spirulina was a stronger inhibitor than chlorella."

Arthritis

*Evaluation of protective efficacy of Spirulina platensis against collagen-induced **arthritis** in rats.* Kumar N, Singh S, Patro N, Patro I. Inflammopharmacology. 2009 Jun;17(3):181-90. **Key Finding:** "Spirulina platensis (400 mg kg(-1)) significantly normalizes changes observed in arthritic rats to near normal conditions, indicates that S. platensis has promising protection efficacy against collagen-induced arthritis."

*Anti-inflammatory effect of Spirulina fusiformis on adjuvant-induced **arthritis** in mice.* Rasool M, Sabina EP, Lavanya B. Biol Pharm Bull. 2006 Dec;29(12):2483-7. **Key Finding:** "Results of this study clearly indicate that Spirulina fusiformis has promising anti-inflammatory activity against adjuvant-induced arthritic animals."

*Inhibitory effects of Spirulina in zymosan-induced **arthritis** in mice.* Remirez D, Gonzalez R, Merino N, Rodriguez S, Ancheta O. Mediators Inflamm. 2002 Apr;11(2):75-9. **Key Finding:** "The anti-arthritic effect exerted by Spirulina as shown in this model may be at least partly due to the previously reported anti-inflammatory and antioxidative properties of its constituent, phycocyanin. To our knowledge, this is the first report on the anti-inflammatory effect of Spirulina in an experimental model of arthritis."

Atherosclerosis

Biological activities of exogenous polysaccharides via controlling endogenous proteoglycan metabolism in vascular endothelial cells. Sato T, Yamamoto C, Fujiwara Y, Kaji T. Yakugaku Zasshi (Japanese). 2008 May;128(5):717-23. **Key Finding:** "In this review, we describe sodium spirulan, a sulfated polysaccharide obtained from a hot-water extract of the blue-green alga Spirulina platensis, as an exogenous polysaccharide that stimulates the release of proteoglycans from vascular endothelial cells. Further research is required to obtain exogenous polysaccharide-related molecules that exhibit useful biological activities through controlling endothelial proteoglycan for protection against vascular lesions such as **atherosclerosis.**"

Phycobiliprotein C-phycocyanin from Spirulina platensis is powerfully responsible for reducing oxidative stress and NADPH oxidase expression induced by an atherogenic diet in hamsters. Riss J, Decorde K, Sutra T, Delage M, Baccou JC, Jouy N, Brune JP, Oreal H, Cristol JP, Rouanet JM. J Agric Food Chem. 2007 Sep 19;55(19):7962-7. **Key Finding:** "The results indicate that chronic consumption of Se-rich spirulina phycocyanin powerfully prevents the development of **atherosclerosis.** The underlying mechanism is related mainly to inhibiting pro-oxidant factors and at a lesser extent improving the serum lipid profile."

C-phycocyanin ameliorates doxorubicin-induced oxidative stress and apoptosis in adult rat cardiomyocytes. Kahn M, Varadharaj S, Shobha JC, Naidu MU, Parinandi NL, Kutala VK, Kuppusamy P. J Cardiovasc Pharmacol. 2006 Jan;47(1):9-20. **Key Finding:** "This study further supports the crucial role of the antioxidant nature of C-phycocyanin in its **cardio protection** against doxorubicin-induced oxidative stress and apoptosis."

Preventing **dyslipidemia** *by Chlorella pyrenoidosa in rats and hamsters after chronic high fat diet treatment.* Cherng JY, Shih MF. Life Sci. 2005 May 13;76(26):3001-13. **Key Finding:** "Chlorella pyrenoidosa has the ability to prevent dyslipidemia in chronic high-fat fed animals and could be potential to prevent intestinal absorption of redundant lipid from our daily intake and subsequently to prevent **hyperlipidemia** as well as **atherosclerosis.**"

Mechanisms involved in the **antiplatelet** *effect of C-phycocyanin.* Chiu HF, Yang SP, Kuo YL, Lai YS, Chou TC. Br J Nutr. 2006 Feb;95(2):435-40. **Key Finding:** "These findings strongly demonstrate that C-phycocyanin from Spirulina platensis is an inhibitor of platelet aggregation, which may be associated with mechanisms including inhibition of thromboxane A2 formation, intracellular calcium mobilization and platelet surface glycoprotein IIb/IIIa expression accompanied by increasing cyclic AMP formation and platelet membrane fluidity."

Cancer (breast; colon; leukemia; melanoma; oral)

A case-control study on seaweed consumption and the risk of breast cancer. Yang YJ, Nam SJ, Kong G, Kim MK. Br J Nutr. 2010 May;103(9):1345-53. **Key Finding**: "Gim

(Porphyra sp.) and miyeck (Udaria pinnatifida) are seaweeds most consumed by Koreans. We investigated the association between the intake of gim and miyeck and the risk of **breast cancer** in a case-control study of 362 women aged 30-65 years old who were histologically confirmed to have breast cancer. Controls visiting the same hospital were matched to cases according to their age and menopausal status. The daily intake of gim was inversely associated with the risk of breast cancer, whereas miyeck consumption did not have any significant associations. These results suggest that high intake of gim may have decreased the risk of breast cancer."

The mechanism of fucoidan-induced apoptosis in leukemic cells: involvement of ERK1/2, JNK, glutathione, and nitric oxide. Jin JO, Song MG, Kim YN, Et al. Mol Carcinog. 2010 Aug;49(8):771-82. **Key Finding**: "Fucoidan, a sulfated polysaccharide in brown seaweed, has various biological activities including anti-tumor activity. We investigated the effects of fuccoidan on the apoptosis of human promyleoid **leukemic cells** and fucoidan-mediated signaling pathways. Our results suggest that activation of MEKK1, MEK1, ERK1/2, and JNK, depletion of gluta-thione, and production of NO are important mediators in fucoidan-induced apoptosis of human leukemic cells."

Evaluating the possible genotoxic, mutagenic and tumor cell proliferation-inhibition effects of a non-anticoagulant, but antithrombotic algal heterofucan. Almedia-Lima J, Costa LS, Silva NB, Et al. J Appl Toxicol. 2010 Oct;30(7):708-15. **Key Finding**: "Fucan is a term used to denominate a family of sulfated polysaccharides extracted mainly from brown seaweeds. Our research group purified a non-anticoagulant hetero-fucan (fucan A) which displays antithrombotic activity in vivo. **Tumor-cell** (HeLa, PC3, PANC, HL60) proliferation was inhibited. Non-tumor cell lines proliferation were not affected by this molecule."

Chlorella powder inhibits the activities of peptidase cathepsin S, PLA2, cyclooxygenase-2, thromboxane synthase, tyrosine phosphatases, tumor necrosis factor-alpha converting enzyme, calpain and kinases. Cheng FC, Feng JJ, Chen KH, Imanishi H, Fujishima M, Takekoshi H, Naoki Y, Shimoda M. Int J Food Sci Nutr. 2009;60 Suppl 1:89-98. **Key Finding:** "These results reveal important biochemical activities to be developed that, if confirmed by in vivo studies, might be exploited for the prevention or treatment of several serious pathologies, including **inflamma-tory diseases**, immune and **cancer**."

Chlorella vulgaris triggers apoptosis in hepatocarcinogenesis-induced rats. Mohd Azamai ES, Sulaiman S, Mohd Habib SH, Looi ML, Das S, Abdul Hamid NA, Wan

Ngah WZ, Mohd Yusof YA. J Zhejiang Univ Sci B. 2009 Jan;10(1):14-21. **Key Finding:** "Our study shows that Chlorella vulgaris has definite **chemo preventive** effect by inducing apoptosis via decreasing the expression of Bcl-2 and increasing the expression of caspase 8 in hepatocarcinogenesis-induced rats."

Induction of G1 cell cycle arrest and mitochondria-mediated apoptosis in MCF-7 human **breast carcinoma** *cells by selenium-enriched Spirulina extract.* Chen T, Wong YS, Zheng W. Biomed Pharmacother. 2009 Oct 27. (Epub ahead of print). **Key Finding:** "Both selenium and Spirulina have been demonstrated to show anticancer potential. In the present study, we showed that Se-enriched Spirulina platensis extract inhibited the growth of MCF-7 human breast cancer cells through induction of G1 cell cycle arrest and mitochondria-mediated apoptosis."

Anticancer and Antioxidant Activities of the Peptide Fraction from Algae Protein Waste. Sheih IC, Fang TJ, Wu TK, Lin PH. J Agric Food Chem. 2009 Nov 16. (Epub ahead of print). **Key Finding:** "These results demonstrate that inexpensive algae protein waste could be a new alternative to produce **anticancer** peptides."

Long-term effect of Spirulina platensis extract on DMBA-induced hamster buccal pouch carcinogenesis (immunohistochemical study). Grawich ME, Zaher AR, Gaafar AI, Nasif WA. Med Oncol. 2009 Jan 21. (Epub ahead of print). **Key Finding:** "From these results it can be concluded that Spirulina platensis extract has a beneficial role in regression of **cancer** (squamous cell carcinoma) progression."

Chemoprevention of rat liver toxicity and carcinogenesis by Spirulina. Ismail MF, Ali DA, Fernando A, Abdraboh ME, Gaur RL, Ibrahim WM, Raj MH, Ouhtit A. Int J Biol Sc. 2009 Jun 2;5(4):377-87. **Key Finding:** "This is the first report of the in vivo chemo preventive effect of Spirulina platensis against dibutyl nitrosamine induced rat liver cytotoxicity and carcinogenesis, suggesting its potential use in chemoprevention of **cancer**."

Enhancement of **antitumor** *natural killer cell activation by orally administered Spirulina extract in mice.* Akao Y, Ebihara T, Masuda H, Saeki Y, Akazawa T, Hazeki K, Hazeki O, Matsumoto M, Seya T. Cancer Sci. 2009 Aug;100(8):1494-501. **Key Finding:** "Spirulina and BCG-cell wall skeleton synergistically augmented IFN-gamma production and antitumor potential in the B16D8 versus C57BL/6 system. We infer from these results that NK activation by Spirulina has some advantage in combinational use with BCG-cell wall skeleton for developing adjuvant-based antitumor immunotherapy."

*Antiproliferative effects of carotenoids extracted from Chlorella ellipsoidea and Chlorella vulgaris on human **colon cancer** cells.* Cha KH, Koo SY, Lee DU. J Agric Food Chem. 2008 Nov 26;56(22):10521-6. **Key Finding:** "C. ellipsoidea extract produced an apoptosis-inducing effect almost 2.5 times stronger than that of the C. vulgaris extract. These results indicate that bioactive xanthophyll of C. ellipsoidea might be useful functional ingredients in the prevention of human cancers."

Effects of Spirulina platensis extract on Syrian hamster cheek pouch mucosa painted with 7,12-dimethylbenz{a}anthracene. Grawish ME. Oral Oncol. 2008 Oct;44(10):956-62. **Key Finding:** "In this **cancer** study, 30 male golden Syrian hamsters were divided into three equal groups; the right buccal pouches of the hamster rats in group one were painted with 0.5% solution of 7,12-dimethylbenz{a}anthracene three times a week until sacrificed. The same pouches of group two were also painted with DMBA, but received an additional 10mg/daily Spirulina platensis extract. The hamster rats in group three received neither DMBA nor S. platensis extract and were the control group. An overall significant difference among the three groups was indicated. The pAgNOR was 10% in group one, 5% in group two (Spirulina group) and 4% in group three (control group.) Consequently, S. platensis is an adjunctive means to inhibit the dysplastic changes occurring in the hamster cheek pouch mucosa."

Chemo protective effect of Spirulina (Arthrospira) against cyclophosphamide-induced mutagenicity in mice. Chamorro-Cevallos G, Garduno-Siciliano L, Barron BL, Madrigal-Bujaidar E, Cruz-Vega DE, Pages N. Food Chem Toxicol. 2008 Feb; 45(2):567-74. **Key Finding:** "Our results illustrate protective effects of Spirulina in relation to cyclophosphamide-induced genetic damage to germ cells in male and female mice."

In vitro antioxidant and antiproliferative activities of selenium-containing phycocyanin from selenium-enriched Spirulina platensis. Chen T, Wong YS. J Agric Food Chem. 2008 Jun 25;56(12):4352-8. **Key Finding:** "Our findings suggest that selenium-containing phycocyanin is a promising organic Se species with potential applications in **cancer** chemoprevention."

*Alteration of mitochondrial membrane potential by Spirulina platensis c-phycocyanin induces apoptosis in the doxorubicin resistant human hepatocellular-**carcinoma** cell line HepG2.* Roy KR, Arunasree KM, Reddy NP, Dheeraj B, Reddy GV, Reddanna P. Biotechnol Appl Biochem. 2007 Jul;47(Pt 3):159-67. **Key Finding:** "C-phycocyanin is a water-soluble biliprotein from the filamentous cyanobacterium Spirulina platensis with potent antioxidant, anti-inflammatory and anticancerous properties. In the present study, the effect of C-PC was tested on the proliferation of doxorubicin-sensitive (S-HepG2) and –resistant (R-HepG2) HCC (hepatocellular carcinoma) cell lines. These studies indicate a 50% decrease in the proliferation of S- and R-HepG2 cells treated with 40 and 50 microM C-PC for 24 h respectively."

Antioxidant *and antiproliferative activities of Spirulina and Chlorella water extracts.* Wu LC, Ho JA, Shieh MC, Lu IW. J Agric Food Chem. 2005 May 18;53(10):4207-12. **Key Finding:** "Liver fibrosis is a chronic liver disease that will further develop to cirrhosis if severe damage continues to form. A potential treatment for liver fibrosis is to inhibit activated hepatic stellate cell (HSC) proliferation and, subsequently, to induce HSC apoptosis. In this study, the aqueous extract of spirulina was chosen as the source of antioxidant to investigate the inhibitory effect on the proliferation of HSC. The growth inhibitory effects of aqueous spirulina and chlorella extract on human **liver cancer** cells, HepG2, were also studied. Results indicated that the total phenol content of spirulina was almost five times greater than that of chlorella. The antioxidant activity of spirulina was higher than chlorella. The aqueous extracts of these two algae both showed antiproliferative effects on HSC and HepG2, but spirulina was a stronger inhibitor than chlorella."

Effects of CD59 on ***antitumoral*** *activities of phycocyanin from Spirulina platensis.* Li B, Zhang X, Gao M, Chu X. Biomed Pharmacother. 2005 Dec;59(10):551-60. **Key Finding:** "The regulatory effect of phycocyanin (PC) from Spirulina platensis on cluster of differentiation 59 (CD59) gene expressions of Hela cells and anti-tumoral mechanism of PC was investigated in this study. Results showed that PC can promote the expression of CD59 protein in Hela cells, hold back repro-ductions of Hela cells, and moreover, a dosage effect was found between them. Namely, with the ascendance of PC concentration, the expression quantities of CD59 protein and apoptosis-inducing Fas protein increased and the multiplica-tion activity of Hel cells declined, whereas PC was of no use to CD59 and Fas protein expression, and reproduction of normal CHO cells as well."

Effects of chlorella on activities of protein tyrosine phosphatases, matrix metalloproteinase, caspases, cytokine release, B and T cell proliferations, and phorbol ester receptor binding. Cheng FC, Lin A, Feng JJ, Mizoguchi T, Takekoshi H, Kubota H, Kato Y, Naoki Y. J Med Food. 2004 Summer;7(2):146-52. **Key Finding:** "These results reveal potential pharmacological activities that, if confirmed by vivo studies, might be exploited for the prevention or treatment of several serious pathologies, including **inflammatory** disease and **cancer**."

Molecular mechanisms in C-Phycocyanin induced apoptosis in human chronic myeloid ***leukemia*** *cell line-K562.* Subhashini J, Mahipal SV, Reddy MC, Mallikarjuna Reddy M, Rachamallu A, Reddanna P. Biochem Parmacol. 2004 Aug 1;68(3):453-62. **Key Finding:** "The present study demonstrates that C-Phycocyanin, the major light harvesting biliprotein from Spirulina platensis, induces apoptosis in K562 cells by cytochrome c release from mitochondria into the cytosol, PARP cleavage and down regulation of Bcl-2."

C-Phycocyanin, a selective cyclooxygenase-2 inhibitor, induces apoptosis in lipopolysaccharide-stimulated RAW 264.7 macrophages. Reddy MC, Subhashini J, Mahipal SV, Bhat VB, Srinivas Reddy P, Kiranmai G, Madyastha KM, Reddanna P. Biochem Biophys Res Commun. 2003 May 2;304(2):385-92. **Key Finding:** "C-Phycocyanin (C-PC) is one of the major biliproteins of Spirulina platensis with antioxidant and radical scavenging properties. It is also known to exhibit anti-**inflammatory** and anti-**cancer** properties. Previously, we have shown that C-PC selectively inhibits cyclooxygenase-2 (COX-2), an inducible isoform that is up-regulated during inflammation and cancer. The present study is undertaken to test the effect of C-PC on LPS stimulated RAW 264.7 mouse macrophage cell line. These studies have shown a dose dependent reduction in the growth and multiplication of macrophage cell line by C-PC."____

*Toll-like receptor 2 is at least partly involved in the **antitumor** activity of glycoprotein from Chlorella vulgaris.* Hasegawa T, Matsuguchi T, Noda K, Tanaka K, Kumamoto S, Shoyama Y, Yoshikai Y. Int Immunopharmacol. 2002 Mar;2(4):579-89. **Key Finding:** "These results suggest that Toll-like receptor signaling is at least partly involved in the antitumor activity of the water-soluble antitumor glycoprotein from C. vulgaris."

*Effect of polysaccharide from Spirulina platensis on hematopoietic cells proliferation, apoptosis and Bcl-2 expression in mice bearing **tumor** treated with chemotherapy.* Liu XM, Zhang HQ. Yao Xue Xue Bao (Chinese). 2002 Aug;37(8):616-20. **Key Finding:** "Spirulina platensis indirectly up-regulated Bcl-2 expression of hematopoietic cells by promoting endogenous cytokines secretion which may be one of the mechanisms by which Spirulina enhanced hematopoietic cell proliferation and inhibited its apoptosis in mice bearing tumor treated with chemotherapy."

Chemomodulation of carcinogen metabolizing enzymes, antioxidant profiles and skin and fore-stomach papillo magenesis by Spirulina platensis. Dasgupta T, Banejee S, Yaday PK, Rao AR. Mol Cell Biochem. 2001 Oct;226(1-2):27-38. **Key Finding:** "There was a significant inhibition of **tumor** burden as well as tumor incidence in both the tumor model systems studied. In the skin tumor studies, tumor burden was reduced in the Swiss albino mice from 4.86 to 1.20 and 1.15 by the low and high dose treatment respectively. In stomach tumor studies, tumor burden was 2.05 and 1.73 by the low and high doses of Spirulina treatment against 3.73 that of control."

Biological activity of Spirulina. Blinkova LP, Gorobets OB, Baturo AP. Zh Mikrobiol Epidemiol Immunobiol (Russian). 2001 Mar-Apr;(2):114-8. **Key Finding:** "Spirulina platensis has been found suitable for use as bioactive additive. SP produces an immuno-stimulating effect by enhancing the resistance of humans, mammals, chickens and fish to **infections**, the capacity of influencing hemopoiesis, stimulating the production of antibodies and cytokines. SP extracts are capable in inhibiting **cancerogenesis.**"

Chlorella vulgaris culture supernatant (CVS) reduces psychological stress-induced apoptosis in thymocytes of mice. Hasegawa T, Noda K, Kumamoto S, Ando Y, Yamada A, Yoshikai Y. Int J Immunopharmacol. 2000 Nov;22(11):877-85. **Key Finding:** "A glycoprotein prepared from Chlorella vulgaris culture is a biological response modifier which exhibits protective activities against **tumor metastasis** and 5-fluorouracil-induced immunosuppression. These results suggest that Chlorella vulgaris prevents psychological stress and maintains homeostasis in the face of external environmental changes."

*Inhibitory potential of Chlorella vulgaris (E-25) on mouse **skin papillo magenesis** and xenobiotic detoxication system.* Singh A, Singh SP, Bamezai R. Anticancer Res. 1999 May-Jun;19(3A):1887-91. **Key Finding:** "The results suggest the chemo preventive potential of Chlorella vulgaris during peri-, post- or peri- and post-initiational stages of murine skin papillo magenesis."

Modulatory potential of Spirulina fusiformis on carcinogen metabolizing enzymes in Swiss albino mice. Mittal A, Kumar PV, Banerjee S, Rao AR, Kumar A. Phytother Res. 1999 Mar;13(2):111-4. **Key Finding:** "The modulatory potential of Spirulina fusiformis was observed on the hepatic and extra hepatic carcinogen metabolizing enzymes in Swiss albino mice at a dose of 800 mg/kg b.w. given orally. A significant reduction in the hepatic cytochrome P-450 content was observed in the group treated with Spirulina compared with the control group."

*A novel glycoprotein obtained from Chlorella vulgaris strain CK22 shows **antimetastatic immunopotentiation**.* Tanaka K, Yamada A, Noda K, Hasegawa T, Okuda M, Shoyama Y, Notmoto K. Cancer Immunol Immunother. 1998 Feb;45(6):313-20. **Key Finding:** "We conclude that a glycoprotein extract derived from Chlorella vulgaris augments antimetastatic immunity through T cell activation in lymphoid organs and enhances recruitment of these cells to the tumor sites. Pre-surgical treatment with Chlorella vulgaris might prevent metastasis or tumor progression."

Inhibitory effect of mast cell-mediated immediate-type allergic reactions in rats by spirulina. Kim HM, Lee EH, Cho HH, Moon YH. Biochem Parmacol. 1998 Apr 1;55(7):1071-6. **Key Finding:** "Spirulina had a significant inhibitory effect on anti-DNP IgE-induced tumor necrosis factor-alpha productions. These results indicate that spirulina inhibits mast cell-mediated immediate-type allergic reactions in vivo and in vitro."

Inhibition of tumor invasion and metastasis by calcium spirulan (Ca-SP), a novel sulfated polysaccharide derived from a blue-green alga, Spirulina platensis. Mishima T, Murata J, Toyoshima M, Fujii H, Nakajima M, Hayashi T, Kato T, Saiki I. Clin Exp Metastasis. 1998 Aug;16(6):541-50. **Key Finding:** "These results suggest that Ca-SP, a novel sulfated polysaccharide, could reduce the lung metastasis of B16-BL6 **melanoma** cells, by inhibiting the tumor invasion of basement membrane probably through the prevention of the adhesion and migration of tumor cells to laminin substrate and of the heparinize activity."

Anti-tumor *promotion with food phytochemicals: a strategy for cancer chemoprevention.* Murakami A, Ohigashi H, Koshimizu K. Biosci Biotechnol. Biochem. 1996 Jan;60(1):1-8. **Key Finding:** In this review, the anti-tumor promoting properties of vegetables, fruits, and edible marine algae are described. "Anti-tumor promotion with food phytochemicals may be characterized as an efficient and reliable strategy for cancer chemoprevention."

Inhibitory effects of sterols isolated from Chlorella vulgaris on 12-0-tetradecanoylphorbol-13-acetate-induced inflammation and tumor promotion in mouse skin. Yasukawa K, Akihisa T, Kanno H, Kaminaga T, Izumida M, Sakoh T, Tamura T, Takido M. Biol Pharm Bull. 1996 Apr;19(4):573-6. **Key Finding:** "Inhibitory activity against 12-0-tetradecanoylphorbol-13-acetate-induced **inflammation** in mice was observed in the methanol extract of Chlorella vulgaris."

Anti-tumor*-promoting glyceroglycolipids from the green alga, Chlorella vulgaris.* Morimoto T, Nagatsu A, Murakami N, Sakakibara J, Tokuda H, Nishino H, Iwashima A. Phytochemistry. 1995 Nov;40(5):1433-7. **Key Finding:** "Two new monogalactosyl diacylglycerols were isolated from the freshwater green alga, Chlorella vulgaris, as anti-tumor promoters, together with three monogalactosyl diacylglycerols and two digalactosyl diacylglycerols. The new monoglactosyl diacylglycerol containing (7Z,10Z)-hexadecadienoic acid showed a more potent inhibitory effect toward tumor promotion than the other glycolipids isolated."

Inhibitive effects of spirulina on aberrant crypts in **colon** *induced by dimethyl hydrazine.* Chen F, Zhang Q. Zhonghua Yu Fang Yi Xue Za Zhi (Chinese). 1995 Jan;29(1):13-7. **Key Finding:** "In the ninth, 13th and 16th week after precancerous pathological changes of colon were induced in Sprague-Dawley rats, the number of aberrant crypts and aberrant crypts foci was significantly less in animals protected by spirulina than in controls."

Evaluation of chemoprevention of **oral cancer** *with Spirulina fusiformis.* Mathew B, Sankaranarayanan R, Nair PP, Varghese C, Somanathan T, Amma BP, Amma NS, Nair MK. Nutr Cancer. 1995;24(2):197-202. **Key Finding:** "We evaluated the chemo preventive activity of spirulina (1 g/day for 12 mos) in reversing oral leukoplakia in pan tobacco chewers in Kerala, India. Complete regression of lesions was observed in 20 of 44 (45%) of subject supplemented with spirulina, as opposed to 3 of 43 (7%) in the placebo arm."

Antitumor *activity of marine algae.* Noda H, Amano H, Arashima K, Nisizawa K. Hydrobiologia. 1990 Sep;204-205(1):577-584. **Key Finding:** "Powdered tissue from 46 species of air-dried marine algae (four green, 21 brown and 21 red algae) were screened for antitumor activity. Significant activity against Ehrlich carcinoma was found in the brown algae *Scytosiphon lomentaria* (69.8% inhibition), *Lessonia nigrescens* (60%), *Laminaria japonica* (57.6%), *Sargassum ringgoldianum* (46.5%), the red algae Porphyra yezoensis (53.2%) and Eucheuma gelatinae (52.1%) and the green algae *Enteromorpha prolifera* (51.7%). Five brown and four red algae showed appreciable antitumor activity against Meth-A fibrosarcoma."

Prevention of experimental **oral cancer** *by extracts of Spirulina–Dunaliella algae.* Schwartz J, Shklar G, Reid S. Trickler D. Nutr Cancer. 1988;11(2):127-34. **Key Finding:** "An extract of Spirulina-Dunaliella algae was shown to prevent tumor development in hamster buccal pouch when a 0.1% solution of 7,12-dimethylbenz{a} anthracene (DMBA) in mineral oil was applied topically three times weekly for 28 weeks. The algae animals presented a complete absence of gross tumors."

Regression of experimental hamster **cancer** *by beta carotene and algae extracts.* Schwartz J, Shklar G. J Oral Maxillofac Surg. 1987 Jun;45(6):510-5. **Key Finding:** "The effect of algae extract on tumor regression was studied using phycotene extract of Spirulina and Dunaliella algae. Total tumor regression was found in 30% of phycotene animals, 20% of beta carotene animals and 15% of canthaxanthin animals after four weeks."

Cataracts

Effect of ambroxol, spirulina and vitamin-E in naphthalene induced **cataract** *in female rats.* Haque SE, Gilani KM. Indian J Physiol Pharmacol. 2005 Jan;49(1):57-64. **Key Finding:** "Lens glutathione, soluble protein and water content profiles revealed the preventive role of Ambroxol, Spirulina and Vitamin E in naphthalene-induced cataract in female rats."

Antioxidant and **anti-cataract** *effects of Chlorella on rats with streptozotocin-induced* **diabetes.** Shibata S, Natori Y, Nishihara T, Tomisaka K, Matsumoto K, Sansawa H, Nguyen VC. J Nutr Sci Vitaminol. 2003 Oct;49(5):334-9. **Key Finding:** "These results indicate that Chlorella has antioxidant activity and may be beneficial for the prevention of diabetic complications such as cataracts."

Cholesterol

Effects of dietary Spirulina on vascular reactivity. Juarez-Oropeza MA, Mascher D, Torres-Duran PV, Farias JM, Paredes-Carbajal MC. J Med Food. 2009 Feb;12(1):15-20. **Key Finding:** "In humans, Spirulina maxima intake decreases **blood pressure** and **plasma lipid** concentrations, especially triacylglycerol and low-density lipoprotein-cholesterol, and indirectly modifies the total cholesterol and high-density lipoprotein-cholesterol values."

A randomized double-blind, placebo-controlled study to establish the effects of spirulina in elderly Koreans. Park HJ, Lee YJ, Ryu HK, Kim MH, Chung HW, Kim WY. Ann Nutr Metab. 2008;52(4):322-8. **Key Finding:** "The results demonstrate that spirulina has favorable effects on **lipid profiles**, immune variables, and antioxidant capacity in healthy, elderly male and female subjects and is suitable as a functional food."

Hypocholesterolemic *mechanism of Chlorella: Chlorella and its indigestible fraction enhance hepatic cholesterol catabolism through up-regulation of cholesterol 7alpha-hydroxylase in rats.* Shibata S, Hayakawa K, Egashira Y, Sanada H. Biosci Biotechnol Biochem. 2007 Apr;71(4):916-25. **Key Finding:** "These results suggest that the hypocholesterolemic effect of Chlorella powder involves enhancement of cholesterol catabolism through up-regulation of hepatic CYP7A1 expression and that chlorella indigestible fraction contributes to the hypocholesterolemic effect."

Antihyperlipemic *and* **antihypertensive** *effects of Spirulina maxima in an open sample of Mexican population: a preliminary report.* Torres-Duran PV, Ferreira-

Hermosillo A, Juarez-Oropeza MA. Lipids Health Dis. 2007 Nov 26;6:33. **Key Finding:** "The purpose of this study was to evaluate the effects of Spirulina maxima orally supplied (4.5g/day, for 6 weeks) to a sample of 36 subjects (16 men and 20 women) with ages between 18-65 years on serum lipids. The Spirulina maxima showed a hypolipemic effect, especially on the **triacylglycerol** and the LDL-C concentrations but indirectly on total **cholesterol** and HDL-C values. It also reduces systolic and diastolic **blood pressure**."

In vitro evaluation of protective effects of ascorbic acid and water extract of Spirulina plantesis (blue green algae) on 5-fluorouracil-induced lipid peroxidation. Ray S, Roy K, Sengupta C. Acta Pol Pharm. 2007 Jul-Aug;64(4):335-44. **Key Finding:** "The present study was designed to evaluate the protective effects of ascorbic acid and water extract of Spirulina plantesis to minimize 5-fluorouracil-induced lipid peroxidation. The results suggest that ascorbic acid and water extract of Spirulina could suppress the 5-FU-induced **lipid peroxidation** to a significant extent."

*Isolation of pancreatic lipase activity-inhibitory component of spirulina platensis and it reduces postprandial **triacylglycerolemia**.* Han LK, Li DX, Xiang L, Gong XJ, Kondo Y, Suzuki I, Okuda H. Yakugaku Zasshi (Japanese). 2006 Jan;126(1):43-9. **Key Finding:** "These results suggest that the inhibitory effects of S. platensis on postprandial triacylglycerolemia may be due in part to the inhibition of pancreatic lipase activity by glycolipid H-b2 and phycocyanin."

A novel protein C-phycocyanin plays a crucial role in the hypocholesterolemic action of Spirulina platensis concentrate in rats. Nagaoka S, Shimizu K, Kaneko H, Shibayama F, Morikawa K, Kanamaru Y, Otsuka A, Hirahashi T, Kato T. J Nutr. 2005 Oct;135(10):2425-30. **Key Finding:** "This study provides the first direct evidence that C-phycocyanin, a novel hypocholesterolemic protein derived from Spirulina platensis, can powerfully influence serum **cholesterol** concentrations and impart stronger hypocholesterolemic activity than Spirulina platensis concentrate in animals."

*A hot water extract of Chlorella pyrenoidosa reduces body weight and **serum lipids** in overiectomized rats.* Hidaka S, Okamoto Y, Arita M. Phytother Res. 2004 Feb;18(2):164-8. **Key Finding:** "These results suggest that a dietary supplement of chlorella growth factor from Chlorella pyrenoidosa may be useful to control the body weight and improve lipid metabolism of menopausal women."

Effects of spirulina on serum lipids, erythrocyte membrane fluidity and vascular endothelial cells in tail-suspended rats. Huang JM, Bai SM, Hu ZX, Yang CL, Zhu DB, Shi JP. Space

Med Med Eng (Beijing). 2003 Jun;16(3):184-6. **Key Finding:** "Spirulina can improve the physiological conditions of erythrocyte membrane fluidity, serum lipid and vascular endothelial cell caused by simulated weightlessness in rats."

Hypocholesterolemic effect of spirulina in patients with **hyperlipidemic** *nephritic syndrome.* Samuels R, Mani UV, Iyer UM, Nayak US. J Med Food. 2002 Summer;5(2):91-6. **Key Finding:** "It can be concluded that spray-dried Spirulina capsules, rich in antioxidants, GLA, amino acids, and fatty acids, helped reduce the increased levels of lipids in patients with hyperlipidemia nephritic syndrome."

Antioxidant activity of different fractions of Spirulina platensis protean extract. Pinero Estrada JE, Bermejo Bescos P, Villar del Fresno AM. Farmaco. 2001 May-Jul;56(5-7):497-500. **Key Finding:** "Previous reports from our laboratory have shown that a protean extract of S. platensis is a potent free-radical scavenger (hydroxyl and peroxyl radicals) and inhibits microsomal **lipid peroxidation**. In this study we observed that an increase in phycocyanin content was related to an increase in the antioxidant activity in different fractions, and therefore phycobiliprotean phycocyanin is the component mainly responsible for the antioxidant activity."

Preventive effect of Spirulina maxima on the fatty liver induced by a fructose-rich diet in the rat, a preliminary report. Gonzalez de Rivera C, Miranda-Zamora R, Diaz-Zagoya JC, Juarez-Oropeza MA. Life Sci. 1993;53(1):57-61. **Key Finding:** "A preventive effect of Spirulina maxima on the fructose-induced increase of the liver **triglycerides** level was observed together with an elevation of the phospholipid concentration in this tissue."

Effects of Spirulina platensis on plasma lipoprotein lipase activity in fructose-induced **hyperlipidemic** *rats.* Iwata K, Inayama T, Kato T. J Nutr Sci Vitaminol. 1990 Apr;36(2):165-71. **Key Finding:** "The dietary hyperlipidemia caused by the high fructose diet was improved by Spirulina feedings, accompanied by a significant increase in the lipoprotein lipase activity in post-heparin plasma."

Cognition

Contribution of supplementation by spirulina to the performance of school children in an introductory course in Dakar (Senegal). Dia AT, Camara MD, Ndiaye P, Faye A, Wone I, Gueye BC, Seck I, Diongue M. Sante Publique (French). 2009 May-Jun;21(3):297-302. **Key Finding:** "The evaluation was conducted comparing school performances of schoolchildren from public elementary schools located in Dakar before supplements, during and after. Supplemental feeding with spirulina was given during two months. Over these 60 days the students took a daily dose of 2 grams of spirulina mixed with 10 g of honey to make the taste acceptable. The sample size was 549 schoolchildren. After two months of supplemental feeding, the academic performance of the children was improved. The average of 2nd quarter marks before supplementation was 5.17 out of 10 IC. After two months of supplementation it was 5.78 out of 10 IC."

Effect of docosahexaenoic acid-fortified Chlorella vulgaris strain CK22 on the radial maze performance in aged mice. Sugimoto Y, Taga C, Nishiga M, Fujiwara M, Knoishi F, Tanaka K, Kamei C. Biol Pharm Bull. 2002 Aug;25(8):1090-2. **Key Finding:** "These results suggest that the intake of DHA-fortified Chlorella oil fraction effectively enhances working memory in maze performance by male ICR mice."

Colitis

*Selenium deficiency and its dietary correction in patients with **irritable bowel syndrome** and chronic catarrhal **colitis**.* Bogatov NV. Vopr Pitan (Russian). 2007;76(3):35-9. **Key Finding:** "Serum selenium levels were measured in 80 patients with chronic catarrhal colitis (CCC) and irritated bowel syndrome (IBS). 78% of patients examined showed selenium insufficiency, which was relatively less pronounced in IBS compared to CCC. Reception of a selenium enriched food supplement based on spirulina led to about a twofold diminishment of patient's number with selenium insufficiency."

*A review of recent clinical trials of the nutritional supplement Chlorella pyrenoidosa in the treatment of **fibromyalgia, hypertension,** and **ulcerative colitis**.* Merchant RE, Andre CA. Alter Ther Health Med. 2001 May-Jun;7(3):79-91. **Key Finding:** "The potential of chlorella to relieve symptoms, improve quality of life, and normalize body functions in patients with fibromyalgia, hypertension, or ulcerative colitis suggests that larger, more comprehensive clinical trials of chlorella are warranted."

Congenital Malformations

Spirulina maxima and its protein extract protect against hydroxyurea-teratogenic insult in mice. Vazquez-Sanchez J, Ramon-Gallegos E, Mojica-Villegas A, Madrigal-Bujaidar E, Perez-Pasten-Borja R, Chamorro-Cevallos G. Food Chem Toxicol. 2009 Nov;47(11):2785-9. **Key Finding:** "Congenital malformations are one of the major causes of child mortality all over the world. In order to prevent them it is necessary to find substances that act as anti-teratogenicity agents. In this study hydroxyurea, an antineoplastic and teratogenicity drug was administered to pregnant mice because one of its major mechanisms of teratogens is the production of reactive oxygen species. Groups tested with Spirulina or its extract, before and after HU exposure, showed a protector effect in a dose-dependent manner."

Corneal diseases

Inhibitory effects of polysaccharide extract from Spirulina platensis on corneal neovascularization. Yang L, Wang Y, Zhou Q, Chen P, Wang Y, Liu T, Xie L. Mol Vis. 2009 Sep 24;15:1951-61. **Key Finding:** "These data suggest that polysaccharide extract from Spirulina platensis is a potent inhibitor of corneal neovascularization and that it may be of benefit in the therapy of **corneal diseases** involving neovascularization and inflammation."

Dementia

*Preventive effects of Chlorella on cognitive decline in age-dependent **dementia** model mice.* Nakashima Y, Ohsawa I, Konishi F, Hasegawa T, Kumamoto S, Suzuki Y, Ohta S. Neurosci Lett. 2009 Oct 30;464(3):193-8. **Key Finding:** "The diet with Chlorella tended to reduce oxidative stress and significantly prevented the decline of cognitive ability. Moreover, consumption of Chlorella decreased the number of activated astrocytes in the DAL101 brain. These findings suggest that the prolonged consumption of Chlorella has the potential to prevent the progression of **cognitive impairment**."

Detoxification

*Protective effects of Chlorella vulgaris on **liver toxicity** in cadmium-administered rats.* Shim JY, Shin HS, Han JG, Park HS, Lim BL, Chung KW, Om AS. J Med Food. 2008 Sep;11(3):479-85. **Key Finding:** "This study suggests that C. vulgaris has a protective effect against (cadmium) Cd-induced liver damage by reducing Cd accumulation and stimulating the expression of MT II in liver."

*Chlorella (Chlorella pyrenoidosa) supplementation **decreases dioxin** and increases immunoglobulin concentrations in breast milk.* Nakano S, Takekoshi H, Nakano M. J Med Food. 2007 Mar;10(1):134-42. **Key Finding:** "The present results suggest that Chlorella supplementation not only reduces dioxin levels in breast milk, but may also have beneficial effects on nursing infants by increasing IgA levels in breast milk."

Effects of spirulina on the number of ovary mast cells in lead-induced toxicity in rats. Karaca T, Simsek N. Phytother Res. 2007 Jan;21(1):44-6. **Key Finding:** "These results indicate that Spirulina decreases the number of mast cells induced by lead in the cortex and medulla of rat ovary."

Evaluation of protective efficacy of Spirulina fusiformis against mercury induced nephrotoxicity in Swiss albino mice. Sharma MK, Sharma A, Kumar A, Kumar M. Food Chem Toxicol. 2007 Jun;45(6):879-87. **Key Finding:** "The results from the present study suggest that S. fusiformis can significantly modify the **renal damages** against mercuric chloride induced toxicity."

Maternal-fetal distribution and transfer of dioxins in pregnant women in Japan, and attempts to reduce maternal transfer with Chlorella (Chlorella pyrenoidosa) supplements. Nakano S, Noguchi T, Takekoshi H, Suzuki G, Nakana M. Chemosphere. 2005 Dec;61(9):1244-55. **Key Finding:** "Total toxic equivalents in breast milk were approximately 30% lower in the Chlorella group than in controls. This finding suggests that maternal transfer of dioxins can be reduced using dietary measures such as Chlorella supplements."

Effect of hexane extract of spirulina in the removal of arsenic from isolated liver tissues of rat. Saha SK, Misbahuddin M, Khatun R, Mamun IR. Mymensingh Med J. 2005 Jul;14(2):191-5. **Key Finding:** "Among the different extracts and residues of spirulina the hexane extract causes highly significant (p<0.001) removal of arsenic. The present study suggests that the active compounds of spirulina are present mostly in its hexane extract."

Protective effect of Spirulina on lead induced deleterious changes in the lipid peroxidation and endogenous antioxidants in rats. Upasani CD, Balaraman R. Phytother Res. 2003 Apr;17(4):330-4. **Key Finding:** "Spirulina had a significant effect on scavenging free radicals, thereby protecting the organs from damage caused by the exposure to lead. Furthermore, Spirulina showed a significant (p<0.05) decrease in the deposition of lead in the brain."

*Chlorophyll derived from Chlorella inhibits dioxin absorption from the gastrointestinal tract and accelerates **dioxin excretion** in rats.* Morita K, Ogata M, Hasegawa T. Environ Health Perspect. 2001 March;109(3):289-294. **Key Finding:** "The amount of polychlorinated dibenzofuran and polychlorinated dibenzo-p-dioxin congeners in rats was remarkably decreased along with the increasing dietary chlorophyll. These findings suggest that chlorophyll is effective for preventing dioxin absorption via foods."

Scavenging of peroxynitrite by phycocyanin and phycocyanobilin from Spirulina platensis: protection against oxidative damage to DNA. Bhat VB, Madyastha KM. Biochem Biophys Res Commun. 2001 Jul 13;285(2):262-6. **Key Finding:** "The platensis and its chromosphere, phycocyanobilin, efficiently scavenge ONOO(-), a potent physiological inorganic toxin."

*Chlorella accelerates **dioxin excretion** in rats.* Morita K, Matsueda T, Iida T, Hasegawa T. J Nutr. 1999 Sep;129(9):1731-6. **Key Finding:** "These findings suggest that the administration of chlorella may be useful in preventing gastrointestinal absorption and for promoting the excretion of dioxin already absorbed into tissues. These findings suggest that chlorella might be useful in the treatment of humans exposed to dioxin."

Diabetes

Algae consumption and risk of type 2 diabetes: Korean National Health and Nutrition Examination Survey in 2005. Lee HJ, Kim HC, Vitek L, Nam CM. J Nutr Sci Vitaminol (Tokyo). 2010;56(1):13-8. **Key Finding**: "Our results suggest that dietary algae consumption may decrease the risk of diabetes mellitus in Korean men."

*Effect of Chlorella vulgaris on **glucose metabolism** in Wistar rats fed high fat diet.* Lee HS, Kim MK. J Med Food. 2009 Oct;12(5):1029-37. **Key Finding:** "10% Chlorella intake was more effective for blood glucose regulation than 5% Chlorella intake in rats fed a high fat diet. Chlorella intake may prevent insulin resistance in Wistar rats fed a high fat diet."

*Alterations in beta-islets of Langerhans in alloxan-induced **diabetic** rats by marine Spirulina platensis.* Muthuraman P, Senthilkumar R, Srikumar K. J Enzyme Inhib Med Chem. 2009 Apr 28. (Epub ahead of print). **Key Finding:** "Treatment with marine Spirulina platensis caused significant alterations in the content of diabetic indicators and therefore in the anti-diabetic capacity of the treated animals compared to control rats."

*Potential **hypoglycemic** effects of Chlorella in streptozotocin-induced **diabetic** mice.* Jong-Yuh C, Mei-Fen S. Life Sci. 2005 Jul 15;77(9):980-90. **Key Finding:** "The current results indicate that Chlorella enhances the hypoglycemic effects of exogenous insulin at a dose which does not produce hypoglycemia in STZ mice, suggesting that insulin sensitivity is increased in these mice."

*Protective effects of polysaccharide of Spirulina platensis and Sargassum thunbeergii on vascular of alloxan induced **diabetic** rats.* Huang ZX, Mei XT, Xu DH, Xu SB, Lu JY. Zhongguo Zhong Yao Za Zhi (Chinese). 2005 Feb;30(3):211-5. **Key Finding:** "Polysaccharide of Spirulina and Sargassum thunbeergii compound could decrease blood glucose and could protect the vascular of alloxan induced diabetic rats."

*Effect of food diet supplements with chromium on the clinical and metabolic parameters in **type 2 diabetic** patients.* Sharafetdinov KH, Meshcheriakova VA, Plotnikova OA, Mazo VK, Gmoshinskii IV, Nechaeva SV. Vopr Pitan (Russian). 2004;73(5):17-20. **Key Finding:** "The influence of food diet supplements with chromium-spirulina was investigated on dynamic of glycaemia, lipid profile, blood pressure and weight in type 2 diabetic patients. The results indicated that the diet has beneficial effects on basal and postprandial glycaemia, the content of **cholesterol** and triglycerides in serum compared with a traditional hypo caloric diet."

*Effect of a zinc-enriched diet on the clinical and metabolic parameters in **type 2 diabetic** patients.* Sharafetdinov KH, Meshcheriakov VA, Plotnikova OA, Mazo VK, Gmoshinskii IV, Aleshko-Ozhevskii IuP, Sheviakova LV, Makhova NN. Vopr Pitan (Russian). 2004;73(4):17-20. **Key Finding:** "Traditional hypo caloric diet was supplemented with zinc-spirulina (7.5 mg zinc per day) in type 2 diabetic patients. The results indicated that a zinc-enriched diet has beneficial effects on basal and postprandial glycaemia, the content of cholesterol and triglycerides in serum compared with a traditional hypo caloric diet."

*Antioxidant and **anti-cataract** effects of Chlorella on rats with streptozotocin-induced **diabetes**.* Shibata S, Natori Y, Nishihara T, Tomisaka K, Matsumoto K, Sansawa H, Nguyen VC. J Nutr Sci Vitaminol. 2003 Oct;49(5):334-9. **Key Finding:** "These results indicate that Chlorella has antioxidant activity and may be beneficial for the prevention of diabetic complications such as cataracts."

*Spirulina maxima prevent fatty liver formation in CD-1 male and female mice with experimental **diabetes**.* Rodriguez-Hernandez A, Ble-Castillo JL, Juarez-Oropeza MA, Diaz-Zagoya JC. Life Sci. 2001 Jul 20;69(9):1029-37. **Key Finding:** "The dietary administration of 5% Spirulina maxima during four weeks to diabetic mice, starting one week after a single dose of alloxan, 250 mg/Kg body weight, prevented fatty liver production in male and female animals. The main action of Spirulina was on triacylglycerol levels in serum and liver."

Role of Spirulina in the Control of Glycaemia and Lipidemia in **Type 2 Diabetes** *Mellitus.* Parikh P, Mani U, Iyer U. J Med Food. 2001 Winter;4(4):193-199. **Key Finding:** "These findings suggest the beneficial effect of Spirulina supplementation in controlling blood glucose levels and in improving the lipid profile of subjects with type 2 diabetes mellitus."

Fibromyalgia

A review of recent clinical trials of the nutritional supplement Chlorella pyrenoidosa in the treatment of **fibromyalgia, hypertension,** *and* **ulcerative colitis**. Merchant RE, Andre CA. Alter Ther Health Med. 2001 May-Jun;7(3):79-91. **Key Finding:** "The potential of chlorella to relieve symptoms, improve quality of life, and normalize body functions in patients with fibromyalgia, hypertension, or ulcerative colitis suggests that larger, more comprehensive clinical trials of chlorella are warranted."

Nutritional supplementation with Chlorella pyrenoidosa for patients with **fibromyalgia** *syndrome: a pilot study.* Merchant RE, Carmack CA, Wise CM. Phytother. Res. 2000 May;14(3):167-73. **Key Finding:** "The results of this pilot study suggest that dietary Chlorella supplementation may help relieve the symptoms of fibromyalgia in some patients."

Hepatic Fibrosis

Genistein and phycocyanobilin may prevent **hepatic fibrosis** *by suppressing proliferation and activation of hepatic stellate cells.* McCarty MF, Barroso-Aranda J. Contreras F. Med Hypotheses. 2009 Mar;72(3):330-2. **Key Finding:** "Joint administration of soy isoflavones and phycocyanobilin from Spirulina in appropriate doses might have considerable potential for prevention of hepatic fibrosis in at-risk subjects."

Hepatitis

Clinical and experimental study of spirulina efficacy in chronic diffuse **liver diseases**. Gorban EM, Orynchak MA, Virstiuk NG, Kuprash LP, Panteleimonova TM, Sharbura LB. Lik Sprava (Ukraine). 2000 Sep;(6):89-93. **Key Finding:** "The results of examination of 60 patients presenting chronic diffuse disorders of the liver and seventy experimental animals with toxic affection of the liver, having been administered spirulina treatments, suggest clinical and laboratory effectiveness. The hepatoprotective properties of spirulina are preferable to its anti-inflammatory, antioxidant, membrane-stabilizing and immunocorrecting actions. In this way the employment of spirulina is believed to be pathogenically validated in chronic diffuse liver conditions, permitting stabilizing the process and preventing the transformation of chronic **hepatitis** into **hepatocirrhosis.**"

Herpes simplex

Nutritional and therapeutic potential of Spirulina. Khan Z, Bhadouria P, Bisen PS. Curr Pharm Biotechnol. 2005 Oct;6(5):373-9. **Key Finding:** "Spirulina preparations influence immune system viz. increase phagocytic activity of macrophages, stimulating the production of antibodies and cytokines, increase accumulation of NK cells into tissue and activation and mobilization of T and B cells. Spirulina have also shown to perform regulatory role on lipid and carbohydrate metabolism by exhibiting glucose and lipid profile correction activity in experimental animals and in diabetic patients. Preparations have been found to be active against several enveloped viruses including **herpes virus, cytomegalovirus, influenza virus** and **HIV.** They are capable to inhibit carcinogenesis due to anti-oxidant properties that protect tissues and also reduce toxicity of liver, kidney and testes."

Antiviral activity of Spirulina maxima against **herpes simplex virus type 2.** Hernandez-Corona A, Nieves I, Meckes M, Chamorro G, Barron BL. Antiviral Res. 2002 Dec;56(3):279-85. **Key Finding:** "This paper presents the antiviral activity found in a hot water extract of Spirulina maxima, studied by a micro plate inhibition assay, using several viruses. The extract inhibited the infection for: herpes simplex virus type 2, pseudo rabies virus, human cytomegalovirus, and herpes simplex-1, and the 50% effective inhibition doses were 0.069, 0.103, 0.142, and 0.333 mg/ml for each virus. For adenovirus the inhibition was less than 20%, and no inhibition was found for measles virus, sub-acute sclerosing panencephalitis virus, vesicular stomatitis virus, poliovirus 1 and rotavirus SA-11."

*A natural sulfated polysaccharide, calcium spirulan, isolated from Spirulina platensis: in vitro and ex vivo evaluation of anti-***herpes simplex virus** *and anti-***human immunodeficiency virus** *activities.* Hayashi K, Hayaski T. KojimaI. AIDS Res Hum Retroviruses. 1996 Oct 10;12(15):1463-71. **Key Finding:** "These data indicate that calcium spirulan, isolated from a sea alga, is a potent antiviral agent against both HIV-1 and HSV-1."

Human Immunodeficiency Virus

Nutritional and therapeutic potential of Spirulina. Khan Z, Bhadouria P, Bisen PS. Curr Pharm Biotechnol. 2005 Oct;6(5):373-9. **Key Finding:** "Spirulina preparations influence immune system viz. increase phagocytic activity of macrophages, stimulating the production of antibodies and cytokines, increase accumulation of NK cells into tissue and activation and mobilization of T and B cells. Spirulina have also shown to perform regulatory role on lipid and carbohydrate metabolism by exhibiting glucose and lipid profile correction activity in experimental animals and in diabetic patients. Preparations have been found to be active against several enveloped viruses including **herpes virus, cytomegalovirus**, **influenza virus** and **HIV**. They are capable to inhibit carcinogenesis due to anti-oxidant properties that protect tissues and also reduce toxicity of liver, kidney and testes."

Nutrition rehabilitation of **HIV-infected** *and HIV-negative* **undernourished** *children utilizing spirulina.* Simpore J, Zongo F, Kabore F, Dansou D, Bere A, Nikiema JB, Pignatelli S, Biondi DM, Ruberto G, Musumeci S. Ann Nutr. Metab. 2005 Nov-Dec;49(6):373-89. **Key Finding:** "Our results confirm that Spirulina platensis is a good food supplement for undernourished children. In particular, rehabilitation with SP also seems to correct **anemia** and weight loss in HIV-infected children, and even more quickly in HIV-negative undernourished children."

*A natural sulfated polysaccharide, calcium spirulan, isolated from Spirulina platensis: in vitro and ex vivo evaluation of anti-***herpes simplex virus** *and anti-***human immunodeficiency virus** *activities.* Hayashi K, Hayaski T. KojimaI. AIDS Res Hum Retroviruses. 1996 Oct 10;12(15):1463-71. **Key Finding:** "These data indicate that calcium spirulan, isolated from a sea alga, is a potent antiviral agent against both HIV-1 and HSV-1."

Inhibition of **HIV-1** *replication by an aqueous extract of Spirulina platensis (Arthrospira platensis).* Ayehunie S, Belay A, Baba TW, Ruprecht RM. J Acquir Immune Defic Syndr Hum Retroviral. 1998 May 1;18(1):7-12. **Key Finding:** "Extract concentrations ranging between 0.3 and 1.2 micro/ml reduced viral production by approximately 50% in peripheral blood mononuclear cells. We conclude that aqueous A platensis extracts contain antiretroviral activity that may be of potential clinical interest."

Hypertension

Anti-hypertensive effect of gamma-amino butyric acid (GABA)-rich Chlorella on high-normal **blood pressure** *and borderline* **hypertension** *in placebo-controlled double blind study.* Shimada M, Hasegawa T, Nishimura C, Kan H, Kanno T, Nakamura T, Matsubayashi T. Clin Exp Hypertens. 2009 Jun;31(4):342-54. **Key Finding:** "These results suggest that GABA-rich Chlorella significantly decreased high-normal blood pressure and borderline hypertension, and is a beneficial dietary supplement for prevention of the development of hypertension."

Effects of dietary Spirulina on vascular reactivity. Juarez-Oropeza MA, Mascher D, Torres-Duran PV, Farias JM, Paredes-Carbajal MC. J Med Food. 2009 Feb;12(1):15-20. **Key Finding:** "In humans, Spirulina maxima intake decreases **blood pressure** and **plasma lipid** concentrations, especially tricyglycerol and low-density lipoprotein-cholesterol, and indirectly modifies the total cholesterol and high-density lipoprotein-cholesterol values."

Antihyperlipemic *and* ***antihypertensive*** *effects of Spirulina maxima in an open sample of Mexican population: a preliminary report.* Torres-Duran PV, Ferreira-Hermosillo A, Juarez-Oropeza MA. Lipids Health Dis. 2007 Nov 26;6:33. **Key Finding:** "The purpose of this study was to evaluate the effects of Spirulina maxima orally supplied (4.5g/day, for 6 weeks) to a sample of 36 subjects (16 men and 20 women) with ages between 18-65 years on serum lipids. The Spirulina maxima showed a hypolipemic effect, especially on the **triacylglycerol** and the LDL-C concentrations but indirectly on total **cholesterol** and HDL-C values. It also reduces systolic and diastolic **blood pressure**."

Nutritional supplementation with Chlorella pyrenoidosa for mild to moderate **hypertension.** Merchant RE, Andre CA, Sica DA. J Med Food. 2002 Fall;5(3):141-52. **Key Finding:** "The results indicate that, for some subjects with mild to moderate hypertension, a daily dietary supplement of Chlorella reduced or kept stable their sitting diastolic blood pressure."

A review of recent clinical trials of the nutritional supplement Chlorella pyrenoidosa in the treatment of **fibromyalgia, hypertension,** *and* **ulcerative colitis**. Merchant RE, Andre CA. Alter Ther Health Med. 2001 May-Jun;7(3):79-91. **Key Finding:** "The potential of chlorella to relieve symptoms, improve quality of life, and normalize body functions in patients with fibromyalgia, hypertension, or ulcerative colitis suggests that larger, more comprehensive clinical trials of chlorella are warranted."

Identification of antihypertensive peptides from peptic digests of two microalgae, Chlorella vulgaris and Spirulina platensis. Suetsuna K, Chen JR. Mar Biotechnol. 2001 Jul;3(4):305-9. **Key Finding:** "The peptidic fractions that inhibited angiotensin I-converting enzyme (ACE) were separated from the peptic digests of 2 microalgae, Chlorella vulgaris and Spirulina platensis, by ion exchange chromatography and gel filtration. Oral administration of peptidic fractions into spontaneously **hypertensive** rats at 200 mg/kg of body weight resulted in marked antihypertensive effects."

Hypoglycemia

Nutrigenomic studies of effects of Chlorella on subjects with high-risk factors for lifestyle-related disease. Mizoguchi T, Takehara I, Masuzawa T, Saito T, Naoki Y. J Med Food. 2008 Sep;11(3):395-404. **Key Finding:** "We conducted blood biochemical tests on 17 subjects over a 16-week period and analyzed gene expression profile in whole blood cells in the peripheral blood before and after Chlorella intake. Chlorella intake resulted in noticeable reductions in body fat percentage, serum total **cholesterol,** and fasting blood glucose levels. There were clear variations in the expression profiles of genes directly related to uptake of glucose resulting from Chlorella intake, indicating that the activation of insulin signaling pathways could be the reason for the **hypoglycemic** effects of Chlorella."

Immune system health

Immunostimulatory *Bioactivity of Algal Polysaccharides from Chlorella pyrenoidosa Activates Macrophages via Toll-Like Receptor 4.* Hsu HY. Jeyashoke N, Yeh CH, Song YJ, Hua KF, Chao LK. J Agric Food Chem. 2009 Nov 16. (Epub ahead of print). **Key Finding:** "Our current results provide support for the possible use of Chlorella pyrenoidosa as a modulation agent of immune responses in humans. This study is the first to report the molecular mechanism of immune-modulated signal transduction in vitro from the polysaccharides of Chlorella pyrenoidosa."

A randomized double-blind, placebo-controlled study to establish the effects of spirulina in elderly Koreans. Park HJ, Lee YJ, Ryu HK, Kim MH, Chung HW, Kim WY. Ann Nutr Metab. 2008;52(4):322-8. **Key Finding:** "The results demonstrate that spirulina has favorable effects on **lipid profiles**, **immune variables, and antioxidant capacity** in healthy, elderly male and female subjects and is suitable as a functional food."

Natural killer cell activation and modulation of chemokine receptor profile in vitro by an extract from the cyanophyta Aphanizomenon flos-aquae. Hart AN, Zaske LA, Patterson KM, Drapeau C, Jensen GS. J Med Food. 2007 Sep;10(3):435-41. **Key Finding:** "We have previously shown, using a double-blind randomized placebo-controlled crossover design, that ingestion of 1.5 g of dried whole A. flos-aquae resulted in a transient reduction in peripheral blood natural killer (NK) cells in 21 healthy human volunteers, suggesting increased NK cell homing into tissue. We have now identified an extract from A. flos-aquae that directly activates NK cells in vitro and modulates the chemokine receptor profile."

*The influence of Spirulina and Selen-Spirulina on some indexes of rat's **immune** status.* Trushina EN, Gladkikh O, Gadzhieva ZM, Mustafina OK, Pozdniakov AL. Vopr Pitan (Russian). 2007;76(2):21-5. **Key Finding:** "The immunostimulatory effect of Spirulina and Selen-Spirulina was confirmed by morphologic and morphometric investigation of rats spleen, also with NBT-test of peritoneal macrophages."

Oral administration of hot water extracts of Chlorella vulgaris increases physical stamina in mice. An HJ, Choi HM, Park HS, Han JG, Lee EH, Park YS, Um JY, Hong SH, Kim HM. Ann Nutr Metab. 2006;50(4):380-6. **Key Finding:** "The results predict a potential benefit of Chlorella vulgaris for enhancing **immune function** and improving physical stamina."

Molecular immune mechanism of C-phycocyanin from Spirulina platensis induces apoptosis in HeLa cells in vitro. Li B, Gao MH, Zhang XC, Chu XM. Biotechnol Appl Biochem. 2006 Mar;43(Pt 3):155-64. **Key Finding:** "In the present study, we first investigated the effect of highly purified C-phycocyanin from Spirulina on growth and proliferation of HeLa cells in vitro. The results indicated that there was a significant decrease in the number of cells that survived for HeLa cells treated with C-PC compared with control cells untreated. Further electron-microscopic studies revealed that C-PC could induce characteristic apoptotic features, including cell shrinkage, microvilli loss, chromatin margination and condensation into dense granules or blocks."

Toll-like receptor 2-dependent activation of monocytes by Spirulina polysaccharide and its immune enhancing action in mice. Balachandran P, Pugh ND, Ma G, Pasco DS. Int Immunopharmacol. 2006 Dec 5;6(12):1808-14. **Key Finding:** "These studies shed light on how a high molecular weight polysaccharide fraction (Immunlina) from Spirulina activates cells of the innate **immune system** and suggests that oral consumption of this polysaccharide can enhance components within both the mucosal and systemic immune systems."

*Activation of the human innate **immune system** by Spirulina: augmentation of interferon production and NK cytotoxicity by oral administration of hot water extract of Spirulina platensis.* Hirahashi T, Matsumoto M, Hazeki K, Saeki Y, Ui M, Seya T. Int Immunopharmacol. 2002 Mar;2(4):423-34. **Key Finding:** "We identified the molecular mechanism of the human immune potentiating capacity of Spirulina by analyzing blood cells of volunteers with pre and post oral administration of hot water extract of Spirulina. These observations indicated that in humans Spirulina acts directly on myeloid lineages and either directly or indirectly on NK cells."

Biological activity of Spirulina. Blinkova LP, Gorobets OB, Baturo AP. Zh Mikrobiol Epidemiol Immunobiol (Russian). 2001 Mar-Apr;(2):114-8. **Key Finding:** "Spirulina platensis has been found suitable for use as bioactive additive. SP produces an immuno-stimulating effect by enhancing the resistance of humans, mammals, chickens and fish to **infections**, the capacity of influencing hemopoiesis, stimulating the production of antibodies and cytokines. SP extracts are capable in inhibiting **cancerogenesis.**"

Effects of Chlorella vulgaris on bone marrow progenitor cells of mice infected with Listeria monocytogenes. Dantas DC, Queiroz ML. Int J Immunopharmacol. 1999 Aug;21(8):499-508. **Key Finding:** "These results demonstrated that Chlorella vulgaris extract produces a significant increase in the resistance of the animals infected with L. monocytogenes, and that this protection is due, at least in part, to increased CFU-GM in the bone marrow of infected animals."

*The effects of Chlorella vulgaris in the protection of mice infected with Listeria monocytogenes. Role of **natural killer cells**.* Dantas DC, Kaneno R, Queiroz ML. Immunopharmacol Immunotoxicol. 1999 Aug;21(3):609-19. **Key Finding:** "Chlorella vulgaris treatment (50 and 500mg/Kg) of mice infected with a dose of 3 x 10(5) bacteria/animal, which was lethal for all the non-treated controls, produced a dose-response protection which led to a 20% and 55% survival, respectively."

The Effects of the Blue Green Algae A.phanizomenon flos-aquae on Human Natural Killer Cells. Manoukian R, Citton M, Huerta P, Rhode B, Drapeau C, Jensen G. IBC Library Series. 1998;vol.1911;Chpt. 3.1. **Key Finding:** A team of medical researchers at Royal Victoria Hospital in Canada examined how Super Blue-Green Algae strengthens the human **immune system**. The double-blind study of 50 people found that after consuming 1.5 grams of this algae, their NK-natural killer cell activity increased significantly, provoking these immune cells to move from the bloodstream into body tissues to scavenge for sick cells and toxic invaders.

*Enhancement of **antibody** production in mice by dietary Spirulina platensis.* Hayashi O, Katoh T, Okuwaki Y. J Nutr Sci Vitaminol. 1994 Oct;40(5):431-41. **Key Finding:** "Mice fed a Spirulina platensis diet showed increased numbers of splenic antibody-producing cells in the primary immune response. These results suggest that Spirulina enhances the immune response, particularly the primary response, by stimulating macrophage functions, phagocytosis, and IL-1 production."

***Immunostimulating** activity of the lipopolysaccharides of blue-green algae.* Besednova NN, Smolina TP, Mikheiskaia LV, Ovodova RG. Zh Mikrobiol Epidemiol Immunobiol (Russian). 1979 Dec;(12):75-9. **Key Finding:** "The whole cells of blue-green algae and lipopolysaccharides isolated from these cells were shown to stimulate the production of macro-(mainly) and microglobulin antibodies in rabbits. The macro- and microphage indices in rabbits increased significantly after the injection of LPS isolated from blue-green algae 24-48 hours before infecting the animals with a virulent Y pseudo tuberculosis strain."

Infectious Agents

Flow cytometric analysis of age-related changes in intestine intraepithelial lymphocyte subsets and their functional preservation after feeding mice on spirulina. Hayashia O, Katayanagi Y, Ishii K, Kato T. J Med Food. 2009 Oct;12(5):982-9. **Key Finding:** "These results suggest that ingestion of SpHW (spirulina) in the aged-SP group may contribute to the functional preservation of the intestinal epithelium as a first line of mucosal barrier against **infectious** agents through retaining the number of certain IELs (intestinal intraepithelial lymphocytes.)"

*Action of Spirulina platensis on **bacterial viruses**.* Gorobets OB, Blinkova LP, Baturo AP. Zh Mikrobiol Epidemiol Immunobiol (Russian). 2002 Nov-Dec;(6):18-21. **Key Finding:** "The impact of the biomass of the blue-green microalga (cyanobacteria) S. platensis on bacteriophage T4 (bacterial virus) has been evaluated. The study revealed that the addition of S. platensis biomass into the agar nutrient medium, followed by sterilization with 2% chloroform and thermal treatment, produced an inhibiting or stimulating effect on the reproduction of the bacteriophage in Escherichia coli B cells, depending on the concentration of S. platensis and the multiplicity of phage infection, as well as on the face whether the microalgae were added during the first cycle of the development of the virus."

Biological activity of Spirulina. Blinkova LP, Gorobets OB, Baturo AP. Zh Mikrobiol Epidemiol Immunobiol (Russian). 2001 Mar-Apr;(2):114-8. **Key Finding:** "Spirulina platensis has been found suitable for use as bioactive additive. SP produces an immuno-stimulating effect by enhancing the resistance of humans, mammals, chickens and fish to **infections**, the capacity of influencing hemopoiesis, stimulating the production of antibodies and cytokines. SP extracts are capable in inhibiting **cancerogenesis**."

Inflammation

Effects of chlorella on activities of protein tyrosine phosphatases, matrix metalloproteinase, caspases, cytokine release, B and T cell proliferations, and phorbol ester receptor binding. Cheng FC, Lin A, Feng JJ, Mizoguchi T, Takekoshi H, Kubota H, Kato Y, Naoki Y. J Med Food. 2004 Summer;7(2):146-52. **Key Finding:** "These results reveal potential pharmacological activities that, if confirmed by vivo studies, might be exploited for the prevention or treatment of several serious pathologies, including **inflammatory** disease and **cancer**."

Attenuating effect of chlorella supplementation on oxidative stress and NFkappaB activation in peritoneal macrophages and liver of C57BL/6 mice fed on an atherogenic diet. Lee HS, Choi CY, Cho C, Song Y. Biosci Biotechnol Biochem. 2003 Oct;67(10):2083-90. **Key Finding:** "These results suggest that chlorella supplementation may attenuate oxidative stress by reducing reactive oxygen production and increasing anti-oxidative processes, thus suppressing **inflammatory** mediatory activation in peritoneal macrophages and liver."

Inhibition of mast cells by algae. Price JA, Sanny C, Shevlin D. J Med Food. 2002 Winter;5(4):205-10. **Key Finding:** "We saw wide phylogenetic dispersion of mast cell inhibition activity, suggesting that this **anti-inflammatory** property is common in algae. This effect was apparently due to multiple activities within the algal extracts."

Role of histamine in the inhibitory effects of phycocyanin in experimental models of allergic **inflammatory** *response.* Remierez D, Ledon N, Gonzalez R. Mediators Inflamm. 2002 Apr;11(2):81-5. **Key Finding:** "The inhibitory effects of phycocyanin, a biliprotein found in Spirulina, were dose dependent. Our results suggest that inhibition of allergic inflammatory response by phycocyanin is mediated, at least in part, by inhibition of histamine release from mast cells."

Anti-inflammatory, analgesic and free radical scavenging activities of the marine microalgae Chlorella stigmatophora and Phaeodactylum tricornutum. Guzman S, Gato A, Calleja JM. Phytother Res. 2001 May;15(3):224-30. **Key Finding:** "Hydro soluble components of Chlorella stigmatophora and Phaeodactylum tricornutum show significant anti-inflammatory, analgesic and free radical scavenging activity. These activities were not detected in the lip soluble fractions."

*Effects of phycocyanin extract on prostaglandin E2 levels in mouse ear **inflammation** test.* Romay C, Ledon N, Gonzalez R. Arzneimittelforschung. 2000 Dec;50(12):1106-9. **Key Finding:** "These results provide the first evidence that the anti-inflammatory effects of phycocyanin may result, at least partially, from inhibition of PGE2 production and a moderate inhibition of PLA2 activity."

Effect of spirulina on the secretion of cytokines from peripheral blood mononuclear cells. Mao TK, Van de Water J, Gershwin ME. J Med Food. 2000 Fall;3(3):135-40. **Key Finding:** "Although Spirulina stimulates several cytokines, it is clearly more effective in the generation of a Thl-type response. This in vitro study offers additional data for consideration of the potential therapeutic benefits of Spirulina."

Influenza

Nutritional and therapeutic potential of Spirulina. Khan Z, Bhadouria P, Bisen PS. Curr Pharm Biotechnol. 2005 Oct;6(5):373-9. **Key Finding:** "Spirulina preparations influence immune system viz. increase phagocytic activity of macrophages, stimulating the production of antibodies and cytokines, increase accumulation of NK cells into tissue and activation and mobilization of T and B cells. Spirulina have also shown to perform regulatory role on lipid and carbohydrate metabolism by exhibiting glucose and lipid profile correction activity in experimental animals and in diabetic patients. Preparations have been found to be active against several enveloped viruses including **herpes virus, cytomegalovirus**, **influenza virus** and **HIV**. They are capable to inhibit carcinogenesis due to anti-oxidant properties that protect tissues and also reduce toxicity of liver, kidney and testes."

Safety and immunoenhancing effect of a Chlorella-derived dietary supplement in health adults undergoing influenza vaccination: randomized, double-blind, placebo-controlled trial. Halperin SA, Smith B, Nolan C, Shay J, Kralovec J. CMAJ. 2003 Jul 22;169(2):111-7. **Key Finding:** "The Chlorella-derived dietary supplement did not have any effect in increasing the antibody response to influenza vaccine in the overall study population, although there was an increase in antibody response among participants aged 50-55 years."

Irritable bowel syndrome

*Selenium deficiency and its dietary correction in patients with **irritable bowel syndrome** and chronic catarrhal **colitis**.* Bogatov NV. Vopr Pitan (Russian). 2007;76(3):35-9. **Key Finding:** "Serum selenium levels were measured in 80 patients with chronic catarrhal colitis (CCC) and irritated bowel syndrome (IBS). 78% of patients examined showed selenium insufficiency, which was relatively less pronounced in IBS compared to CCC. Reception of a selenium enriched food supplement based on spirulina led to about a twofold diminishment of patient's number with selenium insufficiency."

Ischemia

*C-phycocyanin protects against **ischemia**-reperfusion injury of heart through involvement of p38 MAPK and ERK signaling.* Khan M, Varadharaj S, Ganesan LP, Shobha JC, Naidu MU, Parinandi NL, Tridandapani S, Kutala VK, Kuppusamy P. Am J Physiol Heart Circ Physiol. 2006 May;290(5):H2136-45. **Key Finding:** "These results for the first time showed that C-phycocyanin from Spirulina attenuated I/R-induced cardiac dysfunction through its antioxidant and anti-apoptotic actions and modulation of p38 MAPK and ERK1/2."

Dietary supplementation with blueberries, spinach, or spirulina reduces ischemic brain damage. Wang Y, Chang CF, Chou J, Chen HL, Deng X, Harvey BK, Cadet JL, Bickford PC. Exp Neurol. 2005 May;193(1):75-84. **Key Finding:** "Free radicals are involved in neurodegenerative disorders, such as **ischemia** and **aging**. We have previously demonstrated that treatment with diets enriched with blueberry, spinach, or spirulina have been shown to reduce neurodegenerative changes in aged animals. The purpose of this study was to determine if these diets have neuroprotective effects in focal ischemic brain in Sprague-Dawley rats. Animals treated with blueberry, spinach, or spirulina had significantly lower caspase-3 activity in the ischemic hemisphere. In conclusion, our data suggest that chronic treatment with blueberry, spinach, or spirulina reduces ischemia/reperfusion-induced apoptosis and cerebral infarction."

*Use of blue-green micro-seaweed Spirulina platensis for the correction of lipid and hemostatic disturbances in patients with **ischemic heart disease**.* Ionov VA, Basova MM. Vopr Pitan (Russian). 2003;72(6):28-31. **Key Finding:** "Changing in lipid spectrum, immunological state and coagulation in the 68 patients with ischemic heart disease and atherogenic dyslipidemia who were taking biomass microalga Spirulina platensis was investigated. Modification of traditional plan of therapy of IHD when adding Spirulina influences correcting effect to cascade procoagulation and immunopathologic reactions, characteristic of atherosclerosis process."

Jaundice

Administration of Chlorella sp. Microalgae reduces endotoxemia, intestinal oxidative stress and bacterial translocation in experimental biliary obstruction. Bedirli A, Kerem M, Ofluoglu E, Salman B, Katircioglu H, Bedirli N, Yilmazer D, Alper M, Pasaoglu H. Clin Nutr. 2009 Dec;28(6):674-8. **Key Finding:** "Chlorella sp. Microalgae supplemented enteral diet has significant protective effects on intestinal mucosa barrier in **obstructive jaundice**, and reduces intestinal translocation of bacteria and endotoxin."

Liver damage

*Antagonistic effects of Se-rich Spirulina platensis on rat **liver fibrosis**.* Huang Z, Zheng W. Wei Sheng Yan Jiu (Chinese). 2007 Jan;36(1):34-6. **Key Finding:** "The results indicated that Se-SP has detectable antagonistic effects to liver fibrosis, and suggested that enhancement of anti-oxidation level and liver reserve function might be associated with these effects."

Malnutrition

*Nutrition rehabilitation of **undernourished** children utilizing Spirulina and Misola.* Simpore J, Kabore F, Zongo F, Dansou D, Bere A, Pignatelli S, Biondi DM, Buerto G, Musumeci S. Nutr J. 2006 Jan 23;5:3. **Key Finding:** "Our results indicate that Misola, Spirulina plus traditional meals or Spirulina plus Misola are all a good food supplement for undernourished children, but the rehabilitation by Spirulina plus Misola seems to favor the nutrition rehabilitation better than the simple addition of protein and energy intake."

*Nutrition rehabilitation of **HIV-infected** and HIV-negative **undernourished** children utilizing spirulina.* Simpore J, Zongo F, Kabore F, Dansou D, Bere A, Nikiema JB, Pignatelli S, Biondi DM, Ruberto G, Musumeci S. Ann Nutr. Metab. 2005 Nov-Dec;49(6):373-89. **Key Finding:** "Our results confirm that Spirulina platensis is a good food supplement for undernourished children. In particular, rehabilitation with SP also seems to correct **anemia** and weight loss in HIV-infected children, and even more quickly in HIV-negative undernourished children."

Nutritional studies on Spirulina maxima. Maranesi M, Barzanti V, Carenini G, Gentili P. Acta Vitaminol Enzymol. 1984;6(4):295-304. **Key Finding:** "Our research was conducted in young growing rats; it provide confirmation of the validity of Spirulina as a protein source in terms of good weight gain by the animals and freedom from adverse effects; the same research, on the other hand, failed to confirm the effectiveness of these protein materials in reducing caloric intake."

Obesity

Chlorella methanol extract reduces lipid accumulation in and increase the number of apoptotic 3T3-L1 cells. Chon JW, Sung JH, Hwang EJ, Park YK. Ann N Y Acad Sci. 2009 Aug;1171:183-9. **Key Finding:** "Obesity is a fast-growing problem. Chlorella has many biological merits for promoting health, including detoxification, boosting the immune system, and even reversing **cancer**. In this study, we found that methanol extract of Chlorella reduces lipid accumulation in 3T3-L1 adipocytes. It has been postulated that these anti-obesity effects could be a result of reducing **adipogenesis**."

Ethanolic extract of Spirulina maxima alters the vasomotor reactivity of aortic rings from obese rats. Mascher D, Paredes-Carbajal MC, Torres-Duran PV, Zamora-Gonzalez J, Diaz-Zagoya JC, Juarez-Oropeza MA. Arch Med Res. 2006 Jan;37(1):50-7. **Key Finding:** "These results suggest that, in rings from obese rats, the extract, in addition to increasing the synthesis/release of NO, also inhibits the synthesis/release of a cyclooxygenase-dependent vasoconstrictor metabolite of arachidonic acid, which is increased in **obesity**."

Osteoporosis

*Spirulina protects against Rosiglitazone induced **osteoporosis** in insulin resistance rats.* Gupta S, Hrishikeshvan HJ, Sehajpal PK. Diabetes Res Clin Pract. 2009 Nov 4. (Epub ahead of print). **Key Finding:** "These findings suggest that combination therapy of Rosiglitazone with Spirulina reduced the risk of osteoporosis in insulin resistance in rats. Additionally, Spirulina complemented the **anti-hyperglycemic** and **anti-lipidemic** activity of Rosiglitazone."

Parkinson's disease

*Oral phycocyanobilin may diminish the pathogenicity of activated brain microglia in **neurodegenerative disorders**.* McCarty MF, Barroso-Aranda J, Contreras F. Med

Hypotheses. 2009 Jul 1. (Epub ahead of print). **Key Finding:** "There is considerable evidence that activated microglia play a central role in the pathogenesis of many prominent neurodegenerative disorders, including **Parkinson's** and **Alzheimer's** diseases. Phycocyanobilin, a chromophone derived from biliverdin that constitutes up to 1% of the dry weight of Spirulina, has been shown to be a potent inhibitor of NADPH oxidase. Phycocyanobilin supplements may have considerable potential for preventing or slowing the progression of a range of neurodegenerative disorders."

Neuroprotection by Spirulina platensis protean extract and phycocyanin against iron-induced toxicity in SH-SY5Y neuroblastoma cells. Bermejo-Bescos P, Pifiero-Estrada E, Villar del Fresno AM. Toxicol In Vitro. 2008 Sep;22(6):1496-502. **Key Finding:** "These results suggested that S. platensis protean extract is a powerful antioxidant through a mechanism related to antioxidant activity, capable of interfering with radical-mediated cell death. S. platensis may be useful in diseases known to be aggravated by reactive oxygen species and in the development of novel treatments for neurodegenerative disorders as long as iron has been implicated in the neuropathology of several neurodegenerative disorders such as **Alzheimer's** and **Parkinson diseases**."

Spirulina maxima pretreatment partially protects against 1-methyl-4-phenyl-1,2,3,6-tetrahydrophyridine neurotoxicity. Chamorro G, Perez-Albiter M, Serrano-Garcia N, Mares-Samano JJ, Rojas P. Nutr Neurosci. 2006 Oct-Dec;9(5-6):207-12. **Key Finding:** "Spirulina is an alga that has a high nutritional value and some of its biological activities are attributed to the presence of antioxidants. Oxidative stress is involved in **Parkinson's disease**. This study aims at evaluating the neuroprotective role of Spirulina maxima (Sp.) against 1-methyl-4-phenyl-1,2,3,6-tetrahydropyridine (MPTP) neurotoxicity, used as a model of Parkinson's disease. Ninety-six male C-57 black mice were pretreated with Spirulina for 14 days followed by three MPTP administrations. Sp. Pretreatment at 150 mg/kg partially prevented (51%) the DA-depleting effect of MPTP and blocked oxidative stress, suggesting Spirulina could be a possible alternative in experimental therapy."

Blueberry- and spirulina-enriched diets enhance striatal dopamine recovery and induce rapid, transient microglia activation after injury of the rat nigrostriatal dopamine system. Stromberg I, Gemma C, Vila J, Bickford PC. Exp Neurol. 2005 Dec;196(2):298-307. **Key Finding:** "Neuroinflammation plays a critical role in loss of dopamine neurons during brain injury and in **neurodegenerative diseases**. Diets enriched in foods with antioxidant and anti-inflammatory actions may modulate this neuroinflammation. Enhanced striatal dopamine recovery appeared in animals treated with diet enrich in antioxidants and anti-inflammatory phytochemicals (blueberry and spirulina) and coincided with an early, transient increase in OX-6-positive microglia."

Pneumonia

*Experience with a selenium-containing biological active supplement used in children with **pneumonias** in an intensive care unit.* Uglitskikh AK, Tsokova NB, Gmoshionskii IV, Mazo VK, Kon Ha, Ostreikov IF. Anesteziol Reanimatol (Russian). 2006 Jan-Feb;(1):45-8. **Key Finding:** "The findings suggest that the Spirulin-Sochi-Selen is effective as part of therapy for acute pneumonia in children treated in an intensive care unit. There were no signs of selenium deficiency in any case despite the baseline reduction in the average serum levels."

Renal Function

Spirulina platensis protects against gentamicin-induced nephrotoxicity in rats. Karadeniz A, Yildirim A, Simsek N, Kalkan Y, Celebi F. Phytother Res. 2008 Nov;22(11):1506-10. **Key Finding:** "The present study indicates a very important role of reactive oxygen species (ROS) and the relation to **renal dysfunction** and point to the therapeutic potential of Spirulina platensis in gentamicin sulfate induced nephrotoxicity."

*Spirulina platensis protects against **renal injury** in rats with gentamicin-induced acute tubular necrosis.* Avdagic N, Cosovic E, Nakas-Kindic E, Mornjakovic Z, Zaciragic A, Hadzovic-Dzuvo A. Bosn J Basic Med Sci. 2008 Nov;8(4):331-6. **Key Finding:** "The results from the present study suggest that Spirulina platensis has Reno protective potential in gentamicin-induced acute tubular necrosis possibly due to its antioxidant properties."

Protection against cisplatin-induced nephrotoxicity by Spirulina in rats. Mohan IK, Khan M, Shobha JC, Naidu MU, Prayag A, Kuppusamy P, Kutala VK. Cancer Chemother Pharmacol. 2006 Dec;58(6):802-8. **Key Finding:** "Cisplatin-induced nephrotoxicity is associated with the increased generation of reactive oxygen metabolites and lipid peroxidation in kidney, caused by the decreased levels of antioxidants and antioxidant enzymes. Spirulina significantly protected the CP-induced nephrotoxicity through its antioxidant properties."

Effect of Spirulina, blue green algae, on gentamicin-induced oxidative stress and **renal dysfunction** *in rats.* Kuhad A, Tirkey N, Pilkhwal S, Chopra K. Fundam Clin Pharmacol. 2006 Apr;20(2):121-8. **Key Finding:** "The results of present study clearly demonstrate the pivotal role of reactive oxygen species and their relation to renal dysfunction and point to the therapeutic potential of S. fusiformis in GM-induced nephrotoxicity."

Prophylactic role of phycocyanin: a study of oxalate mediated **renal cell injury**. Farooq SM, Asokan D, Kalaiselvi P, Sakthivel R, Varalakshmi P. Chem Biol Interact. 2004 Aug 10;149(1):1-7. **Key Finding:** "The present analysis revealed the antioxidant and antiurolithic potential of phycocyanin thereby projecting it as a promising therapeutic agent against renal cell injury associated with **kidney stone** formation."

Skeletal Muscle Damage

Preventive effects of Spirulina platensis on **skeletal muscle damage** *under exercise-induced oxidative stress.* Lu HK, Hsieh CC, Hsu JJ, Yang YK, Chou HN. Eur J Appl Physiol. 2006 Sep;98(2):220-6. **Key Finding:** "The effects of spirulina supplementation on preventing skeletal muscle damage on untrained human beings were examined in 16 student volunteers. Blood samples were taken after finishing the Bruce incremental treadmill exercise before and after treatment. These results suggest that ingestion of S. platensis showed preventive effect of the skeletal muscle damage and that probably led to postponement of the time of exhaustion during the all-out exercise."

Stroke

Effect of chlorella and its fractions on blood pressure, **cerebral stroke** *lesions, and life-span in stroke-prone spontaneously* **hypertensive** *rats.* Sansawa H, Takahashi M, Tsuchikura S, Endo H. J Nutr Sci Vitaminol. 2006 Dec;52(6):457-66. **Key Finding:** "These experimental results suggest that the beneficial effect of Chlorella on stroke-prone spontaneously hypertensive rats are caused by the synergistic action of several ingredients of Chlorella, which play a role in sustention of a vascular function of rats."

Thrombosis

Evaluating the possible genotoxic, mutagenic and tumor cell proliferation-inhibition effects of a non-anticoagulant, but antithrombotic algal heterofucan. Almedia-Lima J, Costa LS, Silva

NB, Et al. J Appl Toxicol. 2010 Oct;30(7):708-15. **Key Finding**: "Fucan is a term used to denominate a family of sulfated polysaccharides extracted mainly from brown seaweeds. Our research group purified a non-anticoagulant hetero-fucan (fucan A) which displays antithrombotic activity in vivo. Tumor-cell (HeLa, PC3, PANC, HL60) proliferation was inhibited. Non-tumor cell lines proliferation were not affected by this molecule."

C-phycocyanin, a very potent and novel platelet aggregation inhibitor from Spirulina platensis. Hsiao G, Chou PH, Shen MY, Chou DS, Lin CH, Sheu JR. J Agric Food Chem. 2005 Oct 5;53(20):7734-40. **Key Finding:** "These results strongly suggest that C-phycocyanin from Spirulina platensis appears to represent a novel and potential antiplatelet agent for treatment of arterial **thromboembolism**."

Tuberculosis

Evaluation of the efficacy of a plant adaptogen (spirulina) in the pathogenic therapy of primary **tuberculosis** *in children.* Kostromina VP, Derkach OV, Symonenkova NV, Riechkina OO, Otroshchenko AO. Lik Sprava (Ukrainian). 2003 Jul-Aug;(5-6):102-5. **Key Finding:** "The use of spirulina and its efficiency have been studied in a comparative aspect as a systemic bio corrector, in a combined treatment of tuberculosis in 26 children. It has been ascertained that application of spirulina as a pathogenic means of remediation permits shortening the intoxication syndrome regression time, reducing the frequency of adverse reactions in administering anti-tuberculosis preparations."

Ulcers

Oral administration of unicellular green algae, Chlorella vulgaris, prevents stress-induced **ulcer.** Tanaka K, Yamada A, Noda K, Shoyama Y, Kubo C, Nomoto K. Planta Med. 1997 Oct;63(5):465-6. **Key Finding:** "Oral administration of dry powder of Chlorella vulgaris showed clear prophylactic effects in water-immersion restraint stress-induced and in cysteamine-induced peptic ulcer models, but not in Shay's rat model. Chlorella vulgaris may prevent ulcer formation mainly through the immune-brain-gut axis and protection of gastric mucosa by its own characteristics."

Almonds (see Nuts)

Apples

STARTING AT LEAST WITH THE BIBLICAL STORY of Adam and Eve, apples have long been a fixture of the human experience of food. It may have been the first domesticated tree, and its fruits have evolved over thousands of years until today there are at least 7,500 known cultivars of apples grown worldwide. China produces about one-third of all the apples on the planet, followed by the United States (with just under 10 percent of the total), even though the tree wasn't brought to the North American continent until the 1600s, when the first orchard appeared near Boston.

Though relatively low in vitamin C compared to other fruits, apples contain numerous phenolic phytochemical antioxidants, primarily quercetin and epicatechin. They also possess more than a dozen vitamins and minerals. Research has demonstrated a wide array of health benefits of consuming apples, including helping to lower weight and cholesterol and reducing the risk of various cancers, cardiovascular disease, and neurodegenerative declines due to aging.

Aging

*Apple juice concentrate prevents oxidative damage and impaired maze performance in **aged** mice.* Tchantchou F, Chan A, Kifle L, Ortiz D, Shea TB. J Alzheimers Dis. 2005 Dec;8(3):283-7. **Key Finding:** "Supplementation with apple juice concentrate prevented neurodegenerative effects. These findings also support the efficacy of antioxidant supplementation, including consumption of antioxidant rich foods such as apples, in preventing the **decline in cognitive performance** that accompanies normal **aging**."

*Apple juice prevents oxidative stress and impaired **cognitive performance** caused by genetic and dietary deficiencies in mice.* Rogers EJ, Milhalik S, Orthiz D, Shea TB. J Nutr Health Aging. 2004;8(2):92-7. **Key Finding:** "Herein, we demonstrate that apple juice concentrate, administered ad libitum in drinking water, can compensate for the increased reactive oxygen species and decline in cognitive performance in maze trials observed when normal and transgenic mice lacking apolipoprotein E are deprived of folate and vitamin E."

*Diets enriched in foods with high **antioxidant** activity reverse age-induced decreases in cerebellar beta-adrenergic function and increases in proinflammatory cytokines.* Gemma C, Mesches MH, Sepesi B, Choo K, Holmes DB, Bickford PC. J Neurosci. 2002 Jul 15;22(14):6114-20. **Key Finding:** "Antioxidants and diets supplemented with foods high in oxygen radical absorbance capacity (ORAC) reverse **age-**related decreases in cerebellar beta-adrenergic receptor function. Aged male Fischer 344 rats were given apple (5 mg dry weight), spirulina (5 mg) or cucumber (5 mg) daily for 14 days. Electro physiologic techniques revealed a significant decrease in beta-adrenergic receptor function in aged control rats. Spirulina reversed this effect. Apple had an intermediate effect, and cucumber (low ORAC) had no effect, indicating that the reversal of beta-adrenergic receptor function decreases might be related to the ORAC dose."

Allergies

Procyanidin C1 from apple extracts inhibits Fc epsilon RI-mediated mast cell activation. Nakano N, Nishiyama C, Tokura T, Nagasako-Akazome Y, Ohtake Y, Okumura K, Ogawa H. Int Arch Allergy Immunol. 2008;147(3):213-21. **Key Finding:** "Polyphenol-enriched fractions extracted from unripe apples (Rosacea, Malus spp.) consisting of procyanidins have an **anti-allergenic** effect. It suppresses Fc epsilon RI-mediated mast cell activation by inhibiting intracellular signaling pathways. These observations provide evidence for the anti-allergenic effects of the procyanidin-enriched apple extract."

***Antiallergic** effect of apple polyphenols on the allergic model mouse.* Akiyama H, Sakushima J, Taniuchi S, Kanda T, Yanagida A, Kokima T, Tshima R, Kobayashi Y, Goda Y, Toyoda M. Biol Pharm Bull. 2000 Nov;23(11):1370-3. **Key Finding:** "These findings suggest that apple condensed tannins have an antiallergic effect on type I allergic symptoms."

Alzheimer's

Effects of banana, orange, and apple on oxidative stress-induced neurotoxicity in PC12 cells. Heo HJ, Choi SJ, CHoi SG, Shin DH, Lee JM, Lee CY. J Food Sci. 2008 Mar;73(2):H28-32. **Key Finding:** "These results suggest that fresh apples, bananas, and oranges in our daily diet along with other fruits may protect neuron cells against oxidative-stress-induced neurotoxicity and may play an important role in reducing the risk of neurodegenerative disorders such as **Alzheimer's** disease."

Antioxidation

*Efficiency of apples, strawberries, and tomatoes for reduction of **oxidative stress** in pigs as a model for humans.* Pajk T, Rezar V, Levart A, Salobir J. Nutrition. 2006 Apr;22(4):376-84. **Key Finding:** "Our findings support the hypothesis that supplementation with apples, strawberries, or tomatoes effectively decreases oxidative stress by decreasing MDA formation in the body and by protecting mononuclear blood cells against increased DNA damage. This effect was particularly pronounced in the group supplemented with a fruit mixture; among the single fruit supplements, the most beneficial effect was obtained with apples."

Effect of apple extracts on NF-kappaB activation in human umbilical vein endothelial cells. Davis PA, Polagruto JA, Valacchi G, Phung A, Soucek K, Keen CL, Gershwin ME. Exp Biol Med. 2006 May;231(5):594-8. **Key Finding:** "We suggest that flavonoid-rich apple extract down regulates NF-kappaB signaling and that this is indicative of an antioxidant effect of the flavonoids present."

Major Phytochemicals in apple cultivars: contribution to peroxyl radical trapping efficiency. Vanzani P, Rossetto M, Rigo A, Vrhovsek U, Mattivi F, D'Amato E, Scarpa M. J Agric Food Chem. 2005 May 4;53(9):3377-82. **Key Finding:** "Forty-one samples of apples (peel plus pulp) obtained from eight cultivars were examined for concentration of some important phytochemicals and for antioxidant activity. The antioxidant efficiency of the apple extracts and of representative pure compounds for each group of phytochemicals (five major polyphenol groups) was measured. The antioxidant efficiency calculated on the basis of the contribution of the pure compounds was lower than the antioxidant efficiency of the apple extracts. The higher efficiency of apples appears to be strictly related to the overwhelming presence of oligomeric proanthocyanidin."

Protection by quercetin and quercetin-rich fruit juice against induction of oxidative DNA damage and formation of BPDE-DNA adducts in human lymphocytes. Wilms LC, Hollman PC, Boots AW, Kleinjans JC. Mutat Res. 2005 Apr 4;582(1-2):155-62. **Key Finding:** "Lymphocytes from female volunteers who consumed a quercetin-rich blueberry/apple juice mixture for four weeks were treated ex vivo with an effective dose of $H(2)O(2)$ and benzo(a)pyrene, respectively, at three different time points during the intervention. Results in vitro; a significant dose-dependent protection by quercetin against both the formation of **oxidative DNA damage** and of BPDE-DNA adducts was observed. Results in vivo; four weeks of juice intervention led to a significant increase in the total antioxidant capacity of plasma. The combination of our findings in vitro and ex vivo provides evidence that quercetin is able to protect against chemically induced DNA damage in human lympho-cytes, which may underlie its suggested anticarcinogenic properties."

Radical scavenging activities of peels and pulps from cv. Golden Delicious apples as related to their phenolic composition. Chinnici F, Bendini A, Gaiani A, Riponi C. J Agric Food Chem. 2004 Jul 28;52(15):4684-9. **Key Finding:** "The relationship between phenolic composition and radical scavenging activity of apple peel and pulp was investigated. A good correlation between the sum of polyphenols and the radical scavenging activities was found. Among the single classes of compounds, procy-anidins (in peel and pulps) and flavonols (in peels) were statistically correlated to the total antioxidant activities."

Apple and pear peel and pulp and their influence on plasma lipids and **antioxidant** *potentials in rats fed* **cholesterol***-containing diets.* Leontowicz M, Gorinstein S, Leontowicz H, Krzeminski R, Lojek A, Katrich E, Ciz M, Martin-Belloso O, Soliva-Fortuny R, Haruenkit R, Trakhtenberg S. J Agric Food Chem. 2003 Sep 10;51(19):5780-5. **Key Finding:** "The aim of this study was to assess the bioactive compounds of apple and pear peel and pulp in vitro and their influence on plasma lipids and antioxidant potentials in vivo. The content of all studied indices in apple and pear peel was significantly higher than in peeled fruits. Diets supplemented with fruit peels exercised a significantly higher positive influence on plasma lipid levels and on plasma antioxidant capacity of rats than diets with fruit pulps."

Diets enriched in foods with high **antioxidant** *activity reverse age-induced decreases in cerebellar beta-adrenergic function and increases in proinflammatory cytokines.* Gemma C, Mesches MH, Sepesi B, Choo K., Holmes DB, Bickford PC. J Neurosci. 2002 Jul 15;22(14):6114-20. **Key Finding:** "Antioxidants and diets supplemented with foods high in oxygen radical absorbance capacity (ORAC) reverse **age-**related decreases in cerebellar beta-adrenergic receptor function. Aged male Fischer 344 rats were given apple (5 mg dry weight), spirulina (5 mg) or cucumber (5 mg) daily for 14 days. Electro physiologic techniques revealed a significant decrease in beta-adrenergic receptor function in aged control rats. Spirulina reversed this effect. Apple had an intermediate effect, and cucumber (low ORAC) had no effect, indicating that the reversal of beta-adrenergic receptor function decreases might be related to the ORAC dose."

Asthma

Dietary intake of flavonoids and **asthma** *in adults.* Garcia V, Arts IC, Sterne JA, Thompson RL, Shaheen SO. Eur Respir J. 2005 Sep;26(3):449-52. **Key**

Finding: "No evidence was found for a protective effect of three major subclasses of dietary flavonoids on asthma. They were catechins, flavonols and flavones. It is possible that other flavonoids or polyphenols present in apples may explain the protective effect of apples on obstructive lung disease."

Food and nutrient intakes and **asthma** *in young adults.* Woods RK, Walters EH, Raven JM, Wolfe R, Ireland PD, Thien FC, Abramson MJ. Am J Clin Nutr. 2003 Sep;78(3):414-21. **Key Finding:** "Apples and pears appeared to protect against current asthma. Intervention studies using whole foods are required to ascertain whether such modifications of food intake could be beneficial in the prevention or amelioration of asthma."

Dietary antioxidants and **asthma** *in adults: population-based case-control study.* Shaheen SO, Sterne JA, Thompson RL, Songhurst CE, Margetts BM, Burney PG. Am J Respir Crit Care Med. 2001 Nov 15;164(10 Pt 1):1823-8. **Key Finding:** "Apple consumption was negatively associated with asthma. The associations between apple and red wine consumption and asthma may indicate a protective effect of flavonoids."

Antioxidant activity of apple peels. Wolfe K, Wu X, Liu RH. J Agric Food Chem. 2003 Jan 29;51(3):609-14. **Key Finding:** "The high content of phenolic compounds, antioxidant activity, and antiproliferative activity of apple peels indicate that they may impart health benefits when consumed and should be regarded as a valuable source of antioxidants."

Antioxidant and antiproliferative activities of common fruits. Sun J, Chu YF, Wu X, Liu RH. J Agric Food Chem. 2002 Dec 4;50(25):7449-54. **Key Finding:** "Consumption of fruits and vegetables has been associated with reduced risk of chronic diseases such as **cardiovascular disease and cancer**. Phytochemicals, especially phenolic, in fruits and vegetables are suggested to be the major bioactive compounds for the health benefits. This study was designed to investigate the profiles of total phenolic. Cranberry had the highest total phenolic content followed by apple. Cranberry had the highest total antioxidant activity followed by apple. Antiproliferation activities were also studied in vitro using HepG(2) human **liver-cancer** cells, and cranberry showed the highest inhibitory effect followed by lemon and apple."

Relative bioavailability of the antioxidant flavonoid quercetin from various foods in man. Hollman PC, Van Triip JM, Buysman MN, Van der Gaag MS, Mengelers MJ, De Vries JH, Katan MB. FEBS Lett. 1997 Nov 24;418(1-2):152-6. **Key Finding:** "We fed nine subjects a single large dose of onions, which contain glucose conjugates of quercetin, apples, which contain glucose and non-glucose quercetin glycosides, or pure quercetin-3-rutinoside, the major quercetin glycoside in tea. Plasma levels were then measured. Bioavailability of quercetin from apples and of pure quercetin rutinoside was both 30% relative to onions. Peak levels were achieved less than 0.7 after ingestion of onions, 2.5 h after apples and 9 h after the rutinoside. Half-lives of elimination were 28 h for onions and 23 h for apples. We conclude that conjugation with glucose enhances absorption from the small gut. Because of the long half-lives of elimination, repeated consumption of quercetin-containing foods will cause accumulation of quercetin in blood."

Atherosclerosis

Effects of apple juice on risk factors of lipid profile, inflammation and coagulation, endothelial markers and **atherosclerotic lesions** *in high cholesterolemic rabbits.* Setorki M, Asgary S, Eidi A, Rohani AH, Esmaceil N. Lipids Health Dis. 2009 Oct 5;8:39. **Key Finding:** "Apple juice can effectively prevent the progress of **atherosclerosis.** This is likely due to antioxidant and anti-inflammatory effect of apple juice."

Phenolics from purple grape, apple, purple grape juice and apple juice prevent early **atherosclerosis** *induced by an atherogenic diet in hamsters.* Decorde K, Teissedre PL, Auger C, Cristol JP, Rouanet JM. Mol Nutr Food Res. 2008 Apr;52(4):400-7. **Key Finding:** "The results show for the first time that long-term consumption of antioxidants supplied by apple and purple grape, especially phenolic compounds, prevents the development of atherosclerosis in hamsters."

Apply polyphenols and fibers attenuate **atherosclerosis** *in apolipoprotein E-deficient mice.* Auclair S, Silberberg M, Gueux E, Morand C, Mazur A, Milenkovic D, Scalbert A. J Agric Food Chem. 2008 Jul 23;56(14):5558-63. **Key Finding:** "Apple constituents supplied at nutritional doses limit the development of atherosclerotic lesions in the aorta of apo E-deficient mice. On the basis of the results, we hypothesize that apple fibers and polyphenols may play a role in preventing atherosclerosis disease by decreasing uric acid plasma level."

Comparative content of some bioactive compounds in apples, peaches and pears and their influence on lipids and antioxidant capacity in rats. Leontowicz H, Gorinstein S, Lojek A, Leontowicz M, Ciz M, Soliva-Fortuny R, Park YS, Jung ST, Trakhtenberg S, Martin-Belloso O. J Nutr Biochem. 2002 Oct;13(10):603-610. **Key Finding:** "Diets supplemented with apples and to a less extent with peaches and pears have improved lipid metabolism and increased the plasma antioxidant potential especially in rats fed with added cholesterol. Apple is preferable for dietary prevention of **atherosclerosis** and other diseases."

Cancer (breast; colon; lung; prostate; skin)

Antiproliferative effects of apple peel extract against cancer cells. Reagan-Shaw S, Eggert D, Mukhtar H, Ahmad N. Nutr Cancer. 2010;62(4):517-24. **Key Finding**: "Our data demonstrated that apple peel extract, obtained from organic Gala apples, imparted significant reduction in the viability of a variety of cancer cell lines. Our data showed a significant decrease in growth and clonogenic survival of human **prostate carcinoma** CWR22Rnu1 and DU145 cells, and **breast carcinoma** Mcf-7 and Mcf-7:Her18 cells. Apple peels should not be discarded from the diet."

*Case-control study on beneficial effect of regular consumption of apples on **colorectal cancer** risk in a population with relatively low intake of fruits and vegetables.* Jedrychowski W, Maugeri U, Popiela T, Et al. Eur J Cancer Prev. 2010 Jan;19(1):42-7. **Key Finding**: "A total of 592 incident cases of colorectal cancer were compared to a group of 765 controls chosen from patients at the same hospital. The reduced risk of colorectal cancer was already observed at the consumption of at least one apple a day, but at the intake of more than one apple a day the risk was reduced by about 50%. The effect may result from their rich content of flavonoid and other polyphenols which can inhibit cancer onset and cell proliferation."

*An apple a day may hold **colorectal cancer** at bay: recent evidence from a case-control study.* Jedrychowski W, Maugeri U. Rev. Environ Health. 2009 Jan-Mar;24(1):59-74. **Key Finding:** "The risk of colorectal cancer was inversely correlated with daily number of apple servings, but the most significant reductions of OR estimates were observed for an intake one or more apple servings daily. No other fruit was significantly associated with altering the risk of colorectal cancer."

*Apple procyanidins activate apoptotic signaling pathway in human **colon adenocarcinoma** cells by a lipid-raft independent mechanism.* Maldonado-Ceils ME, Bousserouel S, Gosse F, Lobstein A, Raul F. Biochem Biophys Res Commun. 2009 Oct 16;388(2):372-6. **Key Finding:** "These results highlight the potential of procyanidins as a direct activator of TRAIL-death receptors in cell membrane even in the absence of lipid rafts."

*Synergistic effect of apple extracts and quercetin 3-beta-d-glucoside combination on antiproliferative activity in MCF-7 human **breast cancer** cells in vitro.* Yang J, Liu RH. J Agric Food Chem. 2009 Sep 23;57(18):8581-6. **Key Finding:** "The results suggest that the apple extracts plus Q3G combination possesses a synergistic effect in

MCF-7 cell proliferation. The two-way combination of apple plus Q3G was conducted. In this two-way combination, the EC(5) values of apple extracts and Q3G were 2- and 4-fold lower, respectively, than those of apple extracts and Q3G alone. The combination index (Ci) values at 50 and 95% inhibition rates were 0.76 +/- 0.39-fold, respectively."

Pentacyclic triterpenes of the lupane, oleanane and ursane group as tools in **cancer** *therapy.* Laszczyk MN. Panta Med. 2009 Dec;75(15):1549-60. **Key Finding:** Apple peels are rich in triterpenes. "Triterpenes are useful to treat cancer by several modes of action. The pharmacological potential of triterpenes of the lupane, oleanane or ursane type for cancer treatment seems high."

Impact of apple polyphenols on GSTT2 gene expression, subsequent protection of DNA and modulation of proliferation using LT97 human colon adenoma cells. Miene C, Klenow S, Veeriah S, Richling E, Glei M. Mol Nutr Food Res. 2009 Oct;53(10):1254-62. **Key Finding:** "Apple extract enhances expression of glutathione S-transferases (e.g. GSTTe) in human colon cells. Storage of apple extract caused changes in phenolic composition along with loss of activity regarding GSTT2 induction and amplified growth inhibition. Apple extract can protect against oxidative induced DNA damage. Nevertheless, chemo preventive effects of apple extract strongly depend on the specific composition, which is modified by storage."

Prevention of **colon carcinogenesis** *by apple juice in vivo: impact of juice constituents and obesity.* Koch TC, Briviba K, Watzl B, Fahndrich C, Bub A, Rechkemmer G, Barth SW. Mol Nutr Food Res. 2009 Oct;53(10):1289-302. **Key Finding:** "The development of colon cancer is positively associated with obesity and inversely associated with the intake of fiber, fruit and vegetables. Apple juice contains a specific spectrum of polyphenols and other components that may reduce the risk of colon cancer. Epidemiologic studies suggest an inverse correlation between apple consumption and colon cancer risk. The present review summarizes the preventive potential of apples juices and different apple constituents on biomarkers related to colon carcinogenesis."

GSTT2, a phase II gene induced by apple polyphenols, protects colon epithelial cells against genotoxic damage. Petermann A, Miene C, Schulz-Raffelt G, Palige K, Holzer J, Glei M, Bohmer FD. Mol Nutr Food Res. 2009 Oct;53(10):1245-53. **Key Finding:** "We found that polyphenolic apple extracts can directly enhance GSTT2 promoter activity. Induction of phase II genes may contribute to primary chemoprevention of **colon cancer** by apple polyphenols."

Ursolic acid attenuates oxidative stress-mediated hepatocellular carcinoma induction by diethylnitrosamine in male Wistar rats. Gayathri R, Priya DK, Gunaseekaran GR, Sakthisekaran D. Asian Pac J Cancer Prev. 2009;10(5):933-8. **Key Finding:** "Ursolic acid is a natural triterpenoid found in apple peel. Since ursolic acid has been found to be a potent antioxidant, it can be suggested as an excellent chemo preventive agent in overcoming diseases like **cancer** which are mediated by free radicals."

*Fresh apples suppress mammary carcinogenesis and proliferative activity and induce apoptosis in **mammary tumors** of the Sprague-Dawley rat.* Liu JR, Dong HW, Chen BQ, Zhao P, Liu RH. J Agric Food Chem. 2009 Jan 14;57(1):297-304. **Key Finding:** "Whole apple extracts possess potent antioxidant activity and antiproliferative activity against cancer cells in vitro. The objections of this study were to determine the anticancer activity of apple extracts in a rat mammary cancer model induced by 7,12-dimtheylbenz (a)anthracene (DMBA) in vivo and to determine if apple extracts inhibited cell proliferation and affected apoptosis in mammary cancer tissues in vivo. These results demonstrate the potent capacity of fresh apples to suppress DMBA-initiated mammary cancers in rats."

Apple polyphenol phloretin potentiates the anticancer actions of paclitaxel through induction of apoptosis in human hep G2 cells. Yang KC, Tsai CY, Wang YJ, Wei PL, Lee CH, Chen JH, Wu CH, Ho YS. Mol Carcinog. 2009 May;48(5):420-31. **Key Finding:** "Phloretin, which can be obtained from apples, apple juice and cider, is a known inhibitor of the type II glucose transporter. In vitro and in vivo studies were performed to assess phoretin antitumor activity when combined with paclitaxel for treatment of human **liver cancer** cells. The Hep G2-xenografted tumor volume was reduced more than fivefold in the Phloretin + paclitaxel treated mice compared to the paclitaxel treated group. These results suggest that Phloretin may be useful for cancer chemotherapy and chemoprevention."

***Cancer** chemo preventive potential of apples, apple juice, and apple components.* Gerhauser C. Planta Med. 2008 Oct;74(13):1608-24. **Key Finding:** "Apple products have been shown to prevent **skin, mammary and colon carcinogenesis** in animal models. Epidemiological observations indicate that regular consumption of one or more apples a day may reduce the risk for **lung and colon cancer**."

Phytochemicals of apple peels: isolation, structure elucidation, and their antiproliferative and antioxidant activities. He X, Liu RH. J Agric Food Chem. 2008 Nov 12;56(21):9905-10. **Key Finding:** "Most tested flavonoids and phenolic compounds had high antioxidant activity when compared to ascorbic acid and might be responsible for the antioxidant activities of apples. These results showed apple peel phyto-chemicals have potent antioxidant and antiproliferative activities."

*Apple phytochemical extracts inhibit proliferation of estrogen-dependent and estrogen-indepen-dent human **breast cancer** cells through cell cycle modulation.* Sun J, Liu RH. J Agric Food Chem. 2008 Dec 24;56(24):11661-7. **Key Finding:** "The data showed that apple phytochemical extracts significantly inhibited human breast cancer MCF-7 and MDA-MB-231 cell proliferation. These results suggest that the anti-proliferative activities of apple phytochemical extracts toward human breast cancer cells might be due to the modulation effects on cell cycle machinery."

*Fractionation of polyphenol-enriched apple juice extracts to identify constituents with **cancer** chemo preventive potential.* Zessner H, Pan L, Will F, Klimo K, Knauft J, Niewoher R, Hummer W, Owen R, Richling E, Frank N, Schreier P, Becker H, Gerhauser C. Mol Nutr Food Res. 2008 Jun;52 Supply 1:528-44. **Key Finding:** Apple juice extract was fractionated to determine which constituents contribute to potential chemo preventive activities. "Overall, apple juice constituents belonging to different structural classes have distinct profiles of biological activity in these in vitro test systems. Since carcinogenesis is a complex process, combination of compounds with complementary activities may lead to enhanced preventive effects."

*Apple procyanidins induce **tumor cell** apoptosis through mitochondrial pathway activa-tion of caspase-3.* Miura T, Chiba M, Kasai K, Nozaka H, Nakamura T, Shoji T, Kanda T, Ohtake Y. Carcinogenesis. 2008 Mar;29(3):585-93. **Key Finding:** "Our results indicate that the oral administration of apple procyanidins inhibits the proliferation of tumor cells by inducing apoptosis through the intrinsic mito-chondrial pathway."

Apple polyphenols modulate expression of selected genes related to toxicological defense and stress response in human colon adenoma cells. Veeriah S, Miene C, Habermann N, Hofmann T, Klenow S, Sauer J, Bohmer F, Wolfl S, Pool-Zobel BL. Int J Cancer. 2008 Jun 15;122(12):2647-55. **Key Finding:** "Apples contain significant amounts of flavonoids that are potentially cancer risk reducing by acting antioxidative or antiproliferative and by favorably modulating gene expression. The purpose of this study was to investigate whether polyphenols from apples modulate expres-sion of genes related to **colon cancer** prevention. The observed altered gene expression patterns in LT97 cells, resulting from apple extract treatment, points to a possible protection of the cells against some toxicological insults."

Effect of selected phytochemicals and apple extracts on NF-kappaB activation in human **breast cancer** *MCF-7 cells.* Yoon H, Liu RH. J Agric Food Chem. 2007 Apr 18;55(8):3167-73. **Key Finding:** "These results suggest that apple extracts and curcumin have the capabilities of inhibiting TNF-alpha-induced NF-kappaB activation of MCF-7 cells by inhibiting the proteasomal activities instead of IkappaB kinase activation."

Annurca apple polyphenols have potent demethylating activity and can reactivate silenced tumor suppressor genes in **colorectal cancer** *cells.* Fini L, Selgard M, Fogliano V, Graziani G, Romano M, Hotchkiss E, Daoud YA, De Val EB, Boland CR, Ricciardiello L. J Nutr. 2007 Dec;137(12):2622-8. **Key Finding:** Annurca apple, a variety of southern Italy, is rich in polyphenols that are associated with anticancer properties. We evaluated the mechanisms of putative anticancer effects of Annurca polyphenol extract in in vitro models of sporadic colorectal cancers. We observed a significant reduction in expression of DNMT proteins after treatment without changes in messenger RNA. In conclusion, Annurca polyphenol have potent demethylating activity through the inhibition of DNMT proteins."

Polyphenols are intensively metabolized in the human gastrointestinal tract after apple juice consumption. Kahle K, Huemmer W, Kempf M, Scheppach W, Erk T, Richline E. J Agric Food Chem. 2007 Dec 26;55(26):10605-14. **Key Finding:** "Polyphenols are secondary plant compounds showing anticarcinogenic effects both in vitro and in animal experiments and may thus reduce the risk of **colorectal cancer** in man. The identification of polyphenol metabolites formed via their passage through the small intestine of healthy ileostomy subjects after apple juice consumption is presented. Ninety percent of the consumed procyanidins were recovered in the ileostomy effluent and therefore would reach the colon under physiologic circumstances. The gastrointestinal passage seems to play an important role in the colonic availability of apple polyphenols."

Effect of apple polyphenol extract on hepatoma proliferation and invasion in culture and on **tumor growth,** *metastasis, and abnormal lipoprotein profiles in hepatoma-bearing rats.* Miura D, Miura Y, Yagasaki K. Biosci Biotechnol Biochem. 2007 Nov;71(11):2743-50. **Key Finding:** "The effect of dietary apple polyphenol extract on growth and the metastasis of AH109A hepatomas were investigated in vivo. Apple polyphenol extract reduced the growth and metastasis of solid hepatomas and significantly suppressed the serum lipid peroxide level in rats transplanted with AH109A. Apple polyphenol extract also suppressed the serum very-low-density lipoprotein + low-density lipoprotein cholesterol level."

Polyphenolic apple juice extracts and their major constituents reduce oxidative damage in human **colon** *cell lines.* Schaefer S, Baum M, Eisenbrand G, Dietrich H, Will F, Janzowski C. Mol Nutr Food Res. 2006 Jan;50(1):24-33. **Key Finding:** "Apple juice extracts distinctly reduce oxidative cell damage in human colon cell lines, an effect, which in part can be accounted for by their major constituents."

Apple flavonoids inhibit growth of HT29 human **colon cancer** *cells and modulate expression of genes involved in the biotransformation of xenobiotics.* Veeriah S, Kautenburger T, Habermann N, Sauer J, Dietrich H, Will F, Pool-Zobel BL. Mol Carcinog. 2006 Mar;45(3):164-74. **Key Finding:** "We conclude that apple flavonoids modulate toxicological defense against colon cancer risk factors. In addition to the inhibition of tumor cell proliferation, this could be a mechanism of cancer risk reduction."

Apples prevent mammary tumors in rats. Liu RH, Liu J, Chen B. J Agric Food Chem. 2005 Mar 23;53(6):2341-3. **Key Finding:** "This study demonstrated that whole apple extracts effectively inhibited **mammary cancer** growth in the rat model; thus, consumption of apples may be an effective therapy for cancer protection."

Does an apple a day keep the oncologist away? Gallus S, Talamini R, Giacosa A, Montella M, Ramazzotti V, Franceschi S, Negri E, La Vecchia C. Ann Oncol. 2005 Nov;16(11):1841-4. **Key Finding:** "We analyzed data from multicenter case-control studies conducted between 1991 and 2002 in Italy. This investigation found a consistent inverse association between apples and risk of various **cancers**."

The relationship between intake of vegetables and fruits and **colorectal adenoma-carcinoma** *sequence.* Lee SY, Choi KY, Kim MK, Kim KM, Lee JH, Meng KH, Lee WC. Korean J Gastroenterol (from Korean). 2005 Jan;45(1):23-33. **Key Finding:** "These findings suggest that the intake of vegetables and fruits may act differently in developmental steps of colorectal adenoma-carcinoma sequence. For this study, 539 cases with histopathologically confirmed incidental colorectal adenoma, 162 cases with colorectal cancer and 2,576 controls were collected. In females, the high intake of raw green and yellow vegetables was found to be negatively associated with the risk of adenoma with mild dysplasia. In male, the high intake of banana, pear, apple and watermelon among fruits were negatively associated with the risk of colorectal cancer."

Chemo preventive properties of apple procyanidins on human **colon cancer**-*derived metastatic SW620 cells and in a rat model of colon carcinogenesis.* Gosse F, Guyot S, Roussi S, Lobstein A, Fischer B, Seiler N, Raul F. Carcinogenesis. 2005 Jul;26(7):1291-5.

Key Finding: "Our results show that apple procyanidins alter intracellular signaling pathways, polyamine biosynthesis and trigger apoptosis in tumor cells. These compounds antagonize cancer promotion in vivo. In contrast with absorbable drugs, these natural, non-toxic, dietary constituents reach the colon where they are able to exert their antitumor effects."

Lung cancer risk among nonsmoking women in relation to diet and physical activity. Kubik A, Zatloukal P, Tomasek L, Pauk N, Petruzelka L, Plesko I. Neoplasma. 2004;51(2):136-43. **Key Finding:** "Excess lung cancer risk was associated with consumption of red meat among nonsmokers. Protective effects were observed for apples among smokers only."

Biological activity of carotenoids in red paprika, Valencia orange and golden delicious apple. Molnar P, Kawase M, Satoh K, Sohara Y, Tanaka T, Tani S, Sakagami H, Nakashima H, Motohashi N, Gyemant N, Molnar J. Phytother Res. 2005 Aug;19(8):700-7. **Key Finding:** "Carotenoid fractions were extracted from red paprika, Valencia orange peel and the peel of Golden delicious apple. Apple showed potent anti-H. Pylori activity. The extracts were inactive against HIV. Apple and orange showed slightly higher cytotoxic activity against three human tumor cells lines (**squamous cell carcinoma HSC-2, HSC-3, submandibular gland carcinoma HSG, and human promyelocytic leukemic HL-60 cells**. Paprika scavenged efficiently. The data suggest the potential importance of carotenoids as possible anti-H. Pylori and multidrug resistance reversal agents."

*Intake of fruits, vegetables and selected micronutrients in relation to the risk of **breast cancer**.* Malin AS, Qi D, Shu XO, Gao YT, Friedman JM, Jin F, Zheng W. Int J Cancer. 2003 Jun 20;105(3):413-8. **Key Finding:** "Intake of fruits, except watermelons and apples, was inversely associated with breast cancer risk. Our study suggests that high intake of certain vegetables and fruits may be associated with a reduced risk of breast cancer."

*Effects of commonly consumed fruit juices and carbohydrates on redox status and **anticancer** biomarkers in female rats.* Breinholt VM, Nielsen SE, Knuthsen P, Lauridsen ST, Daneshvar B, Sorensen A. Nutr Cancer. 2003;45(1):46-52. **Key Finding:** "The results of the present study suggest that commonly consumed fruit juices {apple juice, orange juice, black currant juice} can alter lipid and protein oxidation biomarkers in the blood as well as hepatic quinine reductase activity and that quercetin may not be the major active principle."

Antioxidant and antiproliferative activities of common fruits. Sun J, Chu YF, Wu X, Liu RH. J Agric Food Chem. 2002 Dec 4;50(25):7449-54. **Key Finding:** "Consumption of fruits and vegetables has been associated with reduced risk of chronic diseases such as **cardiovascular disease and cancer**. Phytochemicals, especially phenolics, in fruits and vegetables are suggested to be the major bioactive compounds for the health benefits. This study was designed to investigate the profiles of total phenolics. Cranberry had the highest total phenolic content followed by apple. Cranberry had the highest total antioxidant activity followed by apple. Antiproliferation activities were also studied in vitro using HepG(2) human **liver-cancer** cells, and cranberry showed the highest inhibitory effect followed by lemon and apple."

Evaluation of the immunomodulatory activity of Aronia in combination with apple pectin in patients with **breast cancer** *undergoing postoperative radiation therapy.* Yaneva MP, Botushanova AD, Grigorov LA, Kokov JL, Todorova EP, Krachanova MG. Folia Med (Bulgaria). 2002;44(1-2):22-5. **Key Finding:** "The aim of the present study was to evaluate the immunomodulatory activity of Aronia in combination with apple pectin in patients with breast cancer in the course of postoperative radiation therapy. The study comprised 42 women (19 to 65 years of age) receiving 15 g of apple pectin in combination with 20 ml of Aronia concentrate (Bioactive Substance Laboratory-Plovdiv) twice daily during postoperative radiation. Assays of immunity parameters in the patients receiving Aronia in combination with apple pectin showed that CD4 and CD8 T cell counts increased significantly. In control patients (non-apple pectin) T cell level lowered."

Intake of Flavonoids and **Lung Cancer**. Le Marchand LL, Murphy SP, Hankin JH, Wilkens LR, Kolonel LN. J Natl Cancer Inst. 2000 Jan 19;92(2):154-60. **Key Finding:** "After adjusting for smoking and intakes of saturated fat and B-carotene, we found statistically significant inverse associations between lung cancer risk and the main food sources of the flavonoids quercetin (onions and apples) and naringin (white grapefruit.)"

Diet and its preventive role in **prostatic disease**. Denis L, Morton MS, Griffiths K. Eur Urol. 1999;35(5-6):377-87. **Key Finding:** "Vegetarian men have a lower incidence of prostate cancer than omnivorous males. Apples and onions are excellent sources of flavonoids. These plant compounds can interfere with steroid metabolism and bioavailability, and also inhibit enzymes which are crucial to cellular proliferation."

*Dietary flavonoids and the risk of **lung cancer** and other malignant neoplasms.* Knekt P, Jaryinen R, Seppanen R, Hellovaara M, Teppo L, Pukkaia E, Aromaa A. Am J Epidemiol. 1997 Aug 1;146(3):223-30. **Key Finding:** "Of the major dietary flavonoid sources, the consumption of apples showed an inverse association with lung cancer incidence. The results are in line with the hypothesis that flavonoid intake in some circumstances may be involved in the cancer process, resulting in lowered risks."

*Dietary flavonoids and **cancer** risk in the Zutphen Elderly Study.* Hertog MG, Feskens EJ, Hollman PC, Katan MB, Krombout D. Nutr Cancer. 1994;22(2):175-84. **Key Finding:** "A high intake of flavonoids from vegetables and fruits only was inversely associated with risk of cancer of the alimentary and respiratory tract. These results suggest the presence of other non-vitamin components with anti-carcinogenic potential in these foods. We conclude that intake of flavonoids, mainly from tea, apples and onions, does not predict a reduced risk of all-cause cancer or of cancer of the alimentary and respiratory tract in elderly men. The effect of flavonoids on risk of cancer at specific sites needs further investigation in prospective cohort studies."

Cardiovascular/Coronary Artery Disease

*Flavonoid intake and the risk of **cardiovascular disease** in women.* Sesso HD, Gaziano JM, Liu S, Buring JE. Am J Clin Nutr. 2003 Jun;77(6):1400-6. **Key Finding:** "Women free of CVD and cancer participated in a prospective study using a food frequency questionnaire. Flavonoid intake was not strongly associated with a reduced risk of cardiovascular disease. The insignificant inverse associations for broccoli, apples, and tea with CVD were not mediated by flavonoids and warrant further study."

Antioxidant and antiproliferative activities of common fruits. Sun J, Chu YF, Wu X, Liu RH. J Agric Food Chem. 2002 Dec 4;50(25):7449-54. **Key Finding:** "Consumption of fruits and vegetables has been associated with reduced risk of chronic diseases such as **cardiovascular disease and cancer**. Phytochemicals, especially phenolics, in fruits and vegetables are suggested to be the major bioactive compounds for the health benefits. This study was designed to investigate the profiles of total phenolics. Cranberry had the highest total phenolic content followed by apple. Cranberry had the highest total antioxidant activity followed by apple. Antiproliferation activities were also studied in vitro using HepG(2) human **liver-cancer** cells, and cranberry showed the highest inhibitory effect followed by lemon and apple."

Apple juice consumption reduces plasma low-density lipoprotein oxidation in healthy men and women. Hyson D, Studebaker-Hallman D, Davis PA, Gershwin ME. J Med Food. 2000 Winter;3(4):159-66. **Key Finding:** "Moderate apple juice consumption provides in vivo antioxidant activity. In view of the current understanding of **coronary artery disease**, the observed effect on LDL might be associated with reduced CAD risk and supports the inclusion of apple juice in a healthy human diet."

Dietary catechins in relation to **coronary heart disease** *death among postmenopausal women.* Arts IC, Jacobs DR Jr, Harnack LJ, Gross M, Folsom AR. Epidemiology. 2001 Nov;12(6):668-75. **Key Finding:** Apple catechins were inversely associated with coronary heart disease death. There was a strong inverse association between the intake of (+)-catechin and (-)-epicatechin and coronary heart disease."

Apple juice inhibits human low density lipoprotein oxidation. Pearson DA, Tan CH, German JB, Davis PA, Gershwin ME. Life Sci. 1999;64(21):1913-20. **Key Finding:** "The ability of compounds in apple juices and extracts from fresh apple to protect LDL was assessed. The apple juices and extracts all inhibited **LDL oxidation**. The inhibition by the juices ranged from 9 to 34% and inhibition by apple peel, flesh and whole fresh Red Delicious apple was 21, 34 and 38% respectively. The specific components in the apple juices and extracts that contributed to antioxidant activity have yet to be identified."

Flavonoid intake and **coronary mortality** *in Finland: a cohort study.* Knekt P, Jarvinen R, Reunanen A, Maatela J. BMJ. 1996 Feb 24;312(7029):478-81. **Key Finding:** "The results suggest that people with very low intakes of flavonoids {such as onions and apples} have higher risks of coronary disease."

Dietary antioxidant flavonoids and risk of **coronary heart disease**: *the Zutphen Elderly Study.* Hertog MG, Feskens EJ, Hollman PC, Katan MB, Kromhout D. Lancet. 1993 Oct 23;342(8878):1007-11. **Key Finding:** The flavonoid intake of 805 men aged 65-84 years was measured. The major sources of intake were tea, onions and apples. "Flavonoid intake was significantly inversely associated with mortality from coronary heart disease. Flavonoids in regularly consumed foods may reduce the risk of death from coronary heart disease in elderly men."

Cerebrovascular disease

Quercetin intake and the incidence of **cerebrovascular disease**. Knekt P, Isotupa S, Rissanen H, Heliovaara M, Jarvinen R, Hakkinen S, Aromaa A, Reunanen A. Eur

J Clin Nutr. 2000 May;54(5):415-7. **Key Finding:** "The results suggest that the intake of apples is related to a decreased risk of thrombotic stroke. This association apparently is not due to the presence of the antioxidant flavonoid quercetin."

Cholera

Inhibition by apple polyphenols of ADP-ribosyltransferase activity of **cholera** *toxin and toxin-induced fluid accumulation in mice.* Saito T, Miyake M, Toba M, Okamatsu H, Shimizu S, Noda M. Microbiol Immunol. 2002;46(4):249-55. **Key Finding:** "The results suggest that polymerized catechin compounds in apple polyphenol extract inhibit the biological and enzymatic activities of cholera toxin and can be used in a precautionary and therapeutic manner in the treatment of cholera patients."

Cholesterol

Apple polyphenols inhibit plasma CETP activity and reduce the ratio of non-HDL to HDL **cholesterol.** Lam CK, Zhang Z, Yu H, Tsang SY, Huang Y, Chen ZY. Mol Nutr Food Res. 2008 Aug;52(8):950-8. **Key Finding:** "It was concluded that apply polyphenols favorably improved distribution of cholesterol in lipoproteins, most likely by its inhibition on plasma cholesteryl ester transport protein activity."

Novel low-density lipoprotein (LDL) oxidation model: antioxidant capacity for the inhibition of LDL oxidation. Chu YF, Liu RH. J Agric Food Chem. 2004 Nov 3;52(22):6818-23. **Key Finding:** "All vitamin C and E and apple extract concentrations tested resulted in increasing partial suppression and delay of LDL oxidation."

Apple pectin and a polyphenol-rich apple concentrate are more effective together than separately on cercal fermentation and **plasma lipids** *in rats.* Aprikian O, Ducios V, Guyot S, Besson C, Manach C, Bernalier A, Morand C, Remesy C, Demigne C. J Nutr. 2003 Jun;133(6):1860-5. **Key Finding:** "Apple pectin and the polyphenol-rich fraction were more effective when fed combined together than when fed separately on large intestine fermentations and lipid metabolism, suggesting interactions between fibers and polyphenols of apples."

Diminution of blood and hepatic **cholesterol** *induced by an apple-supplemented diet in the hamster.* Sicart R, Sable-Amplis R, Agid R. CR Seances Soc Biol Fil. (French). **Key Finding:** "Human daily ingestion of apples caused a significant reduction (16%) of **cholesterolemia**."

Chronic Lung Disease

Chronic obstructive pulmonary disease and intake of fatechines, flavonols, and flavones: the MORGEN Study. Tabak C, Arts IC, Smit HA, Heederik D, Kromhout D. Am J Respir Crit Care Med. 2001 Jul 1;164(1):61-4. **Key Finding:** "Flavonoids have been suggested to protect against chronic lung disease. We studied intake of catechins, flavonols and flavones in relation to pulmonary function and chronic obstructive pulmonary disease symptoms in 13,651 adults from three Dutch cities. Tea and apples were the main source of catechins, flavonols and flavones. Total intake was inversely associated with chronic cough and breathlessness, but not chronic phlegm. Solid fruit but no tea intake was beneficially associated with chronic obstructive pulmonary disease."

Diabetes

*Associations of dietary flavonoids with risk of **type 2 diabetes**, and markers of insulin resistance and systemic inflammation in women: a prospective study and cross-sectional analysis.* Song Y, Manson JE, Buring JE, Sesso HD, Liu S. J Am Coll Nutr. 2005 Oct;24(5):376-84. **Key Finding:** "The aim of this study was to examine the association of dietary flavonols and flavone intake with type 2 diabetes, and biomarkers of insulin resistance and systemic inflammation. These results do not support the hypothesis that high intake of flavonols and flavones reduces the development of type 2 diabetes, although we cannot rule out a modest inverse association with intake of apples and tea."

*Dietary fiber in **type II diabetes**.* Asp NG, Agardh CD, Ahren B, Dencker I, Johansson CG, Lundquist I, Nyman M, Sartor G, Schersten B. Acta Med Scand Supple. 1981;656:47-50. **Key Finding:** "The results indicate that foods rich in dietary fiber (such as whole apples) might be useful in the regulation of type II diabetes."

Gastric Disease

Apple polyphenol extracts prevent damage to human gastric epithelial cells in vitro and to rat gastric mucosa in vivo. Garziani G, D'Argenio G, Tuccillo C, Loguercio C, Ritieni A, Morisco F, Del Vecchio Blanco C, Fogliano V, Romano M. Gut. 2005 Feb;54(2):193-200. **Key Finding:** "Apple extracts prevent exogenous damage to human gastric epithelial cells in vitro and to the rat gastric mucosa in vivo. The effect seems to be associated with the antioxidant activity of apple phenolic compounds. A diet rich in apple antioxidants might exert a beneficial effect in the prevention of **gastric diseases**."

Inflammatory bowel disease

Influence of apple polyphenols on inflammatory gene expression. Jung M, Triebel S, Anke T, Richling E, Erkel G. Mol Nutr Food Res. 2009 Oct;53(10):1263-80. **Key Finding:** "Apples and products thereof contain high amounts of polyphenols which show diverse biological activities and may contribute to beneficial health effects, like protecting the intestine against inflammation initiated by chronic **inflammatory bowel disease**. In the present study we investigated the preventive effectiveness of polyphenol juice extracts on inflammatory gene expression in immune-relevant human cell lines."

Reduction of colonic inflammation in HLA-B27 transgenic rats by feeding Marie Menard apples, rich in polyphenols. Castagnini C, Luceri C, Toti S, Bigagli E, Caderni G, Femia AP, Giovanneilli L, Lodovici M, Pitozzi V, Salvadori M, Messerini L, Martin R, Zoetendal EG, Gai S, Eijssen L, Evelo CT, Renard CM, Baron A, Dolara P. Br J Nutr. 2009 Dec;102(11):1620-8. **Key Finding:** "The administration of Marie Menard apples ameliorates colon inflammation in transgenic rats developing spontaneous intestinal inflammation, suggesting the possible use of these and other apple varieties to control inflammation in **inflammatory bowel disease** patients."

*Orally administered apple procyanidins protect against experimental **inflammatory bowel disease** in mice.* Yoshioka Y, Akiyama H, Nakano M, Shoji T, Kanda T, Ohtake Y, Takita T, Matsuda R, Maitani T. Int Immunopharmacol. 2008 Dec 20;8(13-14):1802-7. **Key Finding:** "The combined anti-inflammatory and immunomodulatory effects of apple procyanidins on intestinal epithelial cells and intraepithelial lymphocytes suggest that it may be an effective oral preventive agent for inflammatory bowel diseases."

Muscle injury

*Dietary apple polyphenols have preventive effects against lengthening contraction-induced **muscle injuries**.* Nakazato K, Ochi E, Waga T. Mol Nutr Food Res. 2010 Mar;54(3):364-72. **Key Finding**: "Sixteen male Wistar rats were randomly assigned into the apple polyphenol feeding group and a control group. The animals were subjected to lengthening contractions and electrical stimulation and forced ankle dorsiflexion. We conclude that dietary apple polyphenols have protective effects against lengthening contraction-induced muscle injury."

Dietary apple polyphenols have preventive effects against lengthening contraction-induced **muscle injuries**. Nakazato K, Ochi E, Waga T. Mol Nutr Food Res. 2009 Oct 28. (Epub ahead of print). **Key Finding:** "We examined whether polyphenols from dietary apple have protective effects against exercise-induced muscle strain injury. Sixteen male Wistar rats were randomly assigned into the apple and control group diets. The animals were subject to lengthening contractions with electrical stimulation and forced ankle dorsiflexion. The apple group had significantly lower torque deficits than the control group. The apple group also had significantly higher glutathione-S-transferase alpha1 mRNA levels than the control group. We conclude that dietary apple polyphenols have protective effects against lengthening contraction-induced muscle injury."

Neurodegeneration

Dietary supplementation with apple juice decreases endogenous amyloid-beta levels in murine brain. Chan A, Shea TB. Alzheimers Dis. 2009 Jan;16(1):167-71. **Key Finding:** "Folate deficiency has been associated with age-related **neurodegeneration**. We demonstrate herein that dietary deficiency in folate and vitamin E, coupled pro-oxidant stress induced by dietary iron, increased amyloid-beta levels in normal adult mice. Dietary supplementation with apple juice concentrate in drinking water alleviated the increase in amyloid-beta for both mouse genotypes."

Dietary supplementation with apple juice concentrate alleviates the compensatory increase in glutathione synthase transcription and activity that accompanies dietary- and genetically-induced oxidative stress. Tchantchou F, Graves M, Ortiz D, Rogers E, Shea TB. J Nutr Health Aging. 2004;8(6):492-6. **Key Finding:** "These findings provide further evidence that the antioxidant potential of apple juice concentrate can compensate for dietary and genetic deficiencies that otherwise promote **neuro-degeneration**."

Periodontal disease

Identification of hop polyphenolic components which inhibit prostaglandin E2 production by gingival epithelial cells stimulated with periodontal pathogen. Inaba H, Tagashira M, Honma D, Kanda T, Kou Y, Ohtake Y, Amano A. Biol Pharm Bull. 2008

Mar;31(3):527-30. **Key Finding:** "These results suggest that apple-derived polyphenols is a potent inhibitor of cellular PGE2 production induced by P. gingivalis, and it may be useful for the prevention and attenuation of **periodontitis**."

*Apple- and hop-polyphenols protect **periodontal** ligament cells stimulated with enamel matrix derivative from Porphyromonas **gingivalis**.* Inaba H, Tagashira M, Kanda T, Ohno T, Kawai S, Amano A. J Periodontol. 2005 Dec;76(12):2223-9. **Key Finding:** "Enamel matrix derivative is a tissue regenerative agent used clinically as an adjunct to periodontal surgery. Porphyronan gingivalis, a periodontal pathogen, significantly diminishes the efficacy of EMD. We examined apple and hop-polyphenols to determine their ability to protect periodontal ligament cells from P. gingivalis. Each polyphenol significantly enhanced the viability of periodontal ligament cells infected with P. gingivalis."

Weight Loss

Weight loss associated with a daily intake of three apples or three pears among overweight women. Conceicao de Oliveira M, Sichieri R, Sanchez-Moura A. Nutrtion. 2003 Mar;19(3):253-6. **Key Finding:** "After 12 week follow-up, the fruit group lost 1.22 kg whereas the oat group had a non-significant weight loss of 0.88 kg. The difference between the two groups was statistically significant. Intake of fruits may contribute to weight loss."

Avocados

NATIVE TO SOUTH AMERICA AND THE CARIBBEAN, the avocado tree produces a fruit that is actually a large egg-shaped berry with a sizable seed at its center. Its use among pre-Incan and other ancient Mesoamerican cultures has been dated to about ten thousand years ago by archaeologists. The Aztecs considered avocado to be a fertility booster.

Though dozens of avocado cultivars are harvested, the Hass cultivar accounts for three-fourths of all avocados consumed. Mexico remains by far the biggest producer. Avocados contain much more potassium than bananas, are high in monounsaturated fats and B vitamins, and have a high fiber content. They have proven health benefits in many areas, particularly in lowering levels of harmful LDL and triglycerides and raising levels of beneficial HDL.

Anti-Inflammatory

AV119, a Natural Sugar from Avocado gratissims, Modulates the LPS-Induced Proinflammatory Response in Human Keratinocytes. Donnarumma G, Paoletti I, Buommino E, Et al. Inflammation. 2010 Oct 9 (Epub ahead of print). **Key Finding**: "Our data show that AV119, a patented blend of avocado sugars, is able to modulate significantly the proinflammatory response in human keratinocytes, blocking the NF-kB activation in human keratinocytes."

Atherosclerosis

Hypoglycemia and hypocholesterolemic potential of Persea Americana leaf extracts. Brai BI, Odetola AA, Agomo PU. J Med Food. 2007 Jun;10(2):356-60. **Key Finding:** "These results suggest that aqueous and methanolic leaf extracts of P. Americana (avocado) lower plasma glucose and influence lipid metabolism in hypercholesterolemic rats with consequent lowering of T-CHOL and LDL-CHOL, and a restoration of HDL-CHOL levels. This could represent a protective mechanism against the development of **atherosclerosis.**"

Cancer (oral; prostate)

*Selective induction of apoptosis of human **oral cancer** cell lines by avocado extracts via a ROS-mediated mechanism.* Ding H, Han C, Guo D, Chin YW, Ding Y, Kinghorn AD, D'Ambrosio SM. Nutr Cancer. 2009;61(3):348-56. **Key Finding:** "Avocados have a high content of phytochemicals with potential chemo preventive activity. Previously we reported that phytochemicals extracted from avocado meat selectively induced apoptosis in cancer but not normal, human oral epithelial cell lines. In the present study, we observed that treatment of human oral cancer cell lines containing high levels of reactive oxygen (ROS) with D003 increased ROS levels twofold to threefold and induced apoptosis. These data suggest that perturbing the ROS levels in human oral cancer cell lines may be a key factor in selective apoptosis and molecular targeting for chemoprevention by photochemical."

Chemoproventive characteristics of avocado fruit. Ding H, Chin YW, Kinghorn AD, D'Ambrosio SM. Semin Cancer Biol. 2007 Oct;17(5):386-94. **Key Finding:** "Our recent studies indicate that phytochemicals extracted with chloroform from avocado fruits target multiple signaling pathways and increase intracellular reactive oxygen leading to apoptosis. This review summarizes the reported phytochemicals in avocado fruit and discusses their molecular mechanisms and targets. These studies suggest that individual and combinations of phytochemicals from the avocado fruit may offer an advantageous dietary strategy in **cancer** prevention."

*Inhibition of **prostate cancer** cell growth by an avocado extract: role of lipid-soluble bioactive substances.* Lu QY, Arteaga JR, Zhang Q, Huerta S, Go VL, Heber D. J Nutr Biochem. 2005 Jan;16(1):23-30. **Key Finding:** "Avocado contains numerous bioactive carotenoids. Because the avocado also contains a significant amount of monounsaturated fat, these bioactive carotenoids are likely to be absorbed into the bloodstream, where in combination with other diet-derived phytochemicals they may contribute to the significant cancer risk reduction associated with a diet of fruits and vegetables."

An avocado constituent, persenone A, suppresses expression of inducible forms of nitric oxide synthase and cyclooxygenase in macrophages, and hydrogen peroxide generation in mouse skin. Kim OK, Murakami A, Takahashi D, Nakamura Y, Torikai K, Kim HW, Ohigashi H. Biosci Biotechnol Biochem. 2000 Nov;64(11):2504-7. **Key Finding:** "This study suggests that persenone A, an avocado constituent, is a possible agent to prevent inflammation-associated diseases including **cancer**."

Cholesterol (and Hypercholesterolemia)

High-density lipoproteins (HDL) size and composition are modified in the rat by a diet supplemented with "Hass" avocado (Persea Americana Miller). Perez-Mendez O, Garcia

Hernandez L. Arch Cardiol Mex. (Spanish). 2007 Jan-Mar;77(1):17-24. **Key Finding:** "The inclusion of avocado in the diet decreased plasma triglycerides increased HDL-**cholesterol** plasma levels and modified HDL structure. The latter effect may enhance the antiatherogenic properties of HDL."

Effects of a vegetarian diet vs. a vegetarian diet enriched with avocado in **hypercholesterolemic** *patients.* Carrznza-Madrigal J, Herrera-Abarca JE, Alvizouri-Munoz M, Alvarado-Jimenez MR, Chavez-Carbajal F. Arch Med Res. 1997 Winter;28(4):537-41. **Key Finding:** "All three diets reduced HDL levels. To obtain beneficial effects on lipid profile with avocado, lower amounts of carbohydrates and polyunsaturated fatty acids are probably needed."

Monounsaturated fatty acid (avocado) rich diet for mild **hypercholesterolemia.** Lopez LR, Frati Munari AC, Hernandez Dominguez BC, Cervantes MS, Hernandez Luna MH, Juarez C, Moran LS. Arch Med Res. 1996 Winter;27(4):519-23. **Key Finding:** "High lipid, high MFA-avocado enriched diet can improve lipid profile in healthy and especially in mild hypercholesterolemic patients, even if hypertriglyceridemia (combined hyperlipidemia) is present."

Effects of avocado on the level of **blood lipids** *in patients with phenotype II and IV dyslipidemias.* Carranza J, Alvizouri M, Alvarado MR, Chavez F, Gomez M, Herrera JE. Arch Inst Cardio Mex. (Spanish). 1995 Jul-Aug;65(4):342-8. **Key Finding:** "Avocado is an excellent source of monounsaturated fatty acids in diets designed to treat hypercholesterolemia with some advantages over low-fat diets with a greater amount of carbohydrates."

Carotenoid absorption from salad and salsa by humans is enhanced by the addition of avocado or avocado oil. Unlu NZ, Bohn T, Clinton SK, Schwartz SJ. J Nutr. 2005 Mar;135(3):431-6. **Key Finding:** "Adding avocado fruit can significantly enhance carotenoid absorption from salad and salsa, which is attributed primarily to the lipids present in avocado."

Hypertension

Cardiovascular effects of Persea Americana Mill (Lauraceae) (avocado) aqueous leaf extract in experimental animals. Ojewole JA, Kamadyaapa DR, Gondwe MM, Moodley K, Musabayane CT. Cardiovasc J Afr. 2007 Mar-Apr;18(2):69-76. **Key Finding:** "The findings of this study tend to suggest that P. Americana leaf could be used as a natural supplementary remedy in essential **hypertension** and certain cases of cardiac dysfunctions."

*Effect of an avocado oil-rich diet over an angiotensin II-induced **blood pressure** response.*
Salazar MJ, El Hafidi M, Pastelin G, Ramirez-Ortega MC, Sanchez-Mendoza MA. J Ethnopharmacol. 2005 Apr 26;98(3):335-8. **Key Finding:** "Avocado oil-rich diet modifies the fatty acid content in cardiac and renal membranes in a tissue-specific manner. Diet content can be a key factor in vascular responses."

Osteoarthritis

A potential role for avocado and soybean based nutritional supplements in the management of osteoarthritis: a review. Dinubile NA. Phys Sportsmed. 2010 Jun;38(2):71-81. **Key Finding**: "Basic scientific research studies and a systematic review and meta-analysis of the available high-quality randomized clinical trials indicate that 300 mg of avocado and soybean unsaponifiables per day (with or without glucosamine and chondroitin sulfate) appears to be beneficial for patients with **hip or knee osteoarthritis**."

*Symptomatic efficacy of avocado-soybean unsaponifiables (ASU) in **osteoarthritis** (OA) patients: a meta-analysis of randomized controlled trials.* Christensen R, Bartels EM, Astrup A, Bliddal H. Osteoarthritis Cartilage. 2008 Apr;16(4):399-408. **Key Finding:** "Based on the available evidence, patients may be recommended to give avocado/soybean unsaponifiables a chance for e.g., 3 months. Meta-analysis data support better chances of success in patients with knee OA than in those with hip OA."

*Avocado/soybean unsaponifiables in the treatment of knee and hip **osteoarthritis**.* Angermann P. Ugeskr Laeger (Danish). 2005 Aug 15;167(33):3023-5. **Key Finding:** "These studies indicate that ASU has an effect on the symptoms of knee and hip osteoarthritis but not on the structural changes caused by osteoarthritis."

*Avocado-soybean unsaponifiables (ASU) for **osteoarthritis**—a systematic review.* Ernst E. Clin Rheumatol. 2003 Oct;22(4-5):285-8. **Key Finding:** "The majority of rigorous trial data available to date suggest that avocado/soybean unsaponifiables is effective for the symptomatic treatment of osteoarthritis."

*Structural effect of avocado/soybean unsaponifiables on joint space loss in **osteoarthritis** of the hip.* Lequesne M, Maheu E, Cadet C, Dreiser RL. Arthritis Rheum. 2002 Feb;47(1):50-8. **Key Finding:** "Avocado/soybean unsaponifiables significantly reduced the progression of joint space loss as compared with placebo in the subgroup of patients with advanced joint space narrowing."

*Symptoms modifying effect of avocado/soybean unsaponifiables (ASU) in **knee osteoarthritis**. A double-blind, prospective, placebo-controlled study.* Appelboom T, Schuermans J, Verbruggen G, Henrotin Y, Reginster JY. Scand J Rheumatol. 2001;30(4):242-7. **Key Finding:** "The efficacy of ASU at a dosage of 300mg/day and 600mg/day was consistently superior to that of placebo at all endpoints, with no differences observed between the two doses."

*Modification of articular cartilage and subchondral bone pathology in an ovine meniscetomy model of **osteoarthritis** by avocado and soya unsaponifiables (ASU).* Cake MA, Read RA, Guillou B, Ghosh P. Osteoarthritis Cartilage. 2000 Nov;8(6):404-11. **Key Finding:** "These findings support other studies which have proposed that avocado and soya unsaponifiables may exhibit disease-modifying anti-osteoarthritis activity."

The possible 'chondroprotective' effect of the unsaponifiable constituents of avocado and soya in vivo. Khayyal MT, el-Ghazaly MA. Drugs Exp Clin Res. 1998;24(1):41-50. **Key Finding:** "An experimental in vivo model for studying **cartilage destruction** has been used to study the possible chondroprotective effect of the unsaponifiable constituents of avocado, soya and their combination. The unsaponifiables of both avocado and soya significantly reduced the degenerative changes induced by the granuloma tissue on the implanted cartilage in control animals. The effect was even more marked when animals were treated with the combination of the two unsaponifiables at a 1:2 ratio."

*Efficacy and safety of avocado/soybean unsaponifiables in the treatment of symptomatic **osteoarthritis** of the knee and hip. A prospective, multicenter, three-month, randomized, double-blind, placebo-controlled trial.* Blotman F, Maheu E, Wulwik A, Caspard H, Lopez A. Rev Rhum Engl Ed. 1997 Dec;64(12):825-34. **Key Finding:** "One of the objectives of symptomatic slow-acting drugs for osteoarthritis is to reduce the need for drugs with a less favorable safety profile, mainly analgesics and non-steroidal anti-inflammatory drugs. Avocado/soybean unsaponifiables reduced the need for these drugs in patients with primary femorotibial or hip osteoarthritis. The functional index showed a significantly greater improvement in the active (avocado/soybean) group."

Psoriasis

*Vitamin B(12) cream containing avocado oil in the therapy of plaque **psoriasis**.* Stucker M, Memmel U, Hoffmann M, Hartung J, Altmeyer P. Dermatology. 2001;203(2):141-7.

Key Finding: "The results of this clinical trial provide evidence that the recently developed vitamin B (12) cream containing avocado oil has considerable potential as a well-tolerated, long-term topical therapy of psoriasis."

The effect of various avocado oils on skin collagen metabolism. Werman MJ, Mokady S, Nimni ME, Neeman I. Connect Tissue Res. 1991;26(1-2):1-10. **Key Finding:** "The effects of various avocado oils on collagen metabolism in skin were studied in growing rats. Rats fed the unrefined avocado oil extracted with hexane from the intact fruit, its unsaponifiables or the avocado seed oil, showed significant increases in soluble collagen content in skin."

Schleroderma

Natural remedies for **schleroderma**. Gaby AR. Altern Med Rev. 2006 Sep;11(3):188-95. **Key Finding:** Avocado/soybean extract is a promising natural treatment for scleroderma, an **autoimmune disease** of the connective tissue characterized by fibrosis and thickening of various tissues.

Wounds

Wound healing *activity of Persea Americana (avocado) fruit: a preclinical study on rats.* Nayak BS, Raju SS, Chalapathia Rao AV. J Wound Care. 2008 Mar;17(3):123-6. **Key Finding:** "Avocado oil is rich in nutrient waxes, proteins and minerals, as well as vitamins A, D and E. It is an excellent source of enrichment for dry, damaged or chapped skin. This study aimed to evaluate the wound-healing activity of fruit extract of Persea Americana in rats. Rate of wound contraction, epithelialization time, together with the hydroxyproline content and histological observations, supports the use of Persea Americana in the management of wound healing."

Beans (Legumes)

THE DRIED SEEDS OF LEGUMES, first cultivated in Asia, are high in protein, which has made them valuable crops, especially when meat was in short supply. The word "pulses" is used to refer to the seeds of legumes used for human consumption, which include peas, beans, lentils, chickpeas, and fava beans. Much of the health potential of pulses stems from the bioactivity of their isoflavones, phytosterols, resistant starch, alkaloids, and saponins.

Soy is in the legume family, and in its most commonly consumed form it contains estrogen activation factors. For this reason, many health practitioners recommend avoiding it or limiting consumption due to its potential cancer connection. For this reason, soy extracts and fermented soy products are often used in both clinical studies and clinical practice. These types of soy can provide health benefits without potentially activating estrogen.

Antioxidation

Antioxidant properties of flavonol glycosides from green beans. Plumb GW, Price KR, Williamson G. Redox Rep. 1999;4(3):123-7. **Key Finding:** "We have examined the antioxidant activity of one class of polyphenol compounds in green beans: two novel flavonol glycosides and the corresponding kaempferol. The compounds described herein demonstrate the antioxidant activity of the flavonols present in green beans."

Atherosclerosis

Comparative studies on the antioxidant activities of nine common food legumes against copper-induced human low-density lipoprotein oxidation in vitro. Xu BJ, Yuan SH, Chang SK. Food Sci. 2007 Sep;72(7):5522-7. **Key Finding:** "These results suggest that consuming black beans, lentils, black soybeans and red kidney beans may have potential in preventing the development of **atherosclerosis** from the perspective of inhibiting LDL oxidation."

*Major dietary patterns are related to plasma concentrations of markers of **inflammation** and endothelial dysfunction.* Lopez-Garcia E, Schulze MB, Fung TT, Meigs JB, Rifai N, Manson JE, Hu FB. Am J Clin Nutr. 2004 Oct;80(4):1029-35. **Key Finding:** "Because endothelial dysfunction is an early step in the development of **atherosclerosis**, this study suggests a mechanism (through higher intakes of legumes, etc.) for the role of dietary patterns in the pathogenesis of cardio-vascular disease."

Can food variety add years to your life? Savige GS. Asia Pac J Clin Nutr. 2002;11 Suppl 3:S637-41. **Key Finding:** "Foods for thought include legumes, which are likely to protect older adults against some of the diseases more prevalent with ageing such as **coronary heart disease and cancer**."

*Health benefits of low glycemic index foods, such as pulses, in **diabetic** patients and health individuals.* Rizkalla SW, Bellisle F, Slama G. Br J Nutr. 2002 Dec;88 Suppl 3:S255-62. **Key Finding:** "The results of human studies have been confirmed by animal experiments in the field of diabetes. Diets with low glycemic index value improve the prevention of **coronary heart disease** in diabetic and healthy subjects. In obese or overweight individuals, low-glycemic index meals increase satiety and facilitate the control of food intake. Pulses are foods with very low glycemic-index values and have demonstrated benefits for healthy persons in terms of post-prandial glucose and lipid metabolism."

Phytoestrogens and human health effects: weighing up the current evidence. Humfrey CD. Nat Toxins. 1998;6(2):51-9. **Key Finding:** "Phytoestrogens are present in beans, sprouts, cabbage, spinach, soybean, grains and hops. Epidemiological studies suggest that foodstuffs containing phytoestrogens may have a beneficial role in protecting against a number of chronic diseases and conditions. For **cancer of the prostate, colon, rectum, stomach and lung**, the evidence is most consistent for a protective effect. Soya and linseed may have beneficial effects on the risk of **breast cancer** and may help to alleviate **postmenopausal symptoms**. Soya also appears to have beneficial effects on blood lipids which may help to reduce the risk of **cardiovascular disease and atherosclerosis**."

Cancer (bladder; breast; colon; esophageal; gastric; lung; rectum; stomach)

*Consumption of a legume-enriched, low-glycemic index diet is associated with biomarkers of insulin resistance and inflammation among men at risk for **colorectal cancer**.* Hartman TJ, Albert PS, Zhang Z, Et al. J Nutr. 2010 Jan;140(1):60-7. **Key Finding:** "Healthy dietary changes {a legume-rich, low glycemic diet} can improve biomarkers of insulin resistance and inflammation."

*Soy phytoestrogens modify DNA methylation of GSTP1, RASSF1A, EPH2, and BRCA1 promoter in **prostate cancer** cells.* Vardi A, Bosviel R, Rabiau N, Et al. In Vivo. 2010 Jul-Aug;24(4):393-400. **Key Finding**: "Epigenetic modifications of DNA, such as the promoter CpG island demethylation of tumor suppressor genes, might be related to the protective effect of soy on prostate cancer."

*Isoflavones from phytoestrogens and **gastric cancer** risk: a nested case-control study within the Korean Multicenter Cancer Cohort.* Ko KP, Park SK, Park B, Et al. Cancer Epidemiol Biomarkers Prev. 2010 May;19(5):1292-300. **Key Finding**: "these results from a study population of 131 cases and 393 matched controls suggest a beneficial effect of high soybean product intake for gastric cancer risk."

*Individual and combined soy isoflavones exert differential effects on **metastatic cancer progression**.* Martinze-Montemayor MM, Otero-Franqui E, Martinze J, Et al. Clin Exp Metastasis. 2010 Oct;27(7):465-80. **Key Finding**: "The role of genistein, daidzein and combined soy isoflavones was studied on progression of subcutaneous tumors in nude mice. Results show that daidzein increased while genistein decreased **mammary tumor** growth by 38 and 33% respectively, Daidzein increased lung and heart metastases while genistein decreased **bone and liver** metastases. Combined soy isoflavones did not affect primary tumor growth but increased metastasis in all organs tested, which include lung, liver, heart, kidney and bones."

*Effect of soy saponin on the growth of human **colon cancer** cells.* Tsai CY, Chen YH, Chien YW, Et al. World J Gastroenterol. 2010 Jul 21;16(27):3371-6. **Key Finding:** "WiDr human colon cancer cells were treated with 150, 300, 600 or 1200 ppm of soy saponin to determine the effect on cell growth, cell morphology and other factors. Soy saponin decreased the number of viable cells in a dose-dependent manner. Soy saponin may be effective in preventing colon cancer by affecting cell morphology, cell proliferation enzymes, and cell growth."

*Effect of soy isoflavones on the incidence of 7, 12-dimethylbenz (alpha) anthracene-induced **breast tumors** in rats.* Hu JW, Zhao XH, Zhang YM,Wang PY. Bejing Da Xue Bao. 2010 Jun 18;42(3):288-92. **Key Finding**: "Soy isoflavones of 50 mg/kg and 100 mg/kg could decrease the incidence of breast tumors in normal rats, which may be related to the higher activities of superoxide dismutase induced by soy isoflavones. However, soy isoflavones could not decrease the incidence of breast tumors and inhibit the activities of SOD in overiectomized rats. This may reflect the different basal levels of estrogen in ovariectomized and normal rats."

Effect of soy isoflavones on **breast cancer** *recurrence and death for patients receiving adjuvant endocrine therapy.* Kang X, Zhang Q, Wang S, Et al. CMAJ. 2010 Nov 23;182(17):1857-62. **Key Finding**: "High dietary intake of soy isoflavones was associated with lower risk of recurrence among post-menopausal patients with breast cancer positive for estrogen and progesterone receptor and those who were receiving anastrozole as endocrine therapy."

Meta-analysis of the relationship between soybean product consumption and **gastric cancer**. Tong X, Li W, Qin LQ. Zhonghua Yu Fang Yi Xue Za Zhi {in Chinese}. 2010 Mar;44(3):215-20. **Key Finding**: "A total of 28 independent studies were selected including 16 case-control studies, 10 cohort studies and 2 cross sectional studies. Consumption of soybean products and tofu was inversely associated with gastric cancer, while miso consumption could increase the risk to gastric cancer."

Genistein depletes telomerase activity through cross-talk between genetic and epigenetic mechanisms. Li Y, Liu L, Andrews LG, Tollefsbol TO. Int J Cancer. 2009 Jul 15;125(2):286-96. **Key Finding:** "Genistein, a natural isoflavone found in soybean products, has been reported to down-regulate telomerase activity and that this prevents cancer and contributes to the apoptosis of cancer cells. These findings collectively show that genistein is working, at least in part, through epigenetic mechanisms of telomerase inhibition in breast benign and cancer cells and may facilitate approaches to **breast cancer** prevention and treatment."

Prospective cohort study of soy food intake and **colorectal cancer** *risk to women.* Yang G, Shu XO, Li H, Chow WH, Cai H, Zhang X, Gao YT, Zheng W. Am J Clin Nutr. 2009 Feb;89(2):577-83. **Key Finding:** "This prospective study suggests that consumption of soy foods may reduce the risk of colorectal cancer in post-menopausal women."

Soy, isoflavones, and **prostate cancer.** Jian L. Mol Nutr Food Res. 2009 Feb;53(2):217-26. **Key Finding:** "The association between dietary factors and prostate cancer has been investigated and one explanation for the low incidence of the cancer in Asia might be high consumption of fresh vegetables including soybean and its products."

Soy isoflavones modulate azoxymethane-induced rat **colon carcinogenesis** *exposed pre- and postnatally and inhibit growth of DLD-1 human colon adenocarcinoma cells by increasing the expression of estrogen receptor-beta.* Raju J, Bielecki A, Caldwell D, Lok E, Taylor M, Kapal K, Curran I, Cooke GM, Bird RP, Mehta R. J Nutr. 2009 Mar;139(3):474-81. **Key Finding:** "Soy isoflavones dose-dependently arrested the growth of DLD-1 cells. Our results suggest that pre- and postnatal exposure to dietary soy isoflavones suppresses the growth of colon tumors in male rats."

Reproductive variables, soy intake, and **lung cancer** *risk among nonsmoking women in the Singapore Chinese Health Study.* Seow A, Koh WP, Wang R, Lee HP, Yu MC. Cancer Epidemiol Biomarkers Prev. 2009 Mar;18(3):821-7. **Key Finding:** "Dietary soy isoflavonoid intake was associated with a statistically significant inverse trend among nonsmokers only."

Adolescent and adult soy food intake and **breast cancer** *risk: results from the Shanghai Women's Health Study.* Lee SA, Shu XD, Li H, Yang G, Cai H, Wen W, Ji BT, Gao J, Gao YT, Zheng W. Am J Clin Nutr. 2009 Jun;89(6):1920-6. **Key Finding:** "This large, population-based, prospective cohort study provides strong evidence of a protective effect of soy food intake against premenopausal breast cancer."

Dietary intake of polyphenols, nitrate and nitrite and **gastric cancer** *risk in Mexico City.* Hernandez-Ramirez RU, Galvan-Portillo MV, Ward MH, Agudo A, Gonzalez CA, Oriate-Ocana LF, Herrera-Goepfert R, Palma-Coca O, Lopez-Carrillo L. Int J Cancer. 2009 Sep 15;125(6):1424-30. **Key Finding:** "Our results show, for the first time, a protective effect for gastric cancer because of higher intake of cinnamic acids, secoisolariciresinol and coumestrol, and suggest that these polyphenols reduce gastric cancer risk through inhibition of endogenous nitrosation. The main sources of these polyphenols were pears, mangos and beans for cinnamic acids; beans, carrots and squash for secoisolariciresinol and legumes for coumestrol."

Soy food consumption and risk of **prostate cancer***: a meta-analysis of observational studies.* Hwang YW, Kim SY, Jee SH, Kim YN, Nam CM. Nutr Cancer. 2009;61(5):598-606. **Key Finding:** "Among individual soy foods, only tofu yielded a significant value. Consumption of soybean milk, miso, or natto did not significantly reduce the risk of prostate cancer. Genistein and daidzein were associated with a lower risk of prostate cancer."

Radiation-induced HIF-1alpha cell survival pathway is inhibited by soy isoflavones in **prostate cancer** *cells.* Singh-Gupta V, Zhang H, Banerjee S, Kong D, Rafoul JJ, Sarkar FH, Hillman GG. Int J Cancer. 2009 Apr 1;124(7):1675-84. **Key Finding:** "We previously showed that treatment of prostate cancer cells with soy isoflavones and radiation resulted in greater cell killing in vitro. We extended our studies to investigate the role of HIF-1alpha survival pathway and its upstream Src and STAT3 molecules in isoflavones and radiation interaction. Our novel findings suggest that the increased responsiveness to radiation mediated by soy isoflavones could be due to pleiotropic effects of isoflavones blocking cell survival pathways induced by radiation."

Intake of vegetables, legumes, and fruit, and risk for all-cause, ***cardiovascular, and cancer mortality*** *in a European diabetic population.* Nothlings U, Et al. Nutr. 2008 Apr;138(4):775-81. **Key Finding:** "An increment intake of total vegetables, legumes and fruit of 80 g/d was associated with a reduced risk of death from all causes. Analyzed separately, vegetables and legumes were associated with a significantly reduced risk, whereas non-significant inverse associations for fruit intake were observed."

Soy intake and ***breast cancer*** *risk in Singapore Chinese Health Study.* Wu AH, Koh WP, Wang R, Lee HP, Yu MC. Br J Cancer. 2008 Jul 8;99(1):196-200. **Key Finding:** "These prospective findings suggest that approximately 10 mg of isoflavones per day, obtained in a standard serving of tofu, may have lasting beneficial effects against breast cancer development."

Can the combination of flaxseed and its lignans with soy and its isoflavones reduce the growth stimulatory effect of soy and its isoflavones on established ***breast cancer?*** Power KA, Thompson LU. Mol Nutr Food Res. 2007 Jul;51(7):845-56. **Key Finding:** "If these studies (animal) can be confirmed in clinical trials, then consumption of combined soy and flaxseed, or their phytoestrogens, may reduce the tumor growth stimulatory effect of soy or genistein. This may indicate that if soy is consumed with lignin-rich foods, it may continue to induce its other beneficial health effects, without inducing adverse effect on postmenopausal breast cancer."

An overview of the health effects of isoflavones with an emphasis on ***prostate cancer*** *risk and prostate-specific antigen levels.* Messina M, Kucuk O, Lampe JW. J AOAC Int. 2006 Jul-Aug;89(4):1121-34. **Key Finding:** "The clinical evidence is sufficiently encouraging to justify considering additional Phase II and III clinical trials investigating the efficacy of soy isoflavones in different populations of prostate cancer patients alone and in combination with other treatments."

Soy food intake and ***breast cancer*** *survival: a follow-up of the Shanghai Breast Cancer Study.* Boyapati SM, Shu XO, Ruan ZX, Dai Q, Cai Q, Gao YT, Zheng W. Breast Cancer Res Treat. 2005 Jul;92(1):11-7. **Key Finding:** "We evaluated data from a cohort of 1459 breast cancer patients. Soy food intake was assessed. These data suggest that soy foods do not have an adverse effect on breast cancer survival."

*Effects of a diet rich in phytoestrogens on prostate-specific antigen and sex hormones in men diagnosed with **prostate cancer**.* Dalais FS, Meliala A, Wattanapenpaiboon N, Frydenberg M, Suter DA, Thomson WK, Wahlqvist ML. Urology. 2004 Sep;64(3):510-5. **Key Finding:** "This work provides some evidence to support epidemiologic studies claiming that male populations who consume high phytoestrogen diets have a reduced risk of prostate cancer development and progression."

Effect of chickpea aqueous extracts, organic extracts and protein concentrates on cell proliferation. Giron-Calle J, Vioque J, del Mar Yust M, Pedroche J, Alaiz M, Millan F. J Med Food. 2004 Summer;7(2):122-9. **Key Finding:** "Pulses should be part of a healthy diet and it is also becoming clear that they have health-promoting effects. We have studied cell growth-regulating properties, which may be responsible for **anti-cancer** properties, in chickpea seeds. The cell lines Caco-2 (epithelial intestinal) and J774(macrophages) have been exposed to chickpea seed extracts. Both cell growth-promoting and cell growth-inhibiting effects were found. It is concluded that chickpea seeds are a source of bioactive components and deserve further study for their possible anti-cancer effect."

*Dietary soy and increased risk of **bladder cancer**: a prospective cohort study of men in Shanghai, China.* Sun CL, Yuan JM, Wang XL, Gao YT, Ross RK, Yu MC. Int J Cancer. 2004 Nov 1;112(2):319-23. **Key Finding:** "The soy-bladder cancer risk associations in smokers and non-smokers were comparable. Compared to men consuming soy less than once a week, the relative risks for those who consumed soy 1-<3 times per week, 3-<7 times a week and daily were 2.05, 2.45 and 4.61 respectively. The soy-bladder cancer relationship became stronger when the analysis was restricted to subjects with 2 or more years of follow-up."

Health benefits of soy isoflavonoids and strategies for enhancement: a review. McCue P, Shetty K. Crit Rev Food Sci Nutr. 2004;44(5):361-7. **Key Finding:** "Soybean consumption has been linked to a reduced risk for certain cancers and diseases of **old age**. In this study, we discuss the current state of knowledge concerning soybean isoflavonoids, their chemo preventive actions against **postmenopausal** health problems, **cancer**, and **cardiovascular disease**."

*Soy and isoflavone intake are associated with reduced risk of **ovarian cancer** in southeast China.* Zhang M, Xie X, Lee AH, Binns CW. Nutr Cancer. 2004;49(2):125-30. **Key Finding:** "Intake of soy and isoflavones was inversely related to the risk of ovarian cancer based on a case-control study of 254 patients with histologically confirmed epithelial ovarian cancer and 652 controls."

Phytoestrogens: implications in neurovascular research. Lephart ED, Porter JP, Hedges DW, Lund TD, Setchell KD. Curr Neurovasc Res. 2004 Dec;1(5):455-64. **Key Finding:** "Isoflavone consumption of soy-derived dietary phytoestrogens have received prevalent usage due to their ability to decrease age related disease (**cardiovascular** and **osteoporosis**) hormone-dependent cancers (**breast and prostate**) and peri- and **postmenopausal symptoms**. Dietary phytoestrogens appear to affect certain aspects of vascular, neuroendocrine and cognitive function."

Potential risks and benefits of phytoestrogen-rich diets. Cassidy A. Int J Vitam Nutr Res. 2003 Mar;73(2):120-6. **Key Finding:** "Soya isoflavones can exert hormonal effects. These effects may be of benefit in the prevention of many of the common diseases observed in Western populations (such as **breast cancer, prostate cancer, menopause symptoms, and osteoporosis**)."

Study on the molecular mechanism of apoptosis in **esophageal cancer** *cells induced by soybean isoflavone.* Ma JX, Su JY, Ma JS, Ji HQ, Yan Y. Zhonghua Liu Xing Bing Xue Za Zhi (Chinese). 2003 Nov;24(11):1040-3. **Key Finding:** "Soybean isoflavone seemed to be able to induce the apoptosis in esophageal cancer."

Inhibitive effect of soybean isoflavone on **prostate hyperplasia** *in rats.* Ren GF, Huang YM. Hunan Yi Ke Da Xue Bao (Chinese). 2003 Aug;28(4):343-6. **Key Finding:** "Soybean isoflavone inhibits prostate hyperplasia and the increase of acid phosphatase and prostate-specific acid phosphatase in a dose-dependent manner in rats."

Soy isoflavones increase latency of spontaneous **mammary tumors** *in mice.* Jin Za, MacDonald RS. J Nutr. 2002 Oct;132(10):3186-90. **Key Finding:** "Mammary tumor latency was significantly delayed in mice fed isoflavones compared with the control. Once tumors formed, however, the isoflavones did not reduce the number or size of tumors."

Can food variety add years to your life? Savige GS. Asia Pac J Clin Nutr. 2002;11 Suppl 3:5637-41. **Key Finding:** "Foods for thought include legumes, which are likely to protect older adults against some of the diseases more prevalent with ageing such as **coronary heart disease and cancer**."

Dietary soy and increased risk of **bladder cancer***: the Singapore Chinese Health Study.* Sun CL, Yuan JM, Arakawa K, Low SH, Lee HP, Yu MC. Cancer Epidemiol Biomarkers Prev. 2002 Dec;11(12):1674-7. **Key Finding:** "High intake of soy food was statistically significantly related to an elevated risk of bladder cancer."

Pulses and carcinogenesis: potential for the prevention of **colon, breast and other cancers.** Mathers JC. Br J Nutr. 2002 Dec;88 Suppl 3:5273-9. **Key Finding:** "Pulses contain a rich variety of compounds which, if consumed in sufficient quantities, may help to reduce tumor risk."

Isolation and characterization of an active compound from black soybean {GLycine max (L.) Merr.} and its effect on proliferation and differentiation of human **leukemic** *U937 cells.* Liao HF, Chou CI, Wu SH, Khoo KH, Chen CF, Wang SY. Anticancer Drugs. 2001 Nov;12(10):841-6. **Key Finding:** "Our results suggest that the black soybean may inhibit proliferation and induce differentiation in human leukemic U937 cells by activating the immune response of mononuclear cells."

Prevention of precancerous **colonic lesions** *in rats by soy flakes, soy flour, genistein, and calcium.* Thiagarajan DG, Bennink MR, Bourquin LD, Kavas FA. Am J Clin Nutr. 1998 Dec;68 (6Suppl):1394S-1399S. **Key Finding:** "Eating soybeans and soy flour may reduce the early stages of colon cancer."

Phytoestrogens and human health effects: weighing up the current evidence. Humfrey CD. Nat Toxins. 1998;6(2):51-9. **Key Finding:** "Phytoestrogens are present in beans, sprouts, cabbage, spinach, soyabean, grains and hops. Epidemiological studies suggest that foodstuffs containing phytoestrogens may have a beneficial role in protecting against a number of chronic diseases and conditions. For **cancer of the prostate, colon, rectum, stomach and lung**, the evidence is most consistent for a protective effect. Soya and linseed may have beneficial effects on the risk of **breast cancer** and may help to alleviate **postmenopausal symptoms**. Soya also appears to have beneficial effects on blood lipids which may help to reduce the risk of **cardiovascular disease and atherosclerosis.**"

Curcumin and genistein, plant natural products, show synergistic inhibitory effects on the growth of human **breast cancer** *MCF-7 cells induced by estrogenic pesticides.* Verma SP, Salamone E, Goldin B. Biochem Biophys Res Commun. 1997 Apr 28;233(3):692-6. **Key Finding:** "When curcumin and genistein were added together to MCF-7 cells, a synergistic effect resulting in a total inhibition of the induction of MCF-7 cells by the highly estrogenic activity of endosulfane/chlordane/DDT mixtures was noted. The inclusion of turmeric and soybeans in the diet to prevent hormone related cancers deserves consideration."

Phyto-oestrogens: where are we now? Bingham SA, Atkinson C, Liggins J, Bluck L, Coward A. Br J Nutr. 1998 May;79(5):393-406. **Key Finding:** "Evidence is beginning to accrue that (legumes) may begin to offer protection against a wide range of human conditions, including **breast, bowel, prostate and other cancers, cardiovascular disease, brain function, alcohol abuse, osteoporosis and menopausal symptoms.**"

Cardiovascular disease

The effects of yellow soybean, black soybean, and sword bean on lipid levels and oxidative stress in overietomized rats. Byun JS, Han YS, Lee SS. Int J Vitam Nutr Res. 2010 Apr;80(2):97-106. **Key Finding**: "Our results suggest that consumption of various types of beans may inhibit oxidative stress in postmenopausal women by increasing antioxidant activity and improving lipid profiles. Notably, intake of black soybean resulted in the greatest improvement in risk factors associated with **cardiovascular disease**."

Fruit, vegetable and bean intake and mortality from **cardiovascular disease** *among Japanese men and women: the JACC Study.* Nagura J, Iso H, Watanabe Y, Maruyama K, Date C, Toyoshima H, Yamamoto A, Kikuchi S, Koizumi A, Kondo T, Wada Y, Inaba Y, Tamakoshi A. Br J Nutr. 2009 Jul;102(2):285-92. **Key Finding:** "Fruit intake was inversely associated with mortality from total stroke and total mortality. Vegetable intake was inversely associated with total cardiovascular disease. Bean intake was inversely associated with other cardiovascular disease, total cardiovascular disease, and total mortality."

Intake of vegetables, legumes, and fruit, and risk for all-cause, **cardiovascular, and cancer mortality** *in a European diabetic population.* Nothlings U, Et al. Nutr. 2008 Apr;138(4):775-81. **Key Finding:** "An increment intake of total vegetables, legumes and fruit of 80 g/d was associated with a reduced risk of death from all causes. Analyzed separately, vegetables and legumes were associated with a significantly reduced risk, whereas non-significant inverse associations for fruit intake were observed."

Soybean, a promising health source. Mateos-Aparicio I, Redondo-Cuenca A, Villanueva-Suarez MJ, Zapata-Revilla MA. Nutr Hosp. 2008 Jul-Aug;23(4):305-12. **Key Finding:** "Soybean represents an excellent source of high quality protein, it has a low content in saturated fat, it contains a great amount of dietary fiber and its isoflavone content makes it singular among other legumes. Most of the studies have been focused on soybean protein as a possible source of prevention against **cardiovascular disease**. This positive effect may be due to a decrease in serum cholesterol concentrations."

Cardiovascular consequences of life-long exposure to dietary isoflavones in the rat. Douglas G, Armitage JA, Taylor PD, Lawson JR, Mann GE, Poston L. J Physiol. 2006 Mar 1;571(Pt 2):477-87. **Key Finding:** "This investigation aimed to establish whether the dietary isoflavones in soy protein affect cardiovascular function. In summary, the isoflavone content of soy protein has no influence on blood pressure in healthy rats fed a diet based on soy protein, but influence small artery function (a modest increase in arterial distensibility.)"

Soy protein, isoflavones, and **cardiovascular health**: an American Heart Association Science Advisory for professionals from the Nutrition Committee. Sacks FM, Lichtenstein A, Van Horn L, Harris W, Kris-Etherton P, Winston M. Circulation. 2006 Feb 21;113(7):1034-44. **Key Finding:** "Many soy products should be beneficial to cardiovascular and overall health because of their high content of polyunsaturated fats, fiber, vitamins, and minerals and low content of saturated fat."

Phytoestrogens and **cardiovascular disease**. Cassidy A, Hooper L. J Br Menopause Soc. 2006 Jun;12(2):49-56. **Key Finding:** "Six systematic reviews have assessed the effects of soy isoflavones on lipid levels and suggested that a diet supplemented with soy protein isolate containing isoflavones reduces low-density lipoprotein (LDL) cholesterol, but without clear effects on triglycerides or high-density lipoprotein (HDL) cholesterol. The reduction in total cholesterol may be greater in men than in postmenopausal women. While there is no evidence of beneficial effects of phytoestrogens on blood pressure, arterial compliance or oxidation of LDL cholesterol, there may be beneficial effects on endothelial function in postmenopausal women and on homocysteine concentrations."

Both soybean and kudzu phytoestrogens modify favorably the **blood lipoprotein** profile in ovariectomized and castrated hamsters. Guan L, Yeung SY, Huang Y, Chen ZY. J Agric Food Chem. 2006 Jun 28;54(13):4907-12. **Key Finding:** "It was concluded that both soybean and kudzu phytoestrogens could modify favorably lipoprotein profiles in overiectomized and castrated hamsters."

A meta-analysis of the effect of soy protein supplementation on **serum lipids**. Reynolds K, Chin A, Lees KA, Nguyen A, Bujnowski D, He J. Am J Cardiol. 2006 Sep 1;98(5):633-40. **Key Finding:** "Meta-regression analyses showed a dose-response relation between soy protein and isoflavone supplementation and net changes in serum lipids. These results indicate that soy protein supplementation reduces serum lipids among adults with or without hypercholesterolemia. In conclusion, replacing foods high in saturated fat, trans-saturated fat, and cholesterol with soy protein may have a beneficial effect on **coronary risk** factors."

Soy food consumption is associated with lower risk of **coronary heart disease** *in Chinese women.* Zhang X, Shu XO, Gao YT, Yang G, Li Q, Li H, Jin F, Zheng W. J Nutr. 2003 Sep;133(9):2874-8. **Key Finding:** "This study provides, for the first time; direct evidence that soy food consumption may reduce the risk of coronary heart disease in women."

Phytoestrogens and human health effects: weighing up the current evidence. Humfrey CD. Nat Toxins. 1998;6(2):51-9. **Key Finding:** "Phytoestrogens are present in beans, sprouts, cabbage, spinach, soybean, grains and hops. Epidemiological studies suggest that foodstuffs containing phytoestrogens may have a beneficial role in protecting against a number of chronic diseases and conditions. For **cancer of the prostate, colon, rectum, stomach and lung**, the evidence is most consistent for a protective effect. Soya and linseed may have beneficial effects on the risk of **breast cancer** and may help to alleviate **postmenopausal symptoms**. Soya also appears to have beneficial effects on blood lipids which may help to reduce the risk of **cardiovascular disease and atherosclerosis.**"

Phytoestrogens: where are we now? Bingham SA, Atkinson C, Liggins J, Bluck L, Coward A. Br J Nutr. 1998 May;79(5):393-406. **Key Finding:** "Evidence is beginning to accrue that (legumes) may begin to offer protection against a wide range of human conditions, including **breast, bowel, prostate and other cancers, cardiovascular disease, brain function, alcohol abuse, osteoporosis and menopausal symptoms.**"

Cholesterol

A high legume low glycemic index diet improves serum lipid profiles in men. Zhang Z, Lanza E, Kris-Etherton PM, Et al. Lipids. 2010 Sep;45(9):765-75. **Key Finding:** "This randomized controlled cross-over feeding study of 64 middle-aged men found that a high legume, high fiber, low glycemic index diet improves serum lipid profiles in men, compared to a healthy American diet."

Soy protein reduces serum **cholesterol** *by both intrinsic and food displacement mechanisms.* Jenkins DJ, Mirrahimi A, Srichaikul K, Et al. J Nutr. 2010 Dec;140(12):2302S-2311S. **Key Finding**: "Soy remains one of a few food components that reduce serum cholesterol when added to the diet."

Non-soy legume consumption lowers **cholesterol levels**: *a meta-analysis of randomized controlled trials.* Bazzano LA, Thompson AM, Tees MT, Nguyen CH, Winham DM. Nutr Metab Cardiovasc Dis. 2009 Nov 23 {Epub ahead of print}. **Key**

Finding: "We conducted a meta-analysis of randomized controlled trials evaluating the effects of non-soy legume consumption on blood lipids. Ten randomized clinical trials were selected. These results indicate that a diet rich in legumes other than soy decreases total and LDL cholesterol."

Protective role of chickpea seed coat fiber on N-nitrosodiethylamine-induced toxicity in **hypercholesterolemic** *rats.* Mittal G, Vadhera S, Brar AP, Soni G. Exp Toxicol Pathol. 2009 Jul;61(4):363-70. **Key Finding:** "Chickpea seed coat fiber considerably reduced the peroxidative damage done by NDEA, a carcinogenic nitrosamine frequently present in human environment and food chain that poses a human health hazard."

Effectiveness of a soy-based compared with a traditional low-calorie diet on **weight loss** *and* **lipid levels** *in overweight adults.* Liao FH, Shieh MJ, Yang SC, Lin SH, Chien YW. Nutrition. 2007 Jul-Aug;23(7-8):551-6. **Key Finding:** "Soy-based low-calorie diets significantly decreased serum total cholesterol and low-density lipoprotein cholesterol concentrations and had a greater effect on reducing body weight percentage than traditional low-calorie diets. Thus, soy-based diets have health benefits in reducing weight and blood lipids."

Soy isoflavones lower serum total and LDL **cholesterol** *in humans: a meta-analysis of 11 randomized controlled trials.* Taku K, Umegaki K, Sato Y, Taki Y, Endoh K, Watanabe S. Am J Clin Nutr. 2007 Apr;85(4):1148-56. **Key Finding:** "Soy isoflavones significantly reduced serum total and LDL cholesterol but did not change HDL cholesterol and triacylglycerol. Soy protein that contained enriched or depleted isoflavones also significantly improved lipid profiles. Reductions in LDL cholesterol were larger in hypercholesterolemic than in normocholesterolemic subjects."

Effects of a controlled diet supplemented with chickpeas on **serum lipids**, *glucose tolerance, satiety and bowel function.* Pittaway JK, Ahula KD, Robertson IK, Ball MJ. J Am Coll Nutr. 2007 Aug;26(4):334-40. **Key Finding:** "The small but significant decrease in serum TC and LDL-C during the chickpea diet compared to the equivalent fiber wheat diet was partly due to unintentional changes in macronutrient intake occurring because of chickpea ingestion. If dietary energy and macronutrients were not controlled, chickpea consumption might result in greater benefits via influence on these factors."

Effects of fermented soy milk on the liver lipids under oxidative stress. Lin CY, Tsai ZY, Cheng IC, Lin SH. World J Gastroenterol. 2005 Dec 14;11(46):7355-8. **Key Finding:** "Consumption of fermented soy milk was positive in lowering total

cholesterol and triglyceride accumulation in the liver under CCI(4)-induced oxidative stress."

Combined intervention of soy isoflavone and moderate exercise prevents body fat elevation and bone loss in ovarietcomized mice. Wu J, Wang X, Chiba H, Higuchi M, Nakatani T, Ezaki O, Cui H, Yamada K, Ishimi Y. Metabolism. 2004 Jul;53(7):942-8. **Key Finding:** "These results demonstrate that combined intervention of soybean isoflavone and exercise prevented **body fat** accumulation in the whole body with an increase in lean body mass and restoration of bone mass, and reduced high serum **cholesterol** in ovarietcomized mice."

*Role of isoflavones in the **hypocholesterolemic** effect of soy.* Demonty I, Lamarche B, Jones PJ. Nutr Rev. 2003 Jun;61(6 Pt 1):189-203. **Key Finding:** "Epidemiologic data suggest an inverse relationship between the consumption of soy isoflavones and cardiovascular disease risk. Some studies show a decrease in total cholesterol and low-density lipoprotein concentrations, and an increase in high-density lipoprotein levels, and other investigations fail to show any beneficial effect of soy isoflavones on lipid profiles. There are currently not enough data to recommend the consumption of isoflavone supplements to lower plasma **cholesterol** levels."

*Soy protein in the management of **hyperlipidemia**.* Costa RL, Summa MA. Pharmacother. 2000 Jul-Aug;34(7-8):931-5. **Key Finding:** "Soy can improve blood lipid parameters in both normocholesterolemic and **hypercholesterolemic** subjects."

Cognition

*Soya isoflavone supplementation enhances spatial working **memory** in men.* Thorp AA, Sinn N, Buckley JD, Coates AM, Howe PR. Br J Nutr. 2009 Nov;102(9):1348-54. **Key Finding:** "Isoflavone supplementation in healthy males may enhance cognitive processes which appear dependent on oestrogen activation."

A high soy diet enhances neurotropin receptor and Bcl-XL gene expression in the brains of ovarietcomized female rats. Lovekamp-Swan T, Glendenning ML, Schriehofer DA. Brain Res. 2007 Jul 23;1159:54-66. **Key Finding:** "These results suggest that a high soy diet may provide beneficial effects to the brain similar to low dose chronic estrogen treatment such as that used for postmenopausal hormone replacement."

*Effect of soybean isoflavone on the **cognitive function** in ovariectomized mice.* Zhu JL, Yang GL, Huang YM. Zhong Nan Da Xue Bao Yi Xue Ban (Chinese). 2004

Feb;29(1):81-3. **Key Finding:** "The continuous oral administration of soybean isoflavone can improve the cognitive function of ovariectomized mice."

Phyto-oestrogens: where are we now? Bingham SA, Atkinson C, Liggins J, Bluck L, Coward A. Br J Nutr. 1998 May;79(5):393-406. **Key Finding:** "Evidence is beginning to accrue that (legumes) may begin to offer protection against a wide range of human conditions, including **breast, bowel, prostate and other cancers, cardiovascular disease, brain function, alcohol abuse, osteoporosis and menopausal symptoms.**"

Diabetes

Soy product and isoflavone intakes are associated with a lower risk of **type 2 diabetes** *in overweight Japanese women.* Nanri A, Mizoue T, Takahashi Y, Et al. J Nutr. 2010 Mar;140(3):580-6. **Key Finding**: "Our results suggest that there are no benefits of soy product or isoflavone intake with respect to risk of type 2 diabetes in either men or women. The possible protective associations of soy and isoflavone intakes among overweight women deserve further investigation."

Antidiabetic effects of fermented soybean products on **type 2 diabetes**. Kwon DY, Daily JW, Kim HJ, Park S. Nutr Res. 2010 Jan;30(1):1-13. **Key Finding**: "Several studies revealed improvements in insulin resistance and insulin secretion with the consumption of fermented soy products. Fermented soybean products may help prevent or attenuate the progression of type 2 diabetes. Although the lack of human intervention trials does not permit definitive conclusions, the evidence does suggest that fermented soy products may be better for preventing or delaying the progression of type 2 diabetes compared with non-fermented soybeans."

Kochujang, a Korean fermented red pepper plus soybean paste, improves glucose homeostasis in 90% pancreatectomized **diabetic** *rats.* Kwon DY, Hong SM, Ahn IS, Kim YS, Shin DW, Park S. Nutrition. 2009 Jul-Aug;25(7-8):790-9. **Key Finding:** Kochu-juan, the fermented product of red pepper, and soybeans have been reported to modulate energy and glucose metabolism. "The combination of red pepper and fermented soybeans in kochujang improves glucose homeostasis by reducing insulin resistance."

Multiple mechanisms of soy isoflavones against oxidative stress-induced endothelium injury. Xu SZ, Zhong W, Ghavideldarestani M, Saurabh R, Lindow SW, Atkin SL. Free Radic Biol Med. 2009 Jul 15;47(2):167-75. **Key Finding:** "These findings imply that multiple mechanisms are involved in the beneficial effects of soy isoflavone supplements for **diabetic** endothelial injury."

Soy protein reduces serum LDL cholesterol and the LDL cholesterol:HDL cholesterol and apolipoprotein B:apolipoprotein A-I ratios in adults **with type 2 diabetes.** Pipe EA, Gobert CP, Capes SE, Darlington GA, Lampe JW, Duncan AM. J Nutr. 2009 Sep;139(9):1700-6. **Key Finding:** "These data demonstrate that consumption of soy protein can modulate some serum lipids in a direction beneficial for **cardiovascular disease risk** in adults with type 2 diabetes."

Soy-protein consumption and kidney-related biomarkers among **type 2 diabetics**: *a crossover randomized clinical trial.* Azadbakht L, Esmaillzadeh A. J Ren Nutr. 2009 Nov;19(6):479-86. **Key Finding:** "Renal disease is a major problem among diabetic patients. The type of protein consumed may affect alterations in kidney-related biomarkers in these patients. This study sought to assess the effects of soy-protein consumption on renal-related markers among type 2 diabetic patients with nephropathy. We conclude that soy-protein consumption reduces proteinuria in type 2 diabetes with nephropathy."

Intake of vegetables, legumes, and fruit, and risk for all-cause, **cardiovascular, and cancer mortality** *in a European diabetic population.* Nothlings U, Et al. Nutr. 2008 Apr;138(4):775-81. **Key Finding:** "An increment intake of total vegetables, legumes and fruit of 80 g/d was associated with a reduced risk of death from all causes. Analyzed separately, vegetables and legumes were associated with a significantly reduced risk, whereas non-significant inverse associations for fruit intake were observed."

Beneficial effects of soy protein consumption for renal function. Anderson JW. Asia Pac J Clin Nutr. 2008;17 Suppl 1:324-8. **Key Finding:** "Substituting of soy protein (from soybeans) for animal protein results in less hyper filtration and glomerular **hypertension** with resulting protection from **diabetic** nephropathy."

Vanadium-enriched chickpea sprout ameliorated hyperglycemia and impaired memory in streptozotocin-induced **diabetes** *rats.* Mao X, Zhang L, Xia Q, Sun Z, Zhao X, Cai H, Yang X, Xia Z, Tang Y. Biometals. 2008 Oct;21(5):563-70. **Key Finding:** "Vanadium compounds have been recognized for their hypoglycemic effects; however, potential short and long-term vanadium toxicity has slowed the acceptance for therapeutic use. In the present work, three batches of vanadium-enriched chickpea sprout were prepared. This food was found to ameliorate some hyperglycemic symptoms of the diabetic rats, i.e., improve lipid metabolism, decrease blood glucose level, prevent body weight loss, and reduce impairment of diabetic related spatial learning and memory."

A meal enriched with soy isoflavones increases nitric oxide-mediated vasodilation in healthy postmenopausal women. Hall WL, Formanuik NL, Harnpanich D, Cheung M, Talbot D, Chowienczyk PJ, Sanders TA. J Nutr. 2008 Jul;138(7):1288-92. **Key Finding:** "Regular consumption of soy isoflavones may protect against endothelial dysfunction (which can lead to hypertension and/or diabetes."

Antidiabetic components contained in vegetables and legumes. Tang GY, Li XJ, Zhang HY. Molecules. 2008 May 23;13 (5):1189-94. **Key Finding:** "Epidemiological analyses in a large Chinese population have revealed that consumption of vegetables and legumes is inversely associated with the risk of **type 2 diabetes.**"

Antidiabetic *activity of Mung bean extracts in diabetic KK-Ay mice.* Yao Y, Chen F, Wang M, Wang J, Ren G. J Agric Food Chem. 2008 Oct 8;56(19):8869-73. **Key Finding:** "It was found that mung bean sprout extracts and mung bean seed coat extracts lowered blood glucose, plasma C-peptide, glucagon, total cholesterol, triglyceride, and blood urea nitrogen levels and at the same time markedly improved glucose tolerance and increased insulin immunoreactive levels."

Isolation and activity of an alpha-amylase inhibitor from white kidney beans. Zhang XQ, Yang MY, Ma Y, Tian J, Song JR. Yao Xue Xue Bao. (Chinese). 2007 Dec;42(12):1282-7. **Key Finding:** "The result showed the alpha-Al obtained from white kidney beans had good hypoglycemic effect on alloxan induced diabetic rats and may have high potential pharmaceutical value as regulative digestive-starch degradation in patients suffering from **diabetes.**"

Protective effect of polyphenol-containing azuki bean (Vigna angularis) seed coats on the renal cortex in streptozotocin-induced **diabetic** *rats.* Sato S, Yamate J, Hori Y, Hatai A, Nozawa M, Sagai M. J Nutr Biochem. 2005 Sep;16(9):547-53. **Key Finding:** "Our results suggest that azuki bean seed coat treatments suppress the increased number of infiltrating macrophages and MCP-1 mRNA expression, and attenuated the glomerular expansion in STZ-induced rat diabetic nephropathy."

New legume sources as therapeutic agents. Madar Z, Stark AH. Br J Nutr. 2002 Dec;88 Suppl 3:5287-92. **Key Finding:** "This review evaluates the potential health benefits of three legume sources that rarely appear in Western diets and are often overlooked. Fenugreek (Trigonella foenum graecum) and isolated fenugreek fractions have been shown to act as **hypoglycemic and hypocholesterolaemic** agents in both animal and human studies. Faba beans (Vicia faba) have lipid-lowering effects and may also be a good source of antioxidants and **chemopreventive** factors. Mung beans (Phaseolus aureus, Vigna radiates) are thought to be beneficial as an **antidiabetic,** low glycemic index food, rich in antioxidants. Evidence suggests that these three novel sources of legumes may provide health benefits when included in the daily diet."

Health benefits of traditional corn, beans, and pumpkin: in vitro studies for **hyperglycemia** *and* **hypertension** *management.* Kwon YI, Apostolidis E, Kim YC, Shetty K. J Med Food. 2007 Jun;10(2):266-75. **Key Finding:** "In this study antidiabetic and anti-hypertension relevant potentials of phenolic phytochemicals were confirmed in select important traditional plant foods of indigenous communities such as pumpkin, beans and maize. Pumpkin showed the best overall potential."

Health benefits of low glycemic index foods, such as pulses, in **diabetic** *patients and health individuals.* Rizkalla SW, Bellisle F, Slama G. Br J Nutr. 2002 Dec;88 Suppl 3:5255-62. **Key Finding:** "The results of human studies have been confirmed by animal experiments in the field of diabetes. Diets with low glycemic index value improve the prevention of **coronary heart disease** in diabetic and healthy subjects. In obese or overweight individuals, low-glycemic index meals increase satiety and facilitate the control of food intake. Pulses are foods with very low glycemic-index values and have demonstrated benefits for healthy persons in terms of post-prandial glucose and lipid metabolism."

Hypertension

Effects of soy isoflavone extract supplements on **blood pressure** *in adult humans: systematic review and meta-analysis of randomized placebo-controlled trials.* Taku K, Lin N, Cai D, Et al. J Hypertens. 2010 Oct;28(10):1971-82. **Key Finding**: "Soy isoflavone extracts significantly decreased systolic blood pressure but not diastolic blood pressure in adult humans, and no dose-response relationship was observed."

Polyphenol-containing azuki bean (Vigna angularis) extract attenuates blood pressure elevation and modulates nitric oxide synthase and caveolin-1 expressions in rats with **hypertension.** Mukai Y, Sato S. Nutr Metab Cardiovasc Dis. 2009 Sep;19(7):491-7. **Key Finding:** "Azuki bean extract reduced the elevated blood pressure and increased nitric oxide production in long-term treatment."

A meal enriched with soy isoflavones increases nitric oxide-mediated vasodilation in healthy postmenopausal women. Hall WL, Formanuik NL, Harnpanich D, Cheung M, Talbot D, Chowienczyk PJ, Sanders TA. J Nutr. 2008 Jul;138(7):1288-92. **Key Finding: "**Regular consumption of soy isoflavones may protect against endothelial dysfunction (which can lead to hypertension and/or diabetes."

*Health benefits of traditional corn, beans, and pumpkin: in vitro studies for **hyperglycemia** and **hypertension** management.* Kwon YI, Apostolidis E, Kim YC, Shetty K. J Med Food. 2007 Jun;10(2):266-75. **Key Finding:** "In this study antidiabetic and antihypertension relevant potentials of phenolic phytochemicals were confirmed in select important traditional plant foods of indigenous communities such as pumpkin, beans and maize. Pumpkin showed the best overall potential."

Inflammation

*Positive effect of dietary soy in ESRD patients with systemic **inflammation**—correlation between blood levels of the soy isoflavones and the acute-phase reactants.* Fanti P, Asmis R, Stephenson TJ, Sawaya BP, Franke AA. Nephrol Dial Transplant. 2006 Aug;21(8):2239-46. **Key Finding:** "These data suggest the possibility of beneficial effects of isoflavone rich soy foods on the inflammatory and nutritional status of hemodialysis patients with underlying systemic inflammation."

*Major dietary patterns are related to plasma concentrations of markers of **inflammation** and endothelial dysfunction.* Lopez-Garcia E, Schulze MB, Fung TT, Meigs JB, Rifai N, Manson JE, Hu FB. Am J Clin Nutr. 2004 Oct;80(4):1029-35. **Key Finding:** "Because endothelial dysfunction is an early step in the development of **atherosclerosis**, this study suggests a mechanism (through higher intakes of legumes, etc.) for the role of dietary patterns in the pathogenesis of cardiovascular disease."

Menopausal symptoms

Effect of high-dose isoflavones on cognition, quality of life, androgens, and lipoprotein in post-menopausal women. Basaria S, Wisniewski A, Dupree K, Bruno T, Song MY, Yao F, Ojumu A, John M, Dobs AS. J Endocrinol Invest. 2009 Feb;32(2):150-5. **Key Finding:** "High-dose isoflavones is associated with improved quality of life among women who have become menopausal recently. Hence, the timing of isoflavone supplementation with regards to the onset of menopause appears to be important. The use of isoflavones, as an alternative to estrogen therapy, may be potentially useful and seemingly safe in this group of women who are looking for relief from **menopausal symptoms**."

*Effect of soybeans and soy sauce on vasomotor symptoms during **menopause**.* Gutierrez Martinez MM, Riquelme Raya R, Campos Martinez AM, Lorite Garzon C, Strivens Vilchez H, Ruiz Rodriguez C. Rev Enferm (Spanish). 2006 Jun;29(6):16-22. **Key Finding:** "Up to now the most effective remedy (for menopause symptoms) was hormone treatment, but a study of isoflavones, such as soybean, suggests it is possible to alleviate the disturbances caused by menopause."

Health benefits of soy isoflavonoids and strategies for enhancement: a review. McCue P, Shetty K. Crit Rev Food Sci Nutr. 2004;44(5):361-7. **Key Finding:** "Soybean consumption has been linked to a reduced risk for certain cancers and diseases of **old age**. In this study, we discuss the current state of knowledge concerning soybean isoflavonoids, their chemo preventive actions against **postmenopausal** health problems, **cancer**, and **cardiovascular disease**."

Phytoestrogens: implications in neurovascular research. Lephart ED, Porter JP, Hedges DW, Lund TD, Setchell KD. Curr Neurovasc Res. 2004 Dec;1(5):455-64. **Key Finding:** "Isoflavone consumption of soy-derived dietary phytoestrogens have received prevalent usage due to their ability to decrease age related disease (**cardiovascular** and **osteoporosis**) hormone-dependent cancers (**breast and prostate**) and peri- and **postmenopausal symptoms**. Dietary phytoestrogens appear to affect certain aspects of vascular, neuroendocrine and cognitive function."

Potential risks and benefits of phytoestrogen-rich diets. Cassidy A. Int J Vitam Nutr Res. 2003 Mar;73(2):120-6. **Key Finding:** "Soya isoflavones can exert hormonal effects. These effects may be of benefit in the prevention of many of the common diseases observed in Western populations (such as **breast cancer, prostate cancer, menopause symptoms, and osteoporosis**)."

Soy isoflavones: are they useful in **menopause***?* Vincent A, Fitzpatrick LA. Mayo Clin Proc. 2000 Nov;75(11):1174-84. **Key Finding:** "Studies of soy-based diets evaluating the relation between soy consumption and serum lipid concentrations revealed that soy consumption significantly decreased total cholesterol, LDL cholesterol, and triglyceride levels. Epidemiological studies suggest a protective effect of soy protein on breast tissue as evidenced by the lower rates of breast cancer in East Asian countries where soy is a predominant part of the diet. A few studies reveal a minimal effect of soy on hot flashes. Current data are insufficient to draw definitive conclusion regarding the use of isoflavones as an alternative to estrogen for hormone replacement in postmenopausal women."

Hot flushes and other **menopausal symptoms** *in relation to soy product intake in Japanese women.* Nagata C, Shimizu H, Takami R, Hayashi M, Takeda N, Yasuda K. Climacteric. 1999 Mar;2(1):6-12. **Key Finding:** "The data support a hypothesis that intake of fermented soy products alleviates the severity of hot flushes."

Phytoestrogens and human health effects: weighing up the current evidence. Humfrey CD. Nat Toxins. 1998;6(2):51-9. **Key Finding:** "Phytoestrogens are present in beans, sprouts, cabbage, spinach, soybean, grains and hops. Epidemiological studies suggest that foodstuffs containing phytoestrogens may have a beneficial role in protecting against a number of chronic diseases and conditions. For **cancer of the prostate, colon, rectum, stomach and lung**, the evidence is most consistent for a protective effect. Soya and linseed may have beneficial effects on the risk of **breast cancer** and may help to alleviate **postmenopausal symptoms**. Soya also appears to have beneficial effects on blood lipids which may help to reduce the risk of **cardiovascular disease and atherosclerosis.**"

Effects of dietary phytoestrogens in postmenopausal women. Dalais FS, Rich GE, Wahlqvist ML, Grehan M, Murkies AL, Medley G, Ayton R, Strauss BJ. Climacteric. 1998 Jun;1(2):124-9. **Key Finding:** "The aim of this study was to test the hypothesis that increased dietary intake of phytoestrogens reduces the health impact of **menopause**. To test this hypothesis, a double-blind, randomized, entry-exit, cross-over study was conducted to assess the effects of three dietary manipulations –soy and linseed diets (high in phytoestrogens) and a wheat diet (low in phytoestrogens.) The data obtained from separate analyses suggest that phytoestrogens in soy and linseed may be of use in ameliorating some of the symptoms of menopause."

Phytoestrogens: where are we now? Bingham SA, Atkinson C, Liggins J, Bluck L, Coward A. Br J Nutr. 1998 May;79(5):393-406. **Key Finding:** "Evidence is beginning to accrue that (legumes) may begin to offer protection against a wide range of human conditions, including **breast, bowel, prostate and other cancers, cardiovascular disease, brain function, alcohol abuse, osteoporosis and menopausal symptoms.**"

Myocardial Infarction (heart attack)

*Decreased consumption of dried mature beans is positively associated with urbanization and nonfatal **acute myocardial infarction**.* Kabagambe EK, Baylin A, Ruiz-Navarez E, Siles X, Campos H. J Nutr. 2005 Jul;135(7):1770-5. **Key Finding:** "Compared with non-consumers, intake of 1 serving of beans/d was inversely associated with myocardial infarction in analyses adjusted for smoking, history of diabetes, history of hypertension, abdominal obesity, physical activity, income, intake of alcohol, total energy, saturated fat, trans fat, polyunsaturated fat, and cholesterol. We found that consumption of 1 serving of beans/d is associated with a 38% lower risk of myocardial infarction."

Obesity

The effects of soy isoflavones on **obesity**. Orgaard A, Jensen L. Exp Biol Med (Maywood). 2008 Sep;233(9):1066-80. **Key Finding:** Soybeans and soybean products contain the isoflavones, genistein and daidzein. "Epidemiologic and laboratory data suggest that these compounds could have health benefits in human obesity."

Cereal grains, legumes, and **weight management**: *a comprehensive review of the scientific evidence.* Williams PG, Grafenauer SJ, O-Shea JE. Nutr Rev. 2008 Apr;66(4):171-82. **Key Finding:** "There is strong evidence that a diet high in whole grains and legumes can help reduce weight gain and that significant weight loss is achievable with energy-controlled diets that are high in cereals and legumes."

Effectiveness of a soy-based compared with a traditional low-calorie diet on **weight loss** *and* **lipid levels** *in overweight adults.* Liao FH, Shieh MJ, Yang SC, Lin SH, Chien YW. Nutrition. 2007 Jul-Aug;23(7-8):551-6. **Key Finding:** "Soy-based low-calorie diets significantly decreased serum total cholesterol and low-density lipo-protein cholesterol concentrations and had a greater effect on reducing body weight percentage than traditional low-calorie diets. Thus, soy-based diets have health benefits in reducing weight and blood lipids."

Combined intervention of soy isoflavone and moderate exercise prevents body fat elevation and bone loss in ovarietcomized mice. Wu J, Wang X, Chiba H, Higuchi M, Nakatani T, Ezaki O, Cui H, Yamada K, Ishimi Y. Metabolism. 2004 Jul;53(7):942-8. **Key Finding:** "These results demonstrate that combined intervention of soybean isoflavone and exercise prevented **body fat** accumulation in the whole body with an increase in lean body mass and restoration of bone mass, and reduced high serum **cholesterol** in ovariectomized mice."

Osteoporosis

Soy protein and **bone mineral density** *in older men and women: a randomized trial.* Newton KM, LaCroix AZ, Levy L, Li SS, Qu P, Potter JD, Lampe JW. Maturitas. 2006 Oct 20;55(3):270-7. **Key Finding:** "Soy protein containing isoflavones showed a modest benefit in preserving spine, but not hip bone mineral density in older women."

Recommended soy and soy products intake to prevent bone fracture and **osteoporosis.** Uenishi K. Clin Calcium (Japanese). 2005 Aug;15(8):1393-8. **Key Finding:** "In this report, we overviewed peer-reviewed papers showing relationship between soy product intake and risks of bone fracture and osteoporosis."

Skeletal benefits of soy isoflavones: a review of the clinical trial and epidemiologic data. Messina M, Ho S, Alekel DL. Curr Opin Clin Nutr Metab Care. 2004 Nov;7(6):649-58. **Key Finding:** "Although soy foods and isoflavones cannot be viewed as substitutes for established anti-**osteoporotic** medications, health professionals can feel justified in encouraging postmenopausal women concerned about **bone health** to incorporate soy foods into their diet."

Phytoestrogens: implications in neurovascular research. Lephart ED, Porter JP, Hedges DW, Lund TD, Setchell KD. Curr Neurovasc Res. 2004 Dec;1(5):455-64. **Key Finding:** "Isoflavone consumption of soy-derived dietary phytoestrogens have received prevalent usage due to their ability to decrease age related disease (**cardiovascular** and **osteoporosis**) hormone-dependent cancers (**breast and prostate**) and peri- and **postmenopausal symptoms**. Dietary phytoestrogens appear to affect certain aspects of vascular, neuroendocrine and cognitive function."

Potential risks and benefits of phytoestrogen-rich diets. Cassidy A. Int J Vitam Nutr Res. 2003 Mar;73(2):120-6. **Key Finding:** "Soya isoflavones can exert hormonal effects. These effects may be of benefit in the prevention of many of the common diseases observed in Western populations (such as **breast cancer, prostate cancer, menopause symptoms, and osteoporosis**)."

The role of phytoestrogens in the prevention and treatment of **osteoporosis** *in ovarian hormone deficiency.* Arjmandi BH. Am Coll Nutr. 2001 Oct;20(5 Suppl):3985-4025. **Key Finding:** "Recent reports support the notion that certain bioactive constituents, e.g., phytoestrogens, in plants play a role in maintaining or improving skeletal health."

Phytoestrogens: where are we now? Bingham SA, Atkinson C, Liggins J, Bluck L, Coward A. Br J Nutr. 1998 May;79(5):393-406. **Key Finding:** "Evidence is beginning to accrue that (legumes) may begin to offer protection against a wide range of human conditions, including **breast, bowel, prostate and other cancers, cardiovascular disease, brain function, alcohol abuse, osteoporosis and menopausal symptoms.**"

Stroke

*Soy consumption reduces risk of **ischemic stroke**: a case-control study in southern China.* Liang W, Lee AH, Binns CW, Huang R, Hu D, Shao H. Neuroepidemiology. 2009;33(2):111-6. **Key Finding:** "The results provided evidence of inverse association between habitual soy food consumption and the risk of ischemic stroke for Chinese adults."

*Fruit and vegetable intake in relation to risk of **ischemic stroke**.* Joshipura KJ, Ascherio A, Manson JE, Stampfer MJ, Rimm EB, Speizer FE, Heennekens CH, Spiegelman D, Willett WC. JAMA. 1999 Oct 6;282(13):1233-9. **Key Finding:** "These data support a protective relationship between consumption of fruit and vegetables—particularly cruciferous and green leafy vegetables and citrus fruit and juice—and **ischemic stroke** risk. Legumes were not associated with lower ischemic stroke risk."

Thyroid Hyperplasia

*Dramatic synergism between excess soybean intake and iodine deficiency on the development of rat **thyroid hyperplasia**.* Ikeda T, Nishikawa A, Imazawa T, Kimura S, Hirose M. Carcinogenesis. 2000 Apr;21(4):707-13. **Key Finding:** "Our results strongly suggest that dietary defatted soybean synergistically stimulates the growth of rat thyroid with iodine deficiency, partly through a pituitary-dependent pathway."

Berries (in General)

(See also Blueberries, Cranberries, Grapes, Raspberries, Resveratrol, Strawberries)

BERRIES ARE SMALL, USUALLY EDIBLE FRUITS THAT CONTAIN SEEDS. Some are sweet tasting, some sour. Their intense distinctive colors, from blue to red, are due to pigments high in polyphenols, which give them a high antioxidant content that may be beneficial to human health.

Blackberries, for instance, native to North and South America, are a group of more than three hundred species that grow wild and contain high levels of polyphenols. The biggest producer of cultivated blackberries is the state of Oregon. Antioxidant activity by blackberries and other types of berries has been demonstrated in numerous science studies, which may explain why they have been proven to help lower the risk for at least eight kinds of cancer, along with hypercholesterolemia and cardiovascular disease.

Aging

Berries: improving human health and **healthy aging**, *and promoting quality life—a review.* Paredes-Lopez O, Et al. Plant Foods Hum Nutr. 2010 Sep;65(3):299-308. **Key Finding**: "Berries are rich sources of a wide variety of phytochemicals. The isolation and characterization of compounds that may delay the onset of aging is receiving intense research attention. Some berry phenolic is being associated with this functional performance."

Dietary compound ellagic acid alleviates **skin wrinkle** *and inflammation induced by UV-B irradiation.* Bae JY, Choi JS, Kang SW, Et al. Exp Dermatol. 2010 Aug;19(8):e182-90. **Key Finding:** "These results demonstrate that ellagic acid present in **berries and pomegranate** prevented collagen destruction and inflammatory responses caused by UV-B. Dietary and pharmacological interventions with ellagic acid may be promising treatment strategies interrupting skin wrinkle and inflammation associated with chronic UV exposure leading to photo aging."

Alzheimer's disease

Oxidative stress and **Alzheimer's disease**: *dietary polyphenols as potential therapeutic agents.* Darvesh AS, Carroll RT, Bishayee A, Geldenhuys WJ, Van der Schyf CJ.

Expert Rev Neurother. 2010 May;10(5):729-45. **Key Finding**: Oxidative stress has been strongly implicated in the pathophysiology of neurodegenerative disorders such as Alzheimer's. This article reviews the antioxidant potential of polyphenol compounds such as anthocyanin from berries, catechins and theaflavins from tea, curcumin from turmeric and resveratrol from grapes.

Withanamides in Withania somnifera fruit protect PC-12 cells from beta-amyloid responsible for **Alzheimer's disease***.* Jayaprakaṣam B, Padmanabhan K, Nair MG. Phytother Res. 2009 Dec 2: (Epub ahead of print.) **Key Finding**: "The beta-amyloid peptide, with 39-42 amino acid residues (BAP) plays a significant role in the development of Alzheimer's disease. Our earlier investigations of the Withanian somnifera fruit (a shrub known as Indian ginseng with a red berry fruit) afforded lipid peroxidation inhibitory withanamides that are more potent than commercial antioxidants. In this study, we have tested two major withanamides A (WA) and C (WC) for their ability to protect the PC-12 cells, rat neuronal cells, from beta-amyloid induced cell damage. Cell death caused by beta-amyloid was negated by withanamide treatment. Molecular modeling studies showed that withanamides A and C uniquely bind to the active motif of beta-amyloid (25-35) and suggest that withanamides have the ability to prevent the fibril formation."

Antioxidation

Antioxidant levels of common fruits, vegetables, and juices versus protective activity against in vitro **ischemia**/*reperfusion.* Bean H, Schuler C, Leggett RE, Levin RM. Int Urol Nephrol. 2009 Sep 19. (Epub ahead of print). **Key Finding:** "An assay was utilized to determine the antioxidant reactivity of a series of fruits, vegetables, and juices, and the results were compared to the protective ability of selected juices in an established in vitro rabbit bladder model of ischemia/reperfusion. The results showed that cranberry juice had the highest level of antioxidant reactivity, blueberry juice had an intermediate activity, and orange juice had the lowest. It was determined, however, that contrary to the hypothesis, the orange juice was significantly more potent in protecting the bladder against ischemia/reperfusion damage than either blueberry or cranberry juice."

Prevention of **oxidative DNA damage** *by bioactive berry components.* Aiyer HS, Kichambare S, Gupta RC. Nutr Cancer. 2008;60 Suppl 1:36-42. **Key Finding:** "The hormone 17ss-estradiol (E(2)) causes oxidative DNA damage via redox cycling of its metabolites. In this study, ACI rats were fed either AIN-93M diet or diets supplemented with 0.5% each of mixed berries (strawberry, blueberry, blackberry, and red and black raspberry), blueberry alone or ellagic acid. Ellagic acid (EA) diet significantly reduced E (2)-induced levels of 8-oxodG. Blueberry alone also significantly reduced the levels. Mixed berries were ineffective. In addition, aqueous extracts of berries (2%) and EA (100 microM) were tested for their efficacy in diminishing oxidative DNA adducts induced by redox cycling of 4E(2) catalyzed by copper chloride in vitro. EA was the most efficacious (90%) followed by extracts of red raspberry (70%), blueberry and strawberry (50% each; $P<0.001$)."

Comparison of antioxidant potency of commonly consumed polyphenol-rich beverages in the United States. Seeram NP, Aviram M, Zhang Y, Henning SM, Feng L, Dreher M, Heber D. J Agric Food Chem. 2008 Feb 27;56(4):1415-22. **Key Finding:** "The present study applied four tests of antioxidant potency. The beverages included several different brands as follows: apple juice, acai juice, black cherry juice, blueberry juice, cranberry juice, Concord grape juice, orange juice, red wines, iced tea beverages, black tea, green tea, white tea, and a major pomegranate juice available in the U.S. market. Pomegranate juice had the greatest antioxidant potency composite index among the beverages tested and was at least 20% greater than any of the other beverages tested."

Characterization of blackberry extract and its antiproliferative and anti-inflammatory properties. Dai J, Patel JD, Mumper RJ. J Med Food. 2007 Jun;10(2):258-65. **Key Finding:** "These results suggest that Hull blackberry extract has potent **antioxidant**, antiproliferative, and anti-inflammatory activates and that HBE-formulated products may have the potential for the treatment and/or prevention of **cancer** and/or other inflammatory diseases."

Anti-angiogenic, antioxidant, *and* ***anti-carcinogenic*** *properties of a novel anthocyanin-rich berry extract formula.* Bagchi D, Sen CK, Bagchi M, Atalay M. Biochemistry. 2004 Jan;69(1):75-80. **Key Finding:** "Six berry extracts (wild blueberry, bilberry, cranberry, elderberry, raspberry seeds and strawberry) were studied for antioxidant efficacy, cytotoxic potential, cellular uptake, and anti-angiogenic (the ability to reduce unwanted growth of blood vessels, which can lead to varicose veins and tumor formation) properties. We evaluated various combinations of edible berry extracts and developed a synergistic formula, OptiBerry IH141, which exhibited high ORAC (Oxygen-Radical Absorbing Capacity) value, low cytotoxicity, and superior anti-angiogenic properties compared to the other combinations tested. Anti-angiogenic approaches to treat cancer represent a priority area in vascular tumor biology. OptiBerry significantly inhibited both H202- and TNF-alpha-induced VEGF (Vascular Endothelial Growth Factor) expression by human keratinocytes. VEGF is a key regulator of tumor angiogenesis. Matrigel assay using human micro vascular endothelial cells showed that OptiBerry impaired angiogenesis. Endothelium cells pretreated with OptiBerry showed a diminished ability to form hemangioma and markedly decreased **tumor** growth by more than 50%."

Oxygen radical absorbing capacity of phenolic in blueberries, cranberries, chokeberries, and lingonberries. Zheng W, Wang SY. J Agric Food Chem. 2003 Jan 15;51(2):502-9. **Key Finding:** "The phenolic constituents and contents among the different berries varied considerably. Anthocyanins were found to be the main components in all these berries. Chlorogenic acid in blueberry, quercetin glycosides in cranberry and lingonberry, and caffeic acid and its derivative in chokeberry were also present in relatively high concentrations. Chlorogenic acid, peonidin 3-galactoside, cyaniding 3-galactoside, and cyaniding 3-galactoside were the most important antioxidants in blueberry, cranberry, wild chokeberry and lingonberry respectively."

Cyclooxygenase inhibitory and **antioxidant** *cyaniding glycosides in cherries and berries.* Seeram NP, Momin RA, Nair MG, Bourquin LD. Phytomedicine. 2001 Sep;8(5):362-9. **Key Finding:** "Anthocyanins from raspberries and sweet cherries demonstrated 45% and 47% cyclooxygenase-I and cyclooxygenase-II inhibitory activities, respectively, when assayed at 125 microg/ml. Anthocyanins 1 and 2 are present in both cherries and raspberry. Fresh blackberries and strawberries contained only anthocyanin 2 in yields of 24 and 22.5 mg/100 g, respectively. Anthocyanins 1 and 2 were not found in bilberries, blueberries, cranberries or elderberries."

Atherosclerosis

Berry anthocyanins as novel antioxidants in human health and disease prevention. Zafra-Stone S, Yasmin T, Bagchi M, Chatterjee A, Vinson JA, Bagchi D. Mol Nutr Food Res. 2007 Jun;51(6):675-83. **Key Finding:** "A novel combination of selected berry extracts known as OptiBerry contains wild blueberry, wild bilberry, cranberry, elderberry, raspberry seeds, and strawberry. Recent studies in our laboratory have demonstrated that OptiBerry exhibits high antioxidant efficacy as shown by its high oxygen radical absorbance capacity values, novel antiangiogenic and **anti-atherosclerotic** activities, and potential cytotoxicity towards Helicobacter pylori, a noxious pathogen responsible for various gastrointestinal disorders including **duodenal ulcer** and **gastric cancer**, as compared to individual berry extracts. OptiBerry also significantly inhibited basal MCP-1 and inducible NF-kappa beta transcriptions as well as the inflammatory biomarker IL-8, and significantly reduced the ability to form hemangioma and markedly decreased EOMA cell-induced tumor growth in anin vivo model."

Cancer (breast; cervical; colon; esophageal; gastric; oral; prostate; stomach)

Recent trends and advances in berry health benefits research. Seeram NP. J Agric Food Chem. 2010 Apr 14;58(7):3869-70: **Key Finding**: "Recent advances have been made in our scientific understanding of how berries promote human health and prevent chronic illnesses such as some **cancers, heart disease, and neuro-degenerative diseases.** Berry bio actives encompass a wide diversity of phytochemicals."

Natural compounds in chemoprevention of **esophageal squamous cell tumors**— *experimental studies.* Szumilo J. Pol Merkur Lekarski. 2009 Feb;26(152):156-61. **Key Finding:** "In esophageal squamous cell carcinoma—this belongs to the group of the most aggressive tumors of digestive system with poor prognosis. Chemo preventive properties of many complex diets and pure natural compounds were evaluated. Most studies were performed on rats exposed to chemical carcino-gens. The best effects were achieved after administration of diallyl sulfide and phenethyl isothiocyanate. Lyophilized black raspberries, blackberries and straw-berries, as well as products obtained from leaves and buds of tea plant, ellagic acid and resveratrol were also very effective."

American ginseng berry enhances chemo preventive effect of 5-FU on human **colorectal cancer** *cells.* Li XL, Wang CZ, Sun S, Mehendale SR, Du W, He TC, Yuan CS. Oncol Rep. 2009 Oct;22(4):943-52. **Key Finding:** "In this study, we investigated the possible synergistic chemo preventive effects of American ginseng berry extract (AGBE) and a chemotherapy agent 5-fluorouracil (5-FU) on human colorectal cancer cell lines, SW-480, HCT-116 and HT-29. The enhancement of S and G2/M phase arrest, rather than cell apoptosis, should be the mechanism of synergistic effects of AGBE on 5-FU. Further in vivo and clinical trial are needed to test AGBE as a valuable chemo-adjuvant."

Berry fruits for **cancer** *prevention: current status and future prospects.* Seeram NP. J Agric Food Chem. 2008 Feb 13;56(3):630-5. **Key Finding:** "Overwhelming evidence suggests that edible small and soft-fleshed berry fruits may have beneficial effects against several types of human cancers. Studies show that the anticancer effects of berry bio actives are partially mediated through their abilities to counteract, reduce, and also repair damage resulting from oxidative stress and inflammation. In addition, berry bio actives also regulate carcinogen and xenobiotic metabolizing enzymes, various transcription and growth factors, inflammatory cytokines, and subcellular signaling pathways of cancer cell proliferation, apoptosis, and tumor angiogenesis."

Berry extracts exert different antiproliferative effects against **cervical** *and* **colon cancer** *cells grown in vitro.* McDougall GJ, Ross HA, Ikeji M, Stewart D. J Agric Food Chem. 2008 May 14;56(9):3016-23. **Key Finding:** "Polyphenol-rich berry extracts were screened for their antiproliferative effectiveness using human cervical cancer (HeLa) cells grown in micro titer plates. Rowan berry, raspberry, lingonberry, cloudberry, arctic bramble, and strawberry extracts were effective, but blueberry, sea buckthorn and pomegranate extracts were considerably less effective. The most effective extracts (strawberry>arctic bramble>cloudberry>lingonberry) gave EC 50 values in the range of 25-40 microg/(mL of phenols). These extracts were also effective against human colon cancer (CaCo-2) cells, which were generally more sensitive at low concentrations but conversely less sensitive at higher concentrations. The strawberry, cloudberry, arctic bramble and the raspberry extracts share common polyphenol constituents, especially the ellagitannins, which have been shown to be effective antiproliferative agents."

Cellular antioxidant activity of common fruits. Wolfe KL, Kang X, He X, Dong M, Zhang Q, Liu RH. J Agric Food Chem. 2008 Sep 24;56(18):8418-26. **Key Finding:** "The objective of this study was to determine the cellular antioxidant activity, total phenolic contents, and oxygen radical absorbance capacity values of 25 fruits commonly consumed in the United States. Pomegranate and berries (wild blueberry, blackberry, raspberry, and blueberry) had the highest cellular antioxidant activity, whereas banana and melons had the lowest. Apple and strawberries were the biggest suppliers of cellular antioxidant activity to the American diet. Increasing fruit consumption is a logical strategy to increase antioxidant intake and decrease oxidative stress and may lead to reduced risk of **cancer.**"

Berry phytochemicals, genomic stability and **cancer**: *evidence for chemo protection at several stages in the carcinogenic process.* Duthie SJ. Mol Nutr Food Res. 2007 Jun;51(6):665-74. **Key Finding:** "There is strong and convincing evidence that berry extracts and berry phytochemicals modulate biomarkers of DNA damage and indicators of malignant transformation in vitro and in vivo. Data from numerous cell culture and animal models indicate that berry components such as the anthocyanin are potent anticarcinogenic agents and are protective against genomic instability at several sites in the carcinogenic pathway."

Cranberry and blueberry: evidence for protective effects against **cancer** *and* **vascular diseases**. Neto CC. Mol Nutr Food Res. 2007 Jun;51(6):652-64. **Key Finding:** "Growing evidence from tissue culture, animal, and clinical models suggests that the flavonoid-rich fruits of the North American cranberry and blueberry have the potential ability to limit the development and severity of certain cancers and vascular diseases including **atherosclerosis, ischemic stroke**, and neurodegenerative **diseases of aging**."

Berry phenolic extracts modulate the expression of p21(WAF1) and Bax but not Bcl-2 in HT-29 **colon cancer** *cells.* Wu QK, Koponen JM, Mykkanen HM, Torronen AR. J Agric Food Chem. 2007 Feb 21;55(4):1156-63. **Key Finding:** "Colon cancer cells were exposed to 0-60 mg/ml of extracts and the cell growth inhibition was determined after 24 h. The degree of cell growth inhibition was as follows: bilberry>black currant>cloudberry>lingonberry>raspberry>strawberry. A 14-fold increase in the expression of p21WAF1, an inhibitors of cell proliferation and a member of the cyclin kinase inhibitors, was seen in cells exposed to cloudberry extract compared to other berry treatments. The pro-apoptosis marker, Bax, was increased 1.3-fold only in cloudberry and bilberry-treated cells. Cloudberry, despite its very low anthocyanin content, was a potent inhibitor of cell proliferation. Therefore, it is concluded that, in addition to anthocyanins, also other phenolic or nonphenolic phytochemicals are responsible for the antiproliferative activity of berries."

Inhibition of **cancer** *cell proliferation and suppression of TNF-induced activation of NFkappaB by edible berry juice.* Boivin D, Blanchette M, Barrette S, Moghrabi A, Beliveau R. Anticancer Res. 2007 Mar-Apr;27(2):937-48. **Key Finding:** "These results illustrate that berry juices have striking differences in their potential chemo preventive activity and that the inclusion of a variety of berries in the diet might be useful for preventing the development of tumors. The growth of various cancer cell lines, including those of **stomach, prostate, intestine and breast**, was strongly inhibited by raspberry, black currant, white currant, gooseberry, velvet leaf blueberry, low-bush blueberry, sea buckthorn and cranberry juice, but not (or only slightly) by strawberry, high-bush blueberry, serviceberry, red currant, or blackberry juice. "

Berry anthocyanins as novel antioxidants in human health and disease prevention. Zafra-Stone S, Yasmin T, Bagchi M, Chatterjee A, Vinson JA, Bagchi D. Mol Nutr Food Res.

2007 Jun;51(6):675-83. **Key Finding:** "A novel combination of selected berry extracts known as OptiBerry contains wild blueberry, wild bilberry, cranberry, elderberry, raspberry seeds, and strawberry. Recent studies in our laboratory have demonstrated that OptiBerry exhibits high antioxidant efficacy as shown by its high oxygen radical absorbance capacity values, novel antiangiogenic and **antiatherosclerotic** activities, and potential cytotoxicity towards Helicobacter pylori, a noxious pathogen responsible for various gastrointestinal disorders including **duodenal ulcer** and **gastric cancer**, as compared to individual berry extracts. OptiBerry also significantly inhibited basal MCP-1 and inducible NF-kappa beta transcriptions as well as the inflammatory biomarker IL-8, and significantly reduced the ability to form hemangioma and markedly decreased EOMA cell-induced tumor growth in anin vivo model."

Characterization of blackberry extract and its antiproliferative and anti-inflammatory properties. Dai J, Patel JD, Mumper RJ. J Med Food. 2007 Jun;10(2):258-65. **Key Finding:** "These results suggest that Hull blackberry extract has potent antioxidant, anti-proliferative, and anti-inflammatory activities and that HBE-formulated product may have the potential for the treatment and/or prevention of **cancer** and/or other inflammatory diseases."

*Blackberry, black raspberry, blueberry, cranberry, red raspberry, and strawberry extracts inhibit growth and stimulate apoptosis of human **cancer** cells in vitro.* Seeram NP, Adams LS, Zhang Y, Lee R, Sand D, Scheuller HS, Heber D. J Agric Food Chem. 2006 Dec 13;54(25):9329-39. **Key Finding:** "The berry extracts were evaluated for their ability to inhibit the growth of human **oral, breast, colon and prostate tumor cell** lines at concentrations ranging from 25 to 200 micro g/ml. With increasing concentration of berry extract, increasing inhibition of cell proliferation in all of the cancer cell lines was observed, with different degrees of potency between cell lines. The berry extracts were also evaluated for their ability to stimulate apoptosis of the COX-2 expressing **colon cancer** cell line, HT-29. Black raspberry and strawberry extracts showed the most significant pro-apoptotic effects against this cell line."

*Protection against **esophageal cancer** in rodents with lyophilized berries: potential mechanisms.* Stoner GD, Chen T, Kresty LA, Aziz RM, Reinemann T, Nines R. Nutr Cancer. 2006;54(1):33-46. **Key Finding:** "Our laboratory has been evaluating the ability of lyophilized (freeze-dried) black raspberries, blackberries and strawberries to inhibit carcinogen-induced cancer in the rodent esophagus. At 25 weeks of the bioassay, all three berry types were found to inhibit the number of esophageal tumors in NMBA-treated animals by 24-56% relative to NMBA controls. Black raspberries and strawberries were also tested in a post initiation scheme and were found to inhibit NMBA-induced esophageal tumorigenesis by 31-64% when administered in the diet following treatment of the animals with NMBA. Berries, therefore, inhibit tumor promotion and progression events as well as tumor initiation."

Anti-angiogenic, antioxidant, and anti-carcinogenic properties of a novel anthocyanin-rich berry extract formula. Bagchi D, Sen CK, Bagchi M, Atalay M. Biochemistry. 2004 Jan;69(1):75-80. **Key Finding:** "Six berry extracts (wild blueberry, bilberry, cranberry, elderberry, raspberry seeds and strawberry) were studied for antioxidant efficacy, cytotoxic potential, cellular uptake, and anti-angiogenic (the ability to reduce unwanted growth of blood vessels, which can lead to varicose veins and tumor formation) properties. We evaluated various combinations of edible berry extracts and developed a synergistic formula, OptiBerry IH141, which exhibited high ORAC (Oxygen-Radical Absorbing Capacity) value, low cytotoxicity, and superior anti-angiogenic properties compared to the other combinations tested. Anti-angiogenic approaches to treat cancer represent a priority area in vascular tumor biology. OptiBerry significantly inhibited both H202- and TNF-alpha-induced VEGF (Vascular Endothelial Growth Factor) expression by human keratinocytes. VEGF is a key regulator of tumor angiogenesis. Madrigal assay using human micro vascular endothelial cells showed that OptiBerry impaired angiogenesis. Endothelium cells pretreated with OptiBerry showed a diminished ability to form hemangioma and markedly decreased **tumor** growth by more than 50%."

Antimutagenic activity of berry extracts. Hope Smith S, Tate PL, Huang G, Magee JB, Meepagala KM, Wedge DE, Larcom LL. J Med Food. 2004 Winter;7(4):450-5. **Key Finding:** "Identification of phytochemicals useful in dietary prevention and intervention of **cancer** is of paramount important. Juice from strawberry, blueberry, and raspberry fruit significantly inhibited **mutagenesis** caused by both carcinogens tested (methyl methanessulfonate and benzo{a}pyrene). Ethanol extracts from freeze-dried fruits of strawberry cultivars (Sweet Charlie and Carlsbad) and blueberry cultivars (Tifblue and Premier) were also tested. Of these, the hydrolysable tannin-containing fraction from Sweet Charlie strawberries was most effective at inhibiting mutations."

Anti-angiogenic property of edible berries. Roy S, Khanna S, Alessio HM, Vider J, Bagchi D, Bagchi M, Sen CK. Free Radic Res. 2002 Sep;36(9):1023-31. **Key Finding:** "Anti-angiogenic approaches to prevent and treat **cancer** represent a priority area in investigative tumor biology. Vascular endothelial growth factor

(VEGF) plays a crucial role for the vascularization of tumors. We sought to test the effects of multiple berry extracts on inducible VEGF expression by human HaCaT keratinocytes. Six berries extract (wild blueberry, bilberry, cranberry, elderberry, raspberry seed, and strawberry) and a grape seed proanthocyanidin extract (GSPE) were studied. Antioxidant activity of the extracts was determined by ORAC. The ORAC values of strawberry powder and GSPE were higher than cranberry, elderberry, or raspberry seed but significantly lower than the other samples studied. Wild bilberry and blueberry extracts possessed the highest ORAC values. Each of the berry samples studied significantly inhibited both H202 as well as TNF alpha induced VEGF expression by the human keratinocytes. Madrigal assay using human dermal micro vascular endothelial cells showed that edible berries impair angiogenesis."

*Anticarcinogenic Activity of Strawberry, Blueberry, and Raspberry Extracts to **Breast and Cervical Cancer** Cells.* Wedge DE, Meepagala KM, Magee JB, Smith SH, Huang G, Larcom LL. J Med Food. 2001 Spring;4(1):49-51. **Key Finding:** "Freeze-dried fruits of two strawberry cultivars, Sweet Charlie and Carlsbad, and two blueberry cultivars, Tifblue and Premier, were sequentially extracted and tested separately for in vitro anticancer activity on cervical and breast cancer cell lines. Ethanol extracts from all four fruits strongly inhibited CaSki and SiHa cervical cancer cell lines and MCF-7 and T47-D breast cancer cell lines. An unfractionated aqueous extract of raspberry and the ethanol extract of Premier blueberry significantly inhibited mutagenesis by both direct-acting and metabolically activated carcinogens."

Cardiovascular Disease

Recent trends and advances in berry health benefits research. Seeram NP. J Agric Food Chem. 2010 Apr 14;58(7):3869-70: **Key Finding**: "Recent advances have been made in our scientific understanding of how berries promote human health and prevent chronic illnesses such as some **cancers, heart disease, and neurodegenerative diseases.** Berry bio actives encompass a wide diversity of phytochemicals."

Berries modify the postprandial plasma glucose response to sucrose in healthy subjects. Torronen R, Sarkkinen E, Tapola N, Hautaniemi E, Kilpi K, Niskanen L. Br J Nutr. 2009 Nov 24;1-4. (Epub ahead of print). **Key Finding:** "Sucrose increases postprandial blood glucose concentrations, and diets with a high glycemic response may be associated with increased risk of **obesity, type 2 diabetes** and **cardiovas-**

cular disease. These results show that berries rich in polyphenols decrease the postprandial glucose response of sucrose in healthy subjects."

Cognition

Recent trends and advances in berry health benefits research. Seeram NP. J Agric Food Chem. 2010 Apr 14;58(7):3869-70: **Key Finding**: "Recent advances have been made in our scientific understanding of how berries promote human health and prevent chronic illnesses such as some **cancers, heart disease, and neuro-degenerative diseases.** Berry bio actives encompass a wide diversity of phytochemicals."

*Recent advances in berry supplementation and **age-related cognitive decline.*** Willis LM. Shukitt-Hale B. Joseph JA. Curr Opin Clin Nutr Metab Care. 2009 Jan;12(1):91-4. **Key Finding:** "Antioxidant-rich berries consumed in the diet can positively impact learning and memory in the aged animal. This effect on cognition is thought to be due to the direct interaction of berry polyphenols with aging neurons, reducing the impact of stress-related cellular signals and increasing the capacity of neurons to maintain proper functioning during aging."

*Effects of blackberries on **motor and cognitive function** in aged rats.* Shukitt-Hale B, Cheng V, Joseph JA. Nutr Neurosci. 2009 Jun;12(3):135-40. **Key Finding:** "Results for the Morris water maze showed that the blackberry-fed rats had significantly greater working, or short-term, memory performance than the control rats."

Behavioral and genoprotective effects of Vaccinium berries intake in mice. Barros D, Amaral OB, Izquierdo I, Geracitano L, do Carmo Bassol Raseira M, Henriques AT, Ramirez MR. Pharmacol Biochem Behav. 2006 Jun;84(2):229-34. **Key Finding:** "These results suggest that supplementation with V. ashei berries to mice improves performance on memory tasks and has a protective effect on DNA damage, possibly due to the antioxidant activity of polyphenols, including anthocyanins."

Diabetes

Berries modify the postprandial plasma glucose response to sucrose in healthy subjects. Torronen R, Sarkkinen E, Tapola N, Hautaniemi E. Kilpi K, Niskanen L. Br J Nutr. 2009 Nov 24;1-4. (Epub ahead of print). **Key Finding:** "Sucrose increases postprandial blood glucose concentrations, and diets with a high glycemic response may be associated with increased risk of **obesity, type 2 diabetes** and **cardiovascular disease.** These results show that berries rich in polyphenols decrease the postprandial glucose response of sucrose in healthy subjects."

Erectile dysfunction

*Oxidative stress in arteriogenic **erectile dysfunction***: *prophylactic role of antioxidants.* Azadzoi KM, Schulman RN, Aviram M, Siroky MB. J Urol. 2005 Jul;174(1):386-93. **Key Finding:** "Arteriogenic erectile dysfunction accumulates oxidative products in erectile tissue, possibly via an intrinsic mechanism. Oxidative stress may be of great important in the pathophysiology of arteriogenic ED. Antioxidant therapy may be a useful prophylactic tool for preventing smooth muscle dysfunction and birosis in ED."

Hypercholesteremia

*Efficiency of pharmacologically-active antioxidant phytomedicine Radical Fruits in treatment **hypercholesteremia** in men.* Abidov M, Jimenez Del Rio M, Ramazanov A, Kalyuzhin O, Chkhikvishvili I. Georgian Med News. 2006 Nov;(140):78-83. **Key Finding:** "Radical Fruits is a dietary supplement that contains standardized extracts and concentrates of prune, pomegranate, apple, grape, raspberry, blueberry, white cherry and strawberry. Forty-four non-obese, non-smoking, non-diabetic hypercholesteremic male volunteers took part in a 4 week double-blind, randomized, placebo-controlled clinical trial. Administration of pharmacologically active antioxidant supplement Radical Fruit in hypercholesteremic men significantly increased plasma HDL and reduced total cholesterol and LDL, and urinary oxidative and inflammatory isoprostanes and thromboxane."

HIV

*Anti-stress, anti-**HIV** and vitamin C-synergized radical scavenging activity of mulberry juice fractions.* Sakagami H, Asano K, Satoh K, Takahashi K, Kobayashi M, Koga N, Takahashi H, Tachikawa R, Tashiro T, Hasegawa A, Kurihara K, Ikarashi T, Kanamoto T, Terakubo S, Nakashima H, Watanabe S, Nakamura W. In Vivo. 2007 May-Jun;21(3):499-505. **Key Finding:** "Anti-stress and anti-HIV activity of mulberry juice were separated by centrifugation. The kinetic study revealed that the anti-stress activity was maintained for 4 hours after cessation of the administration of mulberry juice. The lignin fraction in the precipitate fraction scavenged superoxide and hydroxyl radicals more efficiently than other fractions, in a synergistic fashion with sodium ascorbate. Anti-HIV activity of mulberry juice was concentrated in the lignin fraction, whereas blueberry juice, which has not precipitating fibrous materials, did not show anti-HIV activity. The present study suggests the functionality of mulberry juice as an alternative medicine."

Intestinal Pathogens

*Berry phenolics selectively inhibit the growth of **intestinal pathogens**.* Puupponen-Pimia R, Nohynek L, Hartmann-Schmidlin S, Kahkonen M, Heinonen M, Maatta-Riihinen K, Oksman-Caldentey KM. J Appl Microbiol. 2005;98(4):991-1000. **Key Finding:** "Berries and their phenolics selectively inhibit the growth of human pathogenic bacteria. Cloudberry and raspberry were the best inhibitors, and Staphylococcus and Salmonella the most sensitive bacteria."

Bioactive berry compounds—novel tools against human pathogens. Puuuponen-Pimia R, Nohynek L, Alakomi HL, Oksman-Caldentey KM. Appl Microbiol Biotechnol. 2005 Apr;67(1):8-18. **Key Finding:** "Among different berries and berry phenolics, cranberry, cloudberry, raspberry, strawberry and bilberry especially possess clear antimicrobial effects against, e.g. **Salmonella** and **Staphylococcus**. Complex phenolic polymers, like ellagitannins, are strong antibacterial agents present in cloudberry and raspberry."

*Gastro protective effect of red pigments in black chokeberry fruit (Aronia melanocarpa Elliot) on acute **gastric hemorrhagic** lesions in rats.* Matsumoto M, Hara H, Chiji H, Kasai T. J Agric Food Chem. 2004 Apr 21;52(8):2226-9. **Key Finding:** "The black chokeberry extract and its hydro lysate administered at 2 b/kg of body weight each had nearly the same protective effect as quercetin administered at 100 mg/kg of body weight in suppressing the area of gastric mucosal damage cause by the subsequent application of ethanol to <30% compared to the control group. The black chokeberry red pigment fraction had a similarly significant protective effect on gastric mucosa in a dose-dependent manner when administered at 30-300 mg/kg of body weight, and the administration of 30 mg/kg of body weight could suppress ethanol-induced gastric mucosal damage by approximately 50% (ID(50)=30 mg/kg of body weight)."

*Inhibition of **Heliobacter pylori** in vitro by various berry extracts, with enhanced susceptibility to clarithromycin.* Chatterjee A, Yasmin T, Bagchi D, Stohs SJ. Mol Cell Biochem. 2004 Oct;265(1-2):19-26. **Key Finding:** "Extracts of six berries – raspberry, strawberry, cranberry, elderberry, blueberry, bilberry and OptiBerry, a blend of the six berries, were exposed to Pylori culture strain 49503. All berry extracts significantly (p<0.05) inhibited Pylori, compared with controls, and also increased susceptibility of H.pylori to clarithromycin, with OptiBerry demonstrating maximal effects."

Obesity

Berries modify the postprandial plasma glucose response to sucrose in healthy subjects. Torronen R, Sarkkinen E, Tapola N, Hautaniemi E, Kilpi K, Niskanen L. Br J Nutr. 2009 Nov 24;1-4. (Epub ahead of print). **Key Finding:** "Sucrose increases postprandial blood glucose concentrations, and diets with a high glycemic response may be associated with increased risk of **obesity, type 2 diabetes** and **cardiovascular disease.** These results show that berries rich in polyphenols decrease the postprandial glucose response of sucrose in healthy subjects."

Ulcers

Berry anthocyanins as novel antioxidants in human health and disease prevention. Zafra-Stone S, Yasmin T, Bagchi M, Chatterjee A, Vinson JA, Bagchi D. Mol Nutr Food Res. 2007 Jun;51(6):675-83. **Key Finding:** "A novel combination of selected berry extracts known as OptiBerry contains wild blueberry, wild bilberry, cranberry, elderberry, raspberry seeds, and strawberry. Recent studies in our laboratory have demonstrated that OptiBerry exhibits high antioxidant efficacy as shown by its high oxygen radical absorbance capacity values, novel antiangiogenic and **antiatherosclerotic** activities, and potential cytotoxicity towards Helicobacter pylori, a noxious pathogen responsible for various gastrointestinal disorders including **duodenal ulcer** and **gastric cancer**, as compared to individual berry extracts. OptiBerry also significantly inhibited basal MCP-1 and inducible NF-kappa beta transcriptions as well as the inflammatory biomarker IL-8, and significantly reduced the ability to form hemangioma and markedly decreased EOMA cell-induced tumor growth in anin vivo model."

Vascular disease

Direct vasoactive and vasoprotective properties of anthocyanin-rich extracts. Bell DR, Gochenaur K. J Appl Physiol. 2006 Apr;100(4):1164-70. **Key Finding:** "Anthocyanin-enhanced extracts from chokeberry, bilberry or elderberry produce endothelium-dependent relaxation in porcine coronary arteries. Extract concentrations too low to directly alter coronary vascular tone protect coronary arteries from reactive oxygen species without altering vasorelaxation to endogenous or exogenous NO. These results suggest that such extracts could have significant beneficial effects in **vascular disease**."

Blackberries (see Berries)

Blueberries

WHILE MANY SPECIES OF WILD BLUEBERRY ARE FOUND WORLDWIDE, most of the common species originated in North America. The state of Maine is currently the largest producer of blueberries.

Blueberries are a good source of nearly two dozen vitamins and minerals, with one cup containing 36 percent of the USDA daily recommended allowance of vitamin K for adults and 25 percent of the recommended manganese. Some species contain the phytochemical resveratrol in amounts equal to grapes. Studies have documented a wide range of health benefits from blueberry consumption, including alleviating cognitive decline from aging and disease, lowering cholesterol and blood pressure, and helping reduce the risk of diabetes and several forms of cancer.

Aging

NT-020, a natural therapeutic approach to optimize spatial memory performance and increase neural progenitor cell proliferation and decrease inflammation in the aged rat. Acosta S, Jemberg J, Sanberg CD, Et al. Rejuvenation Res. 2010 Oct;13(5):581-8. **Key Finding**: "The process of **aging** is linked to oxidative stress, microglial activation, and proinflammatory factors which are known to decrease cell proliferation and limit neuroplasticity. We have shown that natural compounds such as polyphenols from blueberry and green tea and amino acids like carnosine are high in antioxidant and anti-inflammatory activity that decreases the damaging effects of reactive oxygen species in the blood, brain and other tissues of the body."

Age-related toxicity of amyloid-beta associated with increased pERK and pCREB in primary hippocampal neurons: reversal by blueberry extract. Brewer GJ, Torricelli JR, Lindsey AL, Et al. J Nutr Biochem. 2010 Oct;21(10):991-8. **Key Finding**: "These results suggest that the beneficial effects of blueberry extract may involve transient stress signaling and ROS protection that may translate into improved **cognition** in aging rats and APP/PS1 mice given blueberry extract."

Blueberry supplementation attenuates microglial activation in hippocampal intraocular grafts to aged hosts. Willis LM, Freeman L, Bickford PC, Et al. Glia. 2010 Apr 15;58(6):679-90. **Key Finding**: "These studies demonstrate direct effects of blueberry upon microglial activation both during isolated conditions and in the aged host brain and suggest that this nutraceutical can attenuate **age-induced inflammation**."

Grape juice berries, and walnuts affect **brain aging** *and behavior.* Joseph JA, Shukitt-Hale B, Willism LM. J Nutr. 2009 Sep;139(9):1813S-7S. **Key Finding:** "Research from our laboratory has suggested that dietary supplementation with fruit or vegetable extracts high in antioxidants (e.g. blueberries, strawberries, walnuts and Concord grape juice) can decrease the enhanced vulnerability to oxidative stress that occurs in aging and these reductions are expressed as improvements in behavior. Collaborative findings indicate that blueberry or Concord grape juice supplementation in humans with mild **cognitive impairment** increased verbal memory performance, thus translating our animal findings to humans."

Age-related toxicity of amyloid-beta associated with increased pERK and pCREB in primary hippocampal neurons: reversal by blueberry extract. Brewer GJ, Torricelli JR, Lindsey AL, Kunz EZ, Neuman A, Fisher DR, Joseph JA. J Nutr Biochem. 2009 Nov 30. (Epub ahead of print). **Key Finding:** "We conclude that the increased age-related susceptibility of **old-age neurons** to abeta toxicity may be due to higher levels of activation of pERK and pCREB pathways that can be protected by blueberry extract through inhibition of both these pathways through an ROS stress response. These results suggest that the beneficial effects of blueberry extract may involve transient stress signaling and ROS protection that may translate into improved **cognition.**"

Blueberry-enriched diet ameliorates age-related declines in NMDA receptor-dependent LTP. Coultrap SJ, Bickford PC, Browning MD. Age (Dordr). 2008 Dec;30(4):263-72. **Key Finding:** "Supplementation of the diet with blueberry extract elevated long-term potentiation in the hippocampus (63%) in aged animals to levels seen in young. The normalization of LTP may be due to the blueberry diet preventing a decline in synaptic strength. This report provides evidence that dietary alterations later in life may prevent or postpone the **cognitive declines** associated with **aging.**"

Cranberry and blueberry: evidence for protective effects against **cancer** *and* **vascular diseases**. Neto CC. Mol Nutr Food Res. 2007 Jun;51(6):652-64. **Key Finding:** "Growing evidence from tissue culture, animal, and clinical models suggests that the flavonoid-rich fruits of the North American cranberry and blueberry have the potential ability to limit the development and severity of certain cancers and vascular diseases including **atherosclerosis**, **ischemic stroke**, and neurodegenerative **diseases of aging.**"

Beneficial effects of fruit extracts on neuronal function and behavior in a rodent model of accelerated **aging**. Shukitt-Hale B, Carey AN, Jenkins D, Rabin BM, Joseph JA. Neurobiol Aging. 2007 Aug;28(8):1187-94. **Key Finding:** "Previous research has shown that diets supplemented with 2% blueberry or strawberry extracts have the ability to retard and even reverse age-related deficits in behavior and signal transduction in rats. This study evaluated the efficacy of these diets on irradiation-induced deficits in these parameters by maintaining rats on these diets or a control diet from 8 weeks prior to being exposed to whole-body irradiation. The strawberry diet offered better protection against spatial deficits in the maze because strawberry-fed animals were better able to retain place information compared to controls. The blueberry diet, on the other hand, seemed to improve reversal learning, a behavior more dependent on intact striatal function."

Dopamine and Abeta-induced stress signaling and decrements in Ca2+ buffering in primary neonatal hippocampal cells are antagonized by blueberry extract. Joseph JA, Carey A, Brewer GJ, Lau FC, Fisher DR. J Alzheimers Dis. 2007 Jul;11(4):433-46. **Key Finding:** "It appears that at least part of the protective effect of blueberries may involve alterations in stress signaling. Analyses indicated that blueberries may be exerting their protective effects in the hippocampal cells by altering levels of phosphorylated MAPK, PKCgamme, and phosphorylated CREB. We have shown previously that dietary blueberry extract supplementation reverse several parameters of **neuronal** and behavioral **aging** in rodents."

Blueberry supplemented diet reverses age-related decline in hippocampal HSP70 neuroprotection. Galli RL, Bielinski DF, Szprengiel A, Shukitt-Hale B, Josephy JA. Neurobiol Aging. 2006 Feb;27(2):344-50. **Key Finding:** "It appeared that the blueberry diet completely restored the HSP70 response to in vitro inflammatory challenge in the old rats at the 90 and 240 min times. This suggests that a short-term blueberry intervention may result in improved HSP70-mediated protection against a number of **neurodegenerative** processes in the brain."

The effects of antioxidants in the senescent auditory cortex. De Rivera C, Shukitt-Hale B, Joseph JA, Mendelson JR. Neurobiol Aging. 2006 Jul;27(7):1035-44. **Key Finding:** "Results showed that most cells recorded from the blueberry-fed rats responded most vigorously to fast frequency modulated sweeps, similar to that observed in young rats. These results suggest that **age-related changes** in temporal processing speed in A1 may be reversed by dietary supplementation of blueberry phytochemicals."

Blueberry polyphenols increase lifespan and thermotolerance in Caenorhabditis elegans. Wilson MA, Shukitt-Hale B, Kalt W, Ingram DK, Joseph JA, Wolkow CA. Aging Cell. 2006 Feb;5(1):59-68. **Key Finding:** "We report that a complex mixture of blueberry polyphenols increased lifespan and slowed **aging**-related declines in C. elegans. We also found that these benefits did not just reflect antioxidant activity in these compounds."

Dietary supplementation with blueberries, spinach, or spirulina reduces ischemic brain damage. Wang Y, Chang CF, Chou J, Chen HL, Deng X, Harvey BK, Cadet JL, Bickford PC. Exp Neurol. 2005 May;193(1):75-84. **Key Finding:** "Free radicals are involved in neurodegenerative disorders, such as **ischemia** and **aging**. We have previously demonstrated that treatment with diets enriched with blueberry, spinach, or spirulina have been shown to reduce neurodegenerative changes in aged animals. The purpose of this study was to determine if these diets have neuroprotective effects in focal ischemic brain in Sprague-Dawley rats. Animals treated with blueberry, spinach, or spirulina had significantly lower caspase-3 activity in the ischemic hemisphere. In conclusion, our data suggest that chronic treatment with blueberry, spinach, or spirulina reduces ischemia/reperfusion-induced apoptosis and cerebral infarction."

*Oxidative stress protection and vulnerability in **aging**: putative nutritional implications for intervention.* Joseph JA, Denisova NA, Bielinski D, Fisher DR, Shukitt-Hale B. Mech Ageing Dev. 2000 Jul 31;116(2-3):141-53. **Key Finding:** "Among the most effective agents that antagonized cellular oxidative stress were the combination of polyphenols found in fruits (e.g. blueberry extract) with high antioxidant activity. Subsequent experiments using dietary supplementation with fruit (strawberry) or vegetable (spinach) extracts have shown that such extracts are also effective in forestalling and reversing the deleterious effects of behavioral aging in F344 rats."

*The beneficial effects of fruit polyphenols on **brain aging**.* Lau FC, Shukitt-Hale B, Joseph JA. Neurobiol Aging. 2005 Dec;26 Suppl 1:128-32. **Key Finding:** "Research from our laboratory has shown that nutritional antioxidants, such as the polyphenols found in blueberries, can reverse age-related declines in neuronal signal transduction as well as cognitive and motor deficits. Furthermore, we have shown that short-term blueberry supplementation increases hippocampal plasticity."

*Reversals of age-related declines in neuronal signal transduction, **cognitive**, and **motor behavioral deficits** with blueberry, spinach, or strawberry dietary supplementation.* Joseph JA, Shukitt-Hale B, Denisvoa NA, Bielinski D, Martin A, McEwen JJ, Bickford PC. J Neurosci. 1999 Sep 15;19(18):8114-21. **Key Finding:** "Our previous study had shown that rats given dietary supplements of fruits and vegetable extracts with high antioxidant activity for 8 months beginning at 6 months of age retarded age-related declines in neuronal and cognitive function. The present study showed that such supplements (strawberry, spinach or blueberry) fed for 8 weeks to 19-month-old Fischer 344 rats were also effective in reversing age-related deficits in several ne enough data to recommend the consumption of isoflavone supplements to lower plasma uronal and behavioral parameters. These findings suggest that, in addition to their known beneficial effects on **cancer** and **heart disease,** phytochemicals present in antioxidant-rich foods may be beneficial in reversing the course of neuronal and behavioral **aging.**"

*Membrane and receptor modifications of oxidative stress vulnerability in **aging**. Nutritional considerations.* Joseph JA, Denisova N, Fisher D, Shukitt-Hale B, Bickford P, Prior R, Cao G. Ann N Y Acad Sci. 1998 Nov 20;854:268-76. **Key Finding:** "Evidence suggests that oxidative stress may contribute to the pathogenesis of age-related decrements in **neuronal function** and that OS vulnerability increases as a function of age. In studies attempts have been made to determine whether increased OS protection via nutritional increases in antioxidant levels in rats (strawberry extracts, dried aqueous extract, spinach, or blueberry extracts) would protect against exposure to 100% O2 (a model of accelerated neuronal aging.) Results indicated that these diets were effective in preventing OS-induced decrements in several parameters, suggesting that although there maybe increases in OS vulnerability in aging, phytochemicals present in antioxidant-rich foods may be beneficial in reducing or retarding the functional central nervous system deficits seen in aging or oxidative insult."

Alzheimer's disease

Blueberry opposes beta-amyloid peptide-induced microglial activation via inhibition of p44/42 mitogen-activation protein kinase. Zhu Y, Bickford PC, Sanberg P, Giunta B, Tan J. Rejuvenation Res. 2008 Oct;11(5):891-901. **Key Finding:** "The aggregation of amyloid-beta(a beta) into fibrillar amyloid plaques is a key pathological event in the development of **Alzheimer's disease**. Microglial proinflammatory activation is widely known to cause neuronal and synaptic damage that correlates with cognitive impairment in Alzheimer's disease. We found that blueberries significantly enhances microglial clearance of A beta, inhibits aggregation of A beta and suppresses microglial activation, all via suppression of the p44/42 MAPK module. Thus, these data may explain the previously observed behavior recovery in PSAPP mice given blueberry supplementation."

Effect of lyophilized Vaccinium berries on memory, anxiety and locomotion in adult rats. Ramirez MR, Izquierdo I, do Carmo Bassols Raseira M, Zuanazzi JA, Barros D, Henriques AT. Pharmacol Res. 2005 Dec;52(6):457-62. **Key Finding:** "The present study showed that lyophilized berries significantly enhanced short-term memory, but not long-term memory in the inhibitory avoidance task. These results suggest that lyophilized berries may be beneficial in the prevention of memory deficits, one of the symptoms related to **Alzheimer's disease** and corroborate previous findings showing that flavonoids present effects in several learning paradigms."

Antioxidation

*Antioxidant levels of common fruits, vegetables, and juices versus protective activity against in vitro **ischemia/reperfusion**.* Bean H, Schuler C, Leggett RE, Levin RM. Int Urol Nephrol. 2009 Sep 19. (Epub ahead of print). **Key Finding:** "An assay was utilized to determine the antioxidant reactivity of a series of fruits, vegetables, and juices, and the results were compared to the protective ability of selected juices in an established in vitro rabbit bladder model of ischemia/reperfusion. The results showed that cranberry juice had the highest level of antioxidant reactivity, blueberry juice had an intermediate activity, and orange juice had the lowest. It was determined, however, that contrary to the hypothesis, the orange juice was significantly more potent in protecting the bladder against ischemia/reperfusion damage than either blueberry or cranberry juice."

*Oxidative stress modulation using polyphenol-rich blueberries: application on a human **retinal cell** model.* Dutot M, Rambaux L, Warnet JM, Rat P. J Fr Ophtalmol (French). 2008 Dec;31(10):975-80. **Key Finding:** "Blueberry protected cells against tBHP-induced cytotoxicity. It increased cell viability, decreased oxidative stress and mitochondrial apoptosis. After a 24-hour pre-incubation time, blueberry totally inhibited tBHP-induced cytotoxicity. Blueberry seems to be a potent antioxidant and could be easily added to food complements to prevent or limit ocular pathologies induced by oxidative stress."

*Prevention of **oxidative DNA damage** by bioactive berry components.* Aiyer HS, Kichambare S, Gupta RC. Nutr Cancer. 2008;60 Suppl 1:36-42. **Key Finding:** "The hormone 17ss-estradiol (E(2)) causes oxidative DNA damage via redox cycling of its metabolites. In this study, ACI rats were fed either AIN-93M diet or diets supplemented with 0.5% each of mixed berries (strawberry, blueberry, blackberry, and red and black raspberry), blueberry along or ellagic acid. Ellagic acid (EA) diet significantly reduced E(2)-induced levels of 8-oxodG. Blueberry alone also significantly reduced the levels. Mixed berries were ineffective. In addition, aqueous extracts of berries (2%) and EA (100 microM) were tested for their efficacy in diminishing oxidative DNA adducts induced by redox cycling of 4E(2) catalyzed by copper chloride in vitro. EA was the most efficacious (90%) followed by extracts of red raspberry (70%), blueberry and strawberry (50% each; P<0.001)."

Cellular antioxidant activity of common fruits. Wolfe KL, Kang X, He X, Dong M, Zhang Q, Liu RH. J Agric Food Chem. 2008 Sep 24;56(18):8418-26. **Key Finding:** "The objective of this study was to determine the cellular antioxidant activity, total phenolic contents, and oxygen radical absorbance capacity values of 25 fruits commonly consumed in the United States. Pomegranate and berries (wild blueberry, blackberry, raspberry, and blueberry) had the highest cellular antioxidant activity, whereas banana and melons had the lowest. Apple and strawberries were the biggest suppliers of cellular antioxidant activity to the American diet. Increasing fruit consumption is a logical strategy to increase antioxidant intake and decrease oxidative stress and may lead to reduced risk of **cancer.**"

Prevention of **oxidative DNA damage** *by bioactive berry components.* Aiyer HS, Kichambare S, Gupta RC. Nutr Cancer. 2008;60 Suppl 1:36-42. **Key Finding:** "In this study, ACI rats (8 wk old) were fed either AIN-93M diet or diets supplemented with 0.5% each of mixed berries (strawberry, blueberry, blackberry, and red and black raspberry), blueberry alone, or ellagic acid. Ellagic acid diet significantly reduced E(2)-induced levels of 8-oxodG, P-1, P-2, and PL-1 by 79, 63, 44, and 67% respectively. Blueberry diet also significantly reduced the levels of P-1, P-2, and PL-1 subgroups by 77, 43, and 68% respectively. Mixed berries were, however, ineffective. In addition, aqueous extracts of berries and EA were tested for their efficacy in diminishing oxidative DNA adducts induced by redox cycling of 4E(2) catalyzed by copper chloride in vitro. Ellagic acid was the most efficacious (90%) followed by extracts of red raspberry (70%), blueberry, and strawberry (50% each)."

Impact of multiple genetic polymorphisms on effects of a 4-week blueberry juice intervention on ex vivo induced lymphocytic **DNA damage** *in human volunteers.* Wilms LC, Boots AW, De Boer VC, Maas LM, Pachen DM, Gottschalk RW, Ketelslegers HB, Haenen GR, Van Schooten FJ, Kleinjans JC. Carcinogenesis. 2007 Aug;28(8):1800-6. **Key Finding:** "In the present study, 168 healthy volunteers consumed a blueberry/apple juice that provided 97 mg quercetin and 16 mg ascorbic acid a day. After a 4-week intervention period, plasma concentrations of quercetin and ascorbic acid and trolox equivalent antioxidant capacity were significantly increased. Further, we found 20% protection against ex vivo H(2)O(2)-provoked oxidative DNA damage, measured by comet assay. Statistical analysis of 34 biologically relevant genetic polymorphisms revealed that six significantly influenced the outcome of the intervention."

*Endotoxin- and D-galactosamine-induced **liver injury** improved by the administration of Lactobacillus, Bifidobacterium and blueberry.* Osman N, Adawi D, Ahrne S, Jeppsson B, Molin G. Dig Liver Dis. 2007 Sep;39(9):849-56. **Key Finding:** "Blueberry and probiotics exert protective effects on acute liver injury. They reduce the hepatocytes injury, the inflammation and the pro-inflammatory cytokines, and improve the barrier functions and antioxidant activity."

Dopamine-induced stress signaling in COS-7 cells transfected with selectively vulnerable muscarinic receptor subtypes is partially mediated via the i3 loop and antagonized by blueberry extract. Joseph JA, Fisher DR, Carey AN, Bielinski DF. J Alzheimers Dis. 2006 Dec;10(4):423-37. **Key Finding:** "Results indicated that blueberry reduced oxidative stress sensitivity in response to dopamine in M1-transfected cells. Blueberries were also effective in preventing these Ca2+ buffering deficits in cells transfected with M1 receptors in which the i3 loop had been removed, but only partially enhanced the protect effects of the M3 i3 loop in the M1(M3i3) chimeric. It appears that antioxidants found in blueberries might be targeting additional sites on these chimeric to decrease oxidative stress sensitivity."

Protection by quercetin and quercetin-rich fruit juice against induction of oxidative DNA damage and formation of BPDE-DNA adducts in human lymphocytes. Wilms LC, Hollman PC, Boots AW, Kleinjans JC. Mutat Res. 2005 Apr 4;582(1-2):155-62. **Key Finding:** "Lymphocytes from female volunteers who consumed a quercetin-rich blueberry/apple juice mixture for four weeks were treated ex vivo with an effective dose of H(2)O(2) and benzo(a)pyrene, respectively, at three different time points during the intervention. Results in vitro; a significant dose-dependent protection by quercetin against both the formation of **oxidative DNA damage** and of BPDE-DNA adducts was observed. Results in vivo; four weeks of juice intervention led to a significant increase in the total antioxidant capacity of plasma. The combination of our findings in vitro and ex vivo provides evidence that quercetin is able to protect against chemically induced DNA damage in human lymphocytes, which may underlie its suggested anticarcinogenic properties."

Berry phenolics and their antioxidant activity. Kahkonen MP, Hopia AI, Heinonen M. J Agric Food Chem. 2001 Aug;49(8):4076-82. **Key Finding:** "Phenolic profiles of a total of 26 berry samples, together with 2 apple samples, were analyzed without hydrolysis of glycosides with HPLC. The phenolic contents among different berry genera varied considerably. Anthocyanin was the main phenolic constituents in bilberry, bog whortleberry, and cranberry, but in cowberries, belonging also to the family Ericaceae genus Vaccinium, flavanols and procyanidins predominated. In the family Rosacea genus Rubus (cloudberry and red raspberry) the main phenolic found were ellagitannins, and in genus Fragaria (strawberry) ellagitannins were the second largest group after anthocyanins."

*Oxidative stress protection and vulnerability in **aging:** putative nutritional implications for intervention.* Joseph JA, Denisova NA, Bielinski D, Fisher DR, Shukitt-Hale B. Mech Ageing Dev. 2000 Jul 31;116(2-3):141-53. **Key Finding:** "Among the most effective agents that antagonized cellular oxidative stress were the combination of polyphenols found in fruits (e.g. blueberry extract) with high antioxidant activity. Subsequent experiments using dietary supplementation with fruit (strawberry) or vegetable (spinach) extracts have shown that such extracts are also effective in forestalling and reversing the deleterious effects of behavioral aging in F344 rats."

Polyphenols enhance red blood cell resistance to oxidative stress: in vitro and in vivo. Youdim KA, Shukitt-Hale B, MacKinnon S, Kalt W, Joseph JA. Biochem Biophys Acta. 2000 Sep 1;1523(1):117-22. **Key Finding:** "In this study we investigated the potential antioxidant properties of blueberry polyphenols in vitro and vivo using red blood cell resistance to reactive oxygen species as the model. In vitro incubation with anthocyanins or hydroxycinnamic acids was found to enhance significantly red blood cell resistance to H_2O_2 induced ROS production. This protection was also observed in vivo following oral supplementation to rats at 100 mg/ml. However, only anthocyanin was found to afford protection at a significant level, this at 6 and 24 h post supplementation."

Atherosclerosis

Dietary blueberries attenuate atherosclerosis in Apo lipoprotein E-deficient mice by up regulating antioxidant enzyme expression. Wu X, Kang J, Xie C, Et al. J Nutr. 2010 Sep;140(9):1628-32. **Key Finding**: "These results suggest a protective effectiveness of blueberry against **atherosclerosis** in this mouse model. The potential mechanisms may involve reduction in oxidative stress by both inhibition of lipid peroxidation and enhancement of antioxidant defense."

Cranberry and blueberry: evidence for protective effects against **cancer** *and* **vascular diseases**. Neto CC. Mol Nutr Food Res. 2007 Jun;51(6):652-64. **Key Finding:** "Growing evidence from tissue culture, animal, and clinical models suggests that the flavonoid-rich fruits of the North American cranberry and blueberry have the potential ability to limit the development and severity of certain cancers and vascular diseases including **atherosclerosis**, **ischemic stroke**, and neurodegenerative **diseases of aging**."

Cancer (breast; cervical; colon; leukemia)

Dietary intake of pterostilbene, a constituent of blueberries, inhibits the beta-catenin/p65 downstream signaling pathway and **colon carcinogenesis** *in rats.* Paul S, DeCastro AJ, Lee HJ, Smolarek AK, So JY, Simi B, Wang CX, Zhou R, Rimando AM, Suh N. Carcinogenesis. 2010 Jul;31(7):1272-8. **Key Finding:** "Our data with pterostilbene in suppressing colon tumorigenesis, cell proliferation as well as key inflammatory markers in vivo and in vitro suggest the potential use of pterostilbene for colon cancer prevention."

Blueberry phytochemicals inhibit growth and metastatic potential of MDA-MB-231 **breast cancer** *cells through modulation of the phosphatidylinositol 3-kinase pathway.* Adams LS, Phung S, Yee N, Seeram NP, Li L, Chen S. Cancer Res. 2010 May 1;70(9):3594-605. **Key Finding:** Blueberry phytochemicals have an inhibitory effect on the growth and metastatic potential of MDA-MB-231 breast cancer cell line in blueberry fed mice.

Blueberry anthocyanin and pyruvic acid adducts: anticancer properties in **breast cancer** *cell lines.* Faria A, Pestana D, Teixeira D, Et al. Phytother Res. 2010 Dec;24(12):1862-9. **Key Finding:** "Blueberry anthocyanin and the respective anthocyanin-pyruvic acid adduct demonstrated anticancer properties by inhibiting cancer cell proliferation and by acting as cell anti-invasive factors and chemo inhibitors."

Pterostilbene and tamoxifen show an additive effect against **breast cancer** *in vitro.* Mannal P, McDonald D, McFadden D. Am J Surg. 2010 Nov;200(5):577-80. **Key Finding:** "Pterostilbene is a bioavailable stilbenoid found in blueberries and has been found to inhibit breast cancer growth in vitro. Pterostilbene also shows an additive inhibitory effect on breast cancer cells when combined with tamoxifen, most likely from augmented cancer cell apoptosis."

Oral administration of blueberry inhibits **angiogenic tumor** *growth and enhances survival of mice with endothelial cell neoplasm.* Gordillo G, Fang H, Khanna S, Harper J,

Phillips G, Sen CK. Antiox Redox Signal. 2009 Jan;11(1):47-58. **Key Finding:** "Endothelial cell neoplasms are the most common soft tissue **tumor** in infants. This work provides first evidence demonstrating that blueberry extract can limit tumor formation through antiangiogenic effects and inhibition of JNK and NF-kappaB signaling pathways. Oral administration of blueberry extract represents a potential therapeutic antiangiogenic strategy for treating endothelial cell neoplasms in children."

*Pterostilbene Inhibits **Breast Cancer** In Vitro Through Mitochondrial Depolarization and Induction of Caspase-Dependent Apoptosis.* Alosi JA, McDonald DE, Schneider JS, Privette AR, McFadden DW. J Surg Res. 2009 Aug 18. (Epub ahead of print). **Key Finding:** "Pterostilbene, an analogue of resveratrol found in blueberries, has both antioxidant and antiproliferative properties. Pterostilbene treatment inhibits the growth of breast cancer in vitro through caspase-dependent apoptosis. Further in vitro mechanistic studies and in vivo experiments are warranted to determine its potential for the treatment of breast cancer."

*Pterostilbene Inhibits **Lung Cancer** Through Induction of Apoptosis.* Schnieder JG, Alosi JA, McDonald DE, McFadden DW. J Surg Res. 2009 Jul 21. (Epub ahead of print). **Key Finding:** "We investigated the effects of pterostilbene, an analog of resveratrol found in blueberries, on lung cancer, in vitro. Pterostilbene significantly decreased cell viability in lung cancer cells in a concentration and time-dependent manner. Further in vitro mechanistic studies and in vivo experiments are warranted to determine the potential role for pterostilbene in lung cancer treatment or prevention."

*Dietary berries and ellagic acid diminish estrogen-mediated **mammary tumorigenesis** in ACI rats.* Aiyer HS, Srinivasan C, Gupta RC. Nutr Cancer. 2008;60(2):227-34. **Key Finding:** "We investigated the efficacy of dietary berries and ellagic acid to reduce estrogen-mediated mammary tumorigenesis. Compared with the control group, ellagic acid reduced the tumor volume by 75% and tumor multiplicity by 44%. Black raspberry followed closely with tumor volume diminished by >69% and tumor multiplicity by 37%. Blueberry showed a reduction (40%) only in tumor volume. This is the first report showing the significant efficacy of both ellagic acid and berries in the prevention of solely estrogen-induced mammary tumors."

Cellular antioxidant activity of common fruits. Wolfe KL, Kang X, He X, Dong M, Zhang Q, Liu RH. J Agric Food Chem. 2008 Sep 24;56(18):8418-26. **Key Finding:** "The objective of this study was to determine the cellular antioxidant activity, total phenolic contents, and oxygen radical absorbance capacity values of 25 fruits commonly consumed in the United States. Pomegranate and berries (wild blueberry, blackberry, raspberry, and blueberry) had the highest cellular antioxidant activity, whereas banana and melons had the lowest. Apple and strawberries were the biggest suppliers of cellular antioxidant activity to the American diet. Increasing fruit consumption is a logical strategy to increase antioxidant intake and decrease oxidative stress and may lead to reduced risk of **cancer.**"

Inhibitory effects of various beverages on the sulfoconjugation of 17beta-estradiol in human **colon carcinoma** *Caco-2 cells.* Saruwatari A, Isshiki M, Tamura H. Biol Pharm Bull. 2008 Nov;31(11):2131-6. **Key Finding:** "Among the 35 beverages analyzed, four (aronia, blueberry, coffee and peppermint) exhibited strong inhibitory effects on E2 sulfation within Caco-2 cells IC50 values ranging from 1.9 to 4.4% (v/v). These active beverages also strongly inhibited the cytosolic estrogen SULT activity of Caco-2 cells in vitro (IC50 values ranging from 0.18 to 0.3% (v/v))."

Cranberry and blueberry: evidence for protective effects against **cancer** *and* **vascular diseases**. Neto CC. Mol Nutr Food Res. 2007 Jun;51(6):652-64. **Key Finding:** "Growing evidence from tissue culture, animal, and clinical models suggests that the flavonoid-rich fruits of the North American cranberry and blueberry have the potential ability to limit the development and severity of certain cancers and vascular diseases including **atherosclerosis**, **ischemic stroke**, and neurodegenerative **diseases of aging**."

Inhibition of **cancer** *cell proliferation and suppression of TNF-induced activation of NFkappaB by edible berry juice.* Boivin D, Blanchette M, Barrette S, Moghrabi A, Beliveau R. Anticancer Res. 2007 Mar-Apr;27(2):937-48. **Key Finding:** "These results illustrate that berry juices have striking differences in their potential chemo preventive activity and that the inclusion of a variety of berries in the diet might be useful for preventing the development of tumors. The growth of various cancer cell lines, including those of **stomach, prostate, intestine and breast**, was strongly inhibited by raspberry, black currant, white currant, gooseberry, velvet leaf blueberry, low-bush blueberry, sea buckthorn and cranberry juice, but not (or only slightly) by strawberry, high-bush blueberry, serviceberry, red currant, or blackberry juice. "

Pterostilbene, an active constituent of blueberries, suppresses aberrant crypt foci formation in the azoxymethane-induced colon carcinogenesis model in rats. Suh N, Paul S, Hao X, Simi B, Xiao H, Rimando AM, Reddy BS. Clin Cancer Res. 2007 Jan 1;13(1):350-5. **Key Finding:** "Administration of pterostilbene for 8 weeks significantly suppressed azoxymethane-induced formation of aberrant crypt foci (57% inhibition, P<0.001) and multiple clusters of aberrant crypts (29% inhibition, P<0.01). Importantly, dietary pterostilbene also suppressed azoxymethane-induced colonic cell proliferation and iNOS expression. Inhibition of iNOS expression by pterostilbene was confirmed in cultured human colon cancer cells. The results of the present study suggest that pterostilbene, a compound present in blueberries, is of great interest for the prevention of **colon cancer**."

Selected fruits reduce azoxymethane (AOM)-induced aberrant crypt foci (ACF) in Fisher 344 male rats. Boateng J, Verghese M, Shackelford L, Walker LT, Kahtiwada J, Oguto S, Williams DS, Jones J, Guyton M, Asiamah D, Henderson F, Grant L, DeBruce M, Johnson A, Washington S, Chawan CB. Food Chem Toxicol. 2007 May;45(5):725-32. **Key Finding:** "In this study we investigated the possible effects of blueberries, blackberries, plums, mangoes, pomegranate juice, watermelon juice and cranberry juice on azoxymethane-induced aberrant crypt foci in Fisher 344 male rats. Our findings suggest that among the fruits and fruit juices, blueberries and pomegranate juice contributed to significant reductions in the formation of AOM-induced ACF."

Pterostilbene induces apoptosis and cell cycle arrest in human gastric carcinoma cells. Pan MH, Chang YH, Badmaev V, Nagabhushanam K, Ho CT. J Agric Food Chem. 2007 Sep 19;55(19):7777-85. **Key Finding:** "The induction of apoptosis by pterostilbene, an active constituent of blueberries, may provide a pivotal mechanism of the antitumor effects and for treatment of human **gastric cancer**."

*Blackberry, black raspberry, blueberry, cranberry, red raspberry, and strawberry extracts inhibit growth and stimulate apoptosis of human **cancer** cells in vitro.* Seeram NP, Adams LS, Zhang Y, Lee R, Sand D, Scheuller HS, Heber D. J Agric Food Chem. 2006 Dec 13;54(25):9329-39. **Key Finding:** "The berry extracts were evaluated for their ability to inhibit the growth of human **oral, breast, colon and prostate tumor cell** lines at concentrations ranging from 25 to 200 micro g/ml. With increasing concentration of berry extract, increasing inhibition of cell proliferation in all of the cancer cell lines was observed, with different degrees of potency between cell lines. The berry extracts were also evaluated for their ability to stimulate apoptosis of the COX-2 expressing **colon cancer** cell line, HT-29.

*In vitro **antileukaemic** activity of extracts from berry plant leaves against sensitive and multidrug resistant HL60 cells.* Skupien K, Oszmianski J, Kostrzewa-Kowak D, Tarasiuk J. Cancer Lett. 2006 May 18;236(2):282-91. **Key Finding:** "It was found that the blueberry extract was the most efficient against sensitive HL60 cell line (about 2-fold more active than strawberry and raspberry extracts) but presented much lower activity towards resistant cells. In contrast, strawberry and raspberry extracts exhibited the high cytotoxic activity against sensitive leukemia HL60 cell line as well as its MDR sub lines."

*Inhibition of matrix metalloproteinase activity in DU145 human **prostate cancer** cells by flavonoids from low bush blueberry (Vaccinium angustifolium): possible role for protein kinase C and mitogen-activated protein-kinase-mediated events.* Matchett MD, MacKinnon SL, Sweeney MI, Gottschall-Pass KT, Hurta RA. J Nutr Biochem. 2006 Feb;17(2):117-25. **Key Finding:** "These findings indicate that blueberry flavonoids may use multiple mechanisms in down-regulating MMP activity in DU145 human prostate cancer cells."

*Differential effects of blueberry proanthocyanidins on androgen sensitive and insensitive human **prostate cancer** cell lines.* Schmidt BM, Erdman JW Jr, Lila MA. Cancer Lett. 2006 Jan 18;231(2):240-6. **Key Finding:** "Blueberry proanthocyanidins have an effect primarily on androgen-dependent growth of prostate cancer cells. When 20 microg/ml of a wild blueberry proanthocyanidin fraction was added to LNCaP prostate cancer cell line growth was inhibited to 11% of control. Two similar proanthocyanidin-rich fractions from cultivated blueberries at the same concentration inhibited LNCaP growth to 57 and 26% of control. In DU145 prostate cancer cells the only fraction that significantly reduced growth compared to contract was fraction 4 from cultivated blueberries."

*Phenolic compounds from blueberries can inhibit **colon cancer** cell proliferation and induce apoptosis.* Yi W, Fischer J, Krewer G, Akoh CC. J Agric Food Chem. 2005 Sep 7;53(18):7320-9. **Key Finding:** "Flavonol and tannin fractions from blueberry extract resulted in 50% inhibition of colon cancer cell proliferation at concentrations of 70-100 and 50-100 microg/ml, in HT-29 and Caco-2 cells, respectively. The phenolic acid fraction showed relatively lower bioactivities with 50% inhibition at approximately 1000 microg/ml. The greatest antiproliferation effect among all four fractions was from the anthocyanin fractions. Both HT-29 and Caco-2 cell growth was significantly inhibited by >50% by the anthocyanin fractions at concentrations of 15-50 microg/ml. Anthocyanin fractions also resulted in 2-7 times increases in DNA fragmentation, indicating the induction of apoptosis. These findings suggest that blueberry intake may reduce colon cancer risk."

*Blueberry flavonoids inhibit matrix metalloproteinase activity in DU145 human **prostate cancer** cells.* Matchett MD, MacKinnon SL, Sweeney MI, Gottschall-Pass KT, Hurta RA. Biochem Cell Biol. 2005 Oct;83(5):637-43. **Key Finding:** "These findings indicate that flavonoids from blueberry possess the ability to effectively decrease matrix metalloproteinase activity, which may decrease overall extracellular matrix degradation. This ability may be important in controlling tumor metastasis formation."

Antimutagenic activity of berry extracts. Hope Smith S, Tate PL, Huang G, Magee JB, Meepagala KM, Wedge DE, Larcom LL. J Med Food. 2004 Winter;7(4):450-5. **Key Finding:** "Identification of phytochemicals useful in dietary prevention and intervention of **cancer** is of paramount important. Juice from strawberry, blueberry, and raspberry fruit significantly inhibited **mutagenesis** caused by both carcinogens tested (methyl methanessulfonate and benzo{a}pyrene). Ethanol extracts from freeze-dried fruits of strawberry cultivars (Sweet Charlie and Carlsbad) and blueberry cultivars (Tifblue and Premier) were also tested. Of these, the hydrolysable tannin-containing fraction from Sweet Charlie strawberries was most effective at inhibiting mutations."

Anti-angiogenic property of edible berries. Roy S, Khanna S, Alessio HM, Vider J, Bagchi D, Bagchi M, Sen CK. Free Radic Res. 2002 Sep;36(9):1023-31. **Key Finding:** "The ORAC values of strawberry powder and grape seed proanthocyanidin extract were higher than cranberry, elderberry or raspberry seed. Wild bilberry and blueberry extracts possessed the highest ORAC values. Each of the berry samples studied significantly inhibited both H2O2 as well as TNF alpha induced vascular endothelial growth factor expression by the human keratinocytes. Madrigal assay using human dermal micro vascular endothelial cells showed that edible berries impair **angiogenesis.**

*Anticarcinogenic Activity of Strawberry, Blueberry, and Raspberry Extracts to **Breast and Cervical Cancer** Cells.* Wedge DE, Meepagala KM, Magee JB, Smith SH, Huang G, Larcom LL. J Med Food. 2001 Spring;4(1):49-51. **Key Finding:** "Freeze-dried fruits of two strawberry cultivars, Sweet Charlie and Carlsbad, and two blueberry cultivars, Tifblue and Premier, were sequentially extracted and tested separately for in vitro anticancer activity on cervical and breast cancer cell lines. Ethanol extracts from all four fruits strongly inhibited CaSki and SiHa cervical cancer cell lines and MCF-7 and T47-D breast cancer cell lines. An unfractionated aqueous extract of raspberry and the ethanol extract of Premier blueberry significantly inhibited mutagenesis by both direct-acting and metabolically active carcinogens."

*In vitro anti**cancer** activity of fruit extracts from Vaccinium species.* Bomser J, Madhavi DL, Singletary K, Smith MA. Planta Med. 1996 Jun;62(3):212-6. **Key Finding:**

"Components of the hexane/chloroform fraction of bilberry and of the proanthocyanidin fraction of low bush blueberry, cranberry, and lingonberry exhibit potential anticarcinogenic activity as evaluated by in vitro screening tests. The concentrations of these crude extracts needed to inhibit ornithine decarboxylase activity by 50% were 8.0 (low bush blueberry) 7.0 (cranberry) 9.0 micrograms (lingonberry.)"

Cardiovascular disease

Blueberries decrease **cardiovascular risk** *factors in obese men and women with metabolic syndrome.* Basu A, Du M, Leyva MJ, Et al. J Nutr. 2010 Sep;140(9):1582-7. **Key Finding**: "We examined the effects of blueberry supplementation on features of metabolic syndrome, lipid peroxidation, and inflammation in 48 obese men and women. Our study shows blueberries may improve selected features of metabolic syndrome and related cardiovascular risk factors at dietary achievable doses."

Blueberry-Enriched Diets Reduce **Metabolic Syndrome** *and Insulin Resistance in Rats.* Seymour M, Tanone I, Lewis S, Urcuyo-Llanes D, Bolling SF, Bennink MR. FASEB Journal. 2009 Apr;23(Meeting Abstracts). **Key Finding:** "The results suggest that regular intake of blueberry reduced several key risk factors for **cardiovascular disease** and metabolic syndrome. Furthermore, these benefits were augmented when fed a low fat diet. Finally, blueberry diet conferred tissue changes in several genes related to lipid and glucose metabolism, which could support the in vivo results of greater insulin sensitivity and reduced fat accumulation."

Wild blueberry (Vaccinium angustifolium) consumption affects the composition and structure of glycosaminoglycan in Sprague-Dawley rat aorta. Kalea AZ, Lamari FN, Theocharis AD, Cordopatis P, Schuschke DA, Karamanos NK, Klimis-Zacas DJ. N Nutr Biochem. 2006 Feb;17(2):109-16. **Key Finding:** "It has been documented that increased intake of polyphenols may provide protection against **coronary heart disease** and **stroke**. Blueberries are one of the richest sources of antioxidants among fruits and vegetables. Our results demonstrate for the first time that a diet rich in blueberries results in structural alterations in rat aortic tissue glycosaminoglycan. These changes may affect cellular signal transduction pathways and could have major consequences for the biological function of GAG molecules within the vascular environment."

Cataracts

*Comparison of antioxidants in the ability to prevent **cataract** in prematurely aging OXYS rats.* Kolosova NG, Lebedev PA, Dikalova AE. Bull Exp Biol Med. 2004 Mar;137(3):249-51. **Key Finding:** "Adrusen Zinco, Mirtilene Forte, blueberry extract, and vitamin E possessing antioxidant properties and given with food decreased the number of OXYS rats with cataract."

Cognition

Age-related toxicity of amyloid-beta associated with increased pERK and pCREB in primary hippocampal neurons: reversal by blueberry extract. Brewer GJ, Torricelli JR, Lindsey AL, Et al. J Nutr Biochem. 2010 Oct;21(10):991-8. **Key Finding**: "These results suggest that the beneficial effects of blueberry extract may involve transient stress signaling and ROS protection that may translate into improved **cognition** in aging rats and APP/PS1 mice given blueberry extract."

Cytoprotective effect of blueberry extracts against oxidative damage of rat hippocampal neurons induced by H2O2. Pang W, Jiang JG, Yang HP, Et al. Zhongguo Ying Yong Sheng Li Xue Za Zhi (Chinese). 2010 Feb;26(1):51-4. **Key Finding:** "Proper dose of blueberry extract has remarkable protective effect against oxidative stress in primary cultures of rat hippocampal neurons induced by H2O2. The mechanism may be related to decreasing the neuronal apoptosis and enhancing the antioxidation of hippocampal neurons."

Blueberry supplementation attenuates microglial activation in hippocampal intraocular grafts to aged hosts. Willis LM, Freeman L, Bickford PC, Et al. Glia. 2010 Apr 15;58(6):679-90. **Key Finding**: "These studies demonstrate direct effects of blueberry upon microglial activation both during isolated conditions and in the aged host brain and suggest that this nutraceutical can attenuate **age-induced inflammation**."

*Grape juice, berries, and walnuts affect **brain aging** and behavior.* Joseph JA, Shukitt-Hale B, Willism LM. J Nutr. 2009 Sep;139(9):1813S-7S. **Key Finding:** "Research from our laboratory has suggested that dietary supplementation with fruit or vegetable extracts high in antioxidants (e.g. blueberries, strawberries, walnuts and Concord grape juice) can decrease the enhanced vulnerability to oxidative stress that occurs in aging and these reductions are expressed as improvements in behavior. Collaborative findings indicate that blueberry or Concord grape juice supplementation in humans with mild **cognitive impairment** increased verbal memory performance, thus translating our animal findings to humans."

Effect of a polyphenol-rich wild blueberry extract on **cognitive performance** *of mice, brain antioxidant markers and acetyl cholinesterase activity.* Papandreou MA, Dimako-poulou A, Linardaki ZI, Cordopatis P, Klimis-Zacas D, Margarity M, Lamari FN. Behav Brain Res. 2009 Mar 17;198(2):352-8. **Key Finding:** "The signifi-cant cognitive enhancement observed in adult mice after short-term supplemen-tation with the blueberry extract concentrated in polyphenols, is closely related to higher brain antioxidant properties and inhibition of AChE activity. These findings stress the critical impact of wild blueberry bioactive components on brain function."

A blueberry-enriched diet provides cellular protection against oxidative stress and reduces a kainite-induced learning impairment in rats. Duffy KB, Spangler EL, Devan BD, Guo Z, Bowker JL, Janas AM, Hagepanos A, Minor RK, DeCabo R, Mouton PR, Shukitt-Hale B, Joseph JA, Ingram DK. Neurobiol Aging. 2008 Nov;29(11):1680-9. **Key Finding:** "These findings suggest the blueberry supplementation may protect against **neuro degeneration** and **cognitive impairment** mediated by exci-totoxicity and oxidative stress."

Age-related toxicity of amyloid-beta associated with increased pERK and pCREB in primary hippocampal neurons: reversal by blueberry extract. Brewer GJ, Torricelli JR, Lindsey AL, Kunz EZ, Neuman A, Fisher DR, Joseph JA. J Nutr Biochem. 2009 Nov 30. (Epub ahead of print). **Key Finding:** "We conclude that the increased age-related susceptibility of **old-age neurons** to a beta toxicity may be due to higher levels of activation of pERK and pCREB pathways that can be protected by blueberry extract through inhibition of both these pathways through an ROS stress response. These results suggest that the beneficial effects of blueberry extract may involve transient stress signaling and ROS protection that may trans-late into improved **cognition.**"

Blueberry-induced changes in spatial working **memory** *correlate with changes in hippo-campal CREB phosphorylation and brain-derived neurotropic factor (BDNF) levels.* Williams CM, El Mohsen MA, Vauzour D, Rendeiro C, Butler LT, Ellis JA, Whiteman M, Spencer JP. Free Radic Biol Med. 2008 Aug 1;45(3):295-305. **Key Finding:** "Although causal relationships cannot be made among supplementation, behavior, and biochemical parameters, the measurement of anthocyanin and flavanols in the brain following blueberry supplementation may indicate that changes in spatial working memory in aged animals are linked to the effects of flavonoids on the ERK-CREB-BDNF pathway."

Blueberry-enriched diet ameliorates age-related declines in NMDA receptor-dependent LTP. Coultrap SJ, Bickford PC, Browning MD. Age (Dordr). 2008 Dec;30(4):263-72. **Key Finding:** "Supplementation of the diet with blueberry extract elevated long-term potentiation in the hippocampus (63%) in aged animals to levels seen in young. The normalization of LTP may be due to the blueberry diet preventing a decline in synaptic strength. This report provides evidence that dietary alterations later in life may prevent or postpone the **cognitive declines** associated with **aging**."

Blueberry extract enhances survival of intraocular **hippocampal transplants**. Willis L, Bickford P, Zaman V, Moore A, Granholm AC. Cell Transplant. 2005;14(4):213-23. **Key Finding:** "When middle-aged animals were maintained on a diet supplemented with 2% blueberry extract, hippocampal graft growth was significantly improved and cellular organization of grafts were comparable to that seen in tissue grafted to young host animals. Thus, the data suggest that factors in blueberries may have significant effects on development and organization of this important brain region."

Anthocyanin in **aged** *blueberry-fed rats is found centrally and may enhance* **memory**. Andres-Lacueva C, Shukitt-Hale B, Galli RL, Jauregui O, Lamuela-Raventos RM, Joseph JA. Nutr Neurosci. 2005 Apr;8(2):111-20. **Key Finding:** "These findings are the first to suggest that polyphenol compounds are able to cross the blood brain barrier and localize in various brain regions important for **learning** and memory. Correlational analyses revealed a relationship between Morris water maze performance in blueberry supplemented rats and the total number of anthocyanin compounds found in the cortex. These findings suggest that these compounds may deliver their antioxidant and signaling modifying capabilities centrally."

Effect of lyophilized Vaccinium berries on memory, anxiety and locomotion in adult rats. Ramirez MR, Izquierdo I, do Carmo Bassols Raseira M, Zuanazzi JA, Barros D, Henriques AT. Pharmacol Res. 2005 Dec;52(6):457-62. **Key Finding:** "The present study showed that lyophilized berries significantly enhanced short-term memory, but not long-term memory in the inhibitory avoidance task. These results suggest that lyophilized berries may be beneficial in the prevention of memory deficits, one of the symptoms related to **Alzheimer's disease** and corroborate previous findings showing that flavonoids present effects in several learning paradigms."

*The beneficial effects of fruit polyphenols on **brain aging***. Lau FC, Shukitt-Hale B, Joseph JA. Neurobiol Aging. 2005 Dec;26 Suppl 1:128-32. **Key Finding:** "Research from our laboratory has shown that nutritional antioxidants, such as the polyphenols found in blueberries, can reverse age-related declines in neuronal signal transduction as well as cognitive and motor deficits. Furthermore, we have shown that short-term blueberry supplementation increases hippocampal plasticity."

*Blueberry supplemented diet: effects on object recognition **memory** and nuclear factor-kappa B levels in aged rats*. Goyarzu P, Malin DH, Lau FC, Taglialatela G, Moon WD, Jennings R, Moy E, Moy D, Lippold S, Shukitt-Hale B, Joseph JA. Nutr Neurosci. 2004 Apr;7(2):75-83. **Key Finding:** "Twelve aged rats were fed a 2% blueberry supplemented diet for 4 months prior to testing. Eleven aged rats and twelve young rats had been fed a control diet. The rats were tested for object recognition memory on the visual paired comparison task. Aged control diet rats performed no better than chance. Young rats and aged blueberry diet rats performed significantly better than the aged control diet group."

*Modulation of hippocampal plasticity and **cognitive behavior** by short-term blueberry supplementation in **aged** rats*. Casadesus G, Shukitt-Hale B, Stellwagen HM, Zhu X, Lee HG, Smith MA, Joseph JA. Nutr Neurosci. 2004 Oct-Dec;7(5-6):309-16. **Key Finding:** "Our results show that all parameters of hippocampal neuronal plasticity are increased in supplemented animals and aspects such as proliferation, extracellular receptor kinase activation and IGF-1 and IGF-1R levels correlate with improvements in spatial memory. Therefore, cognitive improvements afforded by polyphenol-rich fruits such as blueberries appear, in part, to be mediated by their effects on hippocampal plasticity."

*Reversals of age-related declines in neuronal signal transduction, **cognitive,** and **motor behavioral deficits** with blueberry, spinach, or strawberry dietary supplementation*. Joseph JA, Shukitt-Hale B, Denisvoa NA, Bielinski D, Martin A, McEwen JJ, Bickford PC. J Neurosci. 1999 Sep 15;19(18):8114-21. **Key Finding:** "Our previous study had shown that rats given dietary supplements of fruits and vegetable extracts with high antioxidant activity for 8 months beginning at 6 months of age retarded age-related declines in neuronal and cognitive function. The present study showed that such supplements (strawberry, spinach or blueberry) fed for 8 weeks to 19-month-old Fischer 344 rats were also effective in reversing age-related deficits in several neuronal and behavioral parameters. These findings suggest that, in addition to their known beneficial effects on **cancer** and **heart disease,** phytochemicals present in antioxidant-rich foods may be beneficial in reversing the course of neuronal and behavioral **aging.**"

Colitis

Probiotics and blueberry attenuate the severity of dextran sulfate sodium (DSS)-induced **colitis.** Osman N, Adawi D, Ahrne S, Jeppsson B, Molin G. Dig Dis Sci. 2008 Sep;53(9):2464-73. **Key Finding:** "We studied the anti-inflammatory properties of probiotic strains and blueberry in a colitis model. The disease activity index was significantly lower on days 9 and 10 in all groups compared to the colitis control. Myeloperoxidase and bacterial translocation to the liver and to the mesenteric lymph nodes decreased significantly in all groups compared to colitis control. Cecal Enterobacteriaceae count decreased significantly in blueberry with and without probiotics compared to the other groups."

Diabetes

*Anti***obesity** *and anti***diabetic** *effects of bio transformed blueberry juice in KKA(y) mice.* Vuong T, Benhaddou-Andaloussi A, Brault A, Harbilas D, Marineau LC, Vallerand D, Ramassamy C, Matar C, Haddad PS. Int J Obes (Lond). 2009 Oct;33(10):1166-73. **Key Finding:** "This study shows that blueberry juice decreases hyperglycemia in diabetic mice, at least in part by reversing adiponectin levels. Blueberry juice also protects young pre-diabetic mice from developing **obesity** and **diabetes.**"

Effect of a dietary supplement containing blueberry and sea buckthorn concentrate on antioxidant capacity in **type 1 diabetic** *children.* Nemes-Nagy E, Szocs-Molnar T, Dunca I, Balogh-Samarghitan V, Hobai S, Morar R, Pusta DL, Craciun EC. Acta Physiol Hung. 2008 Dec;95(4):383-93. **Key Finding:** "Thirty type 1 diabetic children were treated with a blueberry and sea buckthorn concentrate for two months. These results suggest that treatment with this dietary supplement has a beneficial effect in the treatment of type 1 diabetic children and it should be considered as a phytotherapeutic product in the fight against diabetes mellitus."

*Anti-***diabetic** *properties of the Canadian low bush blueberry Vaccinium angustifolium Ait.* Martineau LC, Couture A, Spoor D, Benhaddou-Andaloussi A, Harris C, Meddah B, Leduc C, Burt A, Vuong T, Mai Le P, Prentki M, Bennett SA, Arnason JT, Haddad PS. Phytomedicine. 2006 Nov;13(9-10):612-23. **Key Finding:** "These results demonstrate that V. angustifolium contains active principles with insulin-like and glitazone-like properties, while conferring protection against glucose toxicity. Enhancement of proliferation in beta cells may represent another potential anti-diabetic property. Extracts of the Canadian blueberry thus show promise for use as a complementary anti-diabetic therapy."

Effect of Blueberin on fasting glucose, C-reactive protein and plasma aminotransferases, in female volunteers with **diabetes type 2**: *double-blind, placebo controlled clinical study.* Abidov M, Ramazanov A, Jimenez Del Rio M, Chkhikvishvili I. Georgian Med News. 2006 Dec;(141):66-72. **Key Finding:** "Blueberin, a phytomedicine containing 250 mg Blueberry leaves (Vaccinium arctostaphylos L. Ericaceae) extract was administered with 42 volunteer subjects diagnosed with Type 2 diabetes. During the 4-week trial, the Blueberin supplement was administered three times per day, 15-30 minutes prior to a meal along with 100 ml of water. Results of this trial revealed that the supplementation reduced fasting plasma glucose from 143+/-5,2mg/L to 104+/-5,7 mg/L., whereas there were no statistically significant changes in the Placebo group.The reduction of fasting glucose was correlated with the reduction of serum CRP in the Blueberin group. In addition to anti-diabetes effects, the Blueberin also possess pharmacologically relevant anti-inflammatory properties."

Novel lipid-lowering properties of Vaccinium myrtillus L. leaves, a traditional antidiabetic treatment, in several models of rat dyslipidaemia: a comparison with ciprofibrate. Cignarella A, Nastasi M, Cavalli E, Puglisi L. Thromb Res. 1996 Dec 1;84(5):311-22. **Key Finding:** "Vaccinium myrtillus L. (blueberry) leaf infusions are traditionally used as a folk medicine treatment of diabetes. To further define this therapeutic action, a dried hydro alcoholic extract of the lead was administered orally to streptozotocin-diabetic rats for 4 days. Plasma glucose levels were consistently found to drop by about 26% at two different stages of **diabetes.** Unexpectedly, plasma triglyceride (TG) was also decreased by 39% following treatment."

Heart failure

Blueberry-enriched diet protects rat heart from ischemic damage. Ahmet I, Spangler E, Shukitt-Hale B, Juhaszova M, Sollott SJ, Joseph JA, Ingram DK, Talan M. PLoS One. 2009 Jun 18;4(6):e5954. **Key Finding:** "A blueberry-enriched diet protects the myocardium from induced ischemic damage and demonstrated the potential to attenuate the development of post myocardial infarction **chronic heart failure**."

Survival and cardio protective benefits of long-term blueberry enriched diet in dilated cardiomyopathy following **myocardial infarction** *in rats.* Ahmet I, Spangler E, Shukitt-Hale B, Joseph JA. Ingram DK, Talan M. PLoS One. 2009 Nov 19;4(11):e7975. **Key Finding:** "This is the first experimental evidence that a blueberry-enriched diet has positive effects on the course of chronic **heart failure** and thus warrants consideration for clinical evaluation."

Hepatitis C

*Proanthocyanidin from blueberry leaves suppresses expression of subgenomic **hepatitis C** virus RNA.* Takeshita M, Ishida Y, Akamatsu E, Ohmori Y, Sudoh M, Uto H, Tsubouchi H, Kataoka H. J Biol Chem. 2009 Aug 7;284(32):21165-76. **Key Finding:** "These data suggest that proanthocyanidin isolated from blueberry leaves may have potential usefulness as an anti-Hepatitis C virus compound by inhibiting viral replication."

Hypertension

*A wild blueberry-enriched diet (Vaccinium angustifolium) improves vascular tone in the adult spontaneously **hypertensive** rat.* Kristo AS, Kalea AZ, Schuschke DA, Et al. J Agric Food Chem. 2010 Nov 24;58(22):11600-5. **Key Finding**: "These findings document the potential of wild blueberries to modify major pathways of vasomotor control and improve the vascular tone in the adult SHR with endothelial dysfunction."

*Diets containing blueberry extract lower **blood pressure** in spontaneously **hypertensive stroke**-prone rats.* Shaughnessy KS, Boswall IA, Scanlan AP, Gottschall-Pass KT, Sweeney MI. Nutr Res. 2009 Feb;29(2):130-8. **Key Finding:** "Blueberry fed rats had reduced markers of renal oxidative stress, such as proteinuria and kidney nitrites. Thus, a 3% blueberry diet may be capable of protecting the kidneys from oxidative damage in spontaneously hypertensive stroke-prone rats, thereby reducing the magnitude of hypertension."

*Effect of Vaccinium ashei reade leaves on angiotensin converting enzyme activity in vitro and on systolic **blood pressure** of spontaneously **hypertensive** rats in vivo.* Sakaida H, Nagao K, Higa K, Shirouchi B, Inoue N, Hidaka F, Kai T, Yanagita T. Biosci Biotechnol Biochem. 2007 Sep;71(9):2335-7. **Key Finding:** "Blueberry leaf showed a strong inhibitory effect on angiotensin-converting enzyme activity in vitro. Additionally, feeding of blueberry leaf suppressed the development of essential hypertension in spontaneously hypertensive rats in vivo. These results promise the use of blueberry leaf as a source of dietary hypotensive components."

Immune System health

Effect of blueberry on hepatic and immunological functions in mice. Wang YP, Cheng ML, Zhang BF, Et al. Hepatobiliary Pancreat Dis Int. 2010 Apr;9(2):164-8. **Key**

Finding: "This study examined the effects of blueberry on liver protection and **cellular immune** functions. Blueberry induces expression of Nrf2, HO-1, and Nqo1, which can protect hepatocytes from oxidative stress. In addition, blueberry can modulate T-cell function in mice."

Nutraceuticals synergistically promote proliferation of human stem cells. Bickford PC, Tan J, Shytle RD, Sanberg CD, El-Badri N, Sanberg PR. Stem Cells Dev. 2006 Feb;15(1):118-23. **Key Finding:** "We report here the effects of several natural compounds on the proliferation of human bone marrow and human CD34(+) and CD133(+) cells. A dose-related effect of blueberry, green tea, catechin, carnosine and vitamin D(3) was observed on proliferation with human bone marrow. We further show that combinations of nutrients produce a synergistic effect to promote proliferation of human hematopoietic progenitors. This demonstrates that nutrients can act to promote healing via an interaction with stem cell populations."

Neurodegenerative diseases

Biotransformed blueberry juice protects neurons from hydrogen peroxide-induced oxidative stress and mitogen-activated protein kinase pathway alterations. Vuong T, Matar C, Ramassamy C, Et al. Br J Nutr. 2010 Sep;104(5):656-63. **Key Finding:** "The present studies demonstrate that blueberry juice can protect neurons against oxidative stress possibly by increasing antioxidant enzyme activities. Blueberry juice may represent a novel approach to prevent and to treat **neurodegenerative disorders**."

Cytoprotective effect of blueberry extracts against oxidative damage of rat hippocampal neurons induced by H2O2. Pang W, Jiang JG, Yang HP, Et al. Zhongguo Ying Yong Sheng Li Xue Za Zhi (Chinese). 2010 Feb;26(1):51-4. **Key Finding:** "Proper dose of blueberry extract has remarkable protective effect against oxidative stress in primary cultures of rat hippocampal neurons induced by H2O2. The mechanism may be related to decreasing the neuronal apoptosis and enhancing the antioxidation of hippocampal neurons."

A blueberry-enriched diet provides cellular protection against oxidative stress and reduces a kainite-induced learning impairment in rats. Duffy KB. Spangler EL, Devan BD, Guo Z, Bowker JL, Janas AM, Hagepanos A, Minor RK, DeCabo R, Mouton PR, Shukitt-Hale B, Joseph JA, Ingram DK. Neurobiol Aging. 2008 Nov;29(11):1680-9. **Key Finding:** "These findings suggest the blueberry supplementation may protect against **neuro-degeneration** and **cognitive impairment** mediated by excitotoxicity and oxidative stress."

*Dietary blueberry supplementation affects growth but not vascularization of **neural transplants**.* Willis LM, Small BJ, Bickford PC, Umphlet CD, Moore AB, Granholm AC. J Cereb Blood Flow Metab. 2008 Jun;28(6):1150-64. **Key Finding:** "Transplantation of neural tissue has been attempted as a treatment method for neurodegenerative disorders. Grafted neurons survive to a lesser extent into middle-aged or aged hosts, and survival rates of <10% of grafted neurons is common. Antioxidant diets, such as blueberry, can exert powerful effects on developing neurons and blood vessels in vitro. In this study, we examined the effects of a blueberry diet on survival, growth, and vascularization of fetal hippocampal tissue to the anterior chamber of the eye of young or middle-aged female rats. The blueberry diet did not affect vessel morphology or density of vessel-associated protein markers but gave rise to significantly increased growth capacity, cytoarchitecture, and the final size of hippocampal grafts."

Blueberry polyphenols attenuate kainic acid-induced decrements in cognition and later inflammatory gene expression in rat hippocampus. Shukitt-Hale B, Lau FC, Carey AN, Galli RL, Spangler EL, Ingram DK, Joseph JA. Nutr Neurosci. 2008 Aug;11(4):172-82. **Key Finding:** "Cognitive impairment in age-related neurodegenerative diseases such as **Alzheimer's disease** may be partly due to long-term exposure and increased susceptibility to inflammatory insults. These results indicate that blueberry polyphenols attenuate learning impairments following neurotoxic insult and exert anti-inflammatory actions, perhaps via alteration of gene expression."

Blueberry supplemented diet reverses age-related decline in hippocampal HSP70 neuroprotection. Galli RL, Bielinski DF, Szprengiel A, Shukitt-Hale B, Josephy JA. Neurobiol Aging. 2006 Feb;27(2):344-50. **Key Finding:** "It appeared that the blueberry diet completely restored the HSP70 response to in vitro inflammatory challenge in the old rats at the 90 and 240 min times. This suggests that a short-term blueberry intervention may result in improved HSP70-mediated protection against a number of **neurodegenerative** processes in the brain."

Dietary supplementation with blueberry extract improves survival of transplanted dopamine neurons. McGuire SO, Sortwell CE, Shukitt-Hale B, Joseph JA, Hejna MJ, Collier TJ. Nutr Neurosci. 2006 Oct-Dec;9(5-6):251-8. **Key Finding:** "These findings provide support for the potential of dietary phytochemicals as an easily administered and well-tolerated therapy that can be used to improve the effectiveness of dopamine neuron replacement in cell transplantation for **Parkinson's disease**."

Inhibitory effects of blueberry extract on the production of inflammatory mediators in lipo-polysaccharide-activated BV2 microglia. Lau FC, Bielinski DF, Joseph JA. J Neurosci Res. 2007 Apr;85(5):1010-7. **Key Finding:** "The results suggest that blueberry polyphenols attenuate inflammatory responses of brain microglia and could be potentially useful in modulation of inflammatory conditions in the central nervous system related to **neurodegenerative diseases**."

Blueberry and spirulina-enriched diets enhance striatal dopamine recovery and induce rapid, transient microglia activation after injury of the rat nigrostriatal dopamine system. Stromberg I, Gemma C, Vila J, Bickford PC. Exp Neurol. 2005 Dec;196(2):298-307. **Key Finding:** "Neuroinflammation plays a critical role in loss of dopamine neurons during brain injury and in **neurodegenerative diseases**. Diets enriched in foods with antioxidant and anti-inflammatory actions may modulate this neuro-inflammation. Enhanced striatal dopamine recovery appeared in animals treated with diet enrich in antioxidants and anti-inflammatory phytochemicals (blueberry and spirulina) and coincided with an early, transient increase in OX-6-positive microglia."

Dietary supplementation with blueberries, spinach, or spirulina reduces ischemic brain damage. Wang Y, Chang CF, Chou J, Chen HL, Deng X, Harvey BK, Cadet JL, Bickford PC. Exp Neurol. 2005 May;193(1):75-84. **Key Finding:** "Free radicals are involved in neurodegenerative disorders, such as **ischemia** and **aging**. We have previously demonstrated that treatment with diets enriched with blueberry, spinach, or spirulina have been shown to reduce neurodegenerative changes in aged animals. The purpose of this study was to determine if these diets have neuroprotective effects in focal ischemic brain in Sprague-Dawley rats. Animals treated with blueberry, spinach, or spirulina had significantly lower caspase-3 activity in the ischemic hemisphere. In conclusion, our data suggest that chronic treatment with blueberry, spinach, or spirulina reduces ischemia/reperfusion-induced apoptosis and cerebral infarction."

Obesity

Purified blueberry anthocyanin and blueberry juice alter development of obesity in mice fed an obesogenic high-fat diet. Prior RL, Wilkes S, Rogers R, Et al. J Agric Food Chem. 2010 Apr 14;58(7):3970-6. **Key Finding:** "Blueberry juice was not as effective as the low dose of blueberry anthocyanin in the drinking water in preventing obesity. Additional studies are needed to determine factors responsible for the differing responses of blueberry juice and whole blueberry in preventing the development of **obesity**."

*Bioactives in blueberries improve insulin sensitivity in **obese**, insulin-resistant men and women.* Stull AJ, Cash KC, Johnson WD, Et al. J Nutr. 2010 Oct;140(10):1764-8. **Key Finding**: "Insulin sensitivity was enhanced in the blueberry group (among 32 obese, non-diabetic and insulin resistant subjects) at the end of the study without significant changes in adiposity, energy intake, and inflammatory biomarkers. In conclusion, daily dietary supplementation with bioactives from whole blueberries improved insulin sensitivity in obese, non-diabetic and insulin-resistant participants."

Purified berry anthocyanin but not whole berries normalize lipid parameters in mice fed an obesogenic high fat diet. Prior RL, Wu X, Gu L, Hager T, Hager A, Wilkes S, Howard L. Mol Nutre Food Res. 2009 Nov;53(11):1406-18. **Key Finding:** "Administering purified anthocyanin from blueberry and strawberry via drinking water prevented the development of **dyslipidemia** and obesity in mice, but feeding diets containing whole berries or purple corn ACNs did not alter the development of **obesity.**"

*Anti**obesity** and anti**diabetic** effects of bio transformed blueberry juice in KKA(y) mice.* Vuong T, Benhaddou-Andaloussi A, Brault A, Harbilas D, Martineau LC, Vallerand D, Ramassamy C, Matar C, Haddad PS. Int J Obes (Lond). 2009 Oct;33(10):1166-73. **Key Finding:** "This study shows that blueberry juice decreases hyperglycemia in diabetic mice, at least in part by reversing adiponectin levels. Blueberry juice also protects young pre-diabetic mice from developing **obesity** and **diabetes.**"

Dietary blueberry attenuates whole-body insulin resistance in high fat-fed mice by reducing adipocyte death and its inflammatory sequelae. DeFuria J, Bennett G, Striseel KJ, Perfield JW, Milbury PE, Greenberg AS, Obin MS. J Nutr. 2009 Aug;139(8):1510-6. **Key Finding:** "These results suggest that cytoprotective and anti-inflammatory actions of dietary blueberries can provide metabolic benefits to combat **obesity**-associated pathology."

*Whole berries versus berry anthocyanin: interactions with dietary fat levels in the C57BL/6J mouse model of **obesity**.* Prior RL, Wu X, Gu L, Hager TJ, Hager A, Howard LR. J Agric Food Chem. 2008 Feb 13;56(3):647-53. **Key Finding:** "Male mice were given freeze-dried powders from whole blueberries or strawberries, or purified anthocyanin extracts from the two berries. After 8 weeks, mice fed the 60% calories from fat diet plus purified anthocyanin from blueberry in the drinking water had lower body weight gains and body fat than the controls. Anthocyanin fed as the whole blueberry did not prevent and may have actually increased obesity. However, feeding purified anthocyanin from blueberries or strawberries reduced obesity."

Osteoporosis

Dietary-induced serum phenolic acids promote bone growth via p38 MAPK/B-catenin canonical Wnt signaling. Chen JR, Lazarenko OP, Kang J, Et al. J Bone Miner Res. 2010 Nov;25(11):2399-411. **Key Finding**: "Diet and nutritional status are critical factors that influences bone development. In this report we demonstrate that a mixture of phenolic acids found in the serum of young rats fed **blueberries** significantly stimulated osteoblast differentiation, resulting in significantly increased bone mass. Blueberry phenolic may provide a basis for developing a new treatment to increase peak bone mass and delay degenerative bone disorders such as osteoporosis."

*Blueberry prevents bone loss in ovariectomized rat model of postmenopausal **osteoporosis**.* Devareddy L, Hooshmand S, Collins JK, Lucas EA, Chai SC, Arjmandi BH. J Nutr Biochem. 2008 Oct;19(10):694-9. **Key Finding:** "Our findings indicate that blueberry can prevent bone loss as seen by the increases in bone mineral density and favorable changes in biomarkers of bone metabolism."

Skeletal muscle damage

Blueberry fruit polyphenols suppress oxidative stress-induced skeletal muscle cell damage in vitro. Hurst RD, Wells RW, Hurst SM, Et al. Mol Nutr Food Res. 2010 Mar;54(3):353-63. **Key Finding**: "Skeletal muscle damage can result from disease and unaccustomed or excessive exercise. Muscle dysfunction occurs via an increased level of reactive oxygen species. These in vitro data support the concept that blueberry fruits or derived fruits rich in malvidin glycosides may be beneficial in alleviating **muscle damage** caused by oxidative stress."

*Blueberry fruit polyphenols suppress oxidative stress-induced **skeletal muscle cell damage** in vitro.* Hurst RD, Wells RW, Hurst SM, McGhie TK, Cooney JM, Jensen DJ. Mol Nutr Food Res. 2009 Nov 2. (Epub ahead of print). **Key Finding:** "Skeletal muscle damage can result from disease and unaccustomed or excessive exercise. These in vitro data support the concept that blueberry fruits or derived foods rich in malvidin glycosides may be beneficial in alleviating muscle damage caused by oxidative stress. More research on the benefits of blueberry fruit consumption in human intervention studies is warranted."

Stroke

Dietary supplementation exerts neuroprotective effects in **ischemic stroke** *model.* Yasuhara T, Hara K, Maki M, Masuda T, Sanberg CD, Sanberg PR, Bickford PC, Borlongan CV. Rejuvenation Res. 2008 Feb;11(1):201-14. **Key Finding:** "Two groups of adult male Sprague-Dawley rats initially received NT-020, a proprietary formulation of blueberry, green tea, Vitamin D3, and carnosine or vehicle. Dosing for NT-020 and vehicle consisted of daily oral administration over a 2-week period. On day 14 following the last drug treatment, all animals underwent the stroke surgery. To reveal the functional effects of NT-020, animals were subjected to established behavioral tests just prior to stroke surgery and again on day 14 post-stroke. ANOVA revealed significant treatment effects ($p<0.05$), characterized by reductions of 11.8% and 24.4% in motor asymmetry and neurologic dysfunction, respectively, in NT-020 treated stroke animals compared to vehicle-treated stroke animals. Evaluation of cerebral infarction revealed a significant 75% decrement in mean glial scar area in ischemic striatum of NT-020 treated stroke animals compared to that of vehicle-treated. These data demonstrate the remarkable neuroprotective effects of NT-020 when given prior to stroke."

Cranberry and blueberry: evidence for protective effects against **cancer** *and* **vascular diseases**. Neto CC. Mol Nutr Food Res. 2007 Jun;51(6):652-64. **Key Finding:** "Growing evidence from tissue culture, animal, and clinical models suggests that the flavonoid-rich fruits of the North American cranberry and blueberry have the potential ability to limit the development and severity of certain cancers and vascular diseases including **atherosclerosis**, **ischemic stroke**, and neurodegenerative **diseases of aging**."

Wild blueberry (Vaccinium angustifolium) consumption affects the composition and structure of glycosaminoglycan in Sprague-Dawley rat aorta. Kalea AZ, Lamari FN, Theocharis AD, Cordopatis P, Schuschke DA, Karamanos NK, Klimis-Zacas DJ. N Nutr Biochem. 2006 Feb;17(2):109-16. **Key Finding:** "It has been documented that increased intake of polyphenols may provide protection against **coronary heart disease** and **stroke**. Blueberries are one of the richest sources of antioxidants among fruits and vegetables. Our results demonstrate for the first time that a diet rich in blueberries results in structural alterations in rat aortic tissue glycosaminoglycan. These changes may affect cellular signal transduction pathways and could have major consequences for the biological function of GAG molecules within the vascular environment."

Broccoli

EVOLVING FROM A TYPE OF WILD CABBAGE found in Europe, broccoli became a dietary staple in Italy at least two thousand years ago during the time of the Roman Empire. Not until the early part of the twentieth century did broccoli become known and grown in the United States, thanks to the culinary habits of Italian immigrants.

Three types of broccoli are common in the world. The most popular, Calabrese, is named after the Calabria region of Italy. Broccoli is one of the most nutritious cruciferous vegetables. it contains almost two dozen important vitamins and minerals, with just one cup of raw broccoli providing 149 percent of the average daily nutritional need of vitamin C for adults. It is also replete in healing agents, including generous amounts of the phytochemical compound sulforaphane, which is a proven anticancer agent for at least eleven forms of cancer. Broccoli consumption also helps prevent and reduce the risk of heart disease, high blood pressure, and stroke.

Antioxidation

Antioxidant and antiproliferative activities of common vegetables. Chu YF, Sun J, WuX, Liu RH. J Agric Food Chem. 2002 Nov 6;50(23):6910-6. **Key Finding:** "In this study, 10 common vegetables were selected on the basis of consumption per capita data in the U.S. Broccoli possessed the highest total phenolic content, followed by spinach, yellow onion, red pepper, carrot, cabbage, potato, lettuce, celery, and cucumber. Red pepper had the highest total antioxidant activity, followed by broccoli, carrot, spinach, cabbage, yellow onion, celery, potato, lettuce and cucumber. Antiproliferative activities were also studied in vitro using human liver cancer cells. Spinach showed the highest inhibitory effect, followed by cabbage, red pepper, onion, and broccoli."

Antioxidant capacity of different broccoli, (Brassica oleracea) genotypes using the oxygen radical absorbance capacity (ORAC) assay. Kurilich AC, Jeffery EH, Juvik JA, Wallig MA, Klein BP. J Agric Food Chem. 2002 Aug 28;50(18):5053-7. **Key Finding:** "Ascorbic acid and flavonoid content of the hydrophilic extracts did not explain the total variation in antioxidant capacity of these extracts, suggesting either the presence of other antioxidant components that have yet to be identified or that the known antioxidants are producing synergistic effects."

*Chemoprotective glucosinolates and isothiocyanates of **broccoli sprouts**: metabolism and excretion in humans.* Shapiro TA, Fahey JW, Wade KL, Stephenson KK, Talalay P. Cancer Epidemiol Biomarkers Prev. 2001 May;10(5):501-8. **Key Finding**: "Broccoli sprouts are a rich source of glucosinolates and isothiocyanates that induce phase 2 detoxification enzymes, boost **antioxidant** status, and protect animals against chemically induced **cancer**. When intact broccoli sprouts are chewed rather than swallowed whole, isothiocyanates become more bioavailable."

Atherosclerosis

*Dietary approach to attenuate oxidative stress, **hypertension**, and **inflammation** in the cardiovascular system.* Wu L, Ashraf MHN, Facci M, Wang R, Paterson PG, Ferrie A, Juurlink BH. Proc Natl Acad Sci. 2004 May 4;101(18):7094-7099. **Key Finding:** "We conclude that a diet containing phase 2 protein inducers (from broccoli sprouts) also reduces the risk of developing cardiovascular problems of hypertension and atherosclerosis. "

Cancer (bladder; breast; colon; esophageal; gastric; leukemia; lung; melanoma/skin; ovarian; pancreatic; prostate)

*Sulforaphane induces cell cycle arrest by protecting RB-E2F-1 complex in epithelial **ovarian** cancer cells.* Bryant CS, Kumar S, Chamala S, Et al. Mol Cancer. 2010 Mar 2;9:47. **Key Finding**: "Sulforaphane, a phytochemical present in Brussels sprout and broccoli, induces growth arrest and apoptosis in epithelial ovarian cancer cells. Inhibition of retinoblastoma (RB) phosphorylation and reduction in levels of free E2F-1 appear to play an important role in growth arrest."

*Luteolin inhibits protein kinase C(epsilon) and c-Src activities and UVB-induced **skin** cancer.* Byun S, Lee KW. Jung SK, Et al. Cancer Res. 2010 Mar 15;70(6):2415-23. **Key Finding**: "Luteolin, a flavonoid present in **onion and broccoli**, exerts potent chemo preventive activity against UVB-induced skin cancer mainly by targeting PKC(epsilon) and Src."

Anticancer activity of a broccoli derivative, sulforaphane, in barrett adenocarcinoma: potential use in chemoprevention and as adjuvant in chemotherapy. Qazi A, Pal J, Maitah M, Et al. Transl Oncol. 2010 Dec 1;3(6):389-99. **Key Finding:** "These data indicate that a natural product with antioxidant properties from broccoli has great potential to be used in chemoprevention and treatment of Barrett **esophageal adenocarcinoma**."

A novel mechanism of indole-3-carbinol effects on breast carcinogenesis involves induction of Cdc25A degradation. Wu Y, Feng X, Jin Y, Et al. Cancer Prev Res. 2010 Jul;3(7):818-28. **Key Finding**: "Indole-3-carbinol (I3C) is found in vegetables of the genus Brassica. The present in vitro and in vivo studies together show that I3C-induced activation of the ATM-Chk2 pathway and degradation of Cdc25A represent a novel molecular mechanism of I3C arresting the G(1) cell cycle and inhibiting the growth of **breast cancer** cells."

*3, 3'-Diindolymethane negatively regulates Cdc25A and induces a G2/M arrest by modulation of microRNA 21 in human **breast cancer** cells.* Jin Y, Zou X, Feng X. Anticancer Drugs. 2010 Oct;21(9):814-22. **Key Finding**: "3,3'-Diindolylmethane (DIM) is a phytochemical derived from Brassica vegetables. Our data show that DIM is able to stop the cell cycle progression of human breast cancer cells regardless of their estrogen-dependence and p53 status by differentially modulating cell cycle regulatory pathways."

*Indole-3-carbinol triggers aryl hydrocarbon receptor-dependent estrogen receptor (ER) alpha protein degradation in **breast cancer** cells disrupting an ERalpha-GATA3 transcriptional cross-regulatory loop.* Marconett CN, Sundar SN, Poindexter KM, Et al. Mol Biol Cell. 2010 Apr 1;21(7):1166-77. **Key Finding**: "Estrogen receptor (ER) alpha is a critical target of therapeutic strategies to control the proliferation of hormone-dependent breast cancers. Our preclinical results implicate indole-3-carbinol from Brassica vegetables as a novel anticancer agent in human cancers that coexpress ERalpha, GATA3, and AhR, a combination found in a large percentage of breast cancers."

*Sulforaphane inhibited melanin synthesis by regulating tyrosinase gene expression in B16 mouse **melanoma** cells.* Shirasugi I, Kamada M, Matsui T, Et al. Biosci Biotechnol Biochem. 2010;74(3):579-82. **Key Finding**: "Sulforaphane present in broccoli inhibited melanogensis and tyrosine expression in mouse melanoma cells by affecting the phosphorylated MAP kinase family."

*Dietary glucoraphanin-rich broccoli sprout extracts protect against UV radiation-induced **skin carcinogenesis** in SKH-1 hairless mice.* Dinkova-Kostova AT, Fahey JW, Benedict AL, Et al. Photochem Photobiol Sci. 2010 Apr;9(4):597-600. **Key Finding**: "Feeding broccoli sprout extracts providing daily doses of 10 micromole of glucoraphanin to SKH-1 hairless mice with prior chronic exposure to UV radiation twice a week for 17 weeks inhibited the development of skin tumors during the subsequent 13 weeks; compared to controls, tumor incidence, multiplicity, and volume were reduced by 25, 47, and 70% respectively."

*Sulforaphane inhibits constitutive and interleukin-6-induced activation of signal transducer and activator of transcription 3 in **prostate cancer** cells.* Hahm ER, Singh SV. Cancer Prev Res. 2010 Apr;3(4):484-94. **Key Finding**: "D,L-sulforaphane (SFN), a synthetic analogue of broccoli-derived L-isomer, inhibits viability of human prostate cancer cells and prevents development of prostate cancer and distant site metastasis in a transgenic mouse model. The present study indicates that inhibition of STAT3 partially contributes to the proapoptotic effect of SFN."

*The dietary isothiocyanate sulforaphane modulates gene expression and alternative gene splicing in a PTEN null preclinical murine model of **prostate cancer**.* Traka MH, Spinks CA, Doleman JF, Et al. Mol Cancer. 2010 Jul 13;9:189. **Key Finding**: "Sulforaphane derived from broccoli suppresses transcriptional changes induced by PTEN deletion and induces additional changes in gene expression associated with cell cycle arrest and apoptosis in PTEN null tissue. Comparative analyses of changes in gene expression in mouse and human prostate tissue indicate that similar changes can be induced in humans with a broccoli-rich diet."

*Sulforaphane, a dietary component of broccoli/broccoli sprouts, inhibits **breast cancer** stem cells.* Li Y, Zhang T, Korkaya H, Et al. Clin Cancer Res. 2010 May 1;16(9):2580-90. **Key Finding**: "Sulforaphane inhibits breast cancer stem cells and down regulates the Wnt/beta-caterin self-renewal pathway. These findings support the use of sulforaphane for the chemoprevention of breast cancer stem cells."

*1-Benzyl-indole-3-carbinol is a novel indole-3-carbinol derivative with significantly enhanced potency of anti-proliferative and anti-estrogenic properties in human **breast cancer** cells.* Nguyen HH, Lavrenov SN, Sundar SN, Et al. Chem Biol Interact. 2010 Aug 5;186(3):255-66. **Key Finding**: "Our results implicate 1-benzyl-13C present in broccoli and cabbage as a novel, potent inhibitor of human breast cancer proliferation and estrogen responsiveness that could potentially be developed into a promising therapeutic agent for the treatment of indole-sensitive cancers."

*Dietary polyphenol quercetin targets **pancreatic cancer** stem cells.* Zhou W, Kalifatidis G, Baumann B, Et al. Int J Oncol. 2010 Sep;37(3):551-61. **Key Finding:** "A combination of quercetin with sulforaphane, an isothiocynate enriched in broccoli, had synergistic effects on pancreatic cancer stem cells. Our data suggest that good ingredients complement each other in the elimination of cancer stem cell characteristics. Since carcinogenesis is a complex process, combination of bioactive dietary agents with complementary activities may be most effective."

Sulforaphane inhibits 4-aminobiphenyl-induced DNA damage in bladder cells and tissues. Ding Y, Paoness JD, Randall KL, Et al. Carcinogenesis. 2010 Nov;31(11):1999-

2003. **Key Finding**: "These data suggest that sulforaphane is a highly promising agent for bladder cancer prevention and provides a mechanistic insight into the repeated epidemiological observation that consumption of broccoli is inversely associated with **bladder cancer** risk and mortality."

*Pharmacokinetics and pharmacodynamics of broccoli sprouts on the suppression of **prostate cancer** in transgenic adenocarcinoma of mouse prostate (TRAMP) mice: implication of induction of Nrf2, HO-1 and apoptosis and the suppression of Akt-dependent kinase pathway.* Keum YS, Khor TO, Lin W, Shen G, Kwon KH, Barve A, Li W, Kong AN. Pharm Res. 2009 Oct;26(10):2324-31. **Key Finding:** "Our findings indicate that broccoli sprouts can serve as a good dietary source of sulforaphane in vivo and that they have significant inhibitory effects on prostate tumorigenesis."

*Temporal changes in gene expression induced by sulforaphane in human **prostate cancer** cells.* Bhamre S, Sahoo D, Tibshirani R., Dill DL, Brooks JD. Prostate. 2009 Feb 1;69(2):181-90. **Key Finding:** "Our data suggest that in prostate cells sulforaphane primarily induces cellular defenses and inhibits cell growth by causing G2/M phase arrest. Furthermore, based on the striking similarities in the gene expression patterns induced across experiments in these cells, sulforaphane appears to be the primary bioactive compound present in broccoli sprouts, suggesting that broccoli sprouts can serve as a suitable source for sulforaphane in intervention trials."

*Phenethyl isothiocyanate inhibits STAT3 activation in **prostate cancer** cells.* Gong A, He M, Krishna Vanaja D, Yin P, Karnes RJ, Young CY. Mol Nutr Food Res. 2009 May 12 (Epub ahead of print). **Key Finding**: "PEITC significantly inhibited DU145 cell proliferation in a dose-dependent manner and induced the cell arrest of G2-M phase. Our data demonstrated that PEITC, a natural compound from cruciferous vegetables, exhibits antitumor effect on prostate cancer cells."

Broccoli consumption interacts with GSTM1 to perturb oncogenic signaling pathways in the prostate. Traka M, Gasper AV, Melchini A, Bacon JR, Needs PW, Frost V, Chantry A, Jones AM, Ortori CA, Barrett DA, Ball RY, Mills RD, Mithen RF. PLoS One. 2008 Jul 2;3(7):e2568. **Key Finding:** "Volunteers were randomly assigned to either a broccoli-rich or pea-rich diet. These findings suggest that consuming broccoli interacts with GSTM1 genotype to result in complex changes to signaling pathways associated with inflammation and carcinogenesis of the prostate. This study provides, for the first time, experimental evidence obtained in human to support observational studies that diets rich in cruciferous vegetables may reduce the risk of **prostate cancer** and other chronic disease."

Putative mechanisms of action for indole-3-carbinol in the prevention of **colorectal cancer.** McGrath DR, Spigelman AD. Expert Opin Ther Targets. 2008 Jun;12(6):729-38. **Key Finding:** "Indole-3-carbinol (from broccoli, Brussels sprouts, cabbage) interacts with a multitude of intracellular processes, which may halt tumorigenesis and induce apoptosis."

Inhibition of urinary **bladder carcinogenesis** *by broccoli sprouts.* Munday R, Mhawech-Fauceglia P, Munday CM, Paonessa JD, Tang L, Munday JS, Lister C, Wilson P, Fahey JW, Davis W, Zhang Y. Cancer Res. 2008 Mar 1;68(5):1593-600. **Key Finding:** "Broccoli sprout extract is a highly promising substance for bladder cancer prevention and the isothiocyanates in the extract are selectively delivered to the bladder epithelium through urinary excretion."

Multi-targeted prevention of cancer by sulforaphane. Clarke JD, Dashwood RH, Ho E. Cancer Lett. 2008 Oct 8;269(2):291-304. **Key Finding:** "This review discusses the established **anti-cancer** properties of sulforaphane, an isothiocyanate found especially high in broccoli and broccoli sprouts, with an emphasis on the possible chemoprevention mechanisms. The current status of SFN in human clinical trials also is included, with consideration of the chemistry, metabolism, absorption and factors influencing SFn bioavailability."

Consuming broccoli does not induce genes associated with xenobiotic metabolism and cell cycle control in human gastric mucosa. Gasper AV, Taka M, Bacon JR, Smith JA, Taylor MA, Hawkey CJ, Barrett DA, Mithen RF. J Nutr. 2007 Jul;137(7):1718-24. **Key Finding:** "Consumption of high glucsinolate broccoli resulted in up-regulation of several xenobiotic metabolizing genes, including thioredoxin reductase, aldo-ketoreductases, and glutamate cysteine ligase modifier subunit, which have previously been reported to be induced in cell and animal models after exposure to sulforaphane. The consequences of these results in relation to the potential **anti-carcinogenic** action of broccoli are discussed."

Sulforaphane mobilizes cellular defenses that protect skin against damage by UV radiation. Talalay P, Fahey JW, Healy ZR, Wehage SL, Benedict AL, Min C, Dinkova-Kostova AT. Proc Natl Acad Sci. 2007 Oct 30;104(44):17500-5. **Key Finding:** "Topical application of sulforaphane-rich extracts of 3-day-old broccoli sprouts up-regulated phase 2 enzymes in the mouse and human skin, protected against UVR-induced inflammation and edema in mice, and reduced susceptibility to erythema arising from narrow-band 311-nm UVR in humans. This protection against a carcinogen in humans is catalytic and long lasting." Sulforaphane stimulates the human body's natural anti-cancer ability and the extract made from broccoli sprouts may prevent **skin cancer**.

*Preclinical and clinical evaluation of sulforaphane for chemoprevention in the **breast**.* Cornblatt BS, Ye L, Dinkova-Kostova AT, Fahey EM, Singh NK, Chen MS, Stierer T, Garrett-Mayer E, Argani P, Davidson NE, Talalay P, Kensler TW, Visvanathan K. Carcinogenesis. 2007 Jul;28(7):1485-90. **Key Finding:** "Oral administration of either the isothiocyanate, sulforaphane, or its glucosinolate precursor, glucoraphanin, inhibits mammary carcinogenesis in rats. In this study, we sought to determine whether sulforaphane exerts a direct chemo preventive action on animal and human mammary tissue. Eight healthy women undergoing reduction mammoplasty were given a single dose of a broccoli sprout preparation containing 200 mumol of sulforaphane. Following oral dosing, sulforaphane metabolites were readily measurable in human breast tissue enriched for epithelial cells. These findings provide a strong rationale for evaluating the protective effects of a broccoli sprout preparation in clinical trials of women at risk for **breast cancer**."

*Combinations of tomato and broccoli enhance **antitumor** activity in dunning r3327-h prostate adenocarcinomas.* Canene-Adams K, Lindshield BL, Wang S, Jeffery EH, Clinton SK, Erdman JW Jr. Cancer Res. 2007 Jan 15;67(2):836-43. Epub 2007 Jan 9. **Key Finding:** "The combination of tomato and broccoli was more effective at slowing tumor growth than either tomato or broccoli alone and supports the public health recommendations to increase the intake of a variety of plant components."

*Quantitative combination effects between sulforaphane and 3, 3'-diindolylmethane on proliferation of human **colon cancer** cells in vitro.* Pappa G, Strathmann J, Lowinger M, Bartsch H, Gerhauser C. Carcinogenesis. 2007 Jul;28(7):1471-7. **Key Finding:** "Our results indicate that cytotoxic concentrations of SFN/DIM combinations affect cell proliferation synergistically. At low total concentrations (below 20 microM), which are physiologically more relevant, the combined broccoli compounds showed antagonistic interactions in terms of cell growth inhibition. These data stress the need for elucidating mechanistic interactions for better predicting beneficial health effects of bioactive food components."

Induction of apoptosis in HT-29 cells by extracts from isothiocyanates-rich varieties of Brassica oleracea. Mas S, Crescenti A, Gasso P, Deulofeu R, Molina R, Ballesta A, Kensler TW, Lafuente A. Nutr Cancer. 2007;58(1):107-14. **Key Finding:** "Varieties of Brassica Oleracea are rich sources of isothiocyanates that potently inhibit the growth of **colon cancer** cells by inducting apoptosis. All the extracts showed anticancer activity at ITC concentrations of between 3.54 to 7.08 mug/ ml. which are achievable in vivo."

Sulforaphane induces cell type-specific apoptosis in human **breast cancer** *cell lines.* Pledgie-Tracy A, Sobolewksi MD, Davidson NE. Mol Cancer Ther. 2007 Mar;6(3):1013-21. **Key Finding:** "These data suggest that sulforaphane inhibits cell growth, activates apoptosis, inhibits HDAC activity, and decreases the expression of key proteins involved in breast cancer proliferation in human breast cancer cells. These results support testing sulforaphane in vivo and warrant future studies examining the critical potential of sulforaphane in human breast cancer."

Sulforaphane as a promising molecule for fighting **cancer**. Fimognari C, Hrelia P. Mutat Res. 2007 May-Jun;635(2-3):90-104. **Key Finding:** Sulforaphane is the most characterized isothiocyanate appearing in cruciferous vegetables like broccoli. "Sulforaphane is able to prevent, delay, or reverse preneoplastic lesions, as well as to act on cancer cells as a therapeutic agent. Taking into account this evidence and its favorable toxicological profile, Sulforaphane can be viewed as a conceptually promising agent in cancer prevent and/or therapy."

Induction of the phase 2 response in mouse and human skin by sulforaphane-containing broccoli and broccoli sprout extracts. Dinkova-Kostova AT, Fahey JW, Wade KL, Jenkins SN, Shapiro TA, Fuchs EJ, Kerns ML, Talalay P. Cancer Epidemiol Biomarkers Prev. 2007 Apr;16(4):847-51. **Key Finding**: "The isothiocyanate sulforaphane was isolated from broccoli extracts in a bioactivity-guided fractionation as the principal and very potent inducer of cytoprotective phase 2 enzymes and subsequently shown to inhibit **tumor development** in animal models that involve various carcinogens and target organs."

Prospective study of fruit and vegetable intake and risk of **prostate cancer**. Kirsh VA, Peters U, Mayne ST, Subar AF, Et al. J Natl Cancer Inst. 2007 Aug 1;99(15):1200-9. **Key Finding**: "High intake of broccoli, cauliflower, may be associated with reduced risk of aggressive prostate cancer. We found some evidence that risk of aggressive prostate cancer decreased with increasing spinach consumption."

Indole-3-carbinol in the maternal diet provides chemo protection for the fetus against trans placental **carcinogenesis** *by the polycyclic aromatic hydrocarbon dibenzo[a,l]pyrene.* Yu Z, Mahadevan B, Lohr CV, Fischer KA, Louderback MA, Krueger SK, Pereira CB, Albershardt DJ, Baird WM, Bailey GS, Williams DE. Carcinogenesis. 2006 Oct;27(10):2116-23. **Key Finding:** An experiment with pregnant mice found that those fed Indole-3-carbinol from broccoli passed a protection against **leukemia, lung cancer** and **lymphoma** on to their offspring. The phytochemical seemed to induct enzymes to detoxify carcinogens and can cause mutated cells to commit suicide.

Induction of GST and NQO1 in cultured bladder cells and in the urinary bladders of rats by an extract of broccoli sprouts. Zhang Y, Munday R, Jobson HE, Munday CM, Lister C, Wilson P, Fahey JW, Mhawech-Fauceglia P. J Agric Food Chem. 2006 Dec 13;54(25):9370-6. **Key Finding:** "Broccoli sprout ITC extract is a potent inducer of glutathione S-transferase and NQO1 in the bladder and is a promising agent for prevention of **bladder cancer**."

*Potent activation of mitochondria-mediated apoptosis and arrest in S and M phases of **cancer** cells by a broccoli sprouts extract.* Tang L, Zhang Y, Jobson HE, Li J, Stephenson KK, Wade KL, Fahey JW. Mol Cancer Ther. 2006 Apr;5(4):935-44. **Key Finding:** "These data show that broccoli sprout isothiocyanate extract is a highly promising substance for cancer prevention/treatment and that its antiproliferative activity is exclusively derived from isothiocyanates."

*Protection against UV-light-induced **skin carcinogenesis** in SKY-1 high-risk mice by sulforaphane-containing broccoli sprout extracts.* Dinkova-Kostova AT, Jenkins SN, Fahey JW, Le L, Wehage SL, Liby KT, Stephenson KK, Wade KL, Talalay P. Cancer Lett. 2006 Aug 28;240(2):243-52. **Key Finding:** "Topical application of sulforaphane-containing broccoli sprout extracts is a promising strategy for protecting against skin tumor formation after exposure to UV radiation."

*Current trends and perspectives in nutrition and **cancer** prevention.* Barta I, Smerak P, Polivkova Z, Sestakova H, Langova M, Turek B, Bartova J. Neoplasma. 2006;53(1):19-25. **Key Finding:** "We investigated antigenotoxic and immunomodulatory effects of juices and vegetable homogenates (carrot+cauliflower, cauliflower, red cabbage, broccoli, onion, garlic) on the genotoxicity of AFB1 and pyro lysates of amino acids. All complete vegetable homogenates and substances of plant origin tested showed a clear antimutagenic and immunomodulatory activities on mutagenicity and immunosuppression induced by reference mutagens."

*Activation and potentiation of interferon-gamma signaling by 3,3'-diindolylmethane in MCF-7 **breast cancer** cells.* Riby JE, Xue L, Chatterji U, Bjeldanes EL, Firestone GL, Bjeldanes LF. Mol Pharmacol. 2006 Feb;69(2):430-9. **Key Finding:** "These results reveal novel immune activating and potentiating activities of DIM (from broccoli, cauliflower and Brussels sprouts) in human tumor cells that may contribute to the established effectiveness of this dietary indole against various tumor types."

*Crambene induces **pancreatic** acinar cell apoptosis via the activation of mitochondrial pathway.* Cao Y, Adhikari S, Ang AD, Clement MV, Wallig M, Bhatia M. Am J Physiol Gastrointest Liver Physiol. 2006 Jul;291(1):G95-G101. **Key Finding:** "These results provide evidence for the induction of pancreatic acinar cell apoptosis in vitro by crambene, (found in broccoli, cabbage, cauliflower, kale and Brussel sprouts) and suggest the involvement of mitochondrial pathway in pancreatic acinar cell apoptosis."

*Effect of cruciferous vegetables on **lung cancer** in patients stratified by genetic status: a mendelian randomization approach.* Brennan P, Hsu CC, Moulian N, Szeszenia-Dabrowska N, Lissowska J, Zaridze D, Rudnai P, Fabianova E, Mates D, Bencko V, Foretova L, Janout V, Gernigani F, Chabrier A, Hall J, Hung RJ, Boffetta P, Canzian F. Lancet. 2005 Oct 29-Nov 4;366(9496):1558-60. **Key Finding:** "These data provide strong evidence for a substantial protective effect of cruciferous vegetable consumption on lung cancer."

*Indole-3-carbinol and **prostate cancer**.* Sarkar FH, Li Y. J Nutr. 2004 Dec;134(12 Suppl):3493S-3498S. **Key Finding:** "Our studies have shown that indole-3-carbinol, a common phytochemical in cruciferous vegetables, up regulate the expression of phase I and phase II enzymes and can induce G1 cell cycle arrest and apoptosis in prostate cancer cells. The results from our laboratory and from others provide ample evidence for the benefit of I3C and DIM for the prevention and the treatment of prostate cancer."

The effect of cruciferous and leguminous sprouts on genotoxicity, in vitro and in vivo. Gill CI, Haidar S, Porter S, Matthews S, Sullivan S, Coulter J, McGlynn H, Rowland I. Cancer Epidemiol Biomarkers Prev. 2004 Jul;13(7):1199-205. **Key Finding:** "The results support the theory that consumption of cruciferous vegetables is linked to a reduced risk of **cancer** via decreased damage to DNA."

Cruciferous vegetable consumption alters the metabolism of the dietary carcinogen 2-amino-1-methyl-6-phenylimidazo[4,5-b]pyridine (PhIP) in humans. Walters DG, Young PJ, Agus C, Knize MG, Boobis AR, Gooderham NJ, Lake BG. Carcinogenesis. 2004 Sep;25(9):1659-69. **Key Finding:** "Consumption of red meat is associated with an increased risk of **colorectal cancer**, whereas cruciferous vegetable consumption reduces cancer risk. While the mechanisms remain to be determined, cruciferous vegetables may act by altering the metabolism of carcinogens present in cooked food. This study demonstrates that cruciferous vegetable consumption can induce both the phase I and II metabolism of PHP in humans."

*Sulforaphane inhibits growth of a **colon cancer** cell line.* Frydoonfar HR, McGrath DR, Spigelman AD. Colorectal Dis. 2004 Jan;6(1):28-31. **Key Finding:** "These findings may help explain the epidemiologically proven protective effect of cruciferous vegetables against colon cancer."

*Ingestion of an isothiocyanate metabolite from cruciferous vegetables inhibits growth of human **prostate cancer** cell xenografts by apoptosis and cell cycle arrest.* Chiao JW, Wu H, Ramaswamy G, Conaway CC, Chung FL, Wang L, Liu D. Carcinogenesis. 2004 Aug;25(8):1403-8. **Key Finding:** "This study demonstrates the first in vivo evidence of dietary phenethyl isothiocyanate (PEITC-NAC) inhibiting tumorigenesis of prostate cancer cells. PEITC-NAC may prevent initiation of carcinogenesis and modulates the post-initiation phase by targeting cell cycle regulators and apoptosis induction."

*Potent chemo preventive agents against **pancreatic cancer.*** Nishikawa A, Furukawa F, lee IS, Tankaka T, Hirose M. Curr Cancer Drug Targets. 2004 Jun;4(4):373-84. **Key Finding:** "Phenethyl isothiocyanate, a constituent of cruciferous vegetables, remarkably blocked the initiation phase of pancreatic as well as lung carcinogenesis in hamsters. However, PEITC failed to affect both pancreatic and lung carcinogenesis when given during the post-initiation (promotion) phase of carcinogenesis."

*Indole-3-carbinol induces a G1 cell cycle arrest and inhibits prostate-specific antigen production in human LNCaP **prostate carcinoma** cells.* Zhang J, Hsu BA, Kinseth BA, Bjeldanes LF, Firestone GL. Cancer. 2003 Dec 1;98(11):2511-20. **Key Finding:** "These findings implicate Indole-3-carbinol found in broccoli, cabbage and Brussels sprouts as a potential chemotherapeutic agent for controlling the growth of human prostate carcinoma cells."

*Reduction of **cancer** risk by consumption of selenium-enriched plants: enrichment of broccoli with selenium increases the anticarcinogenic properties of broccoli.* Finley JW. J Med Food. 2003 Spring;6(1):19-26. **Key Finding:** "Selenium from high-selenium broccoli decreased the incidence of aberrant crypts in rats with chemically induced colon cancer by more than 50%, compared with controls. Selenium from high-selenium broccoli also decreased the incidence of mammary tumors in rats treated with DMBA and tumor number and volume in APC(min) mice. These results suggest that development of methods to increase the natural accumulation of selenium in broccoli may greatly enhance its health-promoting properties."

Sulforaphane and 2-oxohexyl isothiocyanate induce cell growth arrest and apoptosis in L-1210 **leukemia** *and ME-18* **melanoma** *cells.* Misiewicz I, Skupinska K, Kasprzycka-Guttman T. Oncol Rep. 2003 Nov-Dec;10(6):2045-50. **Key Finding:** "Our results strongly suggest a chemo preventive activity toward cancer by the induction of apoptosis by sulforaphane and 2-oxohexyl isothiocyanate."

Sulforaphane inhibits extracellular, intracellular, and antibiotic-resistant strains of Helicobacter pylori and prevents benzo[a]pyrene-induced **stomach tumors**. Fahey JW, Haristoy X, Dolan PM, Kensler TW, Scholtus I, Stephenson KK, Talalay P, Lozniewski A. Proc Natl Acad Sci. 2002 May 28;99(11):7610-5. **Key Finding:** "The dual actions of sulforaphane in inhibiting Helicobacter infections and blocking gastric tumor formation offer hope that these mechanisms might function synergistically to provide diet-based protection against **gastric cancer** in humans."

Botanicals in **cancer** *chemoprevention.* Park EJ, Pezzuto JM. Cancer Metastasis Rev. 2002;21(3-4):231-55. **Key Finding:** "In this review, we discuss the cancer chemo preventive activity of cruciferous vegetables such as cabbage and broccoli, Allium vegetables such as garlic and onion, green tea, citrus fruits, tomatoes, berries, ginger and ginseng. Phytochemicals of these types have great potential in the fight against human cancer, and a variety of delivery methods are available as a result of their occurrence in nature."

Chemo protective glucosinolates and isothiocyanates of broccoli sprouts: metabolism and excretion in humans. Shapiro TA, Fahey JW, Wade KL, Stephenson KK, Talalay P. Cancer Epidemiol Biomarkers Prev. 2001 May;10(5):501-8. **Key Finding:** "Broccoli sprouts are a rich source of glucosinolates and isothiocyanates that induce phase 2 detoxication enzymes, boost antioxidant status, and protect animals against chemically induced cancer. When metabolized they are collectively designated dithiocarbamates. We studied the disposition of broccoli sprout glucosinolates and isothiocyanates in healthy volunteers. Dosing preparations included uncooked fresh sprouts (with active myrosinase) as well as boiled sprouts that were devoid of myrosinase activity. Dithiocarbamate excretion was higher when intact sprouts were chewed thoroughly rather than swallowed whole. Thorough chewing of fresh sprouts exposes the glucosinolates to plant myrosinase and significantly increases dithiocarbamate excretion."

Carotenoids and **colon cancer**. Slattery ML, Benson J, Curtin K, Ma KN, Schaeffer D, Potter JD. Am J Clin Nutr. 2000 Feb;71(2):575-82. **Key Finding:** "Lutein was inversely associated with colon cancer in both men and women studied. The major dietary sources of lutein in subjects with colon cancer and in control subjects were spinach, broccoli, lettuce, tomatoes, oranges and orange juice, carrots, celery, and greens. These data suggest that incorporating these foods into the diet may help reduce the risk of developing colon cancer."

Broccoli sprouts: An exceptionally rich source of inducers of enzymes that protect against chemical carcinogens. Fahey JW, Zhang Y, Talalay P. Proc Natl Acad Sci. 1997 Sept 16;94(19):10367-10372. **Key Finding:** Broccoli sprouts contain 30 to 50 times the concentration of isothiocyanates than mature broccoli plants. Isothiocyanates from the broccoli sprouts markedly reduced the incidence, size and number of **mammary tumors** in rats exposed to a standard carcinogen.

*Epidemiological studies on brassica vegetables and **cancer** risk.* Verhoeven DT, Goldbohm RA, Van Poppel G, Verhagen H, van den Brandt PA. Cancer Epidemiol Biomarkers Prev. 1996 Sep;5(9):733-48. **Key Finding:** "It is concluded that a high consumption of brassica vegetables is associated with a decreased risk of cancer. The association appears to be most consistent for lung, stomach, colon, and rectal cancer and least consistent for prostatic, endometrial, and ovarian cancer."

Bioactive organosulfur phytochemicals in Brassica oleracea vegetables – a review. Stoewsand GS. Food Chem Toxicol. 1995 Jun;33(6):537-43. **Key Finding:** "The **cancer chemo preventive** effects of Brassica vegetables that have been shown in human and animal studies may be due to the presence of both types of sulfur-containing phytochemicals (i.e. certain glucosinolates and S-methyl cysteine sulfoxide)."

*Chemo protection against **cancer** by Phase 2 enzyme induction.* Talalay P, Fahey JW, Holtzclaw WD, Prestera T, Zhang Y. Toxicol Lett. 1995 Dec;82-83:173-179. **Key Finding:** "Inducers are widely, but unequally, distributed among edible plants. Search for such inducer activity in broccoli led to the isolation of sulforaphane, an isothiocyanate that is a very potent Phase 2 enzyme inducer and blocks mammary tumor formation in rats."

Cardiovascular disease

Potential health benefits of broccoli—a chemico-biological review. Vasanthi HR, Mukherjee S, Das DK. Mini Rev Med Chem. 2009 Jun;9(6):749-59. **Key Finding:** "This review compiles the evidence for the beneficial role of glucosinolates. It also gives an overview on the chemical and biological characterization of potential bioactive compounds of broccoli including the interaction of phytochemicals on its bioactivity. The molecular basis of the biological activities of the chemicals present in broccoli potentially responsible for health promotion, from **chemoprevention** to **cardio protection**, are outlined based on in vitro and in vivo studies."

Vegetables, fruits and phytoestrogens in the prevention of diseases. Heber D. J Postgrad Med. 2004 Apr-Jun;50(2):145-9. **Key Finding:** "Consumers are advised to ingest one serving of each of the seven color groups daily. For instance, red foods contain lycopene which may be involved in maintaining **prostate** health and which has been linked to a decreased risk of **cardiovascular disease**. Green foods, including broccoli, Brussels sprouts and kale, have been associated with a decreased risk of cancer. White-green foods such as garlic may inhibit cancer cell growth. Grouping plants foods by color provides simplification, but it is also important as a method to help consumers make wise food choices and promote health."

*Flavonoid intake and the risk of **cardiovascular disease** in women.* Sesso HD, Gaziano JM, Liu S, Buring JE. Am J Clin Nutr. 2003 Jun;77(6):1400-6. **Key Finding:** "Women free of CVD and cancer participated in a prospective study using a food frequency questionnaire. Flavonoid intake was not strongly associated with a reduced risk of cardiovascular disease. The non-significant inverse associations for broccoli, apples, and tea with CVD were not mediated by flavonoids and warrant further study."

Gastritis

*Dietary sulforaphane-rich broccoli sprouts reduce colonization and attenuate **gastritis** in Helicobacter pylori-infected mice and humans.* Fahey YA, Fukumoto A, Nakayama M, Inoue S, Zhang S, Tauchi M, Suzuki H, Hyodo I, Yamamoto M. Cancer Prev Res. 2009 Apr;2(4):353-60. **Key Finding:** "Daily intake of sulforaphane-rich broccoli sprouts for 2 months reduces H. pylori colonization in mice and improves the sequelae of infection in infected mice and in humans. This treatment seems to enhance chemo protection of the gastric mucosa against H. pylori-induced oxidative stress."

Helicobacter pylori infection

*Oral **broccoli sprouts** for the treatment of Helicobacter pylori infection: a preliminary report.* Galan MV, Kishan AA, Silverman AL. Dig Dis Sci. 2004 Aug;49(7-8):1088-90. **Key Finding**: "Consumption of oral broccoli sprouts was temporarily associated with eradication of H. pylori infection in three of nine patients. Further studies are needed to determine the optimal dose of broccoli sprouts."

Hypertension

Dietary approach to decrease aging-related **CNS inflammation.** Noyan-Ashraf MH, Sadeghinejad Z, Juurlink BHJ. Nutr Neuro. 2005 Apr;8(2):101-110. **Key Finding:** "A diet of dried broccoli sprouts significantly decreased the aging-related degenerative changes in the **hypertensive stroke-**prone rat."

Dietary approach to attenuate oxidative stress, **hypertension,** *and* **inflammation** *in the cardiovascular system.* Wu L, Ashraf MHN, Facci M, Wang R, Paterson PG, Ferrie A, Juurlink BH. Proc Natl Acad Sci. 2004 May 4;101(18):7094-7099. **Key Finding:** "We conclude that a diet containing phase 2 protein inducers (from broccoli sprouts) also reduces the risk of developing cardiovascular problems of hypertension and atherosclerosis."

Stroke

Dietary approach to decrease aging-related **CNS inflammation.** Noyan-Ashraf MH, Sadeghinejad Z, Juurlink BHJ. Nutr Neuro. 2005 Apr;8(2):101-110. **Key Finding:** "A diet of dried broccoli sprouts significantly decreased the aging-related degenerative changes in the **hypertensive stroke-**prone rat."

Brussels Sprouts

A CULTIVAR OF THE SAME SPECIES AS CABBAGE AND BROCCOLI, brussels sprouts have been eaten at least since the time of ancient Rome, though their popularity throughout Europe can only be traced to the sixteenth century. Cultivation in the U.S. began in the early 1800s, thanks to French settlers in Louisiana.

They contain high levels of vitamin C (about 142% of the daily USDA allowance for adults in a 3.5 ounce serving) along with folate (vitamin B9), iron and phosphorus. Like other members of the cruciferous family, brussels sprouts have been shown in laboratory studies to possess phytochemicals useful in lowering the risks of various types of cancer.

Cancer (colon; lung; ovarian; pancreatic, prostate)

*Sulforaphane induces cell cycle arrest by protecting RB-E2F-1 complex in epithelial **ovarian cancer** cells.* Bryant CS, Kumar S, Chamala S, Et al. Mol Cancer. 2010 Mar 2;9:47. **Key Finding**: "Sulforaphane, a phytochemical present in Brussel sprouts and broccoli, induces growth arrest and apoptosis in epithelial ovarian cancer cells. Inhibition of retinoblastoma (RB) phosphorylation and reduction in levels of free E2F-1 appear to play an important role in growth arrest."

*Crambene induces **pancreatic** acinar cell apoptosis via the activation of mitochondrial pathway.* Cao Y, Adhikari S, Ang AD, Clement MV, Wallig M, Bhatia M. Am J Physiol Gastrointest Liver Physiol. 2006 Jul;291(1):G95-G101. **Key Finding:** "These results provide evidence for the induction of pancreatic acinar cell apoptosis in vitro by crambene, (found in broccoli, cabbage, cauliflower, kale and Brussel sprouts) and suggest the involvement of mitochondrial pathway in pancreatic acinar cell apoptosis."

*Effects of Brussels sprout juice on the cell cycle and adhesion of human **colorectal carcinoma** cells (HT29) in vitro.* Smith TK, Lund EK, Clarke RG, Bennett RN, Johnson IT. J Agric Food Chem. 2005 May 18;53(10):3895-901. **Key Finding:** "A variety of biologically active glucosinolate breakdown products are released by mechanical disruption of raw Brussels sprout tissue, but contrary to previous assumptions, alkyl isothiocyanate is not the main compound responsible for the inhibition of colorectal cell proliferation."

*Effect of cruciferous vegetables on **lung cancer** in patients stratified by genetic status: a mendelian randomization approach.* Brennan P, Hsu CC, Moulian N, Szeszenia-Dabrowska N, Lissowska J, Zaridze D, Rudnai P, Fabianova E, Mates D, Bencko V, Foretova L, Janout V, Gernigani F, Chabrier A, Hall J, Hung RJ, Boffetta P, Canzian F. Lancet. 2005 Oct 29-Nov 4;366(9496):1558-60. **Key Finding:** "These data provide strong evidence for a substantial protective effect of cruciferous vegetable consumption on lung cancer."

*Indole-3-carbinol and **prostate cancer**.* Sarkar FH, Li Y. J Nutr. 2004 Dec;134(12 Suppl):3493S-3498S. **Key Finding:** "Our studies have shown that indole-3-carbinol, a common phytochemical in cruciferous vegetables, up regulate the expression of phase I and phase II enzymes and can induce G1 cell cycle arrest and apoptosis in prostate cancer cells. The results from our laboratory and from others provide ample evidence for the benefit of I3C and DIM for the prevention and the treatment of prostate cancer."

***Chemoprevention** of 2-amino-3-methyllimidazo[4,5-f]quinoline (IQ)-induced colonic and hepatic preneoplastic lesions in the F344 rat by cruciferous vegetables administered simultaneously with the carcinogen.* Kassie F, Uhi M, Rabot S, Grasi-Kraupo B, Verkerk R, Kundi M, Chabicovsky M, Schulte-Hermann R, Knasmuller S. Carcinogenesis. 2003 Feb;24(2):255-61. **Key Finding:** "The induction effect of Brussels sprouts on the activity of UDPGT-2 was more marked than that of the red cabbage cultivars, suggesting that increased glucuronidation of IQ may account for the reduction of the preneoplastic lesions. Our findings support the assumption that Brassica vegetables protect against the carcinogenic effects of heterocyclic amines."

Effects of Brassica vegetable juice on the induction of apoptosis and aberrant crypt foci in rat colonic mucosal crypts in vivo. Smith TK, Mithen R, Johnson IT. Carcinogenesis. 2003 Mar;24(3):491-5. **Key Finding:** "In this study we explored the effects of both raw and thermally processed Brussels sprout tissue on the modulation of crypt cell apoptosis and mitosis, and the frequency of aberrant crypt foci in the colon. Freeze-dried raw and microwave-cooked Brussels sprouts contained high levels of intact glucosinolates, but they were absent from freshly prepared sprout juice. Oral administration of uncooked Brussels sprouts, whether as a juice or as a freeze-dried powder, was associated with significantly enhanced levels of apoptosis and reduced mitosis in the colonic crypts. We conclude that glucosinolate breakdown products derived from Brassica vegetables can exert a profound effect on the balance of **colorectal cell** proliferation and death in an animal model of colorectal neoplasia."

Cardiovascular disease

Vegetables, fruits and phytoestrogens in the prevention of diseases. Heber D. J Postgrad Med. 2004 Apr-Jun;50(2):145-9. **Key Finding:** "Consumers are advised to ingest one serving of each of the seven color groups daily. For instance, red foods contain lycopene which may be involved in maintaining **prostate** health and which has been linked to a decreased risk of **cardiovascular disease**. Green foods, including broccoli, Brussels sprouts and kale, have been associated with a decreased risk of cancer. White-green foods such as garlic may inhibit cancer cell growth. Grouping plants foods by color provides simplification, but it is also important as a method to help consumers make wise food choices and promote health."

Do dietary phytochemicals with cytochrome P-450 enzyme-inducing activity increase high-density lipoprotein concentrations in humans? Nanjee MN, Verhagen H, van Poppel G, Rompelberg CJ, Van Bladeren PJ, Miller NE. Am J Clin Nutr. 1996 Nov;64(5):706-11. **Key Finding:** "Low plasma concentrations of high-density lipoprotein are associated with increased risk of coronary heart disease. To test the hypothesis that phytochemicals with cytochrome P-450-inducing activity may also increase plasma HDL concentrations in humans, two controlled dietary trials were undertaken in healthy nonsmoking males. One study examined the effect of replacing 300 g glucosinolate-free vegetables with 300 g Brussels sprouts for 3 wk. The other study examined the effects of 150 mg eugenol in capsule form. There were no significant increases in plasma apo A-1, apo A-II, HDL cholesterol, or HDL phospholipids. These results suggest that dietary phytochemicals that induce members of the cytochrome P-450 system do not necessarily raise plasma HDL concentrations in humans."

Cabbage

IN THE SAME GENUS AS TURNIPS (*Brassica*), cabbage has been a food staple since the days of ancient Greece and Rome, where it was praised and used for its medicinal properties. It is the primary ingredient in Korean kimchee, German sauerkraut, and coleslaw. Most of the world's cabbage production occurs in China and India.

High in vitamin C and many of the B vitamins, cabbage was traditionally used in European folk medicine to treat all types of inflammation. In the late twentieth century this traditional use was affirmed in experiments that showed cabbage does indeed possess phytochemicals with anti-inflammatory properties useful in fighting cancer. Cabbage juice promotes the healing of peptic ulcers.

Antioxidation

Transcriptional regulation of anthocyanin biosynthesis in red cabbage. Yuan Y, Chiu LW, Li L. Planta. 2009 Nov;230(6):1141-53. **Key Finding**: "The color of red cabbage (Brassica oleracea var. capitata) is due to anthocyanin accumulation. The amount of total anthocyanins in red cabbage was found to be positively correlated with total antioxidant power, implicating the potential health benefit of red cabbage to human health."

Cancer (breast, pancreas, prostate, lung, stomach)

*1-Benzyl-indole-3-carbinol is a novel indole-3-carbinol derivative with significantly enhanced potency of anti-proliferative and anti-estrogenic properties in human **breast cancer** cells.* Nguyen HH, Lavrenov SN, Sundar SN, Et al. Chem Biol Interact. 2010 Aug 5;186(3):255-66. **Key Finding**: "Our results implicate 1-benzl-13C present in broccoli and cabbage as a novel, potent inhibitor of human breast cancer proliferation and estrogen responsiveness that could potentially be developed into a promising therapeutic agent for the treatment of indole-sensitive cancers."

Influence of fermentation conditions on glucosinolates, ascorbigen, and ascorbic acid content in white cabbage (Brassica oleracea var. capitata cv. Taler) cultivated in different seasons. Martinez-Villaluenga C, Penas E, Frias J, Ciska E, Honke J, Piskula MK, Kozlowskia H, Vidal-Valverde C. J Food Sci. 2009 Jan;74(1):C62-7. **Key Finding:** "The selection of cabbages with high glucobrassicin content and the production of low-sodium sauerkrauts may provide enhanced health benefits towards prevention of **chronic disease**."

*Lupeol, a novel anti-inflammatory and **anti-cancer** dietary triterpene.* Saleem M. Cancer Lett. 2009 Nov 28;285(2):109-15. **Key Finding**: "Lupeol, a triterpene found in green pepper, white cabbage, olive, strawberry, mangoes and grapes, was reported to possess beneficial effects as a therapeutic and preventive agent for a range of disorders. Lupeol at its effective therapeutic doses exhibit no toxicity to normal cells and tissues. This mini review provides detailed account of preclinical studies conducted to determine the utility of lupeol as a therapeutic and chemo preventive agent for the treatment of inflammation and cancer."

*Dietary isothiocyanates, glutathione S-transferase M1 (GSTM1), and **lung cancer** risk in African Americans and Caucasians from Los Angeles County, California.* Carpenter CL, Yu MC, London SJ. Nutr Cancer. 2009;61(4):492-9. **Key Finding**: "Isothiocyanates found in cruciferous vegetables such as cabbage and broccoli is anticarcinogenic. Isothiocyanates are protective for lung cancer risk."

*3, 3'-Diindolylmethane (DIM) induces a G (1) arrest in human **prostate cancer** cells irrespective of androgen receptor and p53 status.* Vivar OI, Lin CL, Firestone GL, Bideldanes LF. Biochem Pharmacol. 2009 Sep 1;78(5):469-76. **Key Finding**: "Our results indicate that DIM from Brassica vegetables is able to stop the cell cycle progression of human prostate cancer cells regardless of their androgen-dependence and p53 status, by differentially modulating cell cycle regulatory pathways."

Cancer chemo preventive agents: glucosinolates and their decomposition products in white cabbage (Brassica oleracea var. capitata). Smiechowska A, Bartoszek A, Namiesnik J. Postepy Hig Med Dosw (Polish). 2008 Apr 2;62:125-40. **Key Finding**: "A number of recent epidemiological studies have indicated that high intake of white cabbage may be associated with a lower risk of neoplastic diseases such as **cancer of the pancreas, breast, prostate, stomach and lungs.** The chemo preventive effects of cabbage may be connected with modulation of the activity of phase I and II detoxification enzymes and other mechanisms triggered by glucosinolates and products of their decomposition."

Induction of apoptosis in HT-29 cells by extracts from isothiocyanates-rich varieties of Brassica oleracea. Mas S, Crescenti A, Gasso P, Deulofeu R, Molina R, Ballesta A, Kensler TW, Lafuente A. Nutr Cancer. 2007;58(1):107-14. **Key Finding:** "Our results showed that isothiocyanate concentration and the chemo preventive responses of plant extracts vary among the varieties of Brassica Oleracea and among their cultivars. Purple cabbage extract showed the highest ITC concentration per gram, followed by black cabbage and Romanesque cauliflower. Brussels sprouts showed the strongest effects on cell viability and caspase-3 activity. All the extracts showed anticancer activity at ITC concentrations of between 3.54 to 7.08 mug/ml which are achievable in vivo."

*Current trends and perspectives in nutrition and **cancer** prevention.* Barta I, Smerak P, Polivkova Z, Sestakova H, Langova M, Turek B, Bartova J. Neoplasma. 2006;53(1):19-25. **Key Finding:** "We investigated antigenotoxic and immunomodulatory effects of juices and vegetable homogenates (carrot+cauliflower, cauliflower, red cabbage, broccoli, onion, garlic) on the genotoxicity of AFB1 and pyrolysates of amino acids. All complete vegetable homogenates and substances of plant origin tested showed a clear antimutagenic and immunomodulatory activities on mutagenicity and immunosuppression induced by reference mutagens."

Updates on Cancer Risk & Diet. Tuma RS. Oncology Times. 2006 Feb 10;28(3):29-30. **Key Finding:** "The large case-control Polish Women's Health Study found that women who consumed three or more servings of raw or short-cooked cabbage a week during adolescence had a **breast cancer** risk reduction of 72% relative to women who consumed fewer than 1.5 servings a week."

*Crambene induces **pancreatic** acinar cell apoptosis via the activation of mitochondrial pathway.* Cao Y, Adhikari S, Ang AD, Clement MV, Wallig M, Bhatia M. Am J Physiol Gastrointest Liver Physiol. 2006 Jul;291(1):G95-G101. **Key Finding:** "These results provide evidence for the induction of pancreatic acinar cell apoptosis in vitro by crambene, (found in broccoli, cabbage, cauliflower, kale and Brussel sprouts) and suggest the involvement of mitochondrial pathway in pancreatic acinar cell apoptosis."

Chinese cabbage extracts and sulforaphane can protect H2O2-induced inhibition of gap junctional intercellular communication through the inactivation of ERK1/2 and p38 MAP kinases. Hwang JW, Park JS, Jo EH, Kim SJ, Yoon BS, Kim SH, Lee YS, Kang KS. J Agric Food Chem. 2005 Oct 19;53(21):8205-10. **Key Finding:** "The results suggest that cruciferous vegetables and their components, sulforaphane glucosinolate, may exert the **anticancer** effect by targeting the GJIC (gap junctional intercellular communication) as a functional dietary chemo preventive agent."

*Comparison of lifestyle risk factors by family history for **gastric, breast, lung and colorectal cancer**.* Huang XE, Hirose K, Wakai K, Matsuo K, Ito H, Xiang J, Takezaki T, Tajima K. Asian Pac J Cancer Prev. 2004 Oct-Dec;5(4):419-27.

Key Finding: "Frequent intake of pumpkin, cabbage, lettuce and fruits and raw vegetables were associated with decreased risk for all four sites of cancer—gastric, breast, lung and colon."

*Indole-3-carbinol and **prostate cancer**.* Sarkar FH, Li Y. J Nutr. 2004 Dec;134(12 Suppl):3493S-3498S. **Key Finding:** "Our studies have shown that indole-3-carbinol, a common phytochemical in cruciferous vegetables, up regulate the expression of phase I and phase II enzymes and can induce G1 cell cycle arrest and apoptosis in prostate cancer cells. The results from our laboratory and from others provide ample evidence for the benefit of I3C and DIM for the prevention and the treatment of prostate cancer."

Antioxidant and antiproliferative activities of common vegetables. Chu YF, Sun J, Wu X, Liu RH. J Agric Food Chem. 2002 Nov 6;50(23):6910-6. **Key Finding:** "In this study, 10 common vegetables were selected on the basis of consumption per capita data in the U.S. Broccoli possessed the highest total phenolic content, followed by spinach, yellow onion, red pepper, carrot, cabbage, potato, lettuce, celery, and cucumber. Red pepper had the highest total antioxidant activity, followed by broccoli, carrot, spinach, cabbage, yellow onion, celery, potato, lettuce and cucumber. Antiproliferative activities were also studied in vitro using human liver cancer cells. Spinach showed the highest inhibitory effect, followed by cabbage, red pepper, onion, and broccoli."

*Botanicals in **cancer** chemoprevention.* Park EJ, Pezzuto JM. Cancer Metastasis Rev. 2002;21(3-4):231-55. **Key Finding:** "In this review, we discuss the cancer chemo preventive activity of cruciferous vegetables such as cabbage and broccoli, Allium vegetables such as garlic and onion, green tea, citrus fruits, tomatoes, berries, ginger and ginseng. Phytochemicals of these types have great potential in the fight against human cancer, and a variety of delivery methods are available as a result of their occurrence in nature."

*3,3'-Diindolylmethane (DIM) induces a G(1) cell cycle arrest in human **breast cancer** cells that is accompanied by Sp1-mediated activation of p21(WAF1/CIP1) expression.* Hong C, Kim HA, Firestone GL, Bjeldanes LF. Carcinogenesis. 2002 Aug;23(8):1297-305. **Key Finding**: "Our observations have uncovered an antiproliferative pathway for DIM (from Brassica food plants) that implicates Sp1/Sp3-induced expression of p21 as a target for cell cycle control in human breast cancer cells."

Ulcers

*Rapid Healing Of **Peptic Ulcers** In Patients Fed Fresh Cabbage Juice.* Cheney G. Calif Med. 1949 Jan;70(1):10-15. **Key Finding:** "Thirteen patients with peptic ulcer were treated with fresh cabbage juice, which contains an antipeptic ulcer factor. The average crater healing time for six patients with gastric ulcer treated with cabbage juice was 7.3 days, compared with 42 days, as reported in the literature, for six patient treated with other therapy. The rapid healing of peptic ulcers observed radiologically and gastroscopically with fresh cabbage juice indicates an anti-peptic ulcer dietary factor."

Cinnamon

NATIVE TO SRI LANKA, THE COUNTRY FORMERLY KNOWN AS CEYLON, cinnamon is a spice obtained from the bark of a small evergreen tree. Two similar species are *Cassia* and *Cinnamomum burmannii*, which also go by the name of cinnamon.

Cinnamon has a long culinary history. Numerous mentions of the spice are made in the Old Testament of the Bible, as both a perfume and a spice. It was considered valuable throughout antiquity and was used by the pharaohs in Egypt at least 4,000 years ago, though traders tried to keep its actual source a closely guarded secret to keep demand and price for it high.

Its medicinal value was affirmed in late twentieth century medical studies that showed it to be beneficial in treating diabetes and insulin resistance. It also has value as an immune system booster and treatment for cardiovascular disease and hypertension.

Alzheimer's disease

Cinnamon extract inhibits tau aggregation associated with Alzheimer's disease in vitro. Peterson DW, George RC, Scaramozzino F, LaPointe NE, Anderson RA, Graves DJ, Lew J. Alzheimer's Dis. 2009 Jul;17(3):585-97. **Key Finding**: "This work shows that compounds endogenous to cinnamon may be beneficial to Alzheimer's disease or may guide the discovery of other potential therapeutics if their mechanisms of action can be discerned."

Anti-Inflammatory

Anti-inflammatory *activities of essential oils and their constituents from different provenances of indigenous* ***cinnamon*** *(Cinnamomum osmophloeum) leaves.* Tung YT, Yen PL, Lin CY, Chang ST. Pharm Biol. 2010 Oct;48(10):1130-6. **Key Finding**: "These findings demonstrate that the leaf essential oils and their constituents of C. osmophloeum have excellent anti-inflammatory activities and thus have great potential as a source of natural health products."

Anti-inflammation activities of essential oil and its constituents from indigenous cinnamon (Cinnamomum osmophloeum) twigs. Tung YT, Chua MT, Wang SY, Chang ST. Bioresour Tchnol. 2008 Jun;99(9):3908-13. **Key Finding**: "These findings demonstrated that essential oil of C. osmophloeum twigs have excellent anti-inflammatory activities and thus have great potential to be used as a source for natural health products."

Antioxidation

Antioxidant effects of a cinnamon extract in people with impaired fasting glucose that are over-weight or obese. Roussel AM, Ininger I, Benaraba R, Ziegenfuss TN, Anderson RA. J Am Coll Nutr. 2009 Feb;28(1):16-21. **Key Finding**: "This study supports the hypothesis that the inclusion of water soluble cinnamon compounds in the diet could reduce risk factors associated with diabetes and cardiovascular disease."

Cancer (cervical; colon; leukemia; lymphoma; melanoma)

Cinnamon extract induces tumor cell death through inhibition of NFkappaB and AP1. Kwon HK, Hwang JS, So JS, Et al. BMC Cancer. 2010 Jul 24;10:392. **Key Finding**: "In this study, we tested anti-tumor activity and elucidated action mechanism of **cinnamon** extract using various types of tumor cell lines including **lymphoma, melanoma, cervix cancer and colorectal cancer** in vitro and in vivo mouse melanoma model. Cinnamon extracts strongly inhibited tumor cell proliferation in vitro and induced active cell death of tumor cells."

*Aqueous cinnamon extract (ACE-c) from the bark of Cinnamomum cassia causes apoptosis in human **cervical cancer** cell line (SiHa) through loss of mitochondrial membrane potential.* Koppikar SJ, Choudhari AS, Suryavanshi SA, Et al. BMC Cancer. 2010 May 18;10:210. **Key Finding**: "Cinnamon alters the growth kinetics of SiHa cervical cancer cells in a dose-dependent manner. Cells treated with cinnamon exhibited reduced number of colonies compared to the control cells."

The cinnamon-derived dietary factor cinnamic aldehyde activates the Nrf2-dependent antioxidant response in human epithelial colon cells. Wondrak GT, Villeneuve NF, Lamore SD, Et al. Molecules. 2010 May 7;15(5):3338-55. **Key Finding**: "Taken together our data demonstrate that the cinnamon-derived food factor is a potent activator of the NrF2-orchestrated antioxidant response in cultured human epithelial colon cells. Cinnamon may therefore represent an underappreciated chemo preventive dietary factor targeting **colorectal carcinogenesis.**"

A polyphenol mixture from cinnamon targets p38 MAP kinase-regulated signaling pathways to produce G2/M arrest. Schoene NW, Kelly MA, Polansky MM, Anderson RA.

J Nutr Biochem. 2009 Aug;20(8):614-20. **Key Finding**: "The data provide evidence that aqueous extract of cinnamon significantly modulated two signaling proteins, p38 MAPK and cyclin B, that regulate progression through G2/M in three **leukemic** cell lines."

Cinnamon extract suppresses tumor progression by modulating angiogenesis and the effector function of CD8+cells. Kwon HK, Jeon WK, Hwang JS, Lee CG, So JS, Park JA, Ko BS, Im SH. Cancer Lett. 2009 Jun 18;278(2):174-82. **Key Finding**: "In vitro and in vivo system cinnamon treatment strongly inhibited the expression of pro-angiogenic factors and master regulators of tumor progression not only in **melanoma** cell lines but also in experimental melanoma model."

*The cinnamon-derived Michael acceptor cinnamic aldehyde impairs **melanoma** cell proliferation, invasiveness, and tumor growth.* Cabello CM, Bair WB, Lamore SD, Ley S, Bause AS, Azimian S, Wondrak GT. Free Radic Biol Med. 2009 Jan 15;46(2):220-31. **Key Finding**: "These findings support a previously unrecognized role of a cinnamon-derived dietary as a Michael acceptor with potential anti-cancer activity."

*Growth inhibition of human **colon cancer** cells by plant compounds.* Duessel S, Heuertz RM, Ezekiel UR. Clin Lab Sci. 2008 Summer;21(3):151-7. **Key Finding**: "The purpose of this study was to determine if resveratrol from red grapes, cinnam-aldehyde from cinnamon, and piperine from black pepper has anti-proliferative effects on colon cancer. All phytochemicals displayed anti-proliferative effects on DLD-1 colon cancer cells in culture. These results taken together with everyday dietary availability of concentrations used in this study strongly suggest that regular intake of low doses of these phytochemicals offer preventive effects against colon cancer."

Water-soluble polymeric polyphenols from cinnamon inhibit proliferation and alter cell cycle distribution patterns of hematologic tumor cell lines. Schoene NW, Kelly MA, Polansky MM, Anderson RA. Cancer Lett. 2005 Dec 8;230(1):134-40. **Key Finding**: "To explore possible anti-cancer properties of water-soluble, polymeric poly-phenols from cinnamon, three myeloid cell lines (Jurkat, Wurzburg, and U937) were exposed to increasing concentrations of an aqueous extract prepared from cinnamon for 24h. Cell growth and cell cycle distribution patterns responded in a dose-dependent manner to cinnamon extract."

Antimicrobial and chemo preventive properties of herbs and spices. Lai PK, Roy J. Curr Med Chem. 2004 Jun;11(11):1451-60. **Key Finding:** "A growing body of research has demonstrated that the commonly used herbs and spices such as garlic, black cumin, cloves, cinnamon, thyme, allspices, bay leaves, mustard and rosemary, possess antimicrobial properties that, in some cases, can be used therapeutically. Other spices, such as saffron, turmeric, green or black tea and flaxseed do contain potent phytochemicals, including carotenoids, curcumins, catechins, lignin, which provide significant protection against **cancer.**

Cardiovascular disease

Antioxidant effects of a cinnamon extract in people with impaired fasting glucose that are overweight or obese. Roussel AM, Hininger I, Benaraba R, Ziegenfuss TN, Anderson RA. J Am Coll Nutr. 2009 Feb;28(1):16-21. **Key Finding:** "Twenty-two subjects with impaired fasting blood glucose with BMI ranging from 25 to 45, were enrolled in a double-blind placebo-controlled trial. This study supports the hypothesis that the inclusion of water soluble cinnamon compounds in the diet could reduce risk factors associated with **diabetes** and **cardiovascular disease**."

Effects of a water-soluble cinnamon extract on body composition and features of the metabolic syndrome in pre-diabetic men and women. Ziegenfuss TN, Hofheins JE, Mendel RW, Landis J, Anderson RA. Int Soc Sports Nutr. 2006 Dec 28;3:45-53. **Key Finding:** "These data support the efficacy of Cinnulin (a water-soluble cinnamon extract) on reducing fasting blood glucose and systolic blood pressure and improving body composition in men and women with the metabolic syndrome and suggest that this naturally-occurring spice can reduce risk factors associated with **diabetes** and **cardiovascular diseases**."

Diabetes

Cinnamon*: potential role in the prevention of insulin resistance, metabolic syndrome, and* **type 2 diabetes***.* Qin B, Panickar KS, Anderson RA. J Diabetes Sci Technol. 2010 May 1;2(3):685-93. **Key Finding:** "Metabolic syndrome is associated with insulin resistance, elevated glucose and lipids, inflammation, decreased antioxidant activity, increased weight gain, and increased glycation of proteins. Cinnamon has been shown to improve all of these variables in vitro, animal, and/or human studies. Components of cinnamon may be important in the alleviation and prevention of signs and symptoms of metabolic syndrome, type 2 diabetes, and cardiovascular and related diseases."

Glycated hemoglobin and blood pressure-lowering effect of **cinnamon** *in multi-ethnic* **Type 2 diabetic** *patients in the UK: a randomized, placebo-controlled, double-blind* *clinical trial.* Akilen R, Tsiami A, Devendra D, Robinson N. Diabet Med. 2010 Oct;27(10):1159-67. **Key Finding**: "Intake of 2g of cinnamon for 12 weeks significantly reduces the HbA1c, SBP and DBP among poorly controlled type 2 diabetes patients. Cinnamon supplementation could be considered as an additional dietary supplement option to regulate blood glucose and **blood pressure** levels along with conventional medications to treat type 2 diabetes mellitus."

Effects of 1 and 3 g cinnamon on gastric emptying, satiety, and postprandial blood glucose, insulin, glucose-dependent insulinotropic polypeptide, glucagon-like peptide 1, and ghrelin concentrations in healthy subjects. Hlebowicz J, Hlebowicz A, Lindstedt S, Bjorgell O, Hoglund P, Holst JJ, Darwiche G, Almer LO. Am J Clin Nutr. 2009 Mar;89(3):815-21. **Key Finding:** "Ingestion of 3 g cinnamon reduced postprandial **serum insulin** and increased GLP-1 concentrations without significantly affecting blood glucose, GIP, the ghrelin concentration, satiety, or GER in health subjects. The results indicate a relation between the amount of cinnamon consumed and the decrease in insulin concentration."

Changes in **glucose tolerance and insulin sensitivity** *following 2 weeks of daily cinnamon ingestion in healthy humans.* Solomon TP, Blannin AK. Eur J Appl Physiol. 2009 Apr;105(6):969-76. **Key Finding:** "Eight male volunteers underwent two 14-day intervention involving cinnamon or placebo supplementation. Cinnamon ingestion reduced the glucose response to oral flucose tolerance tests (OGTT) on day 1 (-13.1 +/-6.3% vs. day 0;P<0.05) and day 14 (-5.5 +/- 8.1% vs. day 0 P=0.09). Cinnamon ingestion also reduced insulin responses to OGTT on day 14 as well as improving insulin sensitivity on day 14. These effects were lost following cessation of cinnamon feeding. Cinnamon may improve glycemic control and insulin sensitivity."

Antioxidant effects of a cinnamon extract in people with impaired fasting glucose that are over-weight or obese. Roussel AM, Hininger I, Benaraba R, Ziegenfuss TN, Anderson RA. J Am Coll Nutr. 2009 Feb;28(1):16-21. **Key Finding:** "Twenty-two subjects with impaired fasting blood glucose with BMI ranging from 25 to 45, were enrolled in a double-blind placebo-controlled trial. This study supports the hypothesis that the inclusion of water soluble cinnamon compounds in the diet could reduce risk factors associated with **diabetes** and **cardiovascular disease**."

Effectiveness of cinnamon for lowering hemoglobin A1C in patients with type 2 diabetes: a randomized, controlled trial. Crawford P. J Am Board Fam Med. 2009 Sep-Oct;22(5):507-12. **Key Finding**: "Taking cinnamon could be useful for lowering serum HbA1C in type 2 diabetes with HbA1c>7.0 in addition to usual care."

The potential of cinnamon to reduce blood glucose levels in patients with type 2 diabetes and insulin resistance. Kirkham S, Akilen R, Sharma S, Tsiami A. Diabetes Obes Metab. 2009 Dec;11(12):1100-13. **Key Finding**: "Whilst definitive conclusions cannot be drawn regarding the use of cinnamon as an antidiabetic therapy, it does possess antihyperglycaemic properties and potential to reduce postprandial blood glucose levels."

Cinnamon extract inhibits the postprandial overproduction of apolipoprotein B48-containing lipoproteins in fructose-fed animals. Qin B, Polansky MM, Sato Y, Adeli K, Anderson RA. Nutr Biochem. 2009 Nov;20(11):901-8. **Key Finding**: "We present both in vivo and ex vivo evidence that a cinnamon extract improves the postprandial over-production of intestinal apoB48-containing lipoproteins by ameliorating intestinal insulin resistance and may be beneficial in the control of lipid metabolism"

Hypoglycemic activity of a polyphenolic oligomer-rich extract of Cinnamonum parthenoxylon bark in normal and streptozotocin-induced diabetic rats. Jia Q, Liu X, Wu X, Wang R, Hu X, Li Y, Huang C. Phytomedicine. 2009 Aug;16(8):744-50. **Key Finding**: "Cinnamon bark has been reported to be effective in the alleviation of diabetes through its antioxidant and insulin-potentiating activities. These results suggest that Cinnamomum parthenoxylon polyphenol rich extract could be potentially useful for post-prandial hyperglycemia treatment."

Chromium and polyphenols from cinnamon improve insulin sensitivity. Anderson RA. Proc Nutr Soc. 2008 Feb;67(1):48-53. **Key Finding**: "In a double-blind placebo-controlled study it has been demonstrated that glucose, insulin, cholesterol and HbA1c are all improved in patients with type 2 diabetes following chromium supplementation. It has also been shown that cinnamon polyphenols improve insulin sensitivity in in vitro, animal and human studies. Cinnamon reduces mean fasting serum glucose (18-29%), TAG (23-30%), total cholesterol (12-26%) and LDL-cholesterol (7-27%) in subjects with type 2 diabetes after 40 d of daily consumption of 1-6 g cinnamon. Subjects with the metabolic syndrome who consume an aqueous extract of cinnamon have been shown to have improved fasting blood glucose, systolic blood pressure, and percentage of body fat and increased lean body mass compared with the placebo group. Studies utilizing an aqueous extract of cinnamon, high in type A polyphenols, have also demon-strated improvements in fasting glucose, glucose tolerance and insulin sensitivity in women with insulin resistance associated with the polycystic ovary syndrome."

Effect of cinnamon on glucose control and lipid parameters. Baker WL, Gutierrez-Williams G, White CM, Kluger J, Coleman CI. Diabetes Care. 2008 Jan;31(1):41-3. **Key**

Finding: "A systematic literature search through July 2007 was conducted to identify randomized placebo-controlled trials of cinnamon that reported data on AlC, fasting blood glucose (FBG), or lipid parameters. Five prospective trials were identified. Upon meta-analysis, the use of cinnamon did not significantly alter A1C, FBG, or lipid parameters. Cinnamon does not appear to improve A1C, FBG, or lipid parameters in patients with **type 1 or type 2 diabetes**."

Cinnamon Supplementation in Patients with **Type 2 Diabetes** *Mellitus.* Pham AQ, Kourlas H, Pham DQ. Pharmacotherapy. 2007 Apr;27(4):595-599. **Key Finding:** "We conducted a literature search limited to English-language human studies. We found two prospective, randomized, double-blind, placebo-controlled peer-reviewed clinical trials and one prospective, placebo-controlled, peer-reviewed clinical trial that evaluated the efficacy of cinnamon supplementation in patients with type 2 diabetes. Two of the studies reported modest improvements in lowering blood glucose levels with cinnamon supplementation. One trial showed no significant differences between cinnamon and placebo. Overall, cinnamon was well tolerated. These data suggest that cinnamon has a possible modest effect in lowering plasma glucose levels in patients with poorly controlled type 2 diabetes."

The effect of cinnamon on A1C among adolescents with type 1 **diabetes**. Altschuler JA, Casella SJ, MacKenzie TA, Curtis KM. Diabetes Care. 2007 Apr;30(4):813-6. **Key Finding:** "Cinnamon is not effective for improving glycemic control in adolescents with type 1 diabetes."

Effect of cinnamon on postprandial **blood glucose,** *gastric emptying, and satiety in healthy subjects.* Hlebowicz J, Darwiche G, Bjorgell O, Almer LO. Am J Clin Nutr. 2007 Jun;85(6):1552-6. **Key Finding:** "The intake of 6 g cinnamon with rice pudding reduces postprandial blood glucose and delays gastric emptying without affecting satiety. Inclusion of cinnamon in the diet lowers the postprandial glucose response, a change that is at least partially explained by a delayed gastric emptying rate."

Effects of a cinnamon extract on plasma glucose, HbA1c, and serum lipids in **diabetes mellitus type 2**. Mang B, Wolters M, Schmitt B, Kelb K, Lichtinghagen R, Stichtenoth DO, Hahn A. Eur J Clin Inves. 2006 May;36(5). **Key Finding:** "The cinnamon extract seems to have a moderate effect in reducing fasting plasma glucose concentrations in diabetic patients with poor glycemic control."

Effects of a water-soluble cinnamon extract on body composition and features of the metabolic syndrome in pre-diabetic men and women. Ziegenfuss TN, Hofheins JE, Mendel RW,

Landis J, Anderson RA. Int Soc Sports Nutr. 2006 Dec 28;3:45-53. **Key Finding**: "These data support the efficacy of Cinnulin (a water-soluble cinnamon extract) on reducing fasting blood glucose and systolic blood pressure and improving body composition in men and women with the metabolic syndrome and suggest that this naturally-occurring spice can reduce risk factors associated with **diabetes** and **cardiovascular diseases**."

Cinnamon Improves Glucose and Lipids of People With **Type 2 Diabetes**. Khan A, Safdar M, Ali Khan MM, Khattak KN, Anderson RA. Diabetes Care. 2003 Dec;26(12):3215-8. **Key Finding:** "The results of this study demonstrate that intake of 1,3 or 6 g of cinnamon per day reduces serum glucose, triglyceride, LDL cholesterol, and total cholesterol in people with type 2 diabetes and suggest that the inclusion of cinnamon in the diet will reduce risk factors associated with diabetes and **cardiovascular diseases**."

A Hydroxychalcone Derived from Cinnamon Functions as a Mimetic for Insulin in 3T3-L1 Adipocytes. Jarvill-Taylor KJ, Anderson RA, Graves DJ. Am Coll Nutr. 2001;20(4):327-336. **Key Finding:** "These results demonstrate that the MHCP is an effective mimetic of insulin. MHCP may be useful in the treatment of insulin resistance and in the study of the pathways leading to glucose utilization in cells."

HIV

HIV type-1 entry inhibitors with a new mode of action. Fink RC, Roschek B Jr, Alberte RS. Antivir Chem Chemother. 2009;19(6):243-55. **Key Finding:** "Optimized elderberry, green tea and cinnamon extracts rich in certain flavonoid compounds were shown to block HIV-1 entry and infection in GHOST cells."

Hypertension

Glycated hemoglobin and blood pressure-lowering effect of **cinnamon** *in multi-ethnic* **Type 2 diabetic** *patients in the UK: a randomized, placebo-controlled, double-blind clinical trial.* Akilen R, Tsiami A, Devendra D, Robinson N. Diabet Med. 2010 Oct;27(10):1159-67. **Key Finding**: "Intake of 2g of cinnamon for 12 weeks significantly reduces the HbA1c, SBP and DBP among poorly controlled type 2 diabetes patients. Cinnamon supplementation could be considered as an additional dietary supplement option to regulate blood glucose and **blood pressure** levels along with conventional medications to treat type 2 diabetes mellitus."

Whole cinnamon and aqueous extracts ameliorate sucrose-induced **blood pressure** *elevations in spontaneously hypertensive rats.* Preuss HG, Echard B, Polansky MM, Anderson R. J Am Coll Nutr. 2006 Apr;25(2):144-50. **Key Finding:** "Blood pressure regulation may not only be influenced favorably by limiting the amounts of dietary substances that have negative effects on BP and insulin function, but also by the addition of beneficial ones, such as cinnamon, that have positive effects."

Immune System

Cinnamon polyphenol extract affects immune responses by regulating anti- and proinflammatory and glucose transporter gene expression in mouse macrophages. Cao H, Urban JF Jr, Anderson RA. J Nutr. 2008 May;138(5):833-40. **Key Finding:** "These results suggest that cinnamon polyphenol extract can affect immune responses by regulating anti- and proinflammatory and GLUT gene expression."

Obesity

Targeting inflammation-induced **obesity** *and metabolic diseases by curcumin and other nutraceuticals.* Aggarwal BB. Annu Rev Nutr. 2010 Aug 21;30:173-99. **Key Finding**: "Curcumin-induced alterations reverse insulin resistance, hyperglycemia, hyperlipidemia and other symptoms linked to obesity. Other structurally homologous nutraceuticals, derived from red **chili, cinnamon, cloves, black pepper and ginger**, also exhibit effects against obesity and insulin resistance."

Cranberries

TRADITIONAL THANKSGIVING MENUS IN NORTH AMERICA typically include cranberries, which are produced by low, creeping shrubs that grow wild in acidic bogs. Native Americans are believed to have been the first humans to use cranberries, employing them as both a food source and a medicine. Starting in the early nineteenth century, cranberries were exported to Europe.

Cranberries are typically processed into such products as sauces and juices, which tends to lower their nutrient levels. Raw cranberries, however, possess a wide range of healing phytochemicals and other nutrients which make it one of the top ten super foods for health. At least sixteen health conditions from arthritis to urinary tract infections have been shown in medical science studies to be treatable or preventable by cranberry consumption, including thirteen forms of cancer.

Aging

Prolongevity effects of an oregano and cranberry extract are diet dependent in the Mexican fruit fly (Anastrepha ludens). Zou S, Carey JR, Lideo P, Et al. J Gerontol A Sci Med Sci. 2010 Jan;65(1):41-50. **Key Finding**: "This study reveals the prolongevity effects of oregano and cranberry mixture and supports the emerging view that benefits botanicals on aging."

A double-blinded, placebo-controlled, randomized trial of the neuropsychologic efficacy of cranberry juice in a sample of cognitively intact older adults: pilot study findings. Crews WD, Harrison DW, Griffin ML, Addison K, Yount AM, Giovenco MA, Hazell J. J Altern Complement Med. 2005 Apr;11(2):305-9. **Key Findings:** "The aim of this research was to conduct the first known clinical trial of the short-term (i.e. 6 weeks) efficacy of cranberry juice on the **neuropsychological functioning** of cognitively intact older adults. Taken together, no significant interactions were found between the cranberry and placebo groups and their pretreatment baseline and end-of-treatment phase standardized neuropsychological assessments. A non-significant trend was noted, however, on a subjective, self-report questionnaire where twice as many participants in the cranberry group rated their overall abilities to remember by treatment end as 'improved' compared to placebo controls."

Antioxidation

Antioxidant levels of common fruits, vegetables, and juices versus protective activity against in vitro **ischemia**/*reperfusion.* Bean H, Schuler C, Leggett RE, Levin RM. Int Urol Nephrol. 2009 Sep 19. (Epub ahead of print). **Key Finding:** "An assay was utilized to determine the antioxidant reactivity of a series of fruits, vegetables, and juices, and the results were compared to the protective ability of selected juices in an established in vitro rabbit bladder model of ischemia/reperfusion. The results showed that cranberry juice had the highest level of antioxidant reactivity, blueberry juice had an intermediate activity, and orange juice had the lowest. It was determined, however, that contrary to the hypothesis, the orange juice was significantly more potent in protecting the bladder against ischemia/reperfusion damage than either blueberry or cranberry juice."

Cranberries and cranberry products: powerful in vitro, ex vivo, and in vivo sources of **antioxidants.** Vinson JA, Bose P, Proch J, Al Kharrat H, Samman N. J Agric Food Chem. 2008 Jul 23;56(14):5884-91. **Key Finding:** "We investigated the effect of the consumption of high fructose corn syrup (HFCS) and ascorbate with cranberry juice antioxidants or without cranberry juice (control) given to 10 normal individuals after an overnight fast. Plasma antioxidant capacity, glucose, triglycerides, and ascorbate were measured 6 times over 7 h after the consumption of a single 240 mL serving of the two different beverages. The control HFCS caused a slight decrease in plasma antioxidant capacity at all-time points and thus an oxidative stress in spite of the presence of ascorbate. Cranberry juice produced an increase in plasma antioxidant capacity that was significantly greater than control HFCS at all-time points. Postprandial triglycerides, due to fructose in the beverages, were mainly responsible for the oxidative stress and were significantly correlated with the oxidative stress as measured by the antioxidant capacity."

Cranberry juice increases antioxidant status without affecting **cholesterol** *homeostasis in orchidectomized rats.* Deyhim F, Patil BS, Villarreal A, Lopez E, Garcia K, Rios R, Garcia C, Gonzales C, Mandadi K. J Med Food. 2007 Mar;10(1):49-53. **Key Finding:** "Drinking cranberry juice did not affect cholesterol concentrations in liver and in plasma. Triglyceride concentration in plasma of orchidectomized rats that were drinking cranberry juice increased, but its concentration in liver decreased to the level of shams. The protective effect of cranberry juice from oxidative damage may be mediated by a decrease in nitrate + nitrite and dose-dependent decrease in peroxidation."

Cranberry juice improved antioxidant status without affecting bone quality in orchidectomized male rats. Villarreal A, Stoecker BJ, Garcia C, Garcia K, Rios R, Gonzales C, Mandadi K, Faraji B, Patil BS, Deyhim F. Phytomedicine. 2007 Dec;14(12):815-20. **Key Finding:** "Cranberry juice increases plasma antioxidant status without affecting bone quality."

*Protective effects of cranberries on infection-induced oxidative renal damage in a rabbit model of **vasico-ureteric reflux**.* Han CH, Kim SH, Kang SH, Shin OR, Lee HK, Kim HJ, Cho YH. BJU Int. 2007 Nov;100(5):1172-5. **Key Finding:** "This study shows that cranberries have an anti-inflammatory effect through their anti-oxidant function and might prevent infection-induced oxidative renal damage. Thus, clinically cranberries might be used as a beneficial adjuvant treatment to prevent damage due to pyelonephritis in children with vesico-ureteric reflux."

***Antioxidant** and antiproliferative activities of common fruits.* Sun J, Chu YF, Wu X, Liu RH. J Agric Food Chem. 2002 Dec 4;50(25):7449-54. **Key Finding:** "Phyto-chemicals, especially phenolic, in fruits and vegetables are suggested to be the major bioactive compound for the health benefits associated with reduced risk of chronic diseases such as **cardiovascular disease** and **cancer**. Cranberry had the highest total phenolic content, followed by apple, red grape, strawberry, pineapple, banana, peach, lemon, orange, pear, and grapefruit. Cranberry had the highest total antioxidant activity followed by apple, red grape, strawberry, peach, lemon, pear, banana, orange, grapefruit and pineapple. Antiproliferation activities were also studied in vitro using HepG(2) human liver-cancer cells, and cranberry showed the highest inhibitory effect followed by lemon, apple, straw-berry, red grape, banana, grapefruit and peach."

Effects of blueberry and cranberry juice consumption on the plasma antioxidant capacity of healthy female volunteers. Pedersen CB, Kyle J, Jenkinson AM, Gardner PT, McPhail DB, Duthie GG. Eur J Clin Nutr. 2000 May;54(5):405-8. **Key Finding:** "Consumption of cranberry juice resulted in a significant increase in the ability of plasma to reduce potassium nitrosodisulphonate and Fe(III)-2,4,6-Tri(2-pyridyl)-s-triazine, these measures of antioxidant capacity attaining a maximum after 60-120 min. This corresponded to a 30% increase in vitamin C and a small but significant increase in total phenols in plasma. Consumption of blueberry juice had no such effects."

Antiviral effects

Antiviral effects on bacteriophages and rotavirus by cranberry juice. Lipson SM, Sethi L, Cohen P, Gordon RE, Tan IP, Burdowski A, Stotzky G. Phytomedicine. 2007 Jan;14(1):23-30. **Key Finding:** "The data suggest, for the first time, a non-specific antiviral effect towards unrelated viral species (vis., bacteriophages T2 and T4 and the simian rotavirus SA-11) by a commercially available cranberry fruit juice drink."

Arthritis and (rheumatoid arthritis)

*Natural products as a gold mine for **arthritis** treatment.* Khanna D, Sethi G, Ahn KS, Pandey MK, Kunnumakkara AB, Sung B, Aggarwal A, Aggarwal BB. Curr Opin Pharmacol. 2007 Jun;7(3):344-51. **Key Finding:** "The large numbers of inexpensive natural products that can modulate inflammatory responses, but lack side effects, constitute 'goldmines' for the treatment of arthritis. Numerous agents derived from plants can suppress cell signaling intermediates, including curcumin, resveratrol, cranberries and peanuts, tea polyphenols, genistein, quercetin from onions, silymarin from artichoke."

***Rheumatoid arthritis** is an autoimmune disease triggered by Proteus urinary tract infection.* Ebringer A, Rashid T. Clin Dev. Immunol. 2006 Mar;13(1):41-8. **Key Finding:** "Extensive evidence based on the results of various microbial, immunological and molecular studies from different parts of the world, shows that a strong link exists between Proteus mirabilis microbes and rheumatoid arthritis. We propose that sub-clinical Proteus urinary tract infections are the main triggering factors. Patients with rheumatoid arthritis, especially during the early stages of the disease, could benefit from Proteus anti-bacterial measures including high intake of fruit juices such as cranberry."

***Rheumatoid arthritis**: proposal for the use of anti-microbial therapy in early cases.* Ebringer A, Rashid T, Wilson C. Scand J Rheumatol. 2003;32(1):2-11. **Key Finding:** "Our working hypothesis is that rheumatoid arthritis develops as a result of repeated episodes of Proteus upper urinary tract infections. Antibiotics, high fluid intake, and fruit extracts, such as cranberry juice, have all been found to be effective in the treatment of urinary tract infections. Such measures could be used as possible additional adjuncts to the standard therapy."

Atherosclerosis

Cranberry flavonoids, **atherosclerosis** *and cardiovascular health.* Reed J. Crit Rev Food Sci Nutr. 2002;42(3 Suppl):301-16. **Key Finding:** "This article reviews the literature on the effects of flavonoids on atherosclerosis with an emphasis on the potential effects of the flavonols and proanthocyanidin in cranberries."

Cancer (bladder; brain; breast; colon; esophageal; gastric; lung; lymphoma; oral; ovarian; prostate; skin; stomach)

Proanthocyanidin from the American Cranberry (Vaccinium macrocarpon) inhibit matrix metalloproteinase-2 and matrix metalloproteinase-9 activity in **human prostate cancer** *cells via alterations in multiple cellular signaling pathways.* Deziel BA, Patel K, Neto C, Gottschall-Pass K, Hurta RA. J Cell Biochem. 2010 Oct 15;111(3):742-54. **Key Finding**: "It is believed that an individual's diet affects his risk of developing prostate cancer. In this study we document the effects of proanthocyanidin from the American Cranberry on MMP activity in DU145 human prostate cancer cells. Cranberry decreased cellular viability of DU145 cells at a concentration of 25 ug/ml by 30% after 6 hour of treatment."

Bioactive compounds in cranberries and their biological properties. Cote J, Cailet S, Doyon G, Sylvain JF, Lacroix M. Crit Rev Food Sci Nutr. 2010 Aug;50(7):666-79. **Key Finding**: "Numerous phytochemicals present in cranberries – the anthocyanin, the flavonols, the flaven-3-ols, the proanthocyanidin, and the phenolic acid derivatives. The presence of these phytochemicals appears to be responsible for the cranberry property of preventing many diseases and infections, including **cardiovascular diseases, various cancers, and infections** involving the urinary tract, dental health, and Helicobacter pylori-induced stomach ulcers and cancers."

Cranberry proanthocyanidin are cytotoxic to human cancer cells and sensitize platinum-resistant **ovarian cancer** *cells to paraplatin.* Singh AP, Singh RK, Kim KK, Satyan KS, Nussbaum R, Torres M, Brard L, Vorsa N. Phytother Res. 2009 Aug;23(8):1066-74. **Key Finding:** "Polyphenol extracts of the principal flavonoid classes present in cranberry were screened in vitro for cytotoxicity against solid tumor cell lines, identifying two fractions composed principally of proanthocyanidin with potential anticancer activity."

Cranberry phytochemical extract inhibits SGC-7901 cell growth and human tumor xenografts in Balb/c nu/nu mice. Liu M, Lin LQ, Song BB, Wang LF, Zhang CP, Zhao JL,

Liu JR. J Agric Food Chem. 2009 Jan 28;57(2):762-8. **Key Finding:** "Cranberry extract possesses potent antioxidant capacity and antiproliferative activity against cancer in vitro and in vivo. The objectives of this study were to determine whether the cranberry extract inhibited proliferation of human **gastric cancer** SGC-7901 cells and human gastric tumor xenografts in the Balb/c nu/nu mouse. Cranberry extract at doses of 0, 5, 10, 20, and 40 mg/mL significantly inhibited proliferation of SGC-7901 cells, and this suppression was partly attributed to decreased PCNA expression and apoptosis induction. In a human tumor xenograft model, the time of human gastric tumor xenografts in the mouse was delayed in a dose-dependent manner."

*The effect of a novel botanical agent TBS-101 on invasive **prostate cancer** in animal models.* Evans S, Dizeyi N, Abrahamsson PA, Persson J. Anticancer Res. 2009 Oct;29(10):3917-24. **Key Finding:** "The natural botanical agent TBS-101 (containing Panax ginseng, cranberry, green tea, grape skin, grape seed, Ganoderma lucdum and chamomile) has a good safety profile and significant anti-cancer activities in hormone-refractory PC-3 cells and large aggressive PC-3 tumors in a xenograft mouse model and has great potential for the treatment of aggressive prostate cancer."

*Cranberry proanthocyanidin induce apoptosis and inhibit acid-induced proliferation of human **esophageal adenocarcinoma** cells.* Kresty LA, Howell AB, Baird M. J Agric Food Chem. 2008 Feb 13;56(3):676-80. **Key Finding:** "This study sought to investigate the chemo preventive potential of a cranberry proanthocyanidin rich extract in SEG-1 human esophageal adenocarcinoma cells. The extract pretreatment significantly inhibited the viability and proliferation of EAC cells in a time and dose-dependent manner. Moreover, the extract significantly inhibited acid-induced cell proliferation of SEG-1 cells. Extract treatment induced cell cycle arrest at the G1 checkpoint and significantly reduced the percentage of SEG-1 cells in S-phase following 24 and 48 h of exposure. Extract treatment also resulted in significant induction of apoptosis."

*Effect of cranberry juice concentrate on chemically-induced urinary **bladder cancers**.* Prasain JK, Jones K, Moore R, Barnes S, Leahy M, Roderick R, Juliana MM, Grubbs CJ. Oncol Rep. 2008 Jun;19(6):1565-70. **Key Finding:** "The chemopreventive efficacy of cranberry juice concentrate in an experimental model of urinary bladder cancer was evaluated using female Fischer-344 rats. These data suggest that components of cranberries may be effective in preventing urinary bladder carcinogenesis."

Anticancer activities of cranberry phytochemicals: an update. Neto CC, Amoroso JW, Liberty AM. Mol Nutr Food Res. 2008 Jun;52 Suppl 1:S18-27. **Key Finding:** "Studies employing mainly vitro tumor models show that extract and compounds isolated from cranberry fruit inhibit the growth and proliferation of several types of tumor including **breast, colon, prostate**, and **lung**. Proanthocyanidin oligomers, flavonol and anthocyanin glycosides and triterpenoids are all likely contributors to the observed anticancer properties and may act in a complementary fashion to limit carcinogenesis."

Cranberry juice constituents impair lymphoma growth and augment the generation of anti-lymphoma antibodies in syngeneic mice. Hochman N, Houri-Haddad Y, Koblinski J, Wahl L, Roniger M, Bar-Sinai A, Weiss EI, Hochman J. Nutr Cancer. 2008;60(4):511-7. **Key Finding:** "Here we show that a fraction (nondialyzable material (NDM) of a molecular weight range 12,000-30,000 derived from cranberry juice impairs in vitro growth and invasion through extracellular matrix of Rev-2-T-6 murine lymphoma cells. Furthermore, intraperitoneal injection of this fraction at nontoxic doses both inhibits the growth of Rev-2-T-6 tumors in vivo and enhances the generation of antilymphoma antibodies. These findings demonstrate the in vivo efficacy of cranberry components against **malignant lymphoma** in immune competent hosts."

*Cranberry and Grape Seed Extracts Inhibit the Proliferative Phenotype of **Oral Squamous Cell Carcinomas**.* Chatelain K, Phippen S, McCabe J, Teeters CA, O'Malley S, Kingsley K. Evid Based Complement Alternat Med. 2008 Jul 23. (Epub ahead of print). **Key Finding:** "This study represents one of the first comparative investigations of cranberry and grape seed extracts and their anti-proliferative effects on oral cancers. These observations provide evidence that cranberry and grape seed extracts not only inhibit oral cancer proliferation but also that the mechanism of this inhibition may function by triggering key apoptotic regulators in these cell lines."

*Cranberry and its phytochemicals: a review of in vitro **anticancer** studies.* Neto CC. J Nutr. 2007 Jan;137(1 Suppl):186S-193S. **Key Finding:** "The unique combination of phytochemicals found in cranberry fruit may produce synergistic health benefits. Possible chemo preventive mechanisms of action by cranberry phytochemicals include induction of apoptosis in tumor cells, reduced ornithine decarboxylase activity, decreased expression of matrix metalloproteinase associated with prostate tumor metastasis, and anti-inflammatory activities including inhibition of cyclooxygenases."

*Inhibition of **cancer** cell proliferation and suppression of TNF-induced activation of NFkappaB by edible berry juice.* Boivin D, Blanchette M, Barrette S, Moghrabi A, Beliveau R. Anticancer Res. 2007 Mar-Apr;27(2):937-48. **Key Finding:** "These results illustrate that berry juices have striking differences in their potential chemo preventive activity and that the inclusion of a variety of berries in the diet might be useful for preventing the development of tumors. The growth of various cancer cell lines, including those of **stomach, prostate, intestine and breast**, was strongly inhibited by raspberry, black currant, white currant, gooseberry, velvet leaf blueberry, low-bush blueberry, sea buckthorn and cranberry juice, but not (or only slightly) by strawberry, high-bush blueberry, serviceberry, red currant, or blackberry juice."

Flavonoids and Vitamin E Reduce the Release of the Angiogenic Peptide Vascular Endothelial Growth Factor from Human Tumor Cells. Schindler R, Mentlein R. J Nutr. 2006 Jun;136:1477-1482. **Key Finding:** "The rank order of inhibitory potency on MDA human breast cancer cells was naringin>rutin>a-tocopheryl succinate>lo vastatin>apigenin>genistein>a-tocopherol>kaempferol. Chrysin and curcumin were inactive except at a concentration of 100 umol/L. Overall, the glycosylated flavonoids (i.e. naringin, a constituent of citrus fruits, and rutin, a constituent of cranberries) induced the greatest response to treatment at the lowest concentration in MDA human **breast cancer** cells. Inhibition of VEGF release by flavonoids, tocopherols, and lovastatin suggests a novel mechanism for mammary cancer prevention."

*Blackberry, black raspberry, blueberry, cranberry, red raspberry, and strawberry extracts inhibit growth and stimulate apoptosis of human **cancer** cells in vitro.* Seeram NP, Adams LS, Zhang Y, Lee R, Sand D, Scheuller HS, Heber D. J Agric Food Chem. 2006 Dec 13;54(25):9329-39. **Key Finding:** "The berry extracts were evaluated for their ability to inhibit the growth of human **oral, breast, colon and prostate tumor cell** lines at concentrations ranging from 25 to 200 micro g/ml. With increasing concentration of berry extract, increasing inhibition of cell proliferation in all of the cancer cell lines was observed, with different degrees of potency between cell lines. The berry extracts were also evaluated for their ability to stimulate apoptosis of the COX-2 expressing **colon cancer** cell line, HT-29. Black raspberry and strawberry extracts showed the most significant pro-apoptotic effects against this cell line."

*Cranberry phytochemical extracts induce cell cycle arrest and apoptosis in human MCF-7 **breast cancer** cells.* Sun J, Hai Liu R. Cancer Lett. 2006 Sep 8;241(1):124-

34. **Key Finding:** "These results suggest that cranberry phytochemical extracts possess the ability to suppress the proliferation of human breast cancer MCF-7 cells at doses of 5 to 30mg/ml, and this suppression is at least partly attributed to both the initiation of apoptosis and the G1 phase arrest."

The effects of cranberry juice consumption on antioxidant status and biomarkers relating to **heart disease** *and* **cancer** *in healthy human volunteers.* Duthie SJ, Jenkinson AM, Crozier A, Mullen W, Pirie L, Kyle J, Yap LS, Christen P, Duthie GG. Eur J Nutr. 2006 Mar;45(2):113-22. **Key Finding:** "Cranberry juice consumption did not affect 8-oxo-deoxyguanosine in urine or endogenous or $H(2)O(2)$-induced DNA damage in lymphocytes. Cranberry juice consumption did not alter blood or cellular antioxidant status or several biomarkers of lipid status pertinent to heart disease. Similarly, cranberry juice had no effect on basal or induced oxidative DNA damage. These results show the importance of distinguishing between the in vitro and in vivo antioxidant activities of dietary anthocyanin in relation to human health."

In vivo inhibition of growth of human **tumor** *lines by flavonoid fractions from cranberry extract.* Ferguson PJ, Kurowska EM, Freeman DJ, Chambers AF, Koropatnick J. Nutr Cancer. 2006;56(1):86-94. **Key Finding:** "As model systems for testing cranberry flavonoid activity, human tumor cells lines representative of three malignancies were chosen: glioblastoma multiforme (U87), **colon carcinoma** (HT-29), and androgen-independent **prostate carcinoma** (DU145). A falvonoid-rich fraction 6 (Fr6) and a more purified proanthocyanidin (PAC)-rich fraction were isolated from cranberry press cake and whole cranberry, respectively. Fr6 and PAC each significantly slowed the growth of explant tumors of U87 in vivo, and PAC inhibited growth of HT-29 and DU145 explants, inducing complete regression of two Du145 tumor explants. Flow cytometric analyses of in vitro-treated U87 cells indicated that Fr6 and PAC could arrest cells in G1 phase of the cell cycle ($P<0.05$) and also induce cell death within 24 to 48 h of exposure. These results indicate the presence of a potential anticancer constituent in the flavonoid-containing fractions from cranberry extracts."

Total cranberry extract versus its phytochemical constituents: antiproliferative and synergistic effects against human **tumor cell** *lines.* Seeram NP, Adams LS, Hardy ML, Heber D. J Agric Food Chem. 2004 May 5;52(9):2512-7. **Key Finding:** "All cranberry fractions were evaluated against human **oral, colon, and prostate cancer** cell lines. The total polyphenol fractions was the most effective against all cell lines with 96.1 and 95% inhibition of KB and CAL27 oral cancer cells, respectively. For the colon cancer cells, the antiproliferative activity of this fraction was greater against HCT116 (92.1%) than against HT-29 (61.1%), SW480 (60%) and SW620 (63%). The enhanced antiproliferative activity of total polyphenols compared to total cranberry extract and its individual phytochemicals suggests synergistic or additive antiproliferative interactions of the anthocyanin, proanthocyanidin, and flavonol glycosides within the cranberry extract."

A flavonoid fraction from cranberry extract inhibits proliferation of human tumor cell lines. Ferguson PJ, Kurowska E, Freeman DJ, Chambers AF, Koropatnick DJ. J Nutr. 2004 Jun;134(6):1529-35. **Key Finding:** "Cranberry press cake (the material remaining after squeezing juice from the berries) when fed to mice bearing human **breast tumor** MDA-MB-435 cells, was shown previously to decrease the growth and metastasis of tumors. Further studies were undertaken to isolate the components of cranberry that contributed to this anticancer activity and determine the mechanisms by which they inhibited proliferation. Using standard chromatographic techniques, a warm-water extract of cranberry press cake was fractionated and an acidified methanol eluate (Fraction 6, or Fr6) containing flavonoids demonstrated antiproliferative activity. The extract inhibited proliferation of 8 human tumor cell lines of multiple origins. The androgen-dependent **prostate** cell line LNCaP was the most sensitive of those tested (10 mg/L Fr6 inhibited its growth by 50%.) Other human tumor lines originating from **breast** (MCF-7), **skin** (SK-MEL-5), **colon** (HT-29), **lung** (DMS114), and **brain** (U87) had intermediate sensitivity to Fr6."

A randomized trial of cranberry versus apple juice in the management of **urinary symptoms** *during external beam radiation therapy for* **prostate cancer**. Campbell G, Picles T, D'yachkova Y. Clin Oncol (R Coll Radiol). 2003 Sep;15(6):322-8. **Key Finding:** "One hundred and twelve men with prostate cancer were randomized to either 354 ml cranberry juice or apple juice a day. We observed no significant differences for DRT related to the consumption of cranberry compared with apple juice. However, we found a significant difference between the history of a previous transurethral resection of prostate that was associated with lower values for both end points."

Antioxidant *and antiproliferative activities of common fruits.* Sun J, Chu YF, Wu X, Liu RH. J Agric Food Chem. 2002 Dec 4;50(25):7449-54. **Key Finding:** "Phytochemicals, especially phenolic, in fruits and vegetables are suggested to be the major bioactive compound for the health benefits associated with reduced risk of chronic diseases such as **cardiovascular disease** and **cancer**. Cranberry had the highest total phenolic content, followed by apple, red grape, strawberry, pineapple, banana, peach, lemon, orange, pear, and grapefruit. Cranberry had the highest total antioxidant activity followed by apple, red grape, strawberry, peach, lemon, pear, banana, orange, grapefruit and pineapple. Antiproliferation activities were also studied in vitro using HepG(2) human liver-cancer cells, and cranberry showed the highest inhibitory effect followed by lemon, apple, strawberry, red grape, banana, grapefruit and peach."

Composition of a chemo preventive proanthocyanidin-rich fraction from cranberry fruits responsible for the inhibition of 12-O-tetradecanoyl phorbol-13-acetate (TPA)-induced ornithine decarboxylase (ODC) activity. Kandil FE, Smith MA, Rogers RB, Pepin MF, Song LL, Pezzuto JM, Seigler DS. J Agric Food Chem. 2002 Feb 27;50(5):1063-9. **Key Finding:** "Antioxidant activity was not restricted to a particular class of components in the extract but was found in a wide range of the fractions. Significant chemo preventive activity, as indicated by an ornithine decarboxylase assay, was localized in one particular proanthocyanidin-rich fraction. Further fractionation of the active **anticarcinogenic** fraction revealed the following components: seven flavonoids, mainly quercetin, myricetin, the corresponding 3-O-glycosides, (-)-epicatechin, (+)-catechin, and dimers of both gallocatechin and spigallocatechin types, and a series of oligomeric proanthocyanidin."

*Antioxidant activities and **antitumor** screening of extracts from cranberry fruit (Vaccinium macrocarpon).* Yan X, Murphy BT, Hammond GB, Vinson JA, Neto CC. J Agric Food Chem. 2002 Oct 9;50(21):5844-9. **Key Finding:** "Extracts of whole fruit were assayed for radical-scavenging activity and tumor growth inhibition using seven tumor cell lines. Selective inhibition of K562 and HT-29 cells was observed from a methanolic extract in the range of 16-125 microg/ml. Radical-scavenging activity was greatest in an extract composed primarily of flavonol glycosides. Most of the flavonol glycosides showed antioxidant activity comparable or superior to that of vitamin E."

*In vitro anti**cancer** activity of fruit extracts from Vaccinium species.* Bomser J, Madhavi DL, Singletary K, Smith MA. Planta Med. 1996 Jun;62(3):212-6. **Key Finding:** "Components of the hexane/chloroform fraction of bilberry and of the proanthocyanidin fraction of low bush blueberry, cranberry, and lingonberry exhibit potential anticarcinogenic activity as evaluated by in vitro screening tests. The concentrations of these crude extracts needed to inhibit ornithine decarboxylase activity by 50% were 8.0 (low bush blueberry) 7.0 (cranberry) 9.0 micrograms (lingonberry.)"

Cardiovascular disease

Bioactive compounds in cranberries and their biological properties. Cote J, Cailet S, Doyon G, Sylvain JF, Lacroix M. Crit Rev Food Sci Nutr. 2010 Aug;50(7):666-79. **Key Finding**: "Numerous phytochemicals present in cranberries – the anthoycanins, the flavonols, the flaven-3-ols, the proanthocyanidin, and the phenolic acid derivatives. The presence of these phytochemicals appears to be responsible for the cranberry property of preventing many diseases and infections, including **cardiovascular diseases, various cancers, and infections** involving the urinary tract, dental health, and Helicobacter pylori-induced stomach ulcers and cancers."

Effects of a flavonol-rich diet on select **cardiovascular** *parameters in a Golden Syrian hamster model.* Kalgaonkar S, Gross HB, Yokoyama W, Et al. J Med Food. 2010 Feb;13(1):108-15. **Key Finding**: "Results obtained from this study support the concept that the chronic consumption of a flavonoid-rich diet from cranberries can be beneficial with respect to cardiovascular health."

Low-calorie cranberry juice supplementation reduces plasma oxidized LDL and cell adhesion molecule concentrations in men. Ruel G, Pomerleau S, Couture P, Lemieux S, Lamarche B, Couillard C. Br J Nutr. 2008 Feb;99(2):352-9. **Key Finding:** "Elevated circulating concentrations of oxidized LDl and cell adhesion molecules are considered to be relevant markers of oxidative stress and endothelial activation which are implicated in the development of **cardiovascular disease**. Thirty men consumed increasing daily doses of cranberry juice cocktail (125, 250 and 500 ml/d) over three successive periods of 4 weeks. We noted a significant decrease in plasma OxLDL concentrations following the intervention. We also found that plasma ICAM-1 and VCAM-1 concentrations decreased significantly during the course of the study."

(Vaccinium macrocarpon) and **cardiovascular disease** *risk factors.* **Cranberries** McKay DL, Blumberg JB. Nutr Rev. 2007 Nov;65(11):490-502. **Key Finding:** "A growing body of evidence suggests that polyphenols, including those found in cranberries, may contribute to reducing the risk of cardiovascular disease by increasing the resistance of LDL to oxidation, inhibiting platelet aggregation, reducing blood pressure, and via other anti-thrombotic and anti-inflammatory mechanisms."

Evidence of the cardio protective potential of fruits: the case of cranberries. Ruel G, Couillard C. Mol Nutr Food Res. 2007 Jun;51(6):692-701. **Key Finding:** "Consumption of cranberries or their related products could be of importance not only in the maintenance of health but also in preventing **cardiovascular disease**. This review presents evidence supported for the most part by clinical observations that cranberries can exert potentially healthy effects for your heart."

Cranberry and blueberry: evidence for protective effects against **cancer** *and* **vascular diseases**. Neto CC. Mol Nutr Food Res. 2007 Jun;51(6):652-64. **Key Finding:** "Growing evidence from tissue culture, animal, and clinical models suggests that the flavonoid-rich fruits of the North American cranberry and blueberry have the potential ability to limit the development and severity of certain cancers and vascular diseases including **atherosclerosis**, **ischemic stroke**, and neurode-generative **diseases of aging**."

Cranberries (Vaccinium macrocarpon) and **cardiovascular disease** *risk factors.* McKay DL, Blumberg JB. Nutr Rev. 2007 Nov;65(11):490-502. **Key Finding:** "A growing body of evidence suggests that polyphenols, including those found in cranberries, may contribute to reducing the risk of cardiovascular disease by increasing the resistance of LDL to oxidation, inhibiting platelet aggregation, reducing blood pressure, and via other anti-thrombotic and anti-inflammatory mechanisms."

Evidences of the **card protective** *potential of fruits: the case of cranberries.* Ruel G, Couillard C. Mol Nutr Food Res. 2007 Jun;51(6):692-701. **Key Finding:** "Consumption of cranberries or their related products could be of importance not only in the maintenance of health but also in preventing **cardiovascular disease**. This review presents evidences supported for the most part by clinical observations that cranberries can exert potentially healthy effects for your heart."

Cranberries (Vaccinium macrocarpon) and **cardiovascular disease** *risk factors.* McKay DL, Blumberg JB. Nutr Rev. 2007 Nov;65(11):490-502. **Key Finding:** "A growing body of evidence suggests that polyphenols, including those found in cranberries, may contribute to reducing the risk of cardiovascular disease by increasing the resistance of LDL to oxidation, inhibiting platelet aggregation, reducing blood pressure, and via other anti-thrombotic and anti-inflammatory mechanisms."

Cranberries inhibit **LDL** *oxidation and induce LDL receptor expression in hepatocytes.* Chu YF, Liu RH. Life Sci. 2005 Aug 26;77(15):1892-901. **Key Finding:** "Cranberries were evaluated for their potential roles in dietary prevention of **cardiovascular disease**. Cranberry extracts were found to have potent antioxidant capacity preventing in vitro LDL oxidation with increasing delay and suppression of LDL oxidation in a dose dependent manner. We propose that additive or synergistic effects of phytochemicals in cranberries are responsible for the inhibition of LDL oxidation, the induced expression of LDL receptors, and the increased uptake of cholesterol in hepatocytes."

Changes in plasma antioxidant capacity and oxidized low-density lipoprotein levels in men after short-term cranberry juice consumption. Ruel G, Pomerleau S, Couture P, Lamarche B, Coullard C. Metabolism. 2005 Jul;54(7):856-61. **Key Finding:** "Our results show that short-term cranberry juice supplementation is associated with significant increase in plasma antioxidant capacity and reduction in circulating OxLDL concentrations. Although the physiological relevance of our observations needs to be further examined, our study supports the potential role of antioxidant-rich foods in maintaining health and preventing **cardiovascular disease**."

***Antioxidant** and antiproliferative activities of common fruits.* Sun J, Chu YF, Wu X, Liu RH. J Agric Food Chem. 2002 Dec 4;50(25):7449-54. **Key Finding:** "Phytochemicals, especially phenolics, in fruits and vegetables are suggested to be the major bioactive compound for the health benefits associated with reduced risk of chronic diseases such as **cardiovascular disease** and **cancer**. Cranberry had the highest total phenolic content, followed by apple, red grape, strawberry, pineapple, banana, peach, lemon, orange, pear, and grapefruit. Cranberry had the highest total antioxidant activity followed by apple, red grape, strawberry, peach, lemon, pear, banana, orange, grapefruit and pineapple. Antiproliferation activities were also studied in vitro using HepG(2) human liver-cancer cells, and cranberry showed the highest inhibitory effect followed by lemon, apple, strawberry, red grape, banana, grapefruit and peach."

Cholesterol

*Cranberry juice increases antioxidant status without affecting **cholesterol** homeostasis in orchidectomized rats.* Deyhim F, Patil BS, Villarreal A, Lopez E, Garcia K, Rios R, Garcia C, Gonzales C, Mandadi K. J Med Food. 2007 Mar;10(1):49-53. **Key Finding:** "Drinking cranberry juice did not affect cholesterol concentrations in liver and in plasma. Triglyceride concentration in plasma of orchidectomized rats that were drinking cranberry juice increased, but its concentration in liver decreased to the level of shams. The protective effect of cranberry juice from oxidative damage may be mediated by a decrease in nitrate + nitrite and dose-dependent decrease in peroxidation."

Favorable impact of low-calorie cranberry juice consumption on plasma HDL-cholesterol concentrations in men. Ruel G, Pemerleau S, Couture P, Lemieux S, Lamarche B, Couillard C. Br J Nutr. 2006 Aug;96(2):357-64. **Key Finding:** "The present results show that daily cranberry juice cocktail consumption is associated with an increase in plasma HDL-cholesterol concentrations in abdominally obese men. We hypothesize that polyphenol compounds from cranberries may be responsible for this effect, supporting the notion that the consumption of flavonoid-rich foods can be **cardio protective**."

Cranberries inhibit LDL oxidation and induce LDL receptor expression in hepatocytes. Chu YF, Liu RH. Life Sci. 2005 Aug 26;77(15):1892-901. **Key Finding:** "The antioxidant activity of 100 g cranberries against LDL oxidation was equivalent to 1000 mg vitamin C or 3700 mg vitamin E. Cranberry extracts also significantly induced expression of hepatic LDL receptors and increased intracellular uptake of cholesterol in HepG2 cells in vitro in a dose-dependent manner. This suggests that cranberries could enhance clearance of excessive plasma **cholesterol** in circulation. We propose that additive or synergistic effects of phytochemicals in cranberries are responsible for the inhibition of LDL oxidation, the induced expression of LDL receptors, and the increased uptake of cholesterol in hepatocytes."

Cranberry extract inhibits low density lipoprotein oxidation. Wilson T, Porcari JP, Harbin D. Life Sci. 1998;62(24):PL381-6. **Key Finding:** "The effect of cranberry juice on **heart disease** has not been investigated. We evaluated how a cranberry extract affected low density lipoprotein oxidation. This study suggests that cranberry extracts have the ability to inhibit the oxidative modification of LDL particles."

Colitis

*Preventive effect of a pectic polysaccharide of the common cranberry Vaccinium oxycoccos L. on acetic acid-induced **colitis** in mice.* Popov SV, Markov PA, Nikitina IR, Petrishev S, Smirnov V, Ovodov YS. World J Gastroenterol. 2006 Nov 7;12(41):6646-51. **Key Finding:** "A preventive effect of pectin from the common cranberry, namely oxycoccusan OP, on acetic acid-induced colitis in mice was detected. A reduction of neutrophil infiltration and antioxidant action may be implicated in the protective effect of oxycoccusan."

Diabetes

Glycemic responses to sweetened dried and raw cranberries in humans **with type 2 diabetes**. Wilson T, Luebke JL, Morcomb EF, Et al. J Food Sci. 2010 Oct;75(8):H218-23. **Key Finding**: "This study compares phenolic content and glycemic responses among different cranberry products. Sweetened dried cranberries containing less sugar were associated with a favorable glycemic and insulinemic response in type 2 diabetics."

Potential of cranberry powder for management of hyperglycemia using in vitro models. Pinto MS, Ghaedian R, Shinde R, Shetty K. J Med Food. 2010 Oct;13(5):1036-44. **Key Finding**: "These in vitro results indicate the potential of cranberry powders as dietary supplement and food-based strategies for potential hyperglycemia management."

Human glycemic response and phenolic content of unsweetened cranberry juice. Wilson T, Singh AP, Vorsa N, Goettl CD, Kittleson KM, Roe CM, Kastello GM, Ragsdale FR. J Med Food. 2008 Mar;11(1):46-54. **Key Finding:** "This study suggests that the consumption of low-calorie cranberry juice in previously uncharacterized trimer and heptamer proanthocyanidin is associated with a favorable glycemic response and may be beneficial for persons with **impaired glucose tolerance.**"

Favorable glycemic response of **type 2 diabetics** *to low-calorie cranberry juice.* Wilson T, Meyers SL, Singh AP, Limburg PJ, Vorsa N. J Food Sci. 2008 Nov;73(9):H241-5. **Key Finding:** "Relative to conventionally sweetened preparation, unsweetened low-calorie cranberry juice provides a favorable metabolic response and should be useful for promoting increased fruit consumption among type 2 diabetics."

Effect of cranberry extracts on lipid profiles in subjects with **Type 2 diabetes**. Lee IT, Chan YC, Lin CW, Lee WJ, Sheu WH. Diabet Med. 2008 Dec;25(12):1473-7. **Key Finding:** "Cranberry supplements are effective in reducing atherosclerotic cholesterol profiles, including LDL cholesterol and total cholesterol levels, as well as total HDL cholesterol ratio, and has a neutral effect on glycemic control in Type 2 diabetic subjects taking oral glucose-lowering agents."

Potential of cranberry-based herbal synergies for **diabetes** *and* **hypertension** *management.* Apostolidis E, Kwon YI, Shetty K. Asia Pac J Clin Nutr. 2006;15(3):433-41. **Key Finding:** "Water soluble cranberry-based phytochemical combinations with oregano, rosemary, and Rhodiola rosea were evaluated for total phenolic content, related antioxidant activity and inhibition of diabetes management-related alpha-glucosidase, pancreatic alpha-amylase inhibition, and hypertension-related ACE-I inhibitory activities. The 75% cranberry and 25% oregano combinations had the highest phenolic among all combinations tested; that same combination also had the highest DPPH radical inhibition activity, and the highest ACE-I inhibitory activity. By bringing together synergistic combinations to cranberry, health beneficial functionality was enhanced. This enhanced functionality in terms of high alpha-glycosidase and alpha-amylase inhibitory activities indicate the potential for diabetes management, and high ACE-I inhibitory activity indicates the potential for hypertension management."

Potential of cranberry-based phytochemical synergies for **diabetes** *and* **hypertension** *management.* Kwon YI, Lin YT, Shetty K. Department of Food Science, University of Massachusetts. 2005; http://ift.confex.com/direct/ift/2005/techprogram/paper_29028.htm. **Key Finding:** "There is a synergistic inhibitory effect of various phytochemical combinations on above enzyme activities. These findings indicate that cranberry-based phytochemical synergies have potential as functional ingredients in the dietary management of diabetes and hypertension."

Hypertension

Potential of cranberry-based herbal synergies for **diabetes** *and* **hypertension** *management.* Apostolidis E, Kwon YI, Shetty K. Asia Pac J Clin Nutr. 2006;15(3):433-41. **Key Finding:** "Water soluble cranberry-based phytochemical combinations with oregano, rosemary, and Rhodiola roses were evaluated for total phenolic content, related antioxidant activity and inhibition of diabetes management-related alpha-glycosidase, pancreatic alpha-amylase inhibition, and hypertension-related ACE-I inhibitory activities. The 75% cranberry and 25% oregano combinations had the highest phenolic among all combinations tested; that same combination also had the highest DPPH radical inhibition activity, and the highest ACE-I inhibitory activity. By bringing together synergistic combinations to cranberry, health beneficial functionality was enhanced. This enhanced functionality in terms of high alpha-glycosidase and alpha-amylase inhibitory activities indicate the potential for diabetes management, and high ACE-I inhibitory activity indicates the potential for hypertension management."

Potential of cranberry-based phytochemical synergies for **diabetes** *and* **hypertension** *management.* Kwon YI, Lin YT, Shetty K. Department of Food Science, University of Massachusetts. 2005; http://ift.confex.com/direct/ift/2005/techprogram/paper_29028.htm. **Key Finding:** "There is a synergistic inhibitory effect of various phytochemical combinations on above enzyme activities. These findings indicate that cranberry-based phytochemical synergies have potential as functional ingredients in the dietary management of diabetes and hypertension."

*Cranberry juice induces nitric oxide-dependent vasodilation in vitro and its infusion transiently reduces **blood pressure** in anesthetized rats.* Maher MA, Matacynski H, Stefaniak HM, Wilson T. J Med Food. 2000 Fall;3(3):141-7. **Key Finding:** "We determined that cranberry juice has vasorelaxing properties. This study suggests that it has the capacity to exert in vitro and in vivo vasodilatory effects."

Influenza

*Cranberry juice constituents affect **influenza virus** adhesion and infectivity.* Weiss EI, Houri-Haddad Y, Greenbaum E, Hochman N, Ofek I, Zakay-Rones Z. Antiviral Res. 2005 Apr;66(1):9-12. **Key Finding:** "Our cumulative findings indicate that the inhibitory effect of high molecular weight materials in cranberry juice on influenza virus adhesion and infectivity may have a therapeutic potential."

Kidney stones

*Influence of cranberry juice on the urinary risk factors for calcium oxalate **kidney stone** formation.* McHarg T, Rodgers A, Charlton K. BJC Int. 2003 Nov;92(7):765-8. **Key Finding:** "Cranberry juice has antilithogenic properties and, as such, deserves consideration as a conservative therapeutic protocol in managing calcium oxalate urolithiasis."

Neurodegenerative diseases

*Cranberry and blueberry: evidence for protective effects against **cancer** and **vascular diseases**.* Neto CC. Mol Nutr Food Res. 2007 Jun;51(6):652-64. **Key Finding:** "Growing evidence from tissue culture, animal, and clinical models suggests that the flavonoid-rich fruits of the North American cranberry and blueberry have the potential ability to limit the development and severity of certain cancers and vascular diseases including **atherosclerosis**, **ischemic stroke**, and neurodegenerative **diseases of aging**."

Potential role of dietary flavonoids in reducing micro vascular endothelium vulnerability to oxidative and inflammatory insults (small star, filled). Youdim KA, McDonald J, Kalt W, Joseph JA. J Nutr Biochem. 2002 May;13(5):282-288. **Key Finding:** "Polyphenols isolated from both blueberry and cranberry were able to afford protection to endothelial cells against stressor induced up-regulation of oxidative and inflammatory insults. This may have beneficial actions against the initiation and development of **vascular diseases** and be a contributing factor in the reduction of age-related deficits in **neurological impairments** previously reported by us."

Periodontitis

Anti-Porphyromonas gingivalis and anti-inflammatory activities of A-type cranberry proanthocyanidin. La VD, Howell AB, Grenier D. Antimicrob Agents Chemother. 2010 May;54(5):1778-84. **Key Finding**: "The purpose of this study was to investigate the effects of A-type cranberry proanthocyanidin on various determinants of periodontitis, a destructive disease of tooth-supporting tissues. Our results showed that the proanthocyanidin neutralized all the virulence properties of P. Gingivalis in dose-dependent fashion and did not interfere with growth. These may be potentially valuable bioactive molecules for the development of new strategies to treat and prevent P. gingivalis-associated **periodontal diseases**."

Cranberry proanthocyanidin inhibit MMP production and activity. La VD, Howell AB, Grenier D. J Dent Res. 2009 Jul;88(7):627-32. **Key Finding:** "Matrix metalloproteinase (MMPs) produced by resident and inflammatory cells in response to periodontopathogens play a major role in **periodontal** tissue destruction. Our aim was to investigate the effects of A-type cranberry proanthocyanidin on the production of various MMPs. Our results indicated that A-type cranberry proanthocyanidin inhibited the production of MMPs in a concentration-dependent manner."

Potential oral health benefits of cranberry. Bodet C, Grenier D, Chandad F, Ofek I, Steinberg D, Weiss EI. Crit Rev Food Sci Nutr. 2008 Aug;48(7):672-80. **Key Finding:** "Cranberry components are potential anti-caries agents since they inhibit acid production, attachment, and biofilm formation by Streptococcus mutants. Glucan-binding proteins, extracellular enzymes, carbohydrate production, and bacterial hydrophobicity, are all affected by cranberry components. Regarding **periodontal diseases**, the same cranberry fraction inhibits host inflammatory responses, production, and activity of enzymes that cause the destruction of the extracellular matrix, biofilm formation, and adherence of Porphyromonas gingivalis, and proteolytic activities and coaggregation of periodontopathogens. The above-listed effects suggest that cranberry components, especially those with high molecular weight, could serve as bioactive molecules for the prevention and/or treatment of **oral diseases**."

Cranberry components inhibit interleukin-6, interleukin-8, and prostaglandin E production by lipo-polysaccharide-activated gingival fibroblasts. Bodet C, Chandad F, Grenier D. Eur J Oral Sci. 2007 Feb;115(1):64-70. **Key Finding:** "This study suggests that cranberry juice contains molecules with interesting properties for the development of new host-modulating therapeutic strategies in the adjunctive treatment of **periodontitis.**"

Inhibition of periodontopathogen-derived proteolytic enzymes by a high-molecular weight fraction isolated from cranberry. Bodet C, Piche M, Chandad F, Grenier D. J Antimicrob Chemother. 2006 Apr;57(4):685-90. **Key Finding:** "The aim of this study was to investigate the effect of non-dialyzable material (NDM) prepared from cranberry juice concentrate on the proteolytic activities of P. gingivalis, T. forsythia and T. denticola. These results suggest that NDM has the potential to reduce either the proliferation of P. gingivalis, T. forsythia and T. denticola in periodontal pockets or their proteinase-mediated destructive process occurring in **periodontitis.**"

*Inhibitory effects of cranberry juice on attachment of **oral streptococci** and biofilm formation.* Yamanaka A, Kimizuka R, Kata T, Okuda K. Oral Microbiol Immunol. 2004 Jun;19(3):150-4. **Key Finding:** "The present findings suggest that cranberry juice components can inhibit colonization by oral streptococci to the tooth surface and can thus slow development of dental plaque."

Ulcers (peptic)

Efficacy of cranberry juice on Helicobacter pylori infection: a double-blind, randomized placebo-controlled trial. Zhang L, Ma J, Pan K, Go VL, Chen J, You WC. Helicobacter. 2005 Apr;10(2):139-45. **Key Finding:** "Helicobacter pylori infection is a major cause of **peptic ulcer disease** and **gastric cancer**. Regular consumption of cranberry juice can suppress H. pylori infection in endemically afflicted populations."

Inhibition of Helicobacter pylori and associated unrease by oregano and cranberry phytochemical synergies. Lin YT, Kwon YI, Labbe RG, Shetty K. Appl Environ Microbiol. 2005 Dec;71(12):8558-64. **Key Finding:** "Ulcer-associated dyspepsia is caused by infection with Helicobacter pylori, linked to a majority of **peptic ulcers**. The results indicated that the antimicrobial activity was greater in extract mixtures than in individual extracts of each species. The results also indicate that the synergistic contribution of oregano and cranberry phenolic may be more important for inhibition than any species-specific phenolic concentration."

Urinary tract infections

Inhibitory activity of cranberry extract on the bacterial adhesiveness in the urine of women: an ex-vivo study. Tempera G, Corsello S, Genovese C, Et al. Int J Immunpathol Pharmacol. 2010 Apr-Jun;23(2):611-8. **Key Finding**: "This ex-vivo study showed that the assumption of cranberry extract in suitable amounts can have an anti-adhesive activity on uropathogenic E. coli, which are responsible for approximately 90% of community-acquired, uncomplicated cystitis."

Cytoprotective effect of proanthocyanidin-rich cranberry fraction against bacterial cell wall-mediated toxicity in macrophages and epithelial cells. La VD, Labrecque J, Grenier D. Phytother Res. 2009 Oct;23(10):1449-52. **Key Finding:** "This study suggests that cranberry polyphenols may exert a protective effect for host cells against the toxicity induced by bacterial components."

Cranberry juice for the prevention of recurrent **urinary tract infections***: A randomized controlled trial in children.* Ferrara P, Romaniello L, Vitelli O, Gatto A, Serva M, Cataldi L. Scand J Urol Nephrol. 2009 May 9;1-5. (Epub ahead of print). **Key Finding:** "These data suggest that daily consumption of concentrated cranberry juice can significantly prevent the recurrence of symptomatic urinary tract infections in children."

Interference of cranberry constituents in cell-cell signaling system of Vibrio harveyi. Feldman M, Weiss EI, Ofek I, Steinberg D. Curr Microbiol. 2009 Oct;59(4):469-74. **Key Finding:** "using a model of V. harveyi bacteria, we found an inhibitory effect of cranberry constituents on bacterial signaling system."

Evaluation of cranberry tablets for the prevention of urinary tract infections in spinal cord injured patients with **neurogenic bladder***.* Hess MJ, Hess PE, Sullivan MR, Nee M, Yalla SV. Spinal Cord. 2008 Sep;46(9):622-6. **Key Finding:** "Cranberry extract tablets should be considered for the prevention of **urinary tract infections** in spinal cord injured patients with neurogenic bladder. Patients with a high glomerular filtration rate may receive the most benefit."

Modulation of Helicobacter pylori colonization with cranberry juice and Lactobacillus johnsonii La1 in children. Gotteland M, Andrews M, Toledo M, Munoz L, Caceres P, Anziani A, Wittig E, Speisky H, Salazar G. Nutrition. 2008 May;24(5):421-6. **Key Finding:** "These results suggest that regular intake of cranberry juice or La1 may be useful in the management of asymptomatic children colonized by H. pylori."

Daily cranberry juice for the prevention of asymptomatic bacteriuria in pregnancy: a random-ized, controlled pilot study. Wing DA, Rumney PJ, Preslicka CW, Chung JH. J Urol. 2008 Oct;180(4):1367-72. **Key Finding:** "These data suggest there may be a protective effect of cranberry ingestion against asymptomatic bacteriuria and symptomatic **urinary tract infections** in pregnancy. Further studies are planned to evaluate this effect."

Anti-microbial Activity of Urine after Ingestion of Cranberry: A Pilot Study. Lee YL, Najm WI, Owens J, Thrupp L, Baron S, Shanbrom E, Cesario T. Evid Based Complement Alternat Med. 2008 Jan 16. (Epub ahead of print). **Key Finding:** "This pilot study demonstrates weak **anti-microbial** activity in urine specimens after ingestion of a single dose of commercial cranberry. Anti-microbial activity was noted only against K. pneumonia 2-6 h after ingestion of the cranberry preparation."

*Can a concentrated cranberry extract prevent recurrent **urinary tract infections** in women? A pilot study.* Bailey DT, Dalton C, Daughterty F, Tempesta MS. Phyto-medicine. 2007 Apr;14(4):237-41. **Key Finding:** "Women between the ages of 25 and 70 years old were included with a history of a minimum of 6 urinary tract infections in the preceding year. The women took one capsule twice daily for 12 weeks containing 200 mg of a concentrated cranberry extract standardized to 30% phenolics. During the study none of the 12 subjects had a urinary tract infection. Two years later, eight of the women who continue to take cranberry, continue to be free from urinary tract infections."

Biosafety, antioxidant status, and metabolites in urine after consumption of dried cranberry juice in healthy women: a pilot double-blind placebo-controlled trial. Valentova K, Stejskal D, Bednar P, Vostalova J, Cihalik C, Vecerova R, Koukalova D, Kolar M, Rech-cnbach R, Sknouril L, Ulrichova J, Simanek V. J Agric Food Chem. 2007 Apr 18;55(8):3217-24. **Key Finding:** "This study assessed the effect of an 8 week consumption of dried cranberry juice on 65 healthy young women. A 1200 mg amount per day resulted in a statistically significant decrease in serum levels of advanced oxidation protein products. This specific protective effect against oxidative damage of proteins is described here for the first time. Cranberry fruits are effective not only in the prevention of **urinary tract infection** but also for the prevention of **oxidative stress**."

Cranberry products inhibit adherence of p-fimbriated Escherichia coli to primary cultured bladder and vaginal epithelial cells. Gupta K, Chou MY, Howell A, Wobbe C, Grady R, Stapleton AE. Urol. 2007 Jun;177(6):2357-60. **Key Finding:** "Cranberry products can inhibit E. coli adherence to biologically relevant model systems of primary cultured bladder and vaginal epithelial cells. This effect occurs in a dose dependent relationship. These findings provide further mechanistic evidence and biological plausibility for the role of cranberry products for preventing **urinary tract infection**."

Reduction of **Escherichia coli** *adherence to uroepithelial bladder cells after consumption of cranberry juice: a double-blind randomized placebo-controlled cross-over trial.* Di Martino P, Agniel R, David K, Templer C, Gaillard JL, Denys P, Botto H. World J Urol. 2006 Feb;24(1):21-7. **Key Finding:** "We observed a dose-dependent significant decrease in bacterial adherence associated with cranberry consumption. Adherence inhibition was observed independently from the presence of genes encoding type P pili and antibiotic resistance phenotypes. Cranberry juice consumption provides significant anti-adherence activity against different E. coli uropathogenic strains in the urine compared with placebo."

Use of cranberry in chronic **urinary tract infections**. Bruyere F. Med Mal Infect (French). 2006 Jul;36(7):358-63. **Key Finding:** "Cranberries can inhibit E. coli adhesion to the urothelium and could be useful to treat urinary infections. Clinical studies confirm the probably benefit of this fruit as a prophylactic treatment for female cystitis."

Increased salicylate concentrations in urine of human volunteers after consumption of cranberry juice. Duthie GG, Kyle JA, Jenkinson AM, Duthie SJ, Baxter GJ, Paterson JR. J Agric Food Chem. 2005 Apr 20;53(8):2897-900. **Key Finding:** "Consumption of cranberry juice was associated with a marked increase of salicyluric and salicylic acids in urine within 1 week of the intervention. After 2 weeks, there was also a small but significant increase in salicylic acid in plasma. The regular consumption of cranberry juice results in the increased absorption of salicylic acid, an anti-inflammatory compound that may benefit health."

Does ingestion of cranberry juice reduce symptomatic **urinary tract infections** *in older people in hospital? A double-blind, placebo-controlled trial.* McMurdo ME, Bissett LY, Price RJ, Phillips G, Crombie IK. Age Ageing. 2005 May;34(3):256-61. **Key Finding:** "Despite having the largest sample size of any clinical trial yet to have examined the effect of cranberry juice ingestion, the actual infection rate observed was lower than anticipated, making the study underpowered. This study has confirmed the acceptability of cranberry juice to older people. Larger trials are now required to determine whether it is effective in reducing urinary tract infections in older hospital patients."

*Effect of cranberry juice consumption on **urinary stone** risk factors.* Gettman MT, Ogan K, Brinkley LJ, Adams-Huet B, Pak CY, Pearle MS. J Urol. 2005 Aug;174(2):590-4. **Key Finding:** "Cranberry juice exerts a mixed effect on urinary stone forming propensity. It reduces urinary pH likely by providing an acid load and decreases urinary uric acid perhaps by retarding urate synthesis. Overall cranberry juice increases the risk of calcium oxalate and uric acid stone formation but decreases the risk of brushite stones."

A-type cranberry proanthocyanidin and uropathogenic bacterial anti-adhesion activity. Howell AB, Reed JD, Krueger CG, Winterbottom R, Cunningham DG, Leahy M. Phytochemistry. 2005 Sep;66(18):2281-91. **Key Finding:** "Anti-adhesion activity in human urine was detected following cranberry juice cocktail consumption, but not after consumption of the non-cranberry food products. Results suggest that presence of the A-type linkage in cranberry proanthocyanidin may enhance both in vitro and urinary bacterial anti-adhesion activities and aid in maintaining **urinary tract health**."

Cranberry juice and bacterial colonization in children --- a placebo-controlled randomized trial. Kontiokari T, Salo J, Eerola E, Uhari M. Clin Nutr. 2005 Dec;24(6):1065-72. **Key Finding:** "Cranberry juice was well accepted by the children, but led to no change in either the **bacterial** flora in the nasopharynx or the bacterial fatty acid composition of stool. Thus cranberries seem to have beneficial effect on urinary health only and this is not compromised by other unexpected antimicrobial effects."

*Inhibition of uropathogenic **Escherichia coli** by cranberry juice: a new antiadherence assay.* Turner A, Chen SN, Joike MK, Pendland SL, Pauli GF, Fransworth NR. J Agric Food Chem. 2005 Nov 16;53(23):8940-7. **Key Finding:** "In this assay, a low-polarity fraction of cranberry juice cocktail demonstrated dose-dependent inhibition of E. coli adherence. Reported here, for the first time in V. macrocarpon, are 1-O-methylgalactose, pruning, and phlorizin, identified in an active fraction of cranberry juice concentrate."

Consumption of sweetened dried cranberries versus unsweetened raisins for inhibition of uropathogenic Escherichia coli adhesion in human urine: a pilot study. Greenberg JA, Newmann SJ, Howell AB. J Altern Complement Med. 2005 Oct;11(5):875-8. **Key Finding:** "Data from this pilot study on only five subjects suggest that consumption of a single serving of sweetened dried cranberries may elicit bacterial antiadhesion activity in human urine, whereas consumption of a single serving of raisins does not."

Evaluation of cranberry supplement for reduction of **urinary tract infections** *in individuals with neurogenic bladders secondary to spinal cord injury. A prospective, double-blinded, placebo-controlled, crossover study.* Linsenmeyer TA, Harrison B, Oakley A, Kirshblum S, Stock JA, Millis SR. J Spinal Cord Med. 2004;27(1):29-34. **Key Finding:** "Cranberry tablets were not found to be effective at changing urinary pH or reducing bacterial counts, urinary WBC counts, or UTIs in individuals with neurogenic bladders. Further long-term studies evaluating specific types of bladder management and UTIs will help to determine whether there is any role for the use of cranberries in individuals with neurogenic bladders."

The role of cranberry and probiotics in intestinal and urogenital tract health. Reid G. Crit Rev Food Sci Nutr. 2002;42(3 Suppl):293-300. **Key Finding:** "There is now strong scientific basis for use of cranberries to reduce the risk of E. coli adhesion to bladder cells and the onset of **urinary tract infections**."

Can ingestion of cranberry juice reduce the incidence of **urinary tract infections** *in a department of geriatric medicine?* Kirchhoff M, Renneberg J, Damkjaer K, Pietersen I, Schroll M. Ugeskr Laeger (Danish). 2001 May 14;163(20):2782-6. **Key Finding:** "Cranberry juice in a geriatric department, where the mean stay was 4 weeks, did not influence the incidence of urinary tract infections."

Randomized trial of cranberry-lingonberry juice and Lactobacillus GG drink for the prevention of **urinary tract infections** *in women.* Kontiokari T, Sundqvist K, Nuutinen M, Pokka T, Koskela M, Uhari M. BMJ. 2001 Jun 30;322(7302):1571. **Key Finding:** "150 women with urinary tract infection caused by Escherichia coli were randomly allocated into three groups. The intervention cranberry group experienced a 20% reduction in absolute risk compared to the control group. Regular drinking of cranberry juice but not lactobacillus seems to reduce the recurrence of urinary tract infection."

Efficacy of cranberry in prevention of **urinary tract infection** *in a susceptible pediatric population.* Foda MM, Middlebrook PF, Gatfield CT, Potvin G, Wells G, Schillinger JF. Can J Urol. 1995 Jan;2(1):98-102. **Key Finding:** "Forty cases were enrolled in a randomized single-blind cross-over study. Subjects ingested 15 mL/kg/day of cranberry cocktail or water for six months followed by the reverse for another six months. Twenty one patients completed the study. Fewer infections were observed in nine patients taking cranberry juice and in nine patients given water; no difference was noted in three. Liquid cranberry products, on a daily basis, at the dosage employed, did not have any effect greater than that of water in preventing urinary tract infections in this pediatric neuropathic bladder population."

Reduction of bacteriuria and pyuria after ingestion of cranberry juice. Avorn J, Monane M, Gurwitz JH, Glynn RJ, Choodnovskiy I, Lipsitz LA. JAMA. 1994 Mar 9;271(10):751-4. **Key Finding:** "These findings suggest that use of a cranberry beverage reduces the frequency of bacteriuria with pyuria in older women. Prevalent beliefs about the effects of cranberry juice on the urinary tract may have microbiologic justification."

New support for a folk remedy: cranberry juice reduces bacteriuria and pyuria in elderly women. Fleet JC. Nutr Rev. 1994 May;52(5):168-70. **Key Finding:** "A new study suggests that **bacterial infections** (bacteriuria) and associated influx of white blood cells into the urine (pyuria) can be reduced by nearly 50% in elderly women who drink 300 ml. of cranberry juice cocktail each day over the course of the 6-month study."

*Cranberry juice and its impact on **peri-stomal skin conditions** for urostomy patients.* Tsukada K, Tokunaga K, Iwama T, Mishima Y, Tazawa K, Fujimaki M. Ostomy Wound Manage. 1994 Nov-Dec;40(9):60-2. **Key Finding:** "In urostomy patients, peristomal skin problems are common and may stem from alkaline urine. Cranberry juice appears to acidify urine and has bacteriostatic properties. The authors conclude that while drinking cranberry juice did not appear to acidify the urine as expected in 13 urostomy patients, improvements were still seen in the skin conditions of the study participants, suggesting that drinking cranberry juice does positively impact the incidence of skin complications for these patients."

An examination of the anti-adherence activity of cranberry juice on urinary and nonurinary bacterial isolates. Schmidt DR, Sobota AE. Microbios. 1988;55(224-225):173-81. **Key Finding:** "Cranberry juice cocktail and urine and urinary epithelial cells obtained after drinking the cocktail all demonstrate anti-adherence activity against Gram-negative rods isolated from urine and other clinical sources. Drinking the cocktail may be useful in managing **urinary tract infections** in certain patients."

*Inhibition of bacterial adherence by cranberry juice: potential use for the treatment of **urinary tract infections**.* Sobota AE. J Urol. 1984 May;131(5):1013-6. **Key Finding:** "Fifteen of 22 subjects showed significant antiadherence activity in the urine 1 to 3 hours after drinking 15 ounces of cranberry cocktail. It is concluded that the reported benefits derived from the use of cranberry juice may be related to its ability to inhibit bacterial adherence."

Curcumin (in Turmeric)

CURCUMIN IS ONE OF THE ACTIVE PHYTOCHEMICAL ingredients in the spice turmeric, derived from the rhizome of a member of the ginger plant family. It is a polyphenol and gives turmeric its distinctive yellow color. This flavoring has been a staple in the Indian Ayurvedic medicine tradition for several thousand years. If you have eaten Indian curry, you have probably consumed curcumin.

The first medical science article examining the use of curcumin in human health treatments appeared in 1937 in the British medical journal, the *Lancet.* Since then, an estimated 2,600 research studies have been published in English-language journals analyzing the reputed health and healing properties of curcumin or turmeric. Most of the more important studies have appeared within the last two decades and show an extraordinarily wide range of health benefits from curcumin consumption (twenty-nine health conditions prevented or treated).

Aging

*Curcumin, inflammation, **ageing and age-related diseases**.* Sikora E, Scapagnini G, Barbagallo M. Immun Ageing. 2010 Jan 17;7(1):1. **Key Finding**: "Ageing is manifested by the decreasing health status and increasing probability to acquired age-related disease such as cancer, Alzheimer's disease, atherosclerosis, metabolic disorders and others. They are likely caused by low grade inflammation driven by oxygen stress and manifested by the increased level of pro-inflammatory cytokines. It is believed that ageing is plastic and can be slowed down by **caloric restriction** as well as by some nutraceuticals. Accordingly, slowing down ageing and postponing the onset of age-related diseases might be achieved by blocking the NF-kappaB-dependent inflammation. In this review we consider the possibility of the spice curcumin, a powerful antioxidant and anti-inflammatory agent possibly capable of improving the health status of the elderly."

*The promise of slow down **ageing** may come from **curcumin**.* Sikora E, Bielak-Zmijewska A, Mosieniak G, Et al. Curr Pharm Des. 2010;16(7):884-92. **Key Finding**: "In this review we consider the possibility of the natural spice curcumin, a powerful antioxidant, anti-inflammatory agent and efficient inhibitor of NF-kappaB and the mTOR signaling pathway which overlaps that of NT-kappaB, to slow down ageing."

*Curcumin extends **life span**, improves health span, and modulates the expression of age-associated aging genes in Drosophila melanogaster.* Lee KS, Lee BS, Semnani S, Et al. Rejuvenation Res. 2010 Oct;13(5):561-70. **Key Finding**: "The observed positive effects of curcumin on life span and health span in two different D. melanogaster strains demonstrate a potential applicability of curcumin treatment in mammals. The ability of curcumin to mitigate the expression levels of age-associated genes in young flies suggests that the action of curcumin on these genes is a cause, rather than an effect, of its life span-extending effects."

*Curcumin, resveratrol and flavonoids as **anti-inflammatory**, cyto- and DNA-protective dietary compounds.* Bisht K, Wagner KH, Bulmer AC. Toxicology. 2009 Nov 10. (Epub ahead of print). **Key Finding:** "The polyphenols afford protection against various stress-induced toxicities through modulating intercellular cascades which inhibit inflammatory molecule synthesis, the formation of free radicals, nuclear damage and induce antioxidant enzyme expressions. These responses have the potential to increase **life expectancy**."

Alzheimer's disease

*Oxidative stress and **Alzheimer's disease**: dietary polyphenols as potential therapeutic agents.* Darvesh AS, Carroll RT, Bishayee A, Geldenhuys WJ, Van der Schyf CJ. Expert Rev Neurother. 2010 May;10(5):729-45. **Key Finding**: Oxidative stress has been strongly implicated in the pathophysiology of neurodegenerative disorders such as Alzheimer's. This article reviews the antioxidant potential of polyphenolic compounds such as anthocyanin from berries, catechins and theaflavins from tea, curcumin from turmeric and resveratrol from grapes.

*REVIEW: **Curcumin** and **Alzheimer's disease**.* Hamaguchi T, Ono K, Yamada M. CNS Neurosci Ther. 2010 Oct;16(5):285-97. **Key Finding**: "Findings suggest that curcumin might be one of the most promising compounds for the development of Alzheimer disease therapies. Additional clinical trials are necessary to determine the clinical usefulness of curcumin in the prevention and treatment."

***Curcuminoids** enhance memory in an amyloid-infused rat model of Alzheimer's disease.* Ahmed T, Enam SA, Gilani AH. Neuroscience. 2010 Sep 1;169(3):1296-306. **Key Finding**: "Curcuminoid mixture showed a memory-enhancing effect in rats displaying **Alzheimer's** disease-like neuronal loss only at 30 mg/kg, whereas individual components were effective at 3-30 mg/kg. This suggests these compounds affect multiple target sites with the potential of curcuminoids in spatial memory enhancing and disease modifying in Alzheimer's disease."

Therapeutic potential of dietary polyphenols against brain ageing and neurodegenerative disorders. Scapagnini G, Caruso C, Calabrese V. Adv Exp Med Biol. 2010;698:27-35. **Key Finding**: "The potential role of **curcumin** as a preventive agent against brain aging and neurodegenerative disorders has been recently reinforced by epidemiological studies showing that in India, where this spice is widely used in the daily diet, there is a lower incidence of **Alzheimer's** disease than in the USA."

Grape seed polyphenols and curcumin reduce genomic instability events in a transgenic mouse model for **Alzheimer's disease**. Thomas P, Wang YJ, Zhong JH, Kosaraju S, O'Callaghan NJ, Zhou XF, Fenech M. Mutat Res. 2009 Feb 10;661(1-2):25-34. **Key Finding:** "These results suggest potential protective effects of polyphenols against genomic instability events in different somatic tissues of a transgenic mouse model for Alzheimer's disease."

Inhibitory effect of curcuminoids on acetyl cholinesterase activity and attenuation of scopolamine-induced amnesia may explain medicinal use of turmeric in **Alzheimer's disease**. Ahmed T, Gilani AH. Pharmacol Biochem Behav. 2009 Feb;91(4):554-9. **Key Finding:** "These data indicate that curcuminoids and all individual components except curcumin possess pronounced AChE inhibitory activity. Curcumin was relatively weak in the in-vitro assay and without effect in the ex-vivo AChE model, while equally effective in memory enhancing effect, suggestive of additional mechanisms involved. Thus curcuminoids mixture might possess better therapeutic profile than curcumin for its medicinal use in Alzheimer's disease."

Curcumin improves learning and memory ability and its neuroprotective mechanism in mice. Pan R, Qiu S, Lu DX, Dong J. Chin Med J (Engl). 2008 May 5;121(9):832-9. **Key Finding:** "This study demonstrates that curcumin improves the memory ability of **Alzheimer's disease** mice and inhibits apoptosis in cultured PC12 cells induced by AICI(3). Its mechanism may involve enhancing the level of Bcl-2."

Molecular orbital basis for yellow curry spice curcumin's prevention of **Alzheimer's disease**. Balasubramanian K. J Agric Food Chem. 2006 May 17;54(10):3512-20. **Key Finding:** Curcumin "exhibits unique charge and bonding characteristics that facilitate penetration into the blood-brain barrier and binding to amyloid beta (Abeta). Alzheimer's disease is caused by Abeta accumulation in the brain cells combined with oxidative stress and inflammation. It is shown here that curcumin possesses suitable charge and bonding features to facilitate the binding to Abeta."

Curcumin: getting back to the roots. Shishodia S, Sethi G, Aggarwal BB. Ann NY Acad Sci. 2005 Nov;1056:206-17. **Key Finding:** "Curcumin is now being used to treat **cancer, arthritis, diabetes, Crohn's disease, cardiovascular disease, osteoporosis, Alzheimer's disease, psoriasis**, and other pathologies. Interestingly, 6-gingerol, a natural analog of curcumin derived from the root of ginger (Zingiber officinalis), exhibits a biologic activity profile similar to that of curcumin."

*A review of antioxidants and **Alzheimer's disease**.* Frank B, Gupta S. Ann Clin Psychiatry. 2005 Oct-Dec;17(4):269-86. **Key Finding:** Over 300 articles were reviewed of antioxidants helpful in the prevention of Alzheimer's disease and 187 articles were selected for inclusion. Agents that show promise helping prevent AD include: 1) aged garlic extract, 2) curcumin, 3) melatonin, 4) resveratrol, 5) Ginkgo biloba extract, 6) green tea, 7) vitamin C and 8) vitamin E.

*Prevention of **Alzheimer's disease**: Omega-3 fatty acid and phenolic anti-oxidant interventions.* Cole GM, Lim GP, Yang F, Teter B, Begum A, Ma Q, Harris-White ME, Frautschy SA. Neurobiol Aging. 2005 Dec;26 Suppl 1:133-6. **Key Finding:** "Both DHA (omega-3 fatty acid) and curcumin have favorable safety profiles, epidemiology and efficacy, and may exert general anti-aging benefits (anti-cancer and cardio protective.)"

*A potential role of the curry spice curcumin in **Alzheimer's disease**.* Ringman JM, Frautschy SA, Cole GM, Masterman DL, Cummings JL. Curr Alzheimer Res. 2005 Apr;2(2):131-6. **Key Finding:** Studies in animal models of Alzheimer's disease indicate a direct effect of curcumin in decreasing the amyloid pathology of AD. Curcumin is a promising agent in the treatment and/or prevention of AD.

Antioxidation

Antioxidant activities of curcumin and combinations of this curcuminoid with other phytochemicals. Aftab N, Vieira A. Phytother Res. 2009 Nov 19. (Epub ahead of print). **Key Finding:** "The main goal of the present study was to compare antioxidant activities of curcumin with those of resveratrol. Combinations of the two were examined for potential synergism in a heme-enhanced oxidation reaction. Curcumin and resveratrol together (5 muM each) resulted in a synergistic antioxidant effect: 15.5 +/- 1.7% greater than an average of individual activities. This synergy was significantly greater than that of curcumin together with the flavonol quercetin."

Antioxidant activities of curcumin and combinations of this curcuminoid with other phyto-chemicals. Aftab N, Vieira A. Phytother Res. 2009 Nov 19. (Epub ahead of print.) **Key Finding:** "Curcumin shows significantly greater synergism with resveratrol than with quercetin. Curcumin and resveratrol together (5 muM each) resulted in a synergistic antioxidant effect: 15.5 +/- 1.7% greater than an average of individual activities. This synergy was significantly greater (p<0.05; about 4-fold) than that of curcumin together with the flavonol quercetin."

Antioxidant and anti-inflammatory properties of curcumin. Menon VP, Sudheer AR. Adv Exp Med Biol. 2007;595:105-25. **Key Finding:** "The past few decades have witnessed intense research devoted to the antioxidant and anti-inflammatory properties of curcumin. In this review, we describe antioxidant and anti-inflammatory properties of curcumin, the mode of action of curcumin, and its therapeutic usage against different pathological conditions."

Turmeric and curcumin enriched beverages for reducing the risk for oxidation linked chronic diseases. Vattem D, Crixell S. Texas State University Office of Sponsored Programs. 2005. Posted http://ecommons.txstate.edu/osp_regs/61. **Key Finding:** "Results strongly suggest that the functionality of fruit extracts can be significantly increased by creating novel synergies with turmeric. We were able to show that **antioxidant** activity of these synergies was significantly higher than the pure extracts alone."

*Modulation of cyclophosphamide-induced early lung injury by curcumin, an anti-inflammatory **antioxidant**.* Venkatesan N, Chandrakasan G. Mol Cell Biochem. 1995 Jan 12;142(1):79-87. **Key Finding:** Oral administration of curcumin in male Wistar rats was performed daily for 7 days prior to cyclophosphamide intoxication. Increased levels of lipid peroxidation and decreased levels of glutathione and ascorbic acid were seen in serum, lung tissue and lavage cells of cyclophosphamide groups.

Studies on the inhibitory effects of curcumin and eugenol on the formation of reactive oxygen species and the oxidation of ferrous iron. Pulla Reddy AC, Lokesh BR. Molecular and Cellular Biochemistry. 1994 Aug; vol 137, no 1:1-8. **Key Finding:** "The effect of curcumin and eugenol (from cloves) on the generation of reactive oxygen species in model systems was investigated. Both curcumin and eugenol inhibited superoxide anion generation in xanthine-xanthine oxidase system to an extent of 40% and 50% respectively. Curcumin and eugenol also inhibited the generation of hydroxyl radicals to an extent of 76% and 70% as measured by deoxybribose degradation."

Effect of dietary turmeric (Curcuma longa) on iron-induced lipid peroxidation in the rat liver. Reddy AC, Lokesh BR. Food Chem Toxicol. 1994 Mar;32(3):279-83. **Key Finding:** "These studies indicate that dietary turmeric lowers lipid peroxidation by enhancing the activities of **antioxidant** enzymes."

Effect of turmeric on xenobiotic metabolizing enzymes. Goud VK, Polasa K, Krishnaswamy K. Plant Foods for Human Nutrition. 1993 July; vol 44, no 1:87-92. **Key Finding:** "The results suggest that turmeric may increase detoxification systems in addition to its **antioxidant** properties. Turmeric used widely as a spice would probably mitigate the effects of several dietary carcinogens."

Studies on curcumin and curcuminoids. XXII. Curcumin as a reducing agent and as a radical scavenger. Hjorth TH, Greenhill JV. International Journal of Pharmaceutics. 1992; vol 87, no 1-3: 79-87. **Key Finding:** "The function of curcumin in the reduction of $Fe3+$ to $Fe2+$ and in oxygen radical reactions is discussed. The presence of the diketone moiety in the curcumin molecule seems to be essential both in redox reactions and in the scavenging of oxygen radicals."

*Studies on spice principles as **antioxidants** in the inhibition of lipid peroxidation of rat liver microsomes.* Reddy AC, Lokesh BR. Mol Cell Biochem. 1992 Apr;111(1-2):117-24. **Key Finding:** "Polyunsaturated fatty acids (PUFA) are vulnerable to peroxidative attack. Protecting PUFA from peroxidation is essential to utilize their beneficial effects in health and in preventing disease. The antioxidants vitamin E inhibited ascorbate/Fe(2+)-induced lipid peroxidation in rat liver microsomes. In addition, a number of spice principles, for example, curcumin (5-50 microM) from turmeric inhibited lipid peroxidation in a dose-dependent manner."

Cytotoxic and Cytoprotective activities of curcumin. Effects on paracetamol-induced cytotoxicity, lipid peroxidation and glutathione depletion in rat hepatocytes. Donatus IA, Sardjoko, Vermeulen NP. Biochem Pharmacol. 1990 Jun 15;39(12):1869-75. **Key Finding:** "It has been concluded that the observed cytoprotective and cytotoxic activities of curcumin may be explained by a strong **antioxidant** capacity of curcumin and the capability of curcumin to conjugate with GSH. Furthermore, it has been concluded that lipid peroxidation is not playing a causal role in cell-death induced by paracetamol or by curcumin."

*In vitro antimutagenicity of curcumin against environmental **mutagens**.* Nagabhushan M, Amonkar AJ, Bhide SV. Food Chem Toxicol. 1987 Jul;25(7):545-7. **Key Finding:** "Our observations indicate that curcumin may alter the metabolic activation and **detoxification** of mutagens."

Arthritis

*Natural products as a gold mine for **arthritis** treatment.* Khanna D, Sethi G, Ahn KS, Pandey MK, Kunnumakkara AB, Sung B, Aggarwal A, Aggarwal BB. Curr Opin Pharmacol. 2007 Jun;7(3):344-51. **Key Finding:** "The large numbers of inexpensive natural products that can modulate inflammatory responses, but lack side effects, constitute 'goldmines' for the treatment of arthritis. Numerous agents derived from plants can suppress cell signaling intermediates, including curcumin, resveratrol, cranberries and peanuts, tea polyphenols, genistein, quercetin from onions, silymarin from artichoke."

Curcumin: getting back to the roots. Shishodia S, Sethi G, Aggarwal BB. Ann NY Acad Sci. 2005 Nov;1056:206-17. **Key Finding:** "Curcumin is now being used to treat **cancer, arthritis, diabetes, Crohn's disease, cardiovascular disease, osteoporosis, Alzheimer's disease, psoriasis**, and other pathologies. Interestingly, 6-gingerol, a natural analog of curcumin derived from the root of ginger (Zingiber officinalis), exhibits a biologic activity profile similar to that of curcumin."

Suppression of the nuclear factor-kappaB activation pathway by spice-derived phytochemicals: reasoning for seasoning. Aggarwal BB, Shishodia S. Ann N Y Acad Sci. 2004 Dec;1030:434-41. **Key Finding:** "The activation of nuclear transcription factor kappaB has now been linked with a variety of inflammatory disease, including **cancer, atherosclerosis, myocardial infarction, diabetes, allergy, asthma, arthritis, Crohn's disease, multiple sclerosis, Alzheimer's disease, osteoporosis, psoriasis, septic shock, and AIDS**. Extensive research in the last few years has shown that the pathway that activates this transcription factor can be interrupted by phytochemicals derived from spices such as turmeric (curcumin), red pepper (capsaicin), cloves (eugenol), ginger (gingerol), cumin, anise, and fennel (anethol), basil and rosemary (ursolic acid), garlic (diallyl sulfide, S-allylmercaptocysteine, ajoene), and pomegranate (ellagic acid). For the first time, therefore, research provides 'reasoning for seasoning.'"

Asthma

Suppression of the nuclear factor-kappaB activation pathway by spice-derived phytochemicals: reasoning for seasoning. Aggarwal BB, Shishodia S. Ann N Y Acad Sci. 2004 Dec;1030:434-41. **Key Finding:** "The activation of nuclear transcription factor kappaB has now been linked with a variety of inflammatory disease, including cancer, **atherosclerosis**, **myocardial infarction**, **diabetes**, **allergy**, **asthma**, **arthritis**, **Crohn's disease**, **multiple sclerosis**, **Alzheimer's disease**, **osteoporosis**, **psoriasis**, **septic shock**, **and AIDS**. Extensive research in the last few years has shown that the pathway that activates this transcription factor can be interrupted by phytochemicals derived from spices such as turmeric (curcumin), red pepper (capsaicin), cloves (eugenol), ginger (gingerol), cumin, anise, and fennel (anethol), basil and rosemary (ursolic acid), garlic (diallyl sulfide, S-allylmercaptocysteine, ajoene), and pomegranate (ellagic acid). For the first time, therefore, research provides 'reasoning for seasoning.'"

Atherosclerosis

Suppression of the nuclear factor-kappaB activation pathway by spice-derived phytochemicals: reasoning for seasoning. Aggarwal BB, Shishodia S. Ann N Y Acad Sci. 2004 Dec;1030:434-41. **Key Finding:** "The activation of nuclear transcription factor kappaB has now been linked with a variety of inflammatory disease, including **cancer**, **atherosclerosis**, **myocardial infarction**, **diabetes**, **allergy**, **asthma**, **arthritis**, **Crohn's disease**, **multiple sclerosis**, **Alzheimer's disease**, **osteoporosis**, **psoriasis**, **septic shock**, **and AIDS**. Extensive research in the last few years has shown that the pathway that activates this transcription factor can be interrupted by phytochemicals derived from spices such as turmeric (curcumin), red pepper (capsaicin), cloves (eugenol), ginger (gingerol), cumin, anise, and fennel (anethol), basil and rosemary (ursolic acid), garlic (diallyl sulfide, S-allylmercaptocysteine, ajoene), and pomegranate (ellagic acid). For the first time, therefore, research provides 'reasoning for seasoning.'"

Inhibitory effect of curcumin, an anti-inflammatory agent, on vascular smooth muscle cell proliferation. Huang HC, Jan TR, Yeh SF. Eur J Pharmacol. 1992 Oct 20;221(2-3):381-4. **Key Finding:** "Curcumin may be useful as a new template for the development of better remedies for the prevention of the pathological changes of **atherosclerosis** and **restenosis**."

Autoimmune disorders

Heat-solubilized curry spice **curcumin** *inhibits antibody-antigen interaction in in vitro studies: a possible therapy to alleviate* **autoimmune disorders**. Kurien BT, D'Souza A, Scofield RH. Mol Nutr Food Res. 2010 Aug;54(8):1202-9. **Key Finding**: "We suggest that the multifaceted heat-solubilized curcumin can ameliorate autoimmune disorders."

'Spicing up' of the immune system by curcumin. Jagetia GC, Aggarwal BB. J Clin Immunol. 2007 Jan;27(1):19-35. **Key Finding:** Curcumin's reported beneficial effects "might be due in part to its ability to modulate the immune system. Together, these findings warrant further consideration of curcumin as a therapy for **immune disorders**."

Cancer (brain; breast; cervical; colon; endometrial; gastrointestinal; head; leukemia; lung; melanoma; neck; oral; ovarian; prostate)

Curcumin inhibits carcinogen and nicotine-induced Mammalian target of rapamycin pathway activation in **head and neck squamous cell carcinoma**. Clark CA, McEachem MD, Shah SH, Et al. Cancer Prev Res. 2010 Dec;3(12):1586-95. **Key Finding:** "This is the first study to demonstrate that curcumin inhibits the adverse effects of nicotine by blocking nicotine-induced activation of the AKT/MTOR pathway in head and neck squamous cell carcinoma, which retards cell migration. These studies indicate that inhibiting the AKT/MTOR pathway with curcumin may be useful as an oral chemo preventive agent."

Curcumin up regulates insulin-like growth factor binding protein-5 (IGFBP-5) and C/EBPalpha during **oral cancer** *suppression.* Chang KW, Hung PS, Lin IY, Et al. Int J Cancer. 2010 Jul 1;127(1):9-20. **Key Finding**: "We conclude that curcumin activates p38, which, in turn, activates the C/EBPalpha trans activator by interacting with binding elements in the IGFBP-5 promoter. The consequential up regulation of C/EBPalpha and IGFBP-5 by curcumin is crucial to the suppression of oral carcinogenesis."

Curcumin suppresses constitutive activation of STAT-3 by up-regulating protein inhibitor of activated STAT-3 (PIAS-3) in **ovarian and endometrial cancer** *cells.* Saydmohammed M, Joseph D, Syed V. J Cell Biochem. 2010 May 15;110(2):447-56. **Key Finding**: "Curcumin suppresses JAK-STAT signaling in ovarian and endometrial cancers via activation of PIAS-3, thus attenuating STAT-3 phosphorylation and tumor cell growth."

Curcumin *induces chemo/radio-sensitization in ovarian cancer cells and curcumin nanoparticles inhibit* **ovarian cancer** *cell growth.* Yallapu MM, Maher DM, Sundram V, Et al. J Ovarian Res. 2010 Apr 29;3:11. **Key Finding**: "Curcumin pre-treatment enhances chemo/radio-sensitization in A2780CP ovarian cancer cells through multiple molecular mechanisms. A targeted PLGA nanoparticles formulation of curcumin is feasible and may improve the in vivo therapeutic efficacy of curcumin."

Curcumin targeted signaling pathways: basis for anti-photo aging and anti-carcinogenic therapy. Heng MC. Int J Dermatol. 2010 Jun;49(6):608-22. **Key Finding**: "Curcumin has been shown to protect against the deleterious effects of skin injury from solar radiation by attenuating oxidative stress and suppressing inflammation. The ability of curcumin to block multiple targets on these pathways serve as a basis for the potential use of this phytochemical in photo aging skin and photo carcinogenesis (**melanoma**)."

Curcumin induces cell death in human unveil **melanoma** cells through mitochondrial pathway. Lu C, Song E, Hu DN, Et al. Curr Eye Res. 2010 Apr;35(4):352-60. **Key Finding**: "Curcumin has selectively potent cytotoxic effects on cultured human unveil melanoma cells. This effect is associated with the release of cytochrome c from the mitochondria and the activation of caspase-9 and caspase-3 in unveil melanoma cells after treatment with curcumin."

Curcumin-induced apoptosis in **ovarian carcinoma** *cells are p53-independent and involve p38 mitogen-active protein kinase activation and down regulation of Bcl-2 and surviving expression and Akt signaling.* Watson JL, Greenshields A, Hill R, Et al. Mol Carcinog. 2010 Jan;49(1):13-24. **Key Finding**: "These data provide a mechanistic rationale for the potential use of curcumin in the treatment of ovarian cancer."

Curcumin causes superoxide anion production and p53-independent apoptosis in human **colon cancer** *cells.* Watson JL, Hill R, Yaffe PB, Et al. Cancer Lett. 2010 Nov 1;297(1):1-8. **Key Finding**: "Our results indicate that, despite p53 up regulation and activation, curcumin-induced apoptosis in colon cancer cells was independent of p53 status and involved oxidative stress. Curcumin may therefore have therapeutic potential in the management of colon cancer."

Distinct combinatorial effects of the plant polyphenols curcumin, carnosic acid, and silibinin on proliferation and apoptosis in acute myeloid **leukemia** *cells.* Pesakhov S, Khanin M, Studzinski GP, Et al. Nutr Cancer. 2010;62(6):811-24. **Key Finding**: "Collectively, these results suggest a mechanistic basis for the potential use of dietary plant polyphenol combinations in the treatment and prevention of acute myeloid leukemia."

Curcumin in cancer chemoprevention: molecular targets, pharmacokinetics, bioavailability, and clinical trials. Shehzad A, Wahid F, Lee YS. Arch Pharm. 2010 Sep;343(9):489-99. **Key Finding**: "Sufficient data has been shown to advocate phase II and phase III clinical trials of curcumin for a variety of cancer conditions including **multiple myeloma, pancreatic, and colon cancer**."

Anti-carcinogenic properties of curcumin on colorectal cancer. Park J, Conteas CN. World J Gastrointest Oncol. 2010 Apr 15;2(4):169-76. **Key Finding**: "We examine the current studies and literature and touch upon many molecular pathways affected by curcumin, and demonstrate the exciting possibility of curcumin as a chemo preventive agent for **colorectal cancer.**"

Curcumin therapeutic promises and bioavailability in **colorectal cancer.** Shehzad A, Khan S, Shehzad O, Lee YS. Drugs Today. 2010 Jul;46(7):523-32. **Key Finding:** "Curcumin, a polyphenol and derivative of turmeric is one of the most commonly used and highly researched phytochemicals. Although curcumin poor absorption and low systemic bioavailability limit its translation into clinics, some of the methods for its use can be approached to enhance the absorption and achieve a therapeutic level of curcumin. Recent clinical trials suggest a potential role for curcumin in regards to colorectal cancer therapy."

Curcumin-*induced apoptosis in PC3* ***prostate carcinoma*** *cells is caspase-independent and involves cellular ceramide accumulation and damage to mitochondria.* Hilchie AL, Furlong SJ, Sutton K, Et al. Nutr Cancer. 2010;62(3):379-89. **Key Finding**: "Curcumin treatment of PC3 prostate carcinoma cells caused time- and dose-dependent induction of apoptosis and depletion of cellular reduced glutathione."

Curcumin *interrupts the interaction between the androgen receptor and WntB-catenin signaling pathway in LNCaP* ***prostate cancer*** *cells.* Choi HY, Lim JE, Hong JH. Prostate Cancer Prostatic Dis. 2010 Dec;13(4):343-9. **Key Finding**: "These findings suggest that curcumin modulates the Wnt/B-catenin signaling pathway and might have a significant role in mediating inhibitory effects on LNCaP prostate cancer cells."

Targeting ***breast*** *stem cells with the* ***cancer*** *preventive compounds curcumin and piperine.* Kakarala M, Brenner DE, Korkaya H, Cheng C, Tazi K, Ginestier C, Lie S, Dontu G, Wicha MS. Breast Cancer Res Treat. 2009 Nov 7 (Epub ahead of print). **Key Finding**: "Curcumin and piperine separately, and in combination, inhibit breast stem cell self-renewal but do not cause toxicity to differentiated cells. These compounds could be potential cancer preventive agents."

Curcumin circumvents chemo resistance in vitro and potentiates the effect of thalidomide and bortezomib against human ***multiple myeloma*** *in nude mice model.* Sung B, Kunnumakkara AB, Sethi G, Anand P, Guha S, Aggarwal BB. Mol Cancer Ther. 2009 Apr;8(4):959-70. **Key Finding:** "Collectively, our results suggest that curcumin overcomes chemo resistance and sensitizes multiple myeloma cells to thalidomide and bortezomib by down-regulating NF-KappaB and NF-kappaB-regulated gene products."

Curcumin blocks CCL2-induced adhesion, motility and invasion, in part, through down-regulation of CCL2 expression and proteolytic activity. Herman JG, Stadelman HL, Roselli CE. Int J Oncol. 2009 May;34(5):1319-27. **Key Finding:** CCL2 is a potent chemotactic factor of **prostate cancer**. "These data indicate a potential mechanism by which curcumin can block the chemotactic effects of CCL2 on PCa. Curcumin exerts potential anti-metastatic effects in bone-derived PCa cells by blocking CCL2 mediated actions on invasion, adhesion and motility, in part through differential regulation of PKC and MMP-9 signaling."

Systemic Delivery of Curcumin: 21st Century Solutions for an Ancient Conundrum. Bisht S, Maitra A. Curr Drug Discov Technol. 2009 Sep 1. (Epub ahead of print). **Key Finding:** "Accumulating experimental evidence suggests that curcumin interferes with a variety of molecular targets and processes involved in **cancer**. This review is intended to provide the reader an update on the bioavailability and pharmacokinetic pitfalls of free curcumin, and a comprehensive cataloging of ongoing approaches that have been undertaken to resolve these issues."

Curcumin induces apoptosis through FAS and FADD, in caspase-3-dependent and –independent pathways in the N18 mouse-rat hybrid retina ganglion cells. Lu HF, Lai KC, Hsu SC, Lin HJ, Yang MD, Chen YL, Fan MJ, Yang JS, Cheng PY, Kup CL, Chung JG. Oncol Rep. 2009 Jul;22(1):97-104. **Key Finding:** Curcumin has broad spectrum of anti-tumor activities against many human **cancer** cells. In this study, curcumin induced apoptosis and caused a marked increase in apoptosis as characterized by DNA fragmentation. Curcumin also induced endoplasmic reticulum stress in N18 cells.

*Curcumin inhibits proliferation and migration by increasing the Bax to Bcl-2 ratio and decreasing NF-kappaBp65 expression in **breast cancer** MDA-MB-231 cells.* Chiu TL, Su CC. Int J Mol Med. 2009 Apr;23(4):469-75. **Key Finding:** The effects of curcumin on human breast cancer MDA-MB-231 cells were evaluated. "Our results show that curcumin inhibits the migratory activity of MDA-MB-231 cells through down-regulating the protein expression of NF-kappaBp65. Accordingly, the therapeutic potential of curcumin for breast cancer deserves further study."

*Curcumin inhibits cell proliferation of MDA-MB-231 and BT-483 **breast cancer** cells mediated by down-regulation of NFkappa B, CyclinD and MMP-1 transcription.* Liu Q, Loo WT, Sze SC, Tong Y. Phytomedicine. 2009 Oct;16(10):916-922. **Key**

Finding: "Our finding extrapolates the antitumor activity of curcumin in mediating the breast cancer cell proliferative rate and invasion by down-regulating the NFkappaB inducing genes."

Synergistic effect of combination of phenethyl isothiocyanate and sulforaphane or curcumin and sulforaphane in the inhibition of inflammation. Cheung KL, Khor TO, Kong AN. Pharm Res. 2009 Jan;26(1):224-31. Epub 2008 Oct 8. **Key Finding:** "Our data suggest that CUR (curcumin) **+** SFN (sulforaphane) and PEITC (phenethyl isothiocyanate) **+** SFN combinations could be more effective than used alone in preventing **inflammation** and possibly its associated diseases including **cancer**."

Curcumin in combination with visible light inhibits tumor growth in a xenograft tumor model. Dujic J, Kippenberger S, Ramirez-Bosca A, Diaz-Alperi J, Bereiter-Hahn J, Kaufman R, Bernd A, Hofmann M. Int J Cancer. 2009 Mar 15;124(6):1422-8. **Key Finding:** "The present findings suggest a combination of curcumin and light as a new therapeutic concept to increase the efficacy of curcumin in the treatment of **cancer**."

*Curcumin inhibits the migration and invasion of human A549 **lung cancer** cells through the inhibition of matrix metalloproteinase-2 and -9 and Vascular Endothelial Growth Factor (VEGF).* Lin SS, Lai KC, Hsu SC, Yang JS, Kuo CL, Lin JP, Ma YS, Wu CC, Chung JG. Cancer Lett. 2009 May 22 (Epub ahead of print). **Key Finding:** "The data shows that the anticancer effect of curcumin is also exist for the inhibition of migration and invasion in lung cancer cells."

Molecular mechanism of curcumin induced cytotoxicity in human cervical carcinoma cells. Singh M, Singh N. Mol Cell Biochem. 2009 May;325(1-2):107-19. **Key Finding:** "Curcumin acts as an anti-inflammatory and anti-proliferative agent by causing down regulation of COX-2, iNOS and cyclin D1 in all the three cells lines of **cervical cancer**, but to a different extent."

*Curcumin synergizes with resveratrol to inhibit **colon cancer**.* Majumdar AP, Banerjee S, Nautiyal J, Patel BB, Patel V, Du J, Yu Y, Elliott AA, Levi E, Sarkar FH. Nutr Cancer. 2009;61(4):544-53. **Key Finding:** "Our current data suggest that the combination of curcumin and resveratrol could be an effective preventive/therapeutic strategy for colon cancer. The combination of curcumin and resveratrol was found to be more effective in inhibiting growth of p53-positive (wt) and p53-negative colon cancer HCT-116 cells in vitro and in vivo in SCID xenografts of colon cancer HCT-116 (wt) cells than either agent alone."

*Curcumin sensitizes human **colorectal cancer** xenografts in nude mice to gamme-radiation by targeting nuclear factor-kappaB-regulated gene products.* Kunnumakkara AB, Diagaradiane P, Guha S, Deorukhkar A, Shentu S, Aggarwal BB, Krishnan S. Clin Cancer Res. 2008 Apr 1;14(7):2128-36. **Key Finding:** "Our results suggest that curcumin potentiates the antitumor effects of radiation therapy in colorectal cancer by suppressing NF-kappaB and NF-kappaB-regulated gene products, leading to inhibition of proliferation and angiogenesis."

*Curcumin inhibits proliferation, invasion, angiogenesis and metastasis of difference **cancers** through interaction with multiple cell signaling proteins.* Kunnumakkara AB, Anand P, Aggarwal BB. Cancer Lett. 2008 Oct 8;269(2):199-225. **Key Finding:** Curcumin has been found to inhibit the proliferation of various tumor cells in culture, prevents carcinogen-induced cancers in rodents, and inhibits the growth of human tumors in xenotransplant or orthotransplant animal models either alone or in combination with chemotherapeutic agents or radiation.

*New mechanisms and therapeutic potential of curcumin for **colorectal cancer**.* Villegas I, Sanchez-Fidalgo S, Alarcon de la Lastra C. Mol Nutr Food Res. 2008 Sept;52(9):1040-61. **Key Finding:** This review provides the reader with an update of the bioavailability and pharmacokinetics of curcumin and describes the recently identified molecular pathways responsible for its anticancer potential in colorectal cancer.

Curcumin sensitizes TRAIL-resistant xenografts: molecular mechanisms of apoptosis, metastasis and angiogenesis. Shankar S, Ganapathy S, Chen Q, Srivastava RK. Mol Cancer. 2008 Jan 29;7:16. **Key Finding:** "The ability of curcumin to inhibit **tumor** growth, metastasis and angiogenesis, and enhance the therapeutic potential of TRAIL suggests that curcumin alone or in combination with TRAIL can be used for prostate cancer prevention and/or therapy."

Anti-cancer effects of curcumin: cycle of life and death. Sa G, Das T. Cell Div. 2008 Oct 3;3:14. **Key Finding:** In this review the authors provide an overview of how curcumin targets cell cycle regulatory molecules to assert anti-proliferative and/or apoptotic effects in **cancer** cells.

*Androgen responsive and refractory **prostate cancer** cells exhibit distinct curcumin regulated transcriptions.* Thangapazham RL, Shaheduzzaman S, Kim KH, Passi N, Tadese A, Vahey M, Dobi A, Srivastava S, Maheshwari RK. Cancer Biol Ther. 2008 Sept;7(9):1427-35. **Key Finding:** "This report for the first time establishes novel features of Cu-GER in prostate cancer cells of varying tumorigenic phenotypes and provides potentially novel read-outs for assessing effectiveness of curcumin in prostate cancer and likely in other cancers. Importantly, new gene-networks identified here further delineate molecular mechanisms of action of curcumin in prostate cancer cells."

Curcumin and cancer: an 'old-age' disease with an 'age-old' solution. Anand P, Sundaram C, Jhurani S, Kunnumakkara AB, Aggarwal BB. Cancer Lett. 2008 Aug 18;267(1):133-64. **Key Finding:** "The activity of curcumin reported against **leukemia and lymphoma, gastrointestinal cancers, genitourinary cancers, breast cancer, ovarian cancer, head and neck squamous cell carcinoma, lung cancer, melanoma, neurological cancers, and sarcoma** reflects its ability to affect multiple targets."

Recent advances in the investigation of curcuminoids. Itokawa H, Shi Q, Akiyama T, Morris-Natschke SL, Lee KH. Chin Med. 2008 Sep 17;3:11. **Key Finding:** "In this article we review the literature between 1976 and mid-2008 on the anti-inflammatory, anti-oxidant, anti-HIV, chemo preventive and anti-**prostate cancer** effects of curcuminoids."

EF24, a novel curcumin analog, disrupts the microtubule cytoskeleton and inhibits HIF-1. Thomas SL, Zhong D, Zhou W, Malik S, Liotta D, Snyder JP, Hamel E, Giannakakou P. Cell Cycle. 2008 Aug;7(15):2409-17. **Key Finding:** "Our study identifies EF24 as a novel curcumin-related compound possessing a distinct mechanism of action, which we believe contributes to the potent **anticancer** activity of this agent and can be further exploited to investigate the therapeutic potential of Ef24."

*Murine **prostate cancer** inhibition by dietary phytochemicals – curcumin and phenyethylisothiocyanate.* Barve A, Khor TO, Hay X, Keum YS, Yang CS, Reddy B, Kong AN. Pharm Res. 2008 Sept;25(9):2181-9. Epub 2008 Apr 25. **Key Finding:** "Our data lucidly evidence the chemo preventive merits of dietary phytochemicals curcumin and PEITC in suppressing prostate adenocarcinoma."

*Curcumin down regulates the constitutive activity of NF-kappaB and induces apoptosis in novel mouse **melanoma** cells.* Marin YE, Wall BA, Wang S, Namkoong J, Martino JJ, Suh J, Lee HJ, Radson AB, Yang CS, Chen S, Ryu JH. Melanoma Res. 2007 Oct;17(5):274-83. **Key Finding:** "Curcumin, a natural and safe compound, inhibits NF-kappaB activity and the expression of its downstream target genes, and also selectively induces apoptosis of melanoma cells but not normal melanocytes. These encouraging in-vitro results support further investigation of curcumin for treatment of melanoma in vivo."

Curcumin suppresses growth and chemo resistance of human gliobastoma cells via AP-1 and NFkappaB transcription factors. Dhandapani KM, Mahesh VB, Brann DW. J Neurochem. 2007 Jul;102(2):522-38. **Key Finding:** Malignant gliomas are a debilitating class of brain tumors that are resistant to radiation. The effect of curcumin on glioma survival was investigated. "These findings support a role for curcumin as an adjunct to traditional chemotherapy and radiation in the treatment of **brain cancer**."

Curcumin potentiates antitumor activity of gemcitabine in an orthotropic model of pancreatic cancer through suppression of proliferation angiogenesis, and inhibition of nuclear factor-kappaB-regulated gene products. Kunnumakkara AB, Guha S, Krishnan S, Diagaradjane P, Gelovania J, Aggarwal BB. Cancer Res. 2007 Apr 15;67(8):3853-61. **Key Finding:** "We investigated whether curcumin can sensitize **pancreatic cancer** to gemcitabine in vitro and in vivo. Overall, our results suggest that curcumin potentiates the antitumor effects of gemcitabine in pancreatic cancer by suppressing proliferation, angiogenesis, NF-kappaB, and NF-kappaB-regulated gene products."

*Curcumin enhances Apo2L/TRAIL-induced apoptosis in chemo resistant **ovarian cancer** cells.* Wahl H, Tan L, Griffith K, Choi M, Liu JR. Gynecol Oncol. 2007 Apr;105(1):104-12. **Key Finding:** "Combined curcumin and Apo2L/TRAIL treatment results in enhanced induction of apoptotic cell death. Because curcumin and Apo2L/TRAIL together can activate both the extrinsic and intrinsic pathways of apoptosis, they may circumvent chemo resistance to conventional chemotherapeutic agents."

Chemo preventive anti-inflammatory activities of curcumin and other phytochemicals mediated by MAP kinase phosphatase-5 in prostate cells. Nonn L, Duong D, Peehl DM. Carcinogenesis. 2007 Jun;28(6):1188-96. **Key Finding:** The mediating anti-inflammatory activities of curcumin, resveratrol and gingerol were examined. "Our findings show direct anti-inflammatory activity of MKP5 in prostate cells and suggest that up-regulation of MKP5 by phytochemicals may contribute to their chemo preventive actions by decreasing **prostatic inflammation**."

Involvement of Bcl-2 family members, phosphatidylinositol 3'-kinase/AKT and mitochondrial p53 in curcumin (diferulolylmethane)-induced apoptosis in prostate cancer. Shankar S, Srivastava RK. Int J Oncol. 2007 Apr;30(4):905-18. **Key Finding:** "Our study establishes a role for AKT in modulating the direct action of p53 on the caspase-dependent mitochondrial death pathway and suggests that these important biological molecules interact at the level of the mitochondria to influence curcumin sensitivity. These properties of curcumin strongly suggest that it could be used as a **cancer** chemo preventive agent."

Curcumin for chemoprevention of **colon cancer**. Johnson JJ, Mukhtar H. Cancer Lett. 2007 Oct 8;255(2):170-81. **Key Finding:** "Overwhelming in vitro evidence and completed clinical trials suggests that curcumin may prove to be useful for the chemoprevention of colon cancer in humans. This review will focus on describing the pre-clinical and clinical evidence of curcumin as a chemo preventive compound in colorectal cancer."

The Chemo preventive Polyphenol Curcumin Prevents Hematogenous **Breast Cancer** *Metastases in Immunodeficient Mice.* Bachmeier B, Nerlich A, Iancu C, Cilli M, Schleicher E, Vene R, Dell Eva R, Jochum M, Albini A, Pfeffer U. Cell Physiol Biochem. 2007;19:137-152. **Key Finding:** "We examined curcumin's effects on the human breast cancer cell line MDA-MB-231 in vitro and in a mouse metastasis model. Curcumin strongly induces apoptosis in MDA-MB-231 cells in correlation with reduced activation of the survival pathway of NFKB, as a consequence of diminished IKB and p65 phosphorylation."

Antioxidant and anti-inflammatory properties of curcumin. Menon VP, Sudheer AR. Adv Exp Med Biol. 2007;595:105-25. **Key Finding:** "The past few decades have witnessed intense research devoted to the antioxidant and anti-inflammatory properties of curcumin. In this review, we describe antioxidant and anti-inflammatory properties of curcumin, the mode of action of curcumin, and its therapeutic usage against different pathological conditions."

Effect of selected phytochemicals and apple extracts on NF-kappaB activation in human **breast cancer** *MCF-7 cells.* Yoon H, Liu RH. J Agric Food Chem. 2007 Apr 18;55(8):3167-73. **Key Finding:** "These results suggest that **apple extracts** and **curcumin** have the capabilities of inhibiting TNF-alpha-induced NF-kappaB activation of MCF-7 cells by inhibiting the proteasome activities instead of IkappaB kinase activation."

Curcumin (diferuloyimethane) down-regulates expression of cell proliferation and antiapoptoic and metastatic gene products through suppression of IkappaBalpha kinase and Akt activation. Aggarwal S, Ichikawa H, Takada Y, Sandur SK, Shishodia S, Aggarwal BB. Mol Pharmacol. 2006 Jan;69(1):195-206. **Key Finding:** "In the present study, we investigated the mechanism by which curcumin manifests its effect on NF-kappaB and NF-kappaB-regulated gene expression. Screening of 20 different analogs of curcumin showed that curcumin was the most potent analog in suppressing the tumor necrosis factor (TNF)-induced NF-kappaB activation. Curcumin inhibited TNF-induced NF-kappaB-dependent reporter gene expression in a dose-dependent manner."

Inhibition of EGFR signaling in human prostate cancer PC-3 cells by combination treatment with beta-phenylethyl isothiocyanate and curcumin. Kim JH, Xu C, Keum YS, Reddy B, Conney A, Kong AN. Carcinogenesis. 2006 Mar;27(3): 475-82. Epub 2005 Nov 19. **Key Finding:** "We conclude that the simultaneous targeting of EGFR, AKt and Nf-kappaB signaling pathways by PEITC and curcumin could be the molecular targets by which PEITC and curcumin exert their additive inhibitory effects on cell proliferation and ultimately lead to programmed cell death of tumor cells."

Combination Treatment with Curcumin and Quercetin of Adenomas in Familial Adenomatous Polyposis. Cruz-Correa M, Shoskes DA, Sanchez P, Zhao R, Hylind LM, Wexner SD, Giardiello FM. Clinical Gastroenterology and Hepatology. 2006 Aug; Vol. 4, No. 8. **Key Finding:** The phytochemical combination of curcumin and quercetin reduced the number of colon polyps in test subjects by 60 percent and caused some polyps to shrink.

Combined inhibitory effects of curcumin and phenethyl isothiocyanate on the growth of human PC-3 prostate xenografts in immunodeficient mice. Khor To, Keum YS, Lin W, Kim JH, Hu R, Shen G, Xu C, Gopalakrishnan A, Reddy B, Zheng X, Conney AH, Kong AN. Cancer Res. 2006 Jan 15;66(2):613-21. **Key Finding:** "Our results show that PEITC and curcumin alone or in combination possess significant **cancer-preventive** activities in the PC-3 prostate tumor xenografts. Furthermore, we found that combination of PEITC and curcumin could be effective in the cancer-therapeutic treatment of prostate cancers."

Curcumin: getting back to the roots. Shishodia S, Sethi G, Aggarwal BB. Ann NY Acad Sci. 2005 Nov;1056:206-17. **Key Finding:** "Curcumin is now being used to treat **cancer, arthritis, diabetes, Crohn's disease, cardiovascular disease, osteoporosis, Alzheimer's disease, psoriasis**, and other pathologies. Interestingly, 6-gingerol, a natural analog of curcumin derived from the root of ginger (Zingiber officinalis), exhibits a biologic activity profile similar to that of curcumin."

Curcumin: the story so far. Sharma RA, Gescher AJ, Steward WP. Eur J Cancer. 2005 Sep;41(13):1955-68. **Key Finding:** "Although curcumin's low systemic bioavailability following oral dosing may limit access of sufficient concentrations for pharmacological effect in certain tissues, the attainment of biologically active levels in the gastrointestinal tract has been demonstrated in animals and humans. Sufficient data currently exist to advocate phase II clinical evaluation of oral curcumin in patients with invasive malignancy or pre-invasive lesions of the gastrointestinal tract, particularly the **colon and rectum**."

Curcumin-induced antiproliferative and proapoptotic effects in **melanoma** *cells are associated with suppression of kappaB kinase and nuclear factor kappaB activity and are independent of the B-Raf/mitogen-activated/extracellular signal-regulated protein kinase pathway and the Akt pathway.* Siwak DR, Shishodia S, Aggarwal BB, Kurzrock R. Cancer. 2005 aug 15;104(4):879-90. **Key Finding:** "Curcumin has potent antiproliferative and proapoptotic effects in melanoma cells. These effects were associated with the suppression of NF-kappaB and IKK activities but were independent of the B-Raf/MEK/ERK and Akt pathways."

Curcumin (diferuloylmethane) inhibits constitutive NF-kappaB activation, induces G1/S arrest, suppresses proliferation, and induces apoptosis in mantle cell **lymphoma**. Shishodia S, Amin HM, Lai R, Aggarwal BB. Biochem Pharmcol. 2005 Sept 1;70(5):700-13. **Key Finding:** "Our results indicate that curcumin inhibits the constitutive NF-kappaB and IKK leading to suppression of expression of NF-kappaB-regulated gene products that result in the suppression of proliferation, cell cycle arrest, and induction of apoptosis in human mantle cell lymphoma, an aggressive B cell non-Hodgkin's lymphoma."

Curcumin confers radio sensitizing effect in **prostate cancer** *cell line PC-3.* Chendil D, Ranga RS, Meigooni D, Sathishkumar S, Ahmed MM. Oncogene. 2004 Feb 26;23(8):1599-607. **Key Finding:** "The natural compound curcumin is a potent radio sensitizer, and it acts by overcoming the effects of radiation-induced prosurvival gene expression in prostate cancer."

Curcumin sensitizes **prostate cancer** *cells to tumor necrosis factor-related apoptosis-inducing ligand/Apo2L by inhibiting nuclear factor-kappaB through suppression of IkappaBalpha phosphorylation.* Deeb D, Jiang H, Gao X, Hafner MS, Wong H, Divine G, Chapman RA, Dulchavsky SA, Gautam SC. Mol Cancer Ther. 2004 Jul;3(7):803-12. **Key Finding:** "We conclude that NF-kappaB mediates resistance of LNCaP cells to TRAIL (tumor necrosis factor-related apoptosis-inducing ligand) and that curcumin enhances the sensitivity of these tumor cells to TRAIL by inhibiting NF-kappaB activation by blocking phosphorylation of IkappaBalpha and its degradation."

Suppression of the nuclear factor-kappaB activation pathway by spice-derived phytochemicals: reasoning for seasoning. Aggarwal BB, Shishodia S. Ann N Y Acad Sci. 2004 Dec;1030:434-41. **Key Finding:** "The activation of nuclear transcription factor kappaB has now been linked with a variety of inflammatory disease, including **cancer, atherosclerosis, myocardial infarction, diabetes, allergy, asthma, arthritis, Crohn's disease, multiple sclerosis, Alzheimer's disease, osteoporosis, psoriasis, septic shock, and AIDS**. Extensive research in the last few years has shown that the pathway that activates this transcription factor can be interrupted by phytochemicals derived from spices such as turmeric (curcumin), red pepper (capsaicin), cloves (eugenol), ginger (gingerol), cumin, anise, and fennel (anethol), basil and rosemary (ursolic acid), garlic (diallyl sulfide, S-allylmercaptocysteine, ajoene), and pomegranate (ellagic acid). For the first time, therefore, research provides 'reasoning for seasoning.'"

Polyphenolic phytochemicals versus non-steroidal anti-inflammatory drugs: which are better cancer chemo preventive agents? Gescher A. J Chemother. 2004 Nov;16 Suppl 4:3-6. **Key Finding:** "As non-steroidal anti-inflammatory drugs possess unwanted side effects, polyphenolic phytochemicals such as curcumin and resveratrol are promising alternatives. They suppress **carcinogenesis** in the ApcMin+ mouse model. Clinical pilot studies of curcumin show that it is safe at doses of up to 3.6g daily, and that the levels of curcumin which can be achieved in the gastrointestinal tract exert pharmacological activity."

*Curcumin (diferuloyl-methane) enhances tumor necrosis factor-related apoptosis-inducing ligand-induced apoptosis in LNCaP **prostate cancer** cells.* Deeb D, Xu YX, Jiang H, Gao X, Janakiraman N, Chapman RA, Gautam SC. Mol Cancer Ther. 2003 Jan;2(1):95-103. **Key Finding:** "These results define a potential use of curcumin to sensitize prostate cancer cells for TRAIL-mediated immunotherapy."

***Anticancer** potential of curcumin: preclinical and clinical studies.* Aggarwal B, Kumar A, Bharti AC. Anticancer Res. 2003 Jan-Feb;23(1A):363-98. **Key Finding:** This review describes in detail the data supporting studies which show curcumin to be a polyphenol that can both prevent and treat cancer.

Curcumin down-regulates the constitutive activation of nuclear factor-kappaB and IkappaBalpha Kinase in human multiple myeloma cells, leading to suppression of proliferation and induction of apoptosis. Bharti AC, Donato N, Singh S, Aggarwal BB. Blood. 2003 Feb 1;101(3):1053-62. **Key Finding:** "Our results indicate that curcumin down-regulates NF-kappaB in human **multiple myeloma** cells, leading to the suppression of proliferation and induction of apoptosis, thus providing the molecular basis for the treatment of MM patients with this pharmacologically safe agent."

Functional properties of spice extracts obtained via supercritical fluid extraction. Leal PF, Braga ME, Sato DN, Carvalho JE, Marques MO, Meireles MA. J Agric Food Chem. 2003 Apr 23;51(9):2520-5. **Key Finding:** "In the present study the antioxidant, **anticancer** and **antimicrobacterial** activities of extracts from ginger, rosemary and turmeric were evaluated. The rosemary extracts exhibited the strongest antioxidant and the lowest antimicrobacterial activities. Turmeric extracts showed the greatest antimicrobacterial activity. Ginger and turmeric extracts showed selected anticancer activities."

Dietary curcumin inhibits chemotherapy-induced apoptosis in models of human **breast cancer.** Somasundaram S, Edmund NA, Moore DT, Small GW, Shi YY, Orlowski RZ. Cancer Res. 2002 Jul 1;62(13):3868-75. **Key Finding:** "These findings support the hypothesis that dietary curcumin can inhibit chemotherapy-induced apoptosis through inhibition of ROS generation and blockade of JNK function, and suggest that additional studies are needed to determine whether breast cancer patients undergoing chemotherapy should avoid curcumin supplementation, and possibly even limit their exposure to curcumin-containing foods."

Curcumin induces apoptosis in human **melanoma** *cells through a Fas receptor/caspase-8 pathway independent of p53.* Bush JA, Cheung KJ, Li G. Exp Cell Res. 2001 Dec 10;271(2):305-14. **Key Finding:** "Since melanoma cells with mutant p53 are strongly resistant to conventional chemotherapy, curcumin may overcome the chemo resistance of these cells and provide potential new avenues for treatment."

Therapeutic potential of curcumin in human **prostate cancer***. III. Curcumin inhibits proliferation, induces apoptosis, and inhibits angiogenesis of LNCaP prostate cancer cells in vivo.* Dorai T, Cao YC, Dorai B, Buttyan R, Katz AE. Prostate. 2001 Jun 1;47(4):293-303. **Key Finding:** "Curcumin could be a potentially therapeutic anti-cancer agent, as it significantly inhibits prostate cancer growth, as exemplified by LNCaP in vivo, and has the potential to prevent the progression of this cancer to its hormone refractory state."

Induction of stress response renders human tumor cells lines resistant to curcumin-mediated apoptosis: role of reactive oxygen intermediates. Khar A, Ali AM, Pardhasaradhi BV, Varalakshmi CH, Anjum R, Kumari AL. Cell Stress Chaperones. 2001 Oct;6(4):368-76. **Key Finding:** "We have shown that different cancer cell lines differ in their sensitivity to curcumin. Cell lines established from malignancies like **leukemia, breast, colon, hepatocellular, and ovarian** carcinomas underwent apoptosis in the presence of curcumin, whereas cell lines from lung, kidney, prostate, cervix, CNS malignancies, and melanomas showed resistance to the cytotoxic effects of curcumin."

Biological Activities of Curcuma longa L. Araujol CAC, Leon LL. Memorias do Instituto Oswaldo Cruz (from Portuguese). 2001 July; vol 96(5):723-728. **Key Finding:** This overview of the pharmacological activities of Curcumin shows its importance for its anti-parasitic, antispasmodic, anti-inflammatory and gastrointestinal effects, as well as inhibiting carcinogenesis and cancer growth.

Therapeutic potential of curcumin in human prostate cancer. II. Curcumin inhibits tyrosine kinase activity of epidermal growth factor receptor and depletes the protein. Dorai T, Gehani N, Katz A. Mol Urol. 2000 Spring;4(1):1-6. **Key Finding:** "These results, taken together with our previous results that curcumin can induce apoptosis in both androgen-dependent and androgen-independent prostate cancer cells, support our view that curcumin may be a novel modality by which one can interfere with the signal transduction pathways of the **prostate cancer** cell and prevent it from progressing to its hormone-refractory state."

Chemo preventive Effect of Curcumin, a Naturally Occurring Anti-Inflammatory Agent, during the Promotion/Progression Stages of Colon Cancer. Kawamori T, Lubet R, Steele VE, Kelloff GJ, Kaskey RB, Rao CV, Reddy BS. Cancer Research. 1999 Feb 1;59:597-601. **Key Finding:** "Chemo preventive activity of curcumin is observed when it is administered prior to, during, and after carcinogen treatment as well as when it is given only during the promotion/progression phase (starting late in premalignant stage) of **colon carcinogenesis**."

Chemoprevention by curcumin during the promotion stage of tumorigenesis of mammary gland in rats irradiated with (gamma)-rays. Inano H, Onoda M, Inafuku N, Kubota M, Kamada Y, Osawa T, Kobayashi H, Wakabayashi K. Carcinogenesis. 1999 June 1;20(6):1011-1018. **Key Finding:** "Whole mounts of the mammary glands showed that curcumin yielded morphologically indistinguishable proliferation and differentiation from the glands of the control rats. These findings suggest that curcumin has a potent preventive activity during the DES-dependent promotion stage of radiation-induced **mammary tumorigenesis**."

Quantitation of chemo preventive synergism between (-)-epigallocatechin-3-gallate and curcumin in normal, premalignant and malignant human oral epithelial cells. Khafif A, Schantz SP, Chou TC, Edelstein D, Sacks PG. Carcinogenesis. 1998; vol 19, no. 3:419-424.

Key Finding: "An in vitro model for **oral cancer** was used to examine the growth inhibitory effects of chemo preventive agents when used singly and in combination. EGCG from green tea was less effective with cell progression. In contrast, curcumin was equally effective regardless of the cell type tested. The combination of both agents showed synergistic interactions in growth inhibition and increased sigmoidicity (steepness) of the dose-effect curves, a response that was dose and cell type dependent."

The Inhibition of the Estrogenic Effects of Pesticides and Environmental Chemicals by Curcumin and Isoflavonoids. Verma SP, Goldin BR, Lin PS. Environmental Health Perspectives. 1998 Dec; vol. 106, no. 12:807-812. **Key Finding:** The inhibitory action of curcumin and a combination of curcumin and isoflavonoids were studied in ER-positive (estrogen receptor-positive) human **breast cancer** cells induced by a pesticide and environmental pollutants. "A combination of curcumin and isoflavonoids was able to inhibit the induced growth of ER-positive cells up to 95%. These data suggest that combinations of natural plant compounds may have preventive and therapeutic applications against the growth of breast tumors induced by environmental estrogens."

Estrogen and progestin bioactivity of foods, herbs, and spices. Zava DT, Dollbaum CM, Blen M. Proc Soc Exp Biol Med. 1998 Mar;217(3):369-78. **Key Finding:** "Over 150 herbs traditionally used by herbalists for treating a variety of health problems were extracted and tested for their relative capacity to compete with estradiol and progesterone binding to intracellular receptors for progesterone (PR) and estradiol (ER) in intact human **breast cancer** cells. The six highest ER-binding herbs that are commonly consumed were soy, licorice, red clover, thyme, turmeric, hops and verbena. The six highest PR-binding herbs and spices commonly consumed were oregano, verbena, turmeric, thyme, red clover and damiana."

Chemo preventive effects of carotenoids and curcumins on mouse **colon carcinogenesis** *after 1,2-dimethylhydrazine initiation.* Kim JM, Araki S, Kim DJ, Park CB, Takasuka N, Baba-Toriyama H, Ota T, Nir Z, Khachik F, Shimidzu N, Tanaka Y, Osawa T, Uraji T, Murakoshi M, Nishino H, Tsuda H. Carcinogenesis. 1998; vol 19, no 1: 81-85. **Key Finding:** "The present study was carried out to examine the chemo preventive effects of carotenoids such as fucoxanthin, lycopene and lutein as well as curcumin and its derivative, tetrahydrocurcumin (THC) on development of putative preneoplastic aberrant crypt foci (ACF) in colons of mice. The results suggest that fucoxanthin, lutein, and THC may have potential as chemo preventive agents against colon carcinogenesis."

Curcumin is an in vivo inhibitor of angiogenesis. Arbiser JL, Klauber N, Rohan R, van Leeuwen R, Huang MT, Fisher C, Flynn E, Byers HR. Mol Med. 1998 Jun;4(6):376-83. **Key Finding:** "These results indicate that curcumin has direct antiangiogenic activity in vitro and in vivo. The activity of curcumin in inhibiting carcinogenesis in diverse organs such as the **skin and colon** may be mediated in part through angiogenesis inhibition."

*Curcumin and genistein, plant natural products, show synergistic inhibitory effects on the growth of human **breast cancer** MCF-7 cells induced by estrogenic pesticides.* Verma SP, Salamone E, Goldin B. Biochem Biophys Res Commun. 1997 Apr 28;233(3):692-6. **Key Finding:** "When curcumin and genistein were added together to MCF-7 cells, a synergistic effect resulting in a total inhibition of the induction of MCF-7 cells by the highly estrogenic activity of endosulfane/chlordane/DDT mixtures was noted. The inclusion of turmeric and soybeans in the diet to prevent hormone related cancers deserves consideration."

Some perspectives on dietary inhibition of carcinogenesis: studies with curcumin and tea. Conney AH, Lou YR, Xie JG, Osawa T, Newmark HL, Liu Y, Chang RL, Huang MT. Proc Soc Exp Biol Med. 1997 Nov;216(2):234-45. **Key Finding:** "Topical application of curcumin inhibits chemically induced carcinogenesis on mouse skin, and oral administration of curcumin inhibits chemically induced **oral, forestomach, duodenal, and colon carcinogenesis**. Although curcumin alone had little or no effect on cellular differentiation in the human promyelocytic HL-60 leukemia cell model system, when it was combined with all-trans retinoic acid or 1alpha,25-dihydroxyvitamin D3 a synergistic effect was observed. It is possible that many dietary chemicals in fruits, vegetables, and other edible plants can prevent cancer by synergizing with endogenously produced stimulators of differentiation."

Inhibitory effects of curcumin on tumorigenesis in mice. Huang MT, Newmark HL, Frenkel K. J Cell Biochem Suppl. 1997;27:26-34. **Key Finding:** Commercial curcumin, pure curcumin, and demethoxycurcumin are about equipotent as inhibitors of TPA-induced tumor promotion in mouse **skin,** whereas bisdemethoxycurcumin is somewhat less active.

Curcumin, a natural plant phenolic food additive, inhibits cell proliferation and induces cell cycle changes in colon adenocarcinoma cell lines by a prostaglandin-independent pathway. Hanif R, Qiao L, Shiff SJ, Rigas B. The Journal of Laboratory and Clinical Medicine. 1997 Dec; vol 130, no 6:576-584. **Key Finding:** "We studied curcumin's role in proliferation and apoptosis in the HT-29 and HCT-15 human **colon cancer** cell lines. Curcumin dose-dependently reduced the proliferation rate of both cell lines, causing a 96% decrease by 48 hours. No apoptosis was detected."

Effects of the phytochemicals, curcumin and quercetin, upon azoxymethane-induced **colon cancer** *and 7, 12-dimethylbenz (a) anthracene-induced mammary cancer in rats.* Pereira MA, Grubbs CJ, Barnes LH, Li H, Olson GR, Eto I, Juliana M, Whitaker LM, Kelloff GJ, Steele VE, Lubet RA. Carcinogenesis. 1996; vol 17, No 6:1305-1311. **Key Finding:** "Curcumin and quercetin were evaluated in rats for their ability to modulate the carcinogenic activity of azoxy-methane (AOM) in the colon and 7, 12-dimethyl-benz (a) anthracene (DMBA) in the mammary gland. While curcumin was highly effective as chemo preventive agent in the colon model, it was only weakly effective in the mammary model. In contrast, quercetin which was also only weakly effective in the mammary model caused a dose-dependent enhancement of tumors induced by AOM in the colon model."

Antimutagenic and **anticarcinogenic** *activity of natural and synthetic curcuminoids.* Anto RJ, George J, Babu KV, Rajasekharan KN, Kuttan R. Mutat Res. 1996 Sep 13;370(2):127-31. **Key Finding:** Five synthetic curcuminoids and three natural curcuminoids were investigated for the antimutagenic and anti-promotional activity. The natural curcuminoids—curcumin I (diferuloylmethane), curcumin II (feruloyl-p-hydroxycinnamoylmethane) and curcumin III (bis-(p-hydroxycin-namoyl) methane) isolated from Curcuma longa were found to be potent inhibitors of mutagenesis and crotean oil-induced tumor promotion. Curcumin III produced 87.6% inhibition, Curcumin II a 70.5%, and Curcumin I a 68.3% inhibition to 2-acetamidofluorene (2-AAF) induced mutagenesis. Salicylcurcuminoid was the most potent anti-carcinogen among the synthetic curcuminoids.

Inhibition of **tumor** *necrosis factor by curcumin, a phytochemical.* Chan MM. Biochem Pharmacol. 1995 May 26;49(11):1551-6. **Key Finding:** "This report shows that, in vitro, curcumin, at 5 microM, inhibited lipopolysaccharide (LPS)-induced production of TNF and IL-1 by a human monocytic macrophage cell lines, Mono Mac 6. In addition, it demonstrates that curcumin, at the corresponding concentration, inhibited LPS-induced activation of nuclear factor kappaB and reduced the biological activity of TNF in L929 fibroblast lytic assay."

Chemoprevention of **colon carcinogenesis** *by dietary curcumin, a naturally occurring plant phenolic compound.* Rao CV, Rivenson A, Simi B, Reddy BS. Cancer Res. 1995 Jan 15;55(2):259-66. **Key Finding:** "Although the precise mechanism by which curcumin inhibits colon tumorigenesis remains to be elucidated, it is likely that the chemo preventive action, at least in part, may be related to the modulation of arachidonic acid metabolism."

Inhibitory Effects of Dietary Curcumin on **Forestomach, Duodenal, and Colon Carcinogenesis** *in Mice.* Huang MT, Lou YR, Ma W, Newmark HL, Reuhl KR, Conney AH. Cancer Research. 1994 Nov 15;54:5841-5847. **Key Finding:** "These results indicate that not only did curcumin inhibit the number of tumors per mouse and the percentage of mice with tumors but it also reduced tumor size. Histopathological examination of the tumors showed that dietary curcumin inhibited the number of papilloma and squamous cell carcinomas of the forestomach as well as the number of adenomas and adenocarcinomas of the duodenum and colon."

Inhibition of 8-hydroxydeoxyguanosine formation by curcumin in mouse fibroblast cells. Shih CA, Lin JK. Carcinogenesis. 1993; vol 14, no 4:709-712. **Key Finding:** "These results suggest that curcumin inhibits the PMA-induced **tumor** promotion by functioning as an OH. Radical scavenger to prevent 8-OH-dG formation within the DNA molecule."

Inhibitory effect of curcumin and some related dietary compounds on **tumor** *promotion and arachidonic acid metabolism in mouse skin.* Conney AH, Lysz T, Ferraro T, Abidi TF, Manchand PS, Laskin JD, Huang MT. Adv Enzyme Regul. 1991;31:385-96. **Key Finding:** "Topical application of curcumin, the major yellow pigment in turmeric and curry, has a potent inhibitory effect on 12-O-tetradecanoylphorbol-13-acetate (TPA)-induced tumor promotion in mouse skin. Examination of the structural features of curcumin required for its biological activity indicates that free hydroxyl groups on the benzene rings are not required for inhibition of TPA-induced ornithine decarboxylase activity and inflammation in mouse skin."

Turmeric (Curcuma longa)-induced reduction in urinary mutagens. Polasa K, Sesikaran B, Krishna TP, Krishnaswamy K. Food Chem Toxicol. 1991 Oct;29(10):699-706. **Key Finding:** "Rats were fed turmeric at various levels in the diet for up to 3 months and then exposed to benzo (a) pyrene (B (a) P) or 3-methylcholanthrene (3-MC) by ip injection. Turmeric fed at 0.5% and above inhibited B (a) P- and 3-MC-mediated **mutagenicity.** These findings are significant in view of the widespread exposure of humans to polycyclic aromatic hydrocarbons."

Studies on the anti-tumor-promoting activity of naturally occurring substances. IV. Pd-II (+) anomalin, (+)praeruptorin B, a seselin-type coumarin, inhibits the promotion of skin tumor formation by 12-O-tetradecanoylphorbol-13-acetate in 7,12-dimtheylbenz(a)anthracene-initiated mice. Nishino H, Okuyama T, Takata M, Shibata S, Tokuda H, Takayasu J, Hasegawa T, Nishino A, Ueyama H, Iwashima A. Carcinogenesis. 1990; vol 11, no 9:1557-1561. **Key Finding:** "Coumarins may be useful in the development of an effective method to prevent **cancer**."

Inhibitory effect of curcumin, chlorogenic acid, caffeic acid, and ferulic acid on **tumor** *promotion in mouse skin by 12-O-tetradecanoylphorbol-13-acetate.* Huang MT, Smart RC, Wong CQ, Conney AH. Cancer Res. 1988 Nov 1;48(21):5941-6. **Key Finding:** "The possibility that curcumin could inhibit the action of arachidonic acid was evaluated by studying the effect of curcumin on arachidonic acid-induced edema of mouse ears. The topical application of 3 or 10 mumol of curcumin 30 min before the application of 1 mumol of arachidonic acid inhibited arachidonic acid-induced edema by 33 or 80% respectively."

Studies on curcumin and curcuminoids IX. Investigation of the photo biological activity of curcumin using bacterial indicator systems. Tonnesen HH, De Vries H, Karlsen J, Van Henegouwen GB. Journal of the Pharmaceutical Sciences. 1987; vol 76, no 5:371-373. **Key Finding:** "On irradiation with visible light, curcumin proves to be phototoxic for Salmonella typhimurium and Escherichia coli, even at very low concentrations. The observed photo toxicity makes curcumin a potential photosensitizing drug which might find application in the phototherapy of, for example, **psoriasis, cancer**, and **bacterial** and **viral diseases**."

Cardiovascular disease

Curcumin inhibits platelet-derived growth factor-stimulated vascular smooth muscle cell function and injury-induced neointima formation. Yang X, Thomas DP, Zhang X, Culver BW, Alexander BM, Murdoch WJ, Rao MN, Tulis DA, Ren J, Sreejayan N. Arterioscier Thromb Vasc Biol. 2006 Jan;26(1):85-90. **Key Finding:** "Vascular smooth muscle cell (VSMC) migration, proliferation, and collagen synthesis are key events involved in the pathogenesis of **cardiovascular disease.** These data suggest that curcumin is a potent inhibitor of key PDGF-stimulated VSMC functions and may play a critical role in regulating these events after vascular injury."

Curcumin: getting back to the roots. Shishodia S, Sethi G, Aggarwal BB. Ann NY Acad Sci. 2005 Nov;1056:206-17. **Key Finding:** "Curcumin is now being used to treat **cancer, arthritis, diabetes, Crohn's disease, cardiovascular disease, osteoporosis, Alzheimer's disease, psoriasis**, and other pathologies. Interestingly, 6-gingerol, a natural analog of curcumin derived from the root of ginger (Zingiber officinalis), exhibits a biologic activity profile similar to that of curcumin."

Cholesterol

Curcumin inhibits cholesterol uptake in Caco-2 cells by down-regulation of NPC1L1 expression. Feng D, Ohlsson L, Duan RD. Lipids Health Dis. 2010 Apr 19;9:40. **Key Finding**: "Curcumin inhibits **cholesterol** uptake through suppression of NPC1L1 expression in the intestinal walls."

Hypocholesterolemic effects of **curcumin** *via up-regulation of cholesterol 7a-hydroxylase in rats fed a high fat diet.* Kim M, Kim Y. Nutr Res Pract. 2010 Jun;4(3):191-5. **Key Finding**: "Male Sprague-Dawley rats were fed a 45% high fat diet, or the same diet supplemented with curcumin for 8 weeks. The curcumin diet significantly decreased serum triglyceride by 27%, total **cholesterol** by 33.8%, and LDL-cholesterol by 56%."

Inhibition of lipid peroxidation and **cholesterol** *levels in mice by curcumin.* Soudamini KK, Unnikrishnan MC, Soni KB, Kuttan R. Indian J Physiol Pharmacol. 1992 Oct;36(4):239-43. **Key Finding:** "Oral administration of curcumin significantly lowered the increased peroxidation of lipids in these tissues produced by these chemicals. Administration of curcumin was also found to lower significantly the serum and tissue cholesterol levels in these animals, indicating that the use of curcumin helps in conditions associated with peroxide induced injury such as liver damage and arterial diseases."

Effect of oral curcumin administration on serum peroxides and **cholesterol** *levels in human volunteers.* Soni KB, Kuttan R. Indian J Physiol Pharmacol. 1992 Oct;36(4):273-5. **Key Finding:** 'The effect of curcumin administration in reducing the serum levels of cholesterol and lipid peroxides was studied in ten healthy human volunteers, receiving 500 me of curcumin per day for 7 days. A significant decrease in the level of serum lipid peroxides (33%), increase in HDL Cholesterol (29%), and a decrease in total serum cholesterol (11.6%) were noted."

Cognition

Curcumin exerts neuro-protective effects against homocysteine intracerebroventricular injection-induced **cognitive impairment** *and oxidative stress in rat brain.* Ataie A, Sabetka-saei M, Haghparast A, Et al. J Med Food. 2010 Aug;13(4):821-6. **Key Finding**: "These results suggest that polyphenol treatment with curcumin improves learning and memory deficits by protecting the nervous system against oxidative stress."

Colitis

Oral Administration of Curcumin Emulsified in Carboxymethyl Cellulose Has a Potent Anti-inflammatory Effect in the IL-10 Gene-Deficient Mouse Model of IBD. Ung VY, Foshaug RR, Macfarlane SM, Churchill TA, Doyle JS, Sydora BC, Fedorak RN. Dig Dis Sci. 2009 Jun 10. (Epub ahead of print). **Key Finding:** "Both oral curcumin and carboxymethyl cellulose appear to have modifying effects on **colitis.** However, curcumin has additional **anti-inflammatory** effects mediated through a reduced production of potent pro-inflammatory mucosal cytokines."

Curcumin, the major component of food flavor turmeric, reduces mucosal injury in trinitrobenzene sulphonic acid-induced **colitis.** Ukil A, Maity S, Karmaker S, Datta N, Vedasiromoni JR, Das PK. Br J Pharmacol. 2003 May;139(2):209-18. **Key Finding:** "These findings suggest that curcumin exerts beneficial effects in experimental colitis and may, therefore, be useful in the treatment of inflammatory bowel disease."

Crohn's disease

Curcumin: getting back to the roots. Shishodia S, Sethi G, Aggarwal BB. Ann NY Acad Sci. 2005 Nov;1056:206-17. **Key Finding:** "Curcumin is now being used to treat **cancer, arthritis, diabetes, Crohn's disease, cardiovascular disease, osteoporosis, Alzheimer's disease, psoriasis**, and other pathologies. Interestingly, 6-gingerol, a natural analog of curcumin derived from the root of ginger (Zingiber officinalis), exhibits a biologic activity profile similar to that of curcumin."

Cystic fibrosis

Curcumin opens cystic fibrosis trans membrane conductance regulator channels by a novel mechanism that requires neither ATP binding nor dimerization of the nucleotide-binding domains. Wang W, Bernard K, Li G, Kirk KL. J Biol Chem. 2007 Feb 16;282(7):4533-44. **Key Finding:** "Loss-of-function mutations in the CFTR gene cause **cystic fibrosis**, thus, there is considerable interest in compounds that improve mutant CFTR function. Curcumin is a useful functional probe of CFTR gating that opens mutant channels by circumventing the normal requirements for ATP binding and NBD heterodimerization."

Curcumin enhances **cystic fibrosis** *trans membrane regulatory expression by down-regulating calreticulin.* Harada K, Okiyoneda T, Hashimoto Y, Oyokawa K, Nakamura K, Suico MA, Shuto T, Kai H. Biochem Biophys Res Commun. 2007 Feb 9;353(2):351-6. **Key Finding:** "Curcumin has been reported to correct cystic fibrosis caused by the DeltaF508 mutation of the cystic fibrosis trans membrane regulator (CFTR) but its mechanistic action remains unclear. Our findings suggest that the positive effect of curcumin on CFTR expression is mediated through the down-regulation of CRT, a negative regulator of CFTR."

Curcumin stimulates **cystic fibrosis** *trans membrane conductance regulator Cl-channel activity.* Berger AL, Randak CO, Ostedgaard LS, Karp PH, Vermeer DW, Welsh MJ. J Biol Chem. 2005 Feb 18;280(7):5221-6. **Key Finding:** "Compounds that enhance either the function or biosynthetic processing of the cystic fibrosis trans membrane conductance regulator (CFTR) Cl(-) channel may be of value in developing new treatments for cystic Fibrosis. We found that curcumin increased the activity of both wild-type and DeltaF508 channels. Adding curcumin also increased Cl(-) transport in differentiated non-CF airway epithelia but not in CF epithelia. These results suggest that curcumin may directly stimulate CFTR Cl(-) channels."

Diabetes

Curcumin improves prostanoid ratio in diabetic mesenteric arteries associated with cyclooxygenase-2 and NF-$_k$B suppression. Rungseesantivanon S, Thengchaisri N, Rungvejvorachai P, Patumraj S. Diabetes Metab Syndr Obes. 2010 Dec 6;3:421-9. **Key Finding**: "These findings show that curcumin can attenuate **diabetes**-induced vascular dysfunction in association with its potential for COX-2 and NF-$_k$B suppression."

Curcumin modulates dopaminergic receptor, CREB and phospholipase C gene expression in the cerebral cortex and cerebellum of streptozotocin induced diabetic rats. Kumar TP, Antony S, Gireesh G, Et al. J Biomed Sci. 2010 May 31;17:43. **Key Finding**: "These results suggest that curcumin holds promise as an agent to prevent or treat complications in **diabetes**."

Curcumin supplementation could improve diabetes-induced endothelial dysfunction associated with decreased vascular superoxide production and PKC inhibition. Rungseesanthivanon S, Thenchaisri N, Ruangvejvorachai P, Patumraj S. BMC Complement Altern Med. 2010 Oct 14;10:57. **Key Finding**: "We propose that curcumin can improve **diabetes**-induced endothelial dysfunction through superoxide reduction."

Heart Failure (myocardial infarction)

The dietary compound curcumin inhibits p300 histone acetyltransferase activity and prevents **heart failure** *in rats.* Morimoto T, Sunagawa Y, Kawamura T, Takaya T, Wada H, Nagasawa A, Komeda M, Fujita M, Shimatsu A, Kita T, Hasegawa K. J Clin Invest. 2008 Mar; 118(3):868-78. **Key Finding:** "The effects of curcumin were examined in vivo in 2 different heart failure models: hypertensive heart disease in salt-sensitive Dahl rats and surgically induced myocardial infarction in rats. In both models, curcumin prevented deterioration of systolic function and heart failure-induced increases in both myocardial wall thickness and diameter. From these results, we conclude that inhibition of p300 HAT activity by the nontoxic dietary compound curcumin may provide a novel therapeutic strategy for heart failure in humans."

Suppression of the nuclear factor-kappaB activation pathway by spice-derived phytochemicals: reasoning for seasoning. Aggarwal BB, Shishodia S. Ann N Y Acad Sci. 2004 Dec;1030:434-41. **Key Finding:** "The activation of nuclear transcription factor kappaB has now been linked with a variety of inflammatory disease, including **cancer, atherosclerosis, myocardial infarction, diabetes, allergy, asthma, arthritis, Crohn's disease, multiple sclerosis, Alzheimer's disease, osteoporosis, psoriasis, septic shock, and AIDS**. Extensive research in the last few years has shown that the pathway that activates this transcription factor can be interrupted by phytochemicals derived from spices such as turmeric (curcumin), red pepper (capsaicin), cloves (eugenol), ginger (gingerol), cumin, anise, and fennel (anethol), basil and rosemary (ursolic acid), garlic (diallyl sulfide, S-allylmercaptocysteine, ajoene), and pomegranate (ellagic acid). For the first time, therefore, research provides 'reasoning for seasoning.'"

Human Immunodeficiency Virus

Suppression of the nuclear factor-kappaB activation pathway by spice-derived phytochemicals: reasoning for seasoning. Aggarwal BB, Shishodia S. Ann N Y Acad Sci. 2004 Dec;1030:434-41. **Key Finding:** "The activation of nuclear transcription factor kappaB has now been linked with a variety of inflammatory disease, including **cancer, atherosclerosis, myocardial infarction, diabetes, allergy, asthma, arthritis, Crohn's disease, multiple sclerosis, Alzheimer's disease, osteoporosis, psoriasis, septic shock, and AIDS**. Extensive research in the last few years has shown that the pathway that activates this transcription factor can be interrupted by phytochemicals derived from spices such as turmeric (curcumin), red pepper (capsaicin), cloves (eugenol), ginger (gingerol), cumin, anise, and fennel (anethol), basil and rosemary (ursolic acid), garlic (diallyl sulfide, S-allylmercaptocysteine, ajoene), and pomegranate (ellagic acid). For the first time, therefore, research provides 'reasoning for seasoning.'"

Inhibition of **human immunodeficiency virus type-1** *integrase by curcumin.* Mazumder A, Raghavan K, Weinstein J, Kohn KW, Pommier Y. Biochem Pharmacol. 1995 Apr 18;49(8):1165-70. **Key Finding:** "These observations suggest new strategies for antiviral drug development that could be based upon curcumin as a lead compound for the development of inhibitors of HIV-1 integrase."

Inflammation

Curcumin prevents and reverses murine cardiac hypertrophy. Li HL, Liu C, de Couto G, Ouzounian M, Sun M, Wang AB, Huang Y, He CW, Shi Y, Chen X, Nghiem MP, Liu Y, Chen M, Dawood F, Fukuoka M, Maekawa Y, Zhang L, Leask A, Ghosh AK, Kirshenbaum LA, Liu PP. J Clin Invest. 2008 Mar;118(3):879-93. **Key Finding:** "Our results indicate that curcumin has the potential to protect against **cardiac hypertrophy, inflammation, and fibrosis** through suppression of p300-HAT activity and downstream GATA4, NF-kappaB, and TGF-beta-Smad signaling pathways."

Inflammatory bowel disease

Curcumin *suppresses p38 mitogen-activated protein kinase activation, reduces IL-1beta and matrix metalloproteinase-3 and enhances IL-10 in the mucosa of children and adults with* **inflammatory bowel disease**. Epstein J, Docena G, MacDonald TT, Sanderson IR. Br J Nutr. 2010 Mar;103(6):824-32. **Key Finding**: "We demonstrate dose-dependent suppression of MMP-3 in CMP with curcumin. We conclude that curcumin holds promise as a novel therapy in inflammatory bowel disease."

Effect of Cyclodextrin Complexation of Curcumin on its Solubility and Antiangiogenic and Anti-inflammatory Activity in Rat Colitis Model. Yadav VR, Suresh S, Devi K, Yadav S. AAPS PharmSciTech. 2009 Jun 3. (Epub ahead of print). **Key Finding:** Curcumin was evaluated for the treatment of **inflammatory bowel disease**. "This study concluded that the degree of colitis caused by administration of DSS was significantly attenuated by CD of curcumin. Being a nontoxic natural dietary product, curcumin could be useful in the therapeutic strategy for IBD patients."

Vascular Cell Adhesion Molecule-1 Expression in Human Intestinal Micro vascular Endothelial Cells is Regulated by Pl3K/Akt/MAPK/NF(kappa)B: Inhibitory Role of Curcumin. Binion DG, Heidemann J, Li MS, Nelson VM, Otterson MF, Rafiee P. Am J Physiol Gastrointest Liver Physiol. 2009 Jun 11. (Epub ahead of print). **Key Finding:** "Curcumin inhibited the expression of VCAM-1in HIMECs through blockade of Akt, p38MAPK and NFkappaB. Curcumin may represent a novel therapeutic agent targeting endothelial activation in **inflammatory bowel disease**."

*Curcumin has bright prospects for the treatment of **inflammatory bowel disease**.* Hanai H, Sugimoto K. Curr Pharm Des. 2009; 15(18):2087-94. **Key Finding:** "The inhibitory effects of curcumin on major inflammatory mechanisms like COX-2, LOX, TNF-alpha, IFN-gamma, NF-kappB and its unrivalled safety profile suggest that it has bright prospects in the treatment of inflammatory bowel disease."

Liver injury

*Curcumin decreased oxidative stress, inhibited NF-kappaB activation, and improved liver pathology in ethanol-induced **liver injury** in rats.* Samuhasaneeto S, Thong-Ngam D, Kulaputana O, Suyasunanont D, Klaikeaw N. J Biomed Biotechnol. 2009 Jul 6;981963. **Key Finding:** "Curcumin treatments resulted in improving of liver pathology, decreasing the elevation of hepatic MDA, and inhibition of NF-kappaB activation."

Multiple Sclerosis

15-deoxy-Delta (12, 14)-prostaglandin J (2) and curcumin modulate the expression of toll-like receptors 4 and 9 in autoimmune T lymphocyte. Chearwae W, Bright JJ. J Clin Immunol. 2008 Sep;28(5):558-70. **Key Finding:** "Although the exact mechanisms are not known, the modulation of TLR expression in T lymphocytes by 15d-PGJ(2) and curcumin suggests new therapeutic targets in the treatment of T cell-mediated autoimmune disease" such as **multiple sclerosis**.

Suppression of the nuclear factor-kappaB activation pathway by spice-derived phytochemicals: reasoning for seasoning. Aggarwal BB, Shishodia S. Ann N Y Acad Sci. 2004 Dec;1030:434-41. **Key Finding:** "The activation of nuclear transcription factor kappaB has now been linked with a variety of inflammatory disease, including **cancer, atherosclerosis, myocardial infarction, diabetes, allergy, asthma, arthritis, Crohn's disease, multiple sclerosis, Alzheimer's**

disease, osteoporosis, psoriasis, septic shock, and AIDS. Extensive research in the last few years has shown that the pathway that activates this transcription factor can be interrupted by phytochemicals derived from spices such as turmeric (curcumin), red pepper (capsaicin), cloves (eugenol), ginger (gingerol), cumin, anise, and fennel (anethol), basil and rosemary (ursolic acid), garlic (diallyl sulfide, S-allylmercaptocysteine, ajoene), and pomegranate (ellagic acid). For the first time, therefore, research provides 'reasoning for seasoning.'"

Curcumin inhibits experimental allergic encephalomyelitis by blocking Il-12 signaling through Janus kinase-STAT pathway in T lymphocytes. Natarajan C, Bright JJ. J Immunol. 2002 Jun 15;168(12):6506-13. **Key Finding:** "These findings highlight the fact that curcumin inhibits EAE by blocking IL-12 signaling in T cells and suggest its use in the treatment of **multiple sclerosis** and other Th1 cell-mediated inflammatory diseases."

Obesity

*Curcumin and **obesity**: evidence and mechanisms.* Alappat L, Awad AB. Nutr Rev. 2010 Dec;68(12):729-38. **Key Finding**: "Evidence suggests curcumin may regulate lipid metabolism, which plays a central role in the development of obesity and its complications. The present review addresses the evidence and mechanisms by which curcumin may play a role in down regulating obesity and reducing the impact of associated problems."

*Targeting inflammation-induced **obesity** and metabolic diseases by curcumin and other nutraceuticals.* Aggarwal BB. Annu Rev Nutr. 2010 Aug 21;30:173-99. **Key Finding**: "Curcumin-induced alterations reverse insulin resistance, hyperglycemia, hyperlipidemia and other symptoms linked to obesity. Other structurally homologous nutraceuticals, derived from red **chili, cinnamon, cloves, black pepper and ginger**, also exhibit effects against obesity and insulin resistance."

Osteoarthritis

Synergistic chondroprotective effects of curcumin and resveratrol in human articular chondrocytes: inhibition of IL-1beta-induced NF-kappaB-mediated inflammation and apoptosis. Csaki C, Mobasheri A, Shakibaei M. Arthritis Res Ther. 2009 Nov 4;11(6):R165. **Key Finding:** "Currently available treatments for **osteoarthritis** are restricted to nonsteroidal anti-inflammatory drugs, which exhibit numerous side effects and are only temporarily effective. Naturally occurring polyphenolic compounds, such as curcumin and resveratrol, are potent agents for modulating inflammation. The aim of this study was to investigate the potential synergistic effects of curcumin and resveratrol on IL-1beta-stimulated human chondrocytes in vitro. Treatment with curcumin and resveratrol suppressed NF-kappaB-regulated gene products involved in inflammation. We propose that combining these natural compounds may be a useful strategy in osteoarthritis therapy as compared with separate treatment with each individual compound."

Treatment of **osteoarthritis** *with a herbomineral formulation: a double-blind, placebo-controlled, cross-over study.* Kulkarni RR, Patki PS, Jog VP, Gandage SG, Patwardhan B. J Ethnopharmacol. 1991 May-Jun;33(1-2):91-5. **Key Finding:** The clinical efficacy of a herbomineral formulation containing roots of Withania somnifera, the stem of Boswellia serrata, rhizomes of Curcuma longa and a zinc complex. "Treatment with the herbomineral formulation produced a significant drop in severity of pain and disability score."

Osteoporosis

Curcumin: getting back to the roots. Shishodia S, Sethi G, Aggarwal BB. Ann NY Acad Sci. 2005 Nov;1056:206-17. **Key Finding:** "Curcumin is now being used to treat **cancer, arthritis, diabetes, Crohn's disease, cardiovascular disease, osteoporosis, Alzheimer's disease, psoriasis**, and other pathologies. Interestingly, 6-gingerol, a natural analog of curcumin derived from the root of ginger (Zingiber officinalis), exhibits a biologic activity profile similar to that of curcumin."

Suppression of the nuclear factor-kappaB activation pathway by spice-derived phytochemicals: reasoning for seasoning. Aggarwal BB, Shishodia S. Ann N Y Acad Sci. 2004 Dec;1030:434-41. **Key Finding:** "The activation of nuclear transcription factor kappaB has now been linked with a variety of inflammatory disease, including **cancer, atherosclerosis, myocardial infarction, diabetes, allergy, asthma, arthritis, Crohn's disease, multiple sclerosis, Alzheimer's disease, osteoporosis, psoriasis, septic shock, and AIDS**. Extensive research in the last few years has shown that the pathway that activates this transcription factor can be interrupted by phytochemicals derived from spices such as turmeric (curcumin), red pepper (capsaicin), cloves (eugenol), ginger (gingerol), cumin, anise, and fennel (anethol), basil and rosemary (ursolic acid), garlic (diallyl sulfide, S-allylmercaptocysteine, ajoene), and pomegranate (ellagic acid). For the first time, therefore, research provides 'reasoning for seasoning.'"

Psoriasis

Curcumin: getting back to the roots. Shishodia S, Sethi G, Aggarwal BB. Ann NY Acad Sci. 2005 Nov;1056:206-17. **Key Finding:** "Curcumin is now being used to treat **cancer, arthritis, diabetes, Crohn's disease, cardiovascular disease, osteoporosis, Alzheimer's disease, psoriasis**, and other pathologies. Interestingly, 6-gingerol, a natural analog of curcumin derived from the root of ginger (Zingiber officinalis), exhibits a biologic activity profile similar to that of curcumin."

Suppression of the nuclear factor-kappaB activation pathway by spice-derived phytochemicals: reasoning for seasoning. Aggarwal BB, Shishodia S. Ann N Y Acad Sci. 2004 Dec;1030:434-41. **Key Finding:** "The activation of nuclear transcription factor kappaB has now been linked with a variety of inflammatory disease, including **cancer, atherosclerosis, myocardial infarction, diabetes, allergy, asthma, arthritis, Crohn's disease, multiple sclerosis, Alzheimer's disease, osteoporosis, psoriasis, septic shock, and AIDS**. Extensive research in the last few years has shown that the pathway that activates this transcription factor can be interrupted by phytochemicals derived from spices such as turmeric (curcumin), red pepper (capsaicin), cloves (eugenol), ginger (gingerol), cumin, anise, and fennel (anethol), basil and rosemary (ursolic acid), garlic (diallyl sulfide, S-allylmercaptocysteine, ajoene), and pomegranate (ellagic acid). For the first time, therefore, research provides 'reasoning for seasoning.'"

Studies on curcumin and curcuminoids IX. Investigation of the photo biological activity of curcumin using bacterial indicator systems. Tonnesen HH, De Vries H, Karlsen J, Van Henegouwen GB. Journal of the Pharmaceutical Sciences. 1987; vol 76, no 5:371-373. **Key Finding:** "On irradiation with visible light, curcumin proves to be phototoxic for Salmonella typhimurium and Escherichia coli, even at very low concentrations. The observed photo toxicity makes curcumin a potential photosensitizing drug which might find application in the phototherapy of, for example, **psoriasis, cancer**, and **bacterial** and **viral diseases**."

Septic shock

Suppression of the nuclear factor-kappaB activation pathway by spice-derived phytochemicals: reasoning for seasoning. Aggarwal BB, Shishodia S. Ann N Y Acad Sci. 2004 Dec;1030:434-41. **Key Finding:** "The activation of nuclear transcription factor kappaB has now been linked with a variety of inflammatory disease, including cancer, atherosclerosis, myocardial infarction, diabetes, allergy, asthma, arthritis, Crohn's disease, multiple sclerosis, Alzheimer's disease, osteoporosis, psoriasis, septic shock, and AIDS. Extensive research in the last few years has shown that the pathway that activates this transcription factor can be interrupted by phytochemicals derived from spices such as turmeric (curcumin), red pepper (capsaicin), cloves (eugenol), ginger (gingerol), cumin, anise, and fennel (anethol), basil and rosemary (ursolic acid), garlic (diallyl sulfide, S-allylmercaptocysteine, ajoene), and pomegranate (ellagic acid). For the first time, therefore, research provides 'reasoning for seasoning.'"

Skin aging

Effects of a turmeric extract (Curcuma longa) on chronic ultraviolet B irradiation-induced skin damage in melanin-possessing hairless mice. Sumiyoshi M, Kimura Y. Phytomedicine. 2009 Jul 3 (Expub ahead of print). **Key Finding:** "Prevention of UVB-induced **skin aging** by turmeric may be due to the inhibition of increases in MMP-2 expression caused by chronic irradiation."

Vascular thrombosis

Effect of curcumin on platelet aggregation and vascular prostacyclin synthesis. Srivastava R, Puri V, Srimal RC, Dhawan BN. Arzneimittelforschung. 1986 Apr;36(4):715-7. **Key Finding:** "Curcumin may be preferable in patients prone to **vascular thrombosis** and requiring antiarthritic therapy."

Fenugreek

LEAVES OF FENUGREEK have traditionally been used as an herb, while the seeds are a spice historically added to cuisines native to India, Ethiopia, and many other countries. Fenugreek seeds were found in the tomb of Tutankhamen and from even earlier archaeological sites dating back six thousand years in present-day Iraq.

Fenugreek is a Latin word meaning "Greek hay," and there is evidence that during the days of the Roman Empire it was fed to cattle along with clover. Indian and Pakistani curries make extensive use of fenugreek. For thousands of years it has been known to have medicinal properties, including for diabetes. Recent medical studies have affirmed its usefulness in preventing and treating diabetes, as well as at least five types of cancer.

Anti-inflammatory

Analgesic and anti-inflammatory activities of Trigonella foenum-graecum (seed) extract. Vyas S, Agrawal RP, Solanki P, Trivedi P. Acta Pol Pharm. 2008 Jul-Aug;65(4):473-6. **Key Finding**: "The results suggest that the water soluble fraction of herbal origin has significant analgesic and anti-inflammatory potential as reflected by the parameters investigated."

Antioxidation

Antioxidant properties of germinated fenugreek seeds. Dixit P, Ghaskadbi S, Mohan H, Devasagayam TP. Phytother Res. 2005 Nov;19(11):977-83. **Key Finding:** "This study reveals significant antioxidant activity in germinated fenugreek seeds which may be due partly to the presence of flavonoids and polyphenols."

Atherosclerosis

Dietary mucilage promotes regression of atheromatous lesions in hypercholesterolemic rabbits. Boban PT, Nambisan B, Sudhakaran PR. Phytother Res. 2009 May;23(5):725-30. **Key Finding**: "The lipid lowering and antiatherogenic effects of mucilage from fenugreek which is used as a food flavoring spice highlights the importance of dietary intervention in the regression of atherosclerosis."

Cancer (breast; colon; leukemia; pancreatic; prostate)

Diosgenin, a steroidal saponin, inhibits STAT3 signaling pathway leading to suppression of proliferation and chemo sensitization of human hepatocellular carcinoma cells. Li F, Fernandez PP, Rajendran P, Et al. Cancer Lett. 2010 Jun 28;292(2):197-207. **Key Finding**: "These results suggest that diosgenin, a steroidal saponin isolated from fenugreek, is a novel blocker of the STAT3 activation pathway with a potential role in the treatment of **hepatocellular carcinoma and other cancers**."

Fenugreek: a naturally occurring edible spice as an anticancer agent. Shabbeer S, Sobolewski M, Anchoori RK, Kachhap S, Hidalgo M, Jimeno A, Davidson N, Carducci MA. Cancer Biol Ther. 2009 Feb; 8(3):272-8. **Key Finding**: "Treatment with 10-14 ug/ml of fenugreek extract for 72h was growth inhibitory to **breast, pancreatic and prostate cancer** cell lines."

*Diosgenin targets Akt-mediated prosurvival signaling in human **breast cancer** cells.* Srinivasan S, Koduru S, Kumar R, Venguswamy G, Kyprianou N, Damodaran C. Int J Cancer. 2009 Aug 15;125(4):961-7. **Key Finding**: "These results suggest that diosgenin (fenugreek) might prove to be a potential chemotherapeutic agent for the treatment of breast cancer."

Fenugreek seeds modulate 1,2-dimethylhydrazine-induced hepatic oxidative stress during **colon carcinogenesis**. Devasena T, Venugopal Menon P. Ital J Biochem. 2007 Mar;56(1):28-34. **Key Finding:** "DMH is a colon carcinogen which undergoes oxidative metabolism in the liver. We have investigated the modulatory effect of fenugreek seeds on colon tumor incidence as well as hepatic lipid peroxidation. We report that fenugreek modulates DMH-induced hepatic oxidative stress during colon cancer."

Differential effects of soybean and fenugreek extracts on the growth of MCF-7 cells. Sebastian KS, Thampan RV. Chem Biol Interact. 2007 Nov 20;170(2):135-43. **Key Finding**: "Our experiments show that while the soybean extract acts as a promoter of MCF-7 (estrogen receptor positive **breast cancer** cell line), the fenugreek extract induces apoptosis."

*Chemo preventive activities of Trigonella foenum graecum (Fenugreek) against **breast cancer**.* Amin A, Alkaabi A, Al-Falasi S, Daoud SA. Cell Biol Int. 2005 Aug;29(8):687-94. **Key Finding**: "This is the first study that suggests significant chemo preventive effects of Fenugreek seeds against breast cancer."

Diosgenin, a steroid saponin of Trigonella Foenum gracum (Fenugreek), inhibits azoxymethane-induced aberrant crypt foci formation in F344 rats and induces apoptosis in HT-29 human **colon cancer** *cells.* Raju J, Patiolla JM, Swamy MV, Rao CV. Cancer Epidemiol Biomarkers Prev. 2004 Aug;13(8):1392-8. **Key Finding**: "Results from the in vitro experiments indicated that diosgenin inhibits cell growth and induces apoptosis in the HT-29 human colon cancer cell line in a dose-dependent manner."

Protodioscin isolated from fenugreek (Trigonella foenumgraecum L.) induces cell death and morphological change indicative of apoptosis in **leukemic cell** *line H-60, but not in gastric cancer cell line KATO III.* Hibasami H, Moteki H, Ishikawa K, Katsuzaki H, Imai K, Yoshioka K, Ishii Y, Komiya T. Int J Mol Med. 2003 Jan;11(1):23-6. **Key Finding**: "These findings suggest that growth inhibition by PD of HL-60 cells (human leukemia) results from the induction of apoptosis by this compound in HL-60 cells."

Enhancement of circulatory antioxidants by fenugreek during 1,2-dimethylhydrazine-induced rat **colon carcinogenesis**. Devasena T, Menon VP. J Biochem Mol Biol Biophys. 2002 Aug;6(4):289-92. **Key Finding**: "We report that fenugreek exert its chemo preventive effect (on colon carcinogenesis) by decreasing circulatory LPO (lipid peroxidation) and enhancing antioxidant levels."

Cholesterol

Lipid-lowering and antioxidant effects of an ethyl acetate extract of fenugreek seeds in high-cholesterol-fed rats. Belguith-Hadriche O, Bouaziz M, Jamoussi K, Et al. J Agric Food Chem. 2010 Feb 24;58(4):2116-22. **Key Finding**: "These results revealed significant **hypocholesterolemic** effects and antioxidant activity in an ethyl acetate extract of fenugreek seeds, which may be partly due to the presence of flavonoids, especially naringenin."

Fenugreek seeds reduce atherogenic diet-induced cholesterol gallstone formation in experimental mice. Reddy RL, Srinivasan K. Indian J Physiol Pharmacol. 2009 Nov;87(11):933-43. **Key Finding**: "Dietary fenugreek significantly lowered the incidence of cholesterol gallstones in mice. Fenugreek seed offers health-beneficial antilithogenic potential by virtue of its favorable influence on cholesterol metabolism."

Dietary fenugreek seed regresses pre-established cholesterol gallstones in mice. Reddy RL, Srinivasan K. Can J Physiol Pharmacol. 2009 Sep;87(9):684-93. **Key Finding:** "The present study provides evidence of the potency of hypolipidemic fenugreek seeds in regressing pre-established cholesterol gallstones and this beneficial antilithogenic effect is attributable to its primary influence on cholesterol levels. This finding is significant in the context of evolving a dietary strategy to address cholesterol gallstones, which could help in preventing the incidence and regression of existing cholesterol gallstones and controlling possible recurrence."

Diabetes

Anti-hyperglycemic compound (GII) from fenugreek (Trigonella foenum-graecum Linn.) seeds, its purification and effect in diabetes mellitus. Moorthy R, Prabhu KM, Murthy PS. Indian J Exp Biol. 2010 Nov;48(11):1111-8. **Key Finding**: "The results suggest that intermittent therapy, instead of daily therapy is possible and GII purified from the water extract of fenugreek seeds has good potential as an oral anti-diabetic drug."

Diosgenin present in fenugreek improves glucose metabolism by promoting adipocyte differentiation and inhibiting inflammation in adipose tissues. Uemura T, Hirai S, Mizoguchi N, Et al. Mol Nutr Food Res. 2010 Nov;54(11):1596-608. **Key Finding**: "These results suggest that fenugreek ameliorated **diabetes** by promoting adipocyte differentiation and inhibiting inflammation in adipose tissues. Fenugreek containing diosgenin may be useful for ameliorating the glucose metabolic disorder associated with **obesity.**"

The effect of fenugreek 4-hydroxyisoleucine on liver function biomarkers and glucose in diabetic and fructose-fed rats. Haeri MR, Izaddoost M, Ardekani MR, Nobar MR, White KN. Phytother Res. 2009 Jan; 23(1):61-4. **Key Finding**: "Fenugreek is a plant traditionally used for the treatment of diabetes. It contains an unusual amino acid, 4-hydroxyisoleucine, demonstrated to have antidiabetic properties in animal models. Here we examine the effect of 4-hydroxyisoleucine on liver function and blood glucose in two rat models of insulin resistance. These findings indicate that it is a useful and well-tolerated treatment for insulin resistance, both directly as a hypoglycemic and also as a protective agent for the liver."

Antihyperglycemic effect of Trigonella foenum-graecum (fenugreek) seed extract in alloxan-induced diabetic rats and its use in diabetes mellitus: a brief qualitative phytochemical and acute toxicity test on the extract. Mowla A, Alauddin M, Rahman MA, Ahmed K. Afr J Tradit Complement Altern Med. 2009 May 7;6(3):255-61. **Key Finding:** "The fenugreek extract showed significant activity against the diabetic state induced by alloxan but the intensity of hypoglycemic effect varied from dose to dose."

Effect of fenugreek seeds on blood glucose and lipid profiles in type 2 diabetic patients. Kassaian N, Azadbakht L, Forghani B, Amini M. Int J Vitamin Nutr Res. 2009 Jan;79(1):34-9. **Key Finding**: "The hypoglycemic and hyplipidemic effects of fenugreek seeds were studied in 24 type 2 diabetic patients. Eleven consumed fenugreek in hot water and the rest in yoghurt. Findings showed that FBS, TG and VLDL-C decreased significantly (25%, 30% and 30.6% respectively) after taking fenugreek seed soaked in hot water whereas there were no significant changes in lab parameters in cases consumed when mixed with yoghurt. This study shows that fenugreek seeds can be used as an adjuvant in the control of type 2 diabetes in the form of soaked in hot water."

Insulin sensitizing actions of fenugreek seed polyphenols, quercetin & metformin in a rat model. Kannappan S, Anuradha CV. Indian J Med Res. 2009 Apr; 129(4):401-8. **Key Finding:** "Our findings indicated that fenugreek seed polyphenolic extract and quercetin improved insulin signaling and sensitivity and thereby promoted the cellular actions of insulin in this model."

*Indigenous drugs in ischemic **heart disease** in patients with **diabetes**.* Dwivedi S, Aggarwal A. J Altern Complement Med. 2009 Nov;15(11):1215-21. **Key Finding**: "The recent evidence that certain medicinal plants possess hypogly-cemic, lipid-lowering and immunomodulation properties on account of their rich flavonoid and/or other glucose-lowering active constituents merits scientific scrutiny in this regard. The present communication aims to give a brief review of those plants that could be used in type 2 diabetes mellitus associated with hypertension, ischemic heart disease, and/or dyslipidemia. Fenugreek has been found to be useful in diabetes associated with ischemic heart disease."

Fenugreek bread: a treatment for diabetes mellitus. Losso JN, Holliday DL, Finley JW, Martin RJ, Rood JC, Yu Y, Greenway FL. J Med Food. 2009 Oct;12(5):1046-9. **Key Finding**: "The bread maintained fenugreek's functional property of reducing insulin resistance. Acceptable baked products can be prepared with added fenugreek, which will reduce insulin resistance and treat type 2 diabetes."

Effect of Trigonella foenum-graecum (fenugreek) extract on blood glucose, blood lipid and hemorhelogical properties in streptozotocin-induced diabetic rats. Xue WL, Li XS, Zhang J, Liu YH, Wang ZL, Zhang RJ. Asia Pac J Clin Nutr. 2007;16 Suppl 1:422-6. **Key Finding:** "It may be concluded that Trigonella foenum-graecum extract can lower kidney/body weight ratio, blood glucose, blood lipid levels and improve hemoheological properties in experimental diabetic rats following repeated treatment for 6 weeks."

Effect of Trigonella foenum-graecum (fenugreek) seeds on glycemic control and insulin resistance in type 2 diabetes mellitus: a double blind placebo controlled study. Gupta A, Gupta R, Lal B. J Assoc Physicians India. 2001 Nov;49:1057-61. **Key Finding:** "Adjunct use of fenugreek seeds improves glycemic control and decreases insulin resistance in mild **type-2 diabetic** patients. There is also a favorable effect on **hypertriglyceridemia**."

Helicobacter pylori infection

*Phenolic, their antioxidant and antimicrobial activity in dark germinated **fenugreek sprouts** in response to peptide and phytochemical elicitors.* Randhir R, Lin YT, Shetty K. Asia Pac J Clin Nutr. 2004;13(3):295-307. **Key Finding**: "High antimicrobial activity against peptic ulcer-linked Helicobacter pylori was observed in the fenugreek sprout extract from control and lactoferrin treatments only. We hypothesized that in fenugreek sprouts, simple free phenolic that are less polymerized have more antimicrobial function."

Liver toxicity

Fenugreek (Trigonella foenum graecum) seed polyphenols protect liver from alcohol toxicity: a role on hepatic detoxification system and apoptosis. Kaviarasan S, Anuradha CV. Pharmazie. 2007 Apr;62(4):299-304. **Key Finding**: "These findings demonstrate that fenugreek seed polyphenol extract acts as a protective agent against ethanol-induced abnormalities in the liver."

Fenugreek (Trigonella Foenum graecum) seed extract prevents ethanol-induced toxicity and apoptosis in Chang liver cells. Kaviarasan S, Ramamurty N, Gunasekaran P, Varalakshmi E, Anuradha CV. Alcohol Alcohol. 2006 May-Jun;41(3):267-73. **Key Finding**: "The findings suggest that the polyphenol compounds of fenugreek seeds can be considered cytoprotective during ethanol-induced liver damage."

Obesity

Diosgenin present in fenugreek improves glucose metabolism by promoting adipocyte differentiation and inhibiting inflammation in adipose tissues. Uemura T, Hirai S, Mizoguchi N, Et al. Mol Nutr Food Res. 2010 Nov;54(11):1596-608. **Key Finding**: "These results suggest that fenugreek ameliorated diabetes by promoting adipocyte differentiation and inhibiting inflammation in adipose tissues. Fenugreek containing diosgenin may be useful for ameliorating the glucose metabolic disorder associated with **obesity**."

*A fenugreek seed extract selectively reduces spontaneous fat intake in **overweight** subjects.* Chevassus H, Gaillard JB, Farret A, Et al. Eur J Clin Pharmacol. 2010 May;66(5):449-55. **Key Finding**: "The repeated administration of fenugreek seed extract slightly but significantly decreased dietary fat consumption in healthy overweight subjects in this short-term study."

Effect of fenugreek fiber and satiety, blood glucose and insulin response and energy intake in obese subjects. Mathern JR, Raatz SK, Thomas W, Slavin JL. Phytother Res. 2009 Nov;23(11):1543-6. **Key Finding**: "Fenugreek fiber (8 g) significantly increased satiety and reduced energy intake at lunch, suggesting it may have short-term beneficial effects in obese subjects."

A fenugreek seed extract selectively reduces spontaneous fat consumption in healthy volunteers. Chevassua H, Molinier N, Costa F, Galtier F, Renard E, Petit P. Eur J Clin Pharmacol. 2009 Dec;65(12):1175-8. **Key Finding**: "Twelve healthy male volunteers completed a double-blind randomized placebo-controlled three-period cross-over trial of two different doses of a fenugreek seed extract. Daily fat consumption was significantly decreased by the higher doses of fenugreek seed extract vs. placebo. The repeated administration of a fenugreek seed extract specifically decreases fat consumption in humans."

Ulcer (gastric)

*Phenolic, their antioxidant and antimicrobial activity in dark germinated **fenugreek sprouts** in response to peptide and phytochemical elicitors.* Randhir R, Lin YT, Shetty K. Asia Pac J Clin Nutr. 2004;13(3):295-307. **Key Finding**: "High antimicrobial activity against **peptic ulcer**-linked Helicobacter pylori was observed in the fenugreek sprout extract from control and lactoferrin treatments only. We hypothesized that in fenugreek sprouts, simple free phenolic that are less polymerized have more antimicrobial function."

Gastro protective effect of fenugreek seeds (Trigonella foenum graecum) on experimental gastric ulcer in rats. Pandian RS, Anuradha CV, Viswanathan P. Ethnopharmacol. 2002 Aug;81(3):393-7. **Key Finding**: "Histological studies revealed that the soluble gel fraction derived from the seeds was more effective than omeprazole in preventing lesion formation. These observations show that fenugreek seeds possess antiulcer potential."

Fruit (in General)

(Cherries, Bananas, Kiwi, Nectarines, Oranges, Peaches, Pears, Pineapple, Plums)

BROADLY SPEAKING, a fruit is that part of a plant or tree that contains its seeds. Animals and humans who consume edible fruits disperse the seeds, serving the evolutionary goals of the plants producing the fruits, since this dispersal helps to ensure the propagation of the species.

The wide variety of medical conditions alleviated by fruits, from Alzheimer's disease to ulcers, provides evidence for the healing properties of their abundant antioxidant phytochemicals, vitamins, and minerals. Consumption of fruits in general has proven beneficial in fighting at least nine types of cancer.

Alzheimer's disease

*Midlife Fruit and Vegetable Consumption and Risk of **Dementia** in Later Life in Swedish Twins.* Hughes TF, Andel R, Small BJ, Borenstein AR, Mortimer JA, Wolk A, Johansson B, Fratiglioni L, Pedersen NL, Gatz M. Am J Geriat Psychiatry. 2009 Nov 10. (Epub ahead of print). **Key Finding:** "A medium or great proportion of fruits and vegetables in the diet, compared with none or small amount, was associated with a decreased risk of dementia and **Alzheimer's disease**. This effect was observed among women and those with angina."

Neuroprotective Effects of Polysaccharides from Wolfberry, the Fruits of Lyceum barbarum, Against Homocysteine-induced Toxicity in Rat Cortical Neurons. Ho YS, Yu MS, Yang XF, So KF, Yuen WH, Chang RC. J Alzheimer's Dis. 2009 Nov 17. (Epub ahead of print). **Key Finding:** "Our data demonstrated that wolfberry exerted neuroprotective effects on cortical neurons exposed to elevated plasma homocysteine. Therefore, wolfberry fruit has the potential to be a disease-modifying agent for the prevention of **Alzheimer's disease**."

Tart cherry juice decrease oxidative stress in healthy older men and women. Traustadottir T, Davies SS, Stock AA, Su Y, Heward CB, Roberts LJ, Harman SM. J Nutr. 2009 Oct;139(10):1896-900. **Key Finding**: "These data suggest that consumption of tart cherry juice improves antioxidant defenses in vivo in older adults." This can reduce susceptibility to **atherosclerosis, cancer, diabetes, and Alzheimer's disease.**

Antifungal effects

Antifungal activity of Morinda citrifolia fruit extract against **Candida albicans**. Jain-kittivong A, Butsarakamruha T, Langlais RP. Oral Surg Oral Med Oral Pathol Oral Radio Endod. 2009 Sep;108(3):394-8. **Key Finding:** "Morinda citrifolia fruit extract had an antifungal effect on C. albicans and the inhibitory effect varied with concentration and contact time."

Antioxidation

Identification and Assessment of **Antioxidant** *Capacity of Phytochemicals from Kiwi Fruits.* Fiorentino A, D'Abrosca B, Pacifico S, Mastellone C, Scognamiglio M, Monaco P. J Agric Food Chem. 2009 Apr 9 (Epub ahead of print). **Key Finding:** "The most common commercially available kiwi fruit is the cultivar 'Hayward,' which belongs to the Actinida deliciosa species. An antioxidative screening of peel and pulp crude extracts was carried out and led to the isolation of vitamin E, 2,8-dimethyl-2-(4,8,12-trimethyltridec-11-enyl)chroman-6-ol, as well as alpha- and delta-tocopherol, 7 sterols, the triterpene ursolic acid, chlorgenic acid, and 11 flavonoids."

Diuretic and **antioxidant** *effects of Cacti-Nea (R), a dehydrated water extract from prickly pear fruit, in rats.* Bisson JF, Daubie S, Hidalgo S, Guillemet D, Linares E. Phyto-ther Res. 2009 Sep 23. (Epub ahead of print). **Key Finding:** "The prickly pear fruit extract Cacti-Nea demonstrated chronic diuretic and antioxidant effects in Wistar rats with respect to the excretion of metabolites."

Antioxidant capacities, phenolic compounds, carotenoids, and vitamin C contents of nectarine, peach, and plum cultivars from California. Gil MI, Tomas-Barberan FA, Hess-Pierce B, Kader AA. J Agric Food Chem. 2002 Aug 14;50(17):4976-82. **Key Finding:** "The contributions of phenolic compounds to antioxidant activity were much greater than those of vitamin C and carotenoids. There was a strong correlation between total phenolic and antioxidant activity of nectarines, peaches, and plums."

Cyclooxygenase inhibitory and **antioxidant** *cyaniding glycosides in cherries and berries.* Seeram NP, Momin RA, Nair MG, Bourquin LD. Phytomedicine. 2001 Sep;8(5):362-9. **Key Finding:** "Anthocyanin from raspberries and sweet cherries demonstrated 45% and 47% cyclooxygenase-I and cyclooxygenase-II inhibitory activities, respectively, when assayed at 125 microg/ml. Anthocyanin 1 and 2 are present in both cherries and raspberry. Fresh blackberries and strawberries contained only anthocyanin 2 in yields of 24 and 22.5 mg/100 g, respectively. Anthocyanin 1 and 2 were not found in bilberries, blueberries, cranberries or elderberries."

Improved antioxidant and anti-inflammatory potential in mice consuming sour cherry juice (Prunus Cerasus cv. Maraska). Saric A, Sobocaner S, Balog T, Kusic B, Sverko V, Dragovic-Uzelac V, Levaj B, Cosic Z, Macak Safranko Z, Marotti T. Plant Foods Hum Nutr. 2009 Dec;64(4):231-7. **Key Finding**: "This study highlights cherry juice as a potent COX-2 inhibitor and **antioxidant** in the liver and blood of mice."

Arthritis

*Effects of alpha-glucosylhesperidin, a bioactive food material, on collagen-induced **arthritis** in mice and **rheumatoid arthritis** in humans.* Komentani T, Fukuda T, Kakuma T, Kawaguchi K, Tamura W, Kumazawa Y, Nagata K. Immunopharmacol Immunotoxicol. 2008;30(1):117-34. **Key Finding**: "Hesperidin, a flavanone in oranges and other citrus fruits, was effective when administered with standard anti-rheumatoid therapy in ameliorating rheumatoid arthritis in mice and humans without any adverse effects."

Atherosclerosis

A study of the comparative effects of hawthorn fruit compound and simvastatin on lowering blood lipid levels. Xu H, Xu HE, Ryan D. Am J Chin Med. 2009;37(5):903-8. **Key Finding**: "The intervention group of atherosclerotic ApoE-deficient mice was fed with a high cholesterol diet and Hawthorn fruit compound (which included Hawthorn and kiwi fruit extract) for eight weeks. There was a significant reduction in triglyceride and in the ratio between low-density lipoprotein cholesterol (LDL-C) and serum cholesterol. Moreover, a reduction of LDL-C was evident. The results indicate that Hawthorn fruit compound can be considered for the treatment of **hyperlipidemia** and prevention of **atherosclerosis.**"

Tart cherry juice decrease oxidative stress in healthy older men and women. Traustadottir T, Davies SS, Stock AA, Su Y, Heward CB, Roberts LJ, Harman SM. J Nutr. 2009 Oct;139(10):1896-900. **Key Finding**: "These data suggest that consumption of tart cherry juice improves antioxidant defenses in vivo in older adults." This can reduce susceptibility to **atherosclerosis, cancer, diabetes, and Alzheimer's disease.**

Cancer (breast; colon; esophageal; gastric; laryngeal; lung; oral; prostate; stomach)

*Fruit and vegetable consumption and risk of **distal gastric cancer** in the Shanghai Women's and Men's Health studies.* Epplein M, Shu XO, Xiang YB, Et al. Am J Epidemiol. 2010 Aug 15;172(4):397-406. **Key Finding**: "Fruit intake is inversely associated with distal gastric cancer risk among men in Shanghai, China."

*Antitumor effects of **Phyllanthus emblica L.**: induction of **cancer cell apoptosis** and inhibition of in vivo tumour promotion and in vitro invasion of human cancer cells.* Ngamkitidechakul C, Jaijoy K, Hansakul P, Et al. Phytother Res. 2010 Sep;24(9):1405-13. **Key Finding**: "These results suggest P. emblica, a medicinal fruit used in many Asian traditional medicine systems exhibits anticancer activity against selected cancer cells and warrants further study as a possible chemo preventive and anti-invasive agent."

*Phenolic composition, antioxidant capacity and in vitro **cancer** cell cytotoxicity of nine **prickly pear** (Opuntia spp.) juices.* Chavez-Santoscoy RA, Gutierrez-Uribe JA, Serna-Saldivar SO. Plant Foods Hum Nutr. 2009 Jun;64(2):146-52. **Key Finding:** "Among cancer line tested, viability of **prostate and colon cells** were the most affected. Moradillo contained the highest flavonoids and diminished both prostate and colon cancer cell viability without affecting mammary or hepatic cancer cells. Rastrero reduced the growth of the four cancer cell lines without affecting normal fibroblast viability. The research shows intervarietal differences among prickly pears in terms of juice properties and phytochemicals that could prevent oxidative stress and cancer."

***Citrus fruit** and **cancer** risk in a network of case-control studies.* Foschi R, Pelucchi C, Dal Maso L, Rossi M, Levi F, Talamini R, Bosetti C, Negri E, Serraino D, Giacosa A, Franceschi S, La Vecchia C. Cancer Causes Control. 2009 Oct 24. (Epub ahead of print). **Key Finding:** "We analyzed data from a series of case-control studies conducted in Italy and Switzerland. Our findings indicate that citrus fruit has a protective role against cancers of the digestive and upper respiratory tract, including **oral, pharyngeal, esophageal, stomach, colorectal and laryngeal.**"

Antioxidant Activity of Limonene on Normal Murine Lymphocytes: Relation to HO Modulation and Cell Proliferation. Roberto D, Micucci P, Sebastian T, Graciela F, Anesini C. Basic Clin Pharmacol Toxicol. 2009 Oct 1. (Epub ahead of print). **Key Finding:**

"Limonene is a monoterpene present in **citrus fruit** and possesses antioxidant activity. Previously, it was demonstrated that limonene exerts anti-proliferative action on a **lymphoma** cell line. In the present study, the effect of limonene on normal lymphocytes proliferation and its relation with H (2) O (2) level modulation was analyzed. In view of the results, it is possible that limonene could protect normal lymphocytes from diseases related to oxidative stress, including **cancer.**"

Fruits and vegetables consumption and the risk of histological subtypes of **lung cancer** *in the European Prospective Investigation into Cancer and Nutrition (EPIC).* Buchner FL, Bueno-de-Mesquita HB, Linseisen J, Boshuizen HC, Kiemeney LA, Ros MM, Overvad K, Hansen L, Tjonneland A, Ranschou-Nielsen O, Et al. Cancer Causes Control. 2009 Nov 19 (Epub ahead of print). **Key Finding:** "We observed inverse associations between the consumption of vegetables and fruits and risk of lung cancer without a clear effect on specific histological subtypes of lung cancer. In current smokers, consumption of vegetables and fruits may reduce lung cancer risk, in particular the risk of squamous cell carcinomas."

Schisantherin A Exhibits **Anti-inflammatory** *Properties by Down-Regulating NF-kappaB and MAPK Signaling Pathways in Lipopolysaccharide-Treated RAW 264.7 Cells.* Ci X, Ren R, Xu K, Li H, Yu Q, Song Y, Wang D, Li R, Deng X. Inflammation. 2009 Nov 14. (Epub ahead of print). **Key Finding:** "Schisantherin A., a dibenzocyclooctadiene legnan isolated from the fruit of **Schisandra sphenathera,** has been used as an antitussive, tonic, and sedative agent under the name of Wuweizi in Chinese traditional medicine. In the present study, we carry out a screening program to identify the anti-inflammatory potentials. We found that it may inhibit TNF-alpha mostly through ERK pathway. It may inhibit LPS-induced production of inflammatory cytokines by blocking NF-kappaB and MAPKs signaling in RAW264.7 cells."

Evaluation of the genotoxic and antigenotoxic effects after acute and sub-acute treatments with **acai pulp** *(Euterpe oleracea Mart.) on mice using the erythrocytes micronucleus test and the comet assay.* Ribeiro JC, Antunes LM, Aissa AF, Darin JD, De Rosso VV, Mercadante AZ, Bianchi MD. Mutat Res. 2009 Nov 3. (Epub ahead of print). **Key Finding:** "Acai, the fruit of a palm native to the Amazonian basin, has polyphenol compounds that have been extensively evaluated. The protective effects of acai pulp were observed in both acute and sub-acute treatments. In general, sub acute treatment provided greater efficiency in protecting against DXR-induced DNA damage in liver and kidney cells. These protective effects can be explained as the result of the phytochemicals present in acai pulp."

Apoptosis-inducing effects of Morinda citrifolia L. and doxorubicin on the Ehrlich ascites tumor in Balb-c mice. Taskin EI, Akgun-Dar K, Kapucu A, Osanc E, Dogruman H, Eraltan H, Ulukaya E. Cell Biochem Funct. 2009 Dec;27(8):542-6. **Key Finding:** "Morinda citrifolia L. (Noni) is an herbal remedy with promising anti-cancer properties. We investigated the cytotoxic potential of noni on Ehrlich ascites tumor grown in female Balb-c mice and also combined it with a potent anti-cancer agent, doxorubicin. We conclude that noni may be useful in the treatment of **breast cancer** either on its own or in combination with doxorubicin."

*Enhancement of **antitumor** activities in sulfated and carboxymethylated polysaccharides of **Ganoderma lucidum**.* Wang J, Zhang l, Yu Y, Cheung PC. J Agric Food Chem. 2009 Nov 25;57(22):10565-72. **Key Finding:** "Water-insoluble polysaccharides extracted from the fruit body of G. Lucidem were prepared and inhibited the in vitro proliferation of Sarcoma 180 (S-180) tumor cells in a dose-dependent manner. They also inhibited the growth of S-180 solid tumors implanted in BALC/c mice, with low toxicity to the animals."

Tart cherry *juice decreases oxidative stress in healthy older men and women.* Traustadottir T, Davies SS, Stock AA, Su Y, Heward CB, Roberts LJ, Harman SM. J Nutr. 2009 Oct;139(10):1896-900. **Key Finding**: "These data suggest that consumption of tart cherry juice improves antioxidant defenses in vivo in older adults." This can reduce susceptibility to **atherosclerosis, cancer, diabetes, and Alzheimer's disease.**

*Tangeretin and nobiletin induce G1 cell cycle arrest but not apoptosis in human **breast and colon cancer** cells.* Morley KL, Ferguson PJ, Koropatnick J. Cancer Lett. 2007 Jun 18;251(1):168-78. **Key Finding**: Tangeretin from **orange** peel and nobiletin from the peels of orange and other citrus fruits "are among the most effective at inhibiting cancer cell growth in vitro and in vivo. Both flavonoids inhibited proliferation of human breast cancer cell lines MDA-MB-435 and MCF-7 and human colon cancer line HT-29 in a dose- and time-dependent manner, and blocked cell cycle progression at G1 in all three cell lines."

*The relationship between intake of vegetables and fruits and **colorectal adenoma-carcinoma** sequence.* Lee SY, Choi KY, Kim MK, Kim KM, Lee JH, Meng KH, Lee WC. Korean J Gastroenterol (from Korean). 2005 Jan;45(1):23-33. **Key Finding:** "These findings suggest that the intake of vegetables and fruits may act differently in developmental steps of colorectal adenoma-carcinoma sequence. For this study, 539 cases with confirmed incidental colorectal adenoma, 162 cases with colorectal cancer and 2,576 controls were collected. In females, the high intake of raw green and yellow vegetables was found to be negatively associated with the risk of adenoma with mild dysplasia. In male, the high intake of **banana, pear, apple and watermelon** among fruits were negatively associated with the risk of colorectal cancer."

Carotenoids and **colon cancer**. Slattery ML, Benson J, Curtin K, Ma KN, Schaeffer D, Potter JD. Am J Clin Nutr. 2000 Feb;71(2):575-82. **Key Finding**: "Data were collected from 1993 case subjects with first primary incident adenocarcinoma of the colon and from 2410 population-based control subjects. These data suggest that incorporating these foods (**oranges and orange juice**) into the diet may help reduce the risk of developing colon cancer."

Cardiovascular disease

Regular **tart cherry** *intake alters abdominal adiposity, adipose gene transcription, and inflammation in obesity-prone rats fed a high fat diet.* Seymour EM, Lewis SK, Urcuyo-Llanes DE, Tanone II, Kirakosyan A, Kaufman PB, Bolling SF. J Med Food. 2009 Oct;12(5):935-42. **Key Finding**: "Tart cherries may reduce the degree or trajectory of metabolic syndrome, thereby reducing risk for the development of **type 2 diabetes** and **heart disease**."

Cardio-protective *mechanisms of Prunus cerasus* **(sour cherry)** *seed extract against ischemia-reperfusion-induced damage in isolated rat hearts.* Bak I, Lekli I, Et al. Am J Physiol Heart Circ Physiol. 2006 Sep;291(3):H1329-36. **Key Finding**: "Sour cherry seed kernel extract significantly improved the postischemic recovery of cardiac function."

Cerebrovascular disease

Plant foods and the risk of **cerebrovascular diseases**: *a potential protection of fruit consumption.* Mizrahi A, Knekt P, Montonen J, Laaksonen MA, Heliovaara M, Jarvinen R. Br J Nutr. 2009 Oct;102(7):1075-83. **Key Finding**: "This cohort study on 3932 men and women was based on data from the Finnish Mobile Clinic Health Examination Survey. The participants were 40-74 years of age and free of cardiovascular diseases at baseline. An inverse association was found between fruit consumption, especially citrus, and the incidence of **cerebrovascular diseases, ischemic stroke and intracerebral hemorrhage**."

Dementia

Midlife Fruit and Vegetable Consumption and Risk of **Dementia** *in Later Life in Swedish Twins.* Hughes TF, Andel R, Small BJ, Borenstein AR, Mortimer JA, Wolk A, Johansson B, Fratiglioni L, Pedersen NL, Gatz M. Am J Geriatr Psychiatry. 2009 Nov 10. (Epub ahead of print). **Key Finding:** "A medium or great proportion of fruits and vegetables in the diet, compared with none or small portion, was associated with a decreased risk of dementia and **Alzheimer's disease**. This effect was observed among women and those with angina."

Diabetes

Hypolipidaemic and antioxidative effects of oligonol, a low-molecular-weight polyphenol derived from **lychee fruit**, *on renal damage in type 2 diabetic mice.* Noh JS, Kim HY, Park CH, Et al. Br J Nutr. 2010 Oct;104(8):1120-8. **Key Finding**: "The present results suggest that oligonol could have Reno protective effects against abnormal lipid metabolism and ROS-related AGE formation in **type 2 diabetes**."

Antidiabetic activity of aqueous fruit extract of **Cucumis trigonus Roxb**. *In strepto-zotocin-induced-diabetic rats.* Salahuddin M, Jalalpure SS. J Ethnopharmacol. 2009 Oct 23. (Epub ahead of print). **Key Finding:** "Cucumis trigonus Roxb. (Cucur-bitaceae) fruit is used in the Indian traditional medicine for the treatment of **diabetes**. Our study indicates a significant increase in the body weight, liver glycogen and serum insulin level and decrease in the blood glucose, glycosyl-ated hemoglobin levels, total cholesterol, and serum triglycerides in STZ-induced diabetic rats. HDL cholesterol level was significantly increased when treated with the extract. The aqueous fruit extract has had beneficial effects in reducing the elevated blood glucose level and lipid profile of STZ-induced-diabetic rats."

Anti-inflammatory and analgesic effects of the aqueous extract of corni fructus in murine RAW 264.7 macrophage cells. Sung YH, Chang HK, Kim SE, Kim YM, Seo JH, Shin MC, Shin MS, Shin DH, Kim H, Kim CJ. Med Food. 2009 Aug;12(4):788-95. **Key Finding:** "Corni fructus is the fruit of **Cornus officinalis Sieb.** Corni fructus has antineoplastic, antioxidative and **antidiabetic** effects. Here we investigated the anti-inflammatory and analgesic effects of an aqueous extract. It exerts anti-inflammatory and analgesic effects by suppressing COX-2 and iNOS expression through the down-regulation of NF-kappaB binding activity."

*Regular **tart cherry** intake alters abdominal adiposity, adipose gene transcription, and inflammation in obesity-prone rats fed a high fat diet.* Seymour EM, Lewis SK, Urcuyo-Llanes DE, Tanone II, Kirakosyan A, Kaufman PB, Bolling SF. J Med Food. 2009 Oct;12(5):935-42. **Key Finding**: "Tart cherries may reduce the degree or trajectory of metabolic syndrome, thereby reducing risk for the development of **type 2 diabetes** and **heart disease**."

***Tart cherry** juice decrease oxidative stress in healthy older men and women.* Traustadottir T, Davies SS, Stock AA, Su Y, Heward CB, Roberts LJ, Harman SM. J Nutr. 2009 Oct;139(10):1896-900. **Key Finding**: "These data suggest that consumption of tart cherry juice improves antioxidant defenses in vivo in older adults." This can reduce susceptibility to **atherosclerosis, cancer, diabetes, and Alzheimer's disease.**

*Altered **hyperlipidemia,** hepatic steatosis, and hepatic peroxisome proliferator-activated receptors in rats with intake of **tart cherry.*** Seymour EM, Singer AA, Kirakosyan A, Urcuyo-Llanes DE, Kaufman PB, Bolling SF. J Med Food. 2008 Jun;11(2):252-9. **Key Finding:** "Physiologically relevant tart cherry consumption reduced several phenotypic risk factors that are associated with risk for **metabolic syndrome** and **Type 2 diabetes**. Tart cherries may represent a whole food research model of the health effects of anthocyanin-rich foods."

Diarrhea

*Studies on the antidiarrheal activity of **Aegle marmelos unripe fruit**: validating its traditional usage.* Brijesh S, Daswani P, Tetali P, Anitia N, Birdi T. BMC Complement Altern Med. 2009 Nov 23;9:47. **Key Finding:** "Aegle marmelos (L.) Correa has been widely used in indigenous systems of Indian medicine due to its various medicinal properties. We evaluated the hot aqueous extract (decoction) of dried unripe fruit pulp of A. marmelos for its antimicrobial activity and effect on various aspects of pathogenicity of infectious diarrhea. We found that it affected the bacterial colonization to gut epithelium and production and action of certain enterotoxins. These observations suggest the varied possible modes of action of A. marmelos in infectious forms of diarrhea thereby validating its mention in the ancient Indian texts for the treatment of **diarrheal diseases**."

Hyperlipidemia

*A study of the comparative effects of **hawthorn fruit** compound and simvastatin on lowering blood lipid levels.* Xu H, Xu HE, Ryan D. Am J Chin Med. 2009;37(5):903-8. **Key Finding**: "The intervention group of atherosclerotic ApoE-deficient mice was fed with a high cholesterol diet and Hawthorn fruit compound (which included Hawthorn and kiwi fruit extract) for eight weeks. There was a significant reduction in triglyceride and in the ratio between low-density lipoprotein cholesterol (LDL-C) and serum cholesterol. Moreover, a reduction of LDL-C was evident. The results indicate that Hawthorn fruit compound can be considered for the treatment of **hyperlipidemia** and prevention of **atherosclerosis**."

*Altered **hyperlipidemia,** hepatic steatosis, and hepatic peroxisome proliferator-activated receptors in rats with intake of tart cherry.* Seymour EM, Singer AA, Kirakosyan A, Urcuyo-Llanes DE, Kaufman PB, Bolling SF. J Med Food. 2008 Jun;11(2):252-9. **Key Finding:** "Physiologically relevant tart cherry consumption reduced several phenotypic risk factors that are associated with risk for **metabolic syndrome** and **Type 2 diabetes**. Tart cherries may represent a whole food research model of the health effects of anthocyanin-rich foods."

Immune function

*Immunomodulatory effects of a standardized **Lycium barbarum fruit** juice in Chinese older health human subjects.* Amagase H, Sun B, Nance DM. J Med Food. 2009 Oct;12(5):1159-65. **Key Finding:** "Lyceum barbarum has been traditionally used in combination with several herbs for medicinal properties. To examine the systematic effects of L. barbarum fruit juice on **immune function**, general well-being, and safety, we tested the effects in a double-blind, placebo-controlled clinical study of 60 older healthy adults (55-72 years old). No adverse reactions, abnormal symptoms or changes in body weight, blood pressure, pulse, visual acuity, urine, stool, or blood biochemistry were seen. Daily consumption of GoChi significantly increased several immunological responses and subjective feelings of general well-being without any adverse reactions."

Inflammation

Consumption of **Bing sweet cherries** *lowers circulating concentrations of* **inflammation** *markers in healthy men and women.* Kelley DS, Rasooly R, Jacob RA, Kader AA, Mackey BE. J Nutr. 2006 Apr;136(4):981-6. **Key Finding:** "Results of the present study suggest a selective modulatory effect of sweet cherries on CRP, NO, and RANTES. Such anti-inflammatory effects may be beneficial for the management and prevention of inflammatory diseases."

Peripheral arterial disease

Supplementation with **orange and blackcurrant juice**, *but not vitamin E, improve inflammatory markers in patients with peripheral arterial disease.* Dalgard C, Nielsen F, Morrow JD, Enghusen-Poulsen H, Jonung T, Horder M, de Maat MP. Br J Nutr. 2009 Jan;101(2):263-9. **Key Finding**: "In this study, orange and blackcurrant juice reduced markers of inflammation, but not markers of endothelial activation, in patients with peripheral arterial disease."

Ulcers

Effect of methanolic extract of **Pongamia pinnata Linn** *seed on gastro-duodenal ulceration and mucosal offensive and defensive factors in rats.* Prabha T, Dorababu M, Goel S, Agarwal PK, Singh A, Joshi VK, Goel RK. Indian J Exp Biol. 2009 Aug;47(8):649-59. **Key Finding:** "Pongamie pinnata has been advocated in Ayurveda for the treatment of various inflammatory conditions and dyspepsia. The present work includes initial phytochemical screening and study of ulcer protective and healing effect of methanolic extract of seeds of P. pinnata in rats. When administered orally it showed dose-dependent ulcer protective effects against **gastric ulcer**."

Garlic

ANCIENT CULTURES SCATTERED ACROSS THE GLOBE used wild and cultivated garlic both as a food and flavoring agent and for medicinal purposes. A close relative of onions, garlic is thought to have first been cultivated in southwestern Asia. China remains the world's primary cultivator, producing three-fourths of the world's output, followed by India.

In terms of disease prevention and healing powers, garlic ranks near the top of the top ten superfoods. Studies have documented at least thirty-two health conditions garlic can help prevent or treat. It has also been shown to reduce risk of at least fifteen types of cancer, making this plant perhaps Nature's greatest cancer fighter.

Aging

Antioxidant health effects of aged garlic extract. Borek C. J Nutr. 2001 Mar;131(3s):1010S-5S. **Key Finding:** "Although additional observations are warranted in humans, compelling evidence supports the beneficial health effects attributed to aged garlic extract, i.e., reducing the risk of **cardiovascular disease, stroke, cancer and aging**, including the oxidant-mediated brain cell damage that is implicated in **Alzheimer's disease**."

New pharmacological activities of garlic and its constituents. Sumiyoshi H. Nippon Yakurigaku Zasshi (Japan). 1997 Oct;110 Suppl 1;93P-97P. **Key Finding:** "Epidemiological studies in China, Italy and USA showed the inverse relationship between **stomach and colon cancer** incidences and dietary garlic intake. Anti-carcinogenic activities of garlic and its constituents including sulfides and S-allyl cysteine, have been demonstrated using several animal models. Garlic preparations has been also shown to lower serum cholesterol and triglyceride levels, which are major risk factors of **cardiovascular diseases**, through inhibition of their bio-synthesis in the liver, and to inhibit oxidation of low density lipoprotein. Furthermore, in vitro and in vivo studies have revealed that aged garlic extract stimulated immune functions, such as proliferation of lymphocyte, cytokine release, NK activity and phagocytosis. More recently, aged garlic extract has been demonstrated to **prolong life span** of senescence accelerated mice and prevent brain atrophy."

Alzheimer's disease

*Garlic reduces **dementia** and **heart-disease** risk.* Borek C. J Nutr. 2006 Mar;136(3 Suppl):810S-812S. **Key Finding:** "Although additional observations are warranted in humans, compelling evidence supports the beneficial health effects attributed to aged garlic extract in helping prevent **cardiovascular and cerebrovascular diseases** and lowering the risk of dementia and **Alzheimer's disease**."

*A review of antioxidants and **Alzheimer's disease**.* Frank B, Gupta S. Ann Clin Psychiatry. 2005 Oct-Dec;17(4):269-86. **Key Finding:** Over 300 articles were reviewed of antioxidants helpful in the prevention of Alzheimer's disease and 187 articles were selected for inclusion. Agents that show promise helping prevent AD include: 1) aged garlic extract, 2) curcumin, 3) melatonin, 4) resveratrol, 5) Ginkgo biloba extract, 6) green tea, 7) vitamin C and 8) vitamin E.

Antioxidant health effects of aged garlic extract. Borek C. J Nutr. 2001 Mar;131(3s):1010S-5S. **Key Finding:** "Although additional observations are warranted in humans, compelling evidence supports the beneficial health effects attributed to aged garlic extract, i.e., reducing the risk of **cardiovascular disease, stroke, cancer and aging**, including the oxidant-mediated brain cell damage that is implicated in **Alzheimer's disease**."

Antibacterial effects

***Antibacterial** potential of garlic-derived allicin and its cancellation by sulfhydryl compounds.* Fujisawa H, Watanabe K, Suma K, Origuchi K, Matsufuji H, Seki T, Ariga T. Biosci Biotechnol Biochem. 2009 Sep;73(9):1948-55. **Key Finding:** "The garlic extract had more potent anti-staphylococcal activity than an equal amount of allicin. The oxygen in the structure of allicin functions to liberate the S-allyl moiety, which might be an offensive tool against bacteria."

Antioxidation

Antioxidant effects of garlic in young and aged rat brain in vitro. Brunetti L, Menghini L, Orlando G, Recinella L, Leone S, Epifano F, Lazzarin F, Chiavaroli A, Ferrante C, Vacca M. J Med Food. 2009 Oct;12(5):1166-9. **Key Finding:** "Garlic supplementation could be effective in preventing **brain oxidative damage** in young animals, whereas the aging brain seems to be resistant to the antioxidant effects of garlic, in vitro."

*Diallyl Trisulfide Protects Rats from Carbon Tetrachloride-Induced **Liver Injury**.* Hosono-Fukao T, Hosono T, Seki T, Ariga T. J Nutr. 2009 Oct 7. (Epub ahead of print). **Key Finding:** "The effects of 6 kinds of alk(en)yl trisulfides, including diallyl trisulfide (DATS) and dipropyl trisulfide, on phase II enzyme activity were examined in rats. Only the allyl group-containing DATS and allyl methyl trisulfide enhanced these activities."

The protective effects of garlic extract against acetaminophen-induced oxidative stress and glutathione depletion. Anoush M, Eghbal MA, Fathiazad F, Hamzeiy H, Kouzehkonani NS. Pak J Biol Sci. 2009 May 15;12(10):765-71. **Key Finding:** "It is concluded that garlic extract has an **antioxidant** effect and can protect hepatocytes from glutathione depletion following NAPQI production."

Cardio protective roles of aged garlic extract, grape seed proanthocyanidin, and hazelnut on doxorubicin-induced cardio toxicity. Demirkaya E, Avci A, Kesik V, Karslioglu Y, Oztas E, Kismet E, Gokcay E, Durak I, Koseoglu V. Can J Physiol Pharmacol. 2009 Aug;87(8):633-40. **Key Finding:** "The positive effects of natural antioxidant foods on the prevention of Doxorubicin-induced **cardiac injury** could not be clearly shown on the basis of antioxidant enzymes. However, the electron microscope changes clearly demonstrated the protective effects of aged garlic extract and grape seed proanthocyanidin. The supplementation of these antioxidant foods over longer periods may show more definitive results. Human studies with different doses are needed to evaluate the effects of these foods on the human heart."

Effects of acute and sub-acute garlic supplement administration on serum total antioxidant capacity and lipid parameters in healthy volunteers. Koseoglu M, Isleten F, Atay A, Kaplan YC. Phytother Res. 2009 Aug 3. (Epub ahead of print). **Key Finding:** "These data suggest that garlic, used as a dietary supplement, may be beneficial in increasing the **antioxidant** capacity of the body."

***Antioxidant** effects of garlic in young and aged rat brain in vitro.* Brunetti L, Menghini L, Orlando G, Recinella L, Leone S, Epifano F, Lazzarin F, Chiavaroli A, Ferrante C, Vacca M. J Med Food. 2009 Oct;12(5):1166-9. **Key Finding:** "In young rats, we observed a concentration-dependent inhibitory effect of the garlic extract on brain 8-iso-PGF(2alpha) production. In aged rats, production was not affected by the garlic extract in the basal state, whereas, after hydrogen peroxide-induced oxidative stimulus, an antioxidant effect of the garlic extract appeared only at the higher concentration tested."

Protective roles of onion and garlic extracts on cadmium-induced changes in sperm characteristics and testicular oxidative damage in rats. Ola-Mudathir KF, Suru SM, Fafunso MA, Obioha UE, Faremi TV. Food Chem Toxicol. 2008 Dec;46(12):3604-11. **Key Finding**: "Our study demonstrated that aqueous extracts of onion and garlic could proffer a measure of protection against Cd-induced **testicular oxidative damage and spermiotoxicity** by possibly reducing lipid peroxidation and increasing the antioxidant defense mechanism in rats."

Black grape and garlic extracts protect against cyclosporine a nephrotoxicity. Durak I, Cetin R, Candir O, Devrim E, Kilicoglu B, Avci A. Immunol Invest. 2007;36(1):105-14. **Key Finding:** "The results suggest that impaired oxidant/antioxidant balance may play part in the CsA-induced nephrotoxicity, and some foods with high antioxidant power may ameliorate this toxicity, in agreement with studies with antioxidant vitamins."

Antioxidant health effects of aged garlic extract. Borek C. J Nutr. 2001 Mar;131(3s):1010S-5S. **Key Finding:** "Although additional observations are warranted in humans, compelling evidence supports the beneficial health effects attributed to aged garlic extract, i.e., reducing the risk of **cardiovascular disease, stroke, cancer and aging**, including the oxidant-mediated brain cell damage that is implicated in **Alzheimer's disease**."

Arthritis

Anti-inflammatory and arthritic effects of thiacremonone, a novel sulfur compound isolated from garlic via inhibition of NF-kappaB. Ban JO, Oh JH, Kim TM, Kim DJ, Jeong HS, Han SB, Hong JT. Arthritis Res Ther. 2009 Sep 30;11(5):R145. **Key Finding:** "The present results suggested that thiacremonone exerted its anti-inflammatory and anti-arthritic properties through the inhibition of NF-kappaB activation via interaction with the sulfhydryl group of NF-kappaB molecules, and thus could be a useful agent for the treatment of **inflammatory and arthritic diseases**."

Suppression of the nuclear factor-kappaB activation pathway by spice-derived phytochemicals: reasoning for seasoning. Aggarwal BB, Shishodia S. Ann N Y Acad Sci. 2004 Dec;1030:434-41. **Key Finding:** "The activation of nuclear transcription factor kappaB has now been linked with a variety of **inflammatory disease, including cancer, atherosclerosis, myocardial infarction, diabetes, allergy, asthma, arthritis, Crohn's disease, multiple sclerosis, Alzheimer's disease, osteoporosis, psoriasis, septic shock, and AIDS**.

Extensive research in the last few years has shown that the pathway that activates this transcription factor can be interrupted by phytochemicals derived from spices such as turmeric (curcumin), red pepper (capsaicin), cloves (eugenol), ginger (gingerol), cumin, anise, and fennel (anethol), basil and rosemary (ursolic acid), garlic (diallyl sulfide, S-allylmercaptocysteine, ajoene), and pomegranate (ellagic acid). For the first time, therefore, research provides 'reasoning for seasoning.'"

Atherosclerosis

Protective effects of Allium sativum against defects of hypercholesterolemia on pregnant rats and their offspring. El-Sayyad HI, Abou-El-Naga AM, Gadallah AA, Bakr IH. Int J Clin Exp Med. 2010 Jun 10;3(2):152-63. **Key Finding**: "Sixty fertile female and male albino rats of Wistar strain were used in the present study. The females were divided into four groups of ten rats each. Group 1 received water and standard feeds for 34 days. Group 2 was fed with a cholesterol-containing diet for two weeks prior to onset of gestation and maintained administration till parturition, produce **atherosclerosis.** Group 3 received trans gastric administration of 100mg homogenate of garlic for three weeks prior to onset of gestation. Group 4 intragastrically administered garlic for one week. Allium sativum-supplementation leads to amelioration of both mother and their offspring as a result of its antioxidant activity. All effects including atherosclerosis were markedly ameliorated by the supplementation."

The influence of raw and processed garlic and onions on plasma classical and non-classical **atherosclerosis** *indices: investigations in vitro and in vivo.* Gorinstein S, Leontowicz H, Leontowicz M, Jastrzebski Z, Najman K, Tashma Z, Katrich E, Heo BG, Cho JY, Park YJ, Trakhtenberg S. Phytother Res. 2009 Oct 13. (Epub ahead of print). **Key Finding:** "Garlic and white and red varieties of onion were subjected to processing by a variety of culinary methods, and bioactive compounds then determined. Blanching for 90 s most fully preserved the bioactive compounds and antioxidant potentials, and hindered the rise in plasma lipid levels and the decrease in plasma antioxidant activity of rats fed cholesterol."

Aged garlic extract supplemented with B vitamins, folic acid and L-arginine retards the progression of subclinical **atherosclerosis**: *a randomized clinical trial.* Budoff MJ, Ahmadi N, Gul KM, Liu ST, Flores FR, Tiano J, Takasu J, Miller E, Tsimikas S. Prev Med. 2009 Aug-Sep;49(2-3):101-7. **Key Finding:** "Aged garlic extract therapy with supplements is associated with a favorable improvement in oxidative biomarkers, vascular function, and reduced progression of atherosclerosis."

Suppression of the nuclear factor-kappaB activation pathway by spice-derived phytochemicals: reasoning for seasoning. Aggarwal BB, Shishodia S. Ann N Y Acad Sci. 2004 Dec;1030:434-41. **Key Finding:** "The activation of nuclear transcription factor kappaB has now been linked with a variety of **inflammatory disease, including cancer, atherosclerosis, myocardial infarction, diabetes, allergy, asthma, arthritis, Crohn's disease, multiple sclerosis, Alzheimer's disease, osteoporosis, psoriasis, septic shock, and AIDS**. Extensive research in the last few years has shown that the pathway that activates this transcription factor can be interrupted by phytochemicals derived from spices such as turmeric (curcumin), red pepper (capsaicin), cloves (eugenol), ginger (gingerol), cumin, anise, and fennel (anethol), basil and rosemary (ursolic acid), garlic (diallyl sulfide, S-allylmercaptocysteine, ajoene), and pomegranate (ellagic acid). For the first time, therefore, research provides 'reasoning for seasoning.'"

Daily supplementation with aged garlic extract, but not raw garlic, protects low density lipoprotein against in vitro oxidation. Munday JS, James KA, Fray LM, Kirkwood SW, Thompson KG. Atherosclerosis. 1999 Apr;143(2):399-404. **Key Finding:** "LDL isolated from subjects given either alpha-tocopherol or aged garlic extract, but not raw garlic, was significantly more resistant to oxidation than LDL isolated from subjects receiving no supplements. These results suggest that if antioxidants are proven to be antiatherogenic, aged garlic extract may be useful in preventing **atherosclerotic disease**."

*The **antiatherosclerotic** effect of Allium sativum.* Koscielny J, Klussendorf D, Latza R, Schmitt R, Radtke H, Siegel G, Kiesewetter H. Atherosclerosis. 1999 May;144(1):237-49. **Key Finding:** "In a randomized, double-blind, placebo-controlled clinical trial, the plaque volumes in both carotid and femoral arteries of 152 people were determined by B-mode ultrasound. Continuous intake of high-dose garlic powder reduced significantly the increases in arteriosclerotic plaque volume by 5-18% or even effected a slight regression within the observational period. These results substantiated that not only a preventive but possibly also a curative role in arteriosclerosis therapy (plaque regression) may be ascribed to garlic remedies."

*Allicin-induced decrease in formation of fatty streaks (**atherosclerosis**) in mice fed a cholesterol-rich diet.* Abramovitz D, Gavri S, Harats D, Levkovitz H, Mirelman D, Miron T, Eilat-Adar S, Rabinkov A, Wilchek M, Eldar M, Vered Z. Coron Artery Dis. 1999 Oct;10(7):515-9. **Key Finding:** "These results indicate that allicin reduces formation of fatty streaks (atherosclerosis) in hyperlipidemic mice. These changes do not seem to occur through an alteration in blood lipid profile."

*Prevention of Hypercholesterolemic **Atherosclerosis** by garlic, an antioxidant.* Prasad K, Mantha SV, Kalra J, Lee P. J Cardiovasc Pharmacol Ther. 1997 Oct; 2(4):309-320. **Key Finding:** "The protection afforded by garlic was associated with decrease in aortic malondialdehyde and chemiluminescence in spite of no change in serum cholesterol. These results suggest that oxygen free radicals are involved in the genesis and maintenance of hypercholesterolemic atherosclerosis and that use of garlic can be useful in preventing the development of hypercholesterolemic atherosclerosis."

*Effect of garlic oil in experimental **cholesterol atherosclerosis**.* Jain RC, Konar DB. Atherosclerosis. 1978 Feb;29(2):125-9. **Key Finding:** "Addition of cholesterol in the diet of male albino rabbits produced hypercholesterolemia, increased tissue cholesterol, and athermanous changes in the aorta. Supplementation of garlic oil along with cholesterol significantly inhibited the hypercholesterolemia, decreased tissue cholesterol and minimized the athermanous changes in the aorta. These results show that the active constituents in garlic responsible for its anti-atherogenic action are present in the oily fraction of garlic."

*Effects of garlic extract and of three pure components isolated from it on human **platelet aggregation**, arachidonate metabolism, release reaction and platelet ultrastructure.* Apitz-Castro R, Cabrera S, Cruz MR, Ledezma E, Jain MK. Thromb Res. 1983 Oct 15;32(2):155-69. **Key Finding:** "We studied the effect of the methanol extract of garlic bulbs and of three pure components isolated from it (F1, F2, F3) on human platelet aggregation induced by ADP, epinephrine, collagen, thrombin, arachidonate, PAF, and the ionosphere A-23187. Incubation of PRP with extract of garlic bulbs, either in methanol or in homologous PPP, inhibits platelet aggregation induced by all of the above mentioned agonists. F1, F2 and F3 also inhibit platelet aggregation; however, F3 was about four times more potent."

Cancer (bladder; breast; colon; endometrial; esophageal; gastric; larynx; leukemia; lung; oral; ovary; melanoma; prostate; renal; stomach)

Diallyl disulfide causes caspase-dependent apoptosis in human cancer cells through a Bax-triggered mitochondrial pathway. Nagaraj NS, Anilakumar KR, Singh OV. J Nutr Biochem. 2010 May;21(5):405-12. **Key Finding**: "Diallyl disulfide (DADS) is an important component of garlic derivative and has been demonstrated to exert a potential molecular target against human cancers. We investigated DADS-induced expressions in **breast, prostate and lung cancer** cells. This study shows clearly that DADS causes caspase-dependent apoptosis in human cancer cells through a Bax-triggered mitochondrial pathway."

*Diallyl trisulfide induces Bcl-2 and caspase-3-dependent apoptosis via down regulation of Akt phosphorylation in human T24 **bladder cancer** cells.* Wang YB, Qin J, Zheng XY, Et al. Phytomedicine. 2010 Apr;17(5):363-8. **Key Finding**: "These findings suggest that the garlic-derived organosulfur compound diallyl trisulfide may be an effective way for treating human bladder and other types of cancers."

Diallylpolysulfides induce growth arrest and apoptosis. Busch C, Jacob C, Anwar A, Et al. Int J Oncol. 2010 Mar;36(3):743-9. **Key Finding**: "Garlic-derived organo sulphur compounds such as diallysulfides provide a significant protection against carcinogenesis and were employed to investigate the influence of these agents on cell viability, cell cycle arrest and induction of apoptosis in HCT116 human **colon cancer c**ells. These results support the therapeutic potential of polysulfide and allow insight into the mechanisms."

*Cytotoxic effect of garlic extract and its fractions on Sk-mel3 **melanoma** cell line.* Hakimzadeh H, Ghazzanfari T, Rahmati B, Naderimanesh H. Immunopharmacol Immunotoxicol. 2010 Sep;32(3):371-5. **Key Finding**: "Garlic extract fractions R100 and R10 have more potential in cytotoxic activities against Sk-mel3 melanoma cells. Garlic appears to be a good candidate as an antitumor agent against melanoma."

*Diallyl sulfide induces growth inhibition and apoptosis of anaplastic **thyroid cancer** cells by mitochondrial signaling pathway.* Shin HA, Cha YY, Park MS, Et al. Oral Oncol. 2010 Apr;46(4):e15-8. **Key Finding**: "Diallyl sulfide from garlic decreased cell proliferation and induced apoptosis via mitochondrial signaling pathway in anaplastic thyroid cancer cells in a dose-dependent manner."

*Anti-invasive activity of diallyl disulfide through tightening of tight junctions and inhibition of matrix metalloproteinase activities in LNCaP **prostate cancer** cells.* Shin DY, Kim GY, Kim JI, Et al. Toxicol In Vitro. 2010 Sep;24(6):1569-76. **Key Finding**: "The present study indicates that tight junctions and matrix metalloproteinase are critical targets of diallyl disulfide-induced anti-invasiveness in human prostate cancer LNCaP cells."

*Allicin induces apoptosis in **gastric cancer** cells through activation of both extrinsic and intrinsic pathways.* Zhang W, Ha M, Gong Y, Et al. Oncol Rep. 2010 Dec;24(6):1585-92. **Key Finding**: "Data from the current study demonstrated that allicin from garlic should be further investigated as a novel cancer preventive or therapeutic agent in control of gastric cancer, with potential uses in other tumor types."

*Garlic intake and **cancer** risk: an analysis using the Food and Drug Administration's evidence-based review system for the scientific evaluation of health claims.* Kim JY, Kwon O. Am J Clin Nutr. 2009 Jan;89(1):257-64. **Key Finding:** "There was no credible evidence to support a relation between garlic intake and a reduced risk of gastric, breast, lung, or endometrial cancer. Very limited evidence supported a relation between garlic consumption and reduced risk of **colon, prostate, esophageal, larynx, oral, ovary or renal cell cancers**."

*Diallyl sulfide inhibits murine WEHI-3 **leukemia** cells in BALB/c mice in vitro and in vivo.* Yu FS, Wu CC, Chen CT, Huang SP, Yang JS, Hsu YM, Wu PP, Lin JP, Lin JG, Chung JG. Hum Exp Toxicol. 2009 Oct 22. (Epub ahead of print). **Key Finding:** "We examined the effects of diallyl sulfide on the cytotoxicity of WEHI-3 cells and results indicated that diallyl sulfide decreased the percentage of viable WEHI-3 cells and these effects are dose-dependent."

*Garlic constituent diallyl trisulfide induced apoptosis in MCF7 human **breast cancer** cells.* Malki A, El-Saadani M, Sultan AS. Cancer Biol Ther. 2009 Nov 22;8(22). **Key Finding:** "The results of the present study show, for the first time, that diallyl trisulfide administration from garlic might offer a novel strategy for the treatment of human breast cancer."

*Diallyl trisulfide induces BcI-2 and caspase-3-dependent apoptosis via down regulation of Akt phosphorylation in human T24 **bladder cancer** cells.* Wang YB, Qin J, Zheng XY, Bai Y, Yang K, Xie LP. Phytomedicine. 2009 Sep 10. (Epub ahead of print). **Key Finding:** "These findings suggest that diallyl trisulfide may be an effective way for treating human bladder and other types of cancers."

*Transcriptional repression and inhibition of nuclear translocation of androgen receptor by diallyl trisulfide in human **prostate cancer** cells.* Stan SD, Singh SV. Clin Cancer Res. 2009 Aug 1;15(15):4895-903. **Key Finding:** "The present study shows, for the first time, that diallyl trisulfide treatment suppresses androgen receptor function in prostate cancer cells."

*The garlic ingredient diallyl sulfide induces Ca(2+) mobilization in Madin-Darby canine **kidney cells**.* Chen CH, Su SJ, Chang KL, Huang MW, Kuo SY. Food Chem Toxicol. 2009 Sep;47(9):2344-50. **Key Finding:** "These findings suggest that diallyl sulfide induced a significant rise in [Ca(2+)](i) in MDCK renal tubular cells by stimulating both extracellular Ca(2+) influx and thapsigargin-sensitive intracellular Ca(2+) release via as yet unidentified mechanisms." .

Thiacremonone augments chemotherapeutic agent-induced growth inhibition in human **colon cancer** *cells through inactivation of nuclear factor-[kappa]B.* Ban JO, Lee HS, Jeong HS, Song S, Hwang BY, Moon DC, Yoondo Y, Han SB, Hong JT. Mol Cancer Res. 2009 Jun;7(6):870-9. **Key Finding:** "Thiacremonone, a novel sulfur compound isolated from garlic, inhibited Nf-kappaB and cancer cell growth with IC(50) values about 100 micrg/mL in colon cancer cells. In the present study, we tested whether thiacremonone could increase susceptibility of cancer cells to chemotherapeutics through inactivation of NF-kappaB. These results warrant carefully designed clinical studies investigating the combination of thiacremonone and commonly used chemotherapeutic agents for the treatment of human cancers."

Diallyl trisulfide-induced apoptosis in human **cancer** *cells is linked to checkpoint kinase 1-mediated mitotic arrest.* Xiao D, Zeng Y, Singh SV. Mol Carcinog. 2009 Nov;48(11):1018-29. **Key Finding:** "The results of the present study indicate that Chk1 dependence of (diallyl trisulfide) DATS-induced mitotic arrest in human cancer cells is not influenced by the p53 status and cells arrested in mitosis upon DATS exposure are driven to apoptotic DNA fragmentation."

Garlic constituent diallyl trisulfide induced apoptosis in MCF7 human **breast cancer** *cells.* Malki A, El-Saadani M, Sultan AS. Cancer Biol Ther. 2009 Nov;8(22):2174-84. **Key Finding:** "The results of the present study show, for the first time, that diallyl trisulfide administration might offer a novel strategy for the treatment of human breast cancer."

Allium vegetables intake and **endometrial cancer** *risk.* Galeone C, Pelucchi C, Dal Maso L, Negri E, Montella M, Zucchetto A, Talamini R, La Vecchia C. Public Health Nutr. 2009 Sep;12(9):1576-9. **Key Finding**: "We analyzed data from a multi-center case-control study of 454 endometrial cancer cases and 908 controls. Our study found a moderate protective role of allium vegetables (onions and garlic) on the risk of endometrial cancer."

Food intake and the occurrence of squamous cell carcinoma in different sections of the esophagus in Taiwanese men. Chen YK, Lee CH, Wu IC, Liu JS, Wu DC, Lee JM, Goan YG, Chou SH, Huang CT, Lee CY, Hung HC, Yang JF, Wu MT. Nutrition. 2009 Jul-Aug;25(7-8):753-61. **Key Finding**: "We found that intake of vegetables, raw onions and raw garlic, and fruits significantly protective against **esophageal squamous cell carcinoma** risk."

Phytochemicals that counteract the cardio toxic side effects of **cancer chemotherapy.** Piasek A, Bartoszek A, Namiesnik J. Postepy Hig Med Dosw (Polish). 2009 Apr 17;63:142-58. **Key Finding**: "Dietary intervention with antioxidants (such as in tomato, garlic, spinach) may be a safe and effective way of alleviating the toxicity of anticancer chemotherapy and preventing **heart failure.**"

Induction of apoptosis by S-allylmercapto-L-cysteine, a bio transformed garlic derivative, on a human **gastric cancer** *cell line.* Lee Y. Int J Mol Med. 2008 Jun;21(6):765-70. **Key Finding:** "Although the bio transformed garlic derivative S-allylmercapto-L-cysteine (SAMC) has been reported to show an inhibitory effect on tumorigenesis, the mechanisms are poorly understood. The present study investigated the effect of SAMC on the growth of human gastric cancer SNU-1 cells. These results suggest that the apoptotic effect of SAMC on gastric cancer SNU-1 cells may be connected with caspase-3 activation through the induction of Bax and p53 rather than Bcl-2 and p21."

Anticancer *effects of diallyl trisulfide derived from garlic.* Seki T, Hosono T, Hosono-Fukao T, Inada K, Tanaka R, Ogihara J, Agriga T. Asia Pac J Clin Nutr. 2008;17 Suppl 1:249-52. **Key Finding:** "These results suggest that diallyl trisulfide is responsible, at least in part, for the epidemiologically proven anticancer effect for garlic eaters."

Multitargeted prevention and therapy of **cancer** *by diallyl trisulfide and related Allium vegetable-derived organosulfur compounds.* Powolny AA, Singh SV. Cancer Lett. 2008 Oct 8;269(2):305-14. **Key Finding:** "The known health benefits of Allium vegetables constituents include **cardiovascular** effects, improvement of the immune function, lowering of blood glucose level, radioprotection, protection against microbial infections, and anti-cancer effects. This article summarizes preclinical and limited clinical data to warrant further clinical evaluation of Allium vegetable constituents for prevention and therapy of human cancers."

Garlic oil inhibits cyclin E expression in gastric adenocarcinoma cells. Liang WJ, Yan X, Zhang WD, Luo RC. Nan Fang Yi Ke Da Xue Xue Bao (China). 2007 Aug;27(8):1241-3. **Key Finding:** "Garlic oil inhibits cyclin E expression in routinely cultured SGC7901 cells and also in TGFalpha-treated ones suggesting that garlic oil can inhibit the TGFalpha autocrine and paracrine loops, which can be one of the pathways of garlic oil to inhibit **cancer** cell proliferation."

Cancer *chemoprevention with garlic and its constituents.* Shukla Y, Kalra N. Cancer Lett. 2007 Mar 18;247(2):167-81. **Key Finding:** "Recent data show that garlic-derived products modulate cell-signaling pathways in a fashion that controls the unwanted proliferation of cells thereby imparting strong cancer chemo preventive as well as cancer therapeutic effects."

Induction of apoptosis and histone hyper acetylation by diallyl disulfide in **prostate cancer** *cell line PC-3.* Arunkumar A, Vijayababu MR, Gunadharini N, Krishnamoorthy G, Arunakaran J. Cancer Lett. 2007 Jun 18;251(1):59-67. **Key Finding:** "It is concluded that diallyl disulfide induces apoptosis by influencing histone acetylation in prostate cancer cells."

S-allylcysteine, a water-soluble garlic derivative, suppresses the growth of a human androgen-independent **prostate cancer** *xenograft, CWR22R, under in vivo conditions.* Chu Q, Lee DT, Tsao SW, Wang X, Wong YC. BJU Int. 2007 Apr;99(4):925-32. **Key Finding:** "These results suggest that this garlic-derived compound might be a potential therapeutic agent for suppressing AI prostate cancer."

Garlic compounds induced calpain and intrinsic caspase cascade for apoptosis in human **malignant neuroblastoma** *SH-SY5Y cells.* Karmakar S, Banik NL, Patel SJ, Ray SK. Apoptosis. 2007 Apr;12(4):671-84. **Key Finding:** "Results strongly suggested that the garlic compounds DAS and DADS suppressed anti-apoptotic factors and activated calpain and intrinsic caspase cascade for apoptosis in SH-SY5Y cells."

Onion and garlic intake and the odds of **benign prostatic hyperplasia**. Galeone C, Pelucchi C, Talamini R, Negri E, Dal Maso L, Montella M, Ramazzotti V, Franceschi S, La Vecchia C. Urology. 2007 Oct; 70(4):672-6. **Key Finding**: "This uniquely large data set from European populations (1369 patients and 1451 controls) showed an inverse association between allium vegetable consumption and benign prostatic hyperplasia."

Diallylsulfide and allylmethylsulfide are uniquely effective among organosulfur compounds in inhibiting CYP2E1 protein in animal models. Wargovich MJ. J Nutr. 2006 Mar;136(3 Suppl):8325-8345. **Key Finding:** "This article summarizes the key findings behind one important mechanism explaining the anticarcinogenic effects of garlic-derived agents in animal models: the inhibition of cytochrome p4502E1, with some commentary on other aspects of carcinogen metabolism modified by these unique phytochemicals."

Current trends and perspectives in nutrition and **cancer** *prevention.* Barta I, Smerak P, Polivkova Z, Sestakova H, Langova M, Turek B, Bartova J. Neoplasma. 2006;53(1):19-25. **Key Finding:** "We investigated antigenotoxic and immunomodulatory effects of juices and vegetable homogenates (carrot+cauliflower, cauliflower, red cabbage, broccoli, onion, garlic) on the genotoxicity of AFB1 and pyro lysates of amino acids. All complete vegetable homogenates and substances of plant origin tested showed a clear antimutagenic and immunomodulatory activities on mutagenicity and immunosuppression induced by reference mutagens."

Crude extract of garlic induced caspase-3 gene expression leading to apoptosis in human **colon cancer** *cells.* Su CC, Chan GW, Tan TW, Lin JG, Chung JG. In Vivo. 2006 Jan-Feb;20(1):85-90. **Key Finding:** "We conclude that crude extract of garlic can induce apoptosis in colon 205 cells through caspase-3 activity, by means of a mitochondrial-dependent mechanism."

Preclinical perspectives on garlic and **cancer.** Milner JA. J Nutr. 2006 Mar;136(3 Suppl):827S-831S. **Key Finding:** "Evidence continues to point to the anti-cancer properties of fresh garlic extracts, aged garlic, garlic oil, and a number of specific organosulfur compounds generated by processing garlic. These anti-carcinogenic and antitumorigenic characteristics appear to arise through both dose- and temporal-related changes in a number of cellular events involved with the cancer process, including those involving drug metabolism, immunocompetence, cell cycle regulation, apoptosis, and angiogenesis. The ability of garlic and related allyl sulfur compounds to block tumors in the colon, lung, breast, and liver suggests general mechanisms that are not tissue specific."

Allyl sulfur compounds from garlic modulate aberrant crypt formation. Ross SA, Finley JW, Milner JA. J Nutr. 2006 Mar;136(3 Suppl):852S-854S. **Key Finding:** "The health benefits of garlic, including inhibition of carcinogenesis, are supported by several epidemiologic and laboratory findings. Garlic's sulfur components have been reported to suppress experimentally induced tumor incidence in several organs, including the colon. Studies in humans also suggest that dietary garlic constituents reduce the risk of colorectal adenomatous polyps, which are considered precursors to **colon cancer.**"

Diallyl disulfide inhibits WEHI-3 **leukemia** *cells in vivo.* Yang JS, Kok LF, Lin YH, Kuo TC, Yang JL, Lin CC, Chen GW, Huang WW, Ho HC, Chung JG. Anticancer Res. 2006 Jan-Feb; 26(1A):219-25. **Key Finding:** "Diallyl disulfide (DADS) a component of garlic, inhibits the proliferation of human blood, colon, lung and skin cancer cells. The present study is focused on the in vivo effects of DADS on WEHI-3 leukemia cells. Apparently, DADS affects WEHI-3 cells both in vitro and in vivo."

Aged garlic extract inhibits angiogenesis and proliferation of **colorectal carcinoma** *cells.* Matsuura N, Miyamae Y, Yamane K, Nagao Y, Hanada Y, Kawaguichi N,

Katsuki T, Hirata K, Sumi S, Ishikawa H. J Nutr. 2006 Mar;136(3 Suppl):842S-846S. **Key Finding:** "These results suggest that aged garlic extract could prevent tumor formation by inhibiting angiogenesis through the suppression of endothelial cell motility, proliferation, and tube formation. AGE would be a good chemo preventive agent for colorectal cancer because of its antiproliferative action on colorectal carcinoma cells and inhibitory activity on angiogenesis."

Induction of apoptosis and transient increase of phosphorylated MAPKs by diallyl disulfide treatment in human **nasopharyngeal carcinoma** *CNE2 cells.* Zhang YW, Wen J, Xiao JB, Talbot SG, Li GC, Xu M. Arch Pharm Res. 2006 Dec; 29(12):1125-31. **Key Finding:** "These results indicate that diallyl disulfide can induce apoptosis in human nasopharyngeal carcinoma cells via, at least partly, S-phase block of the cell cycle, related to a rise in MAPK phosphorylation."

An aqueous garlic extract alleviates water avoidance stress-induced degeneration of the **urinary bladder.** Saglam B, Cikler E, Zeybek A, Cetinel S, Sener G, Ercan F. BJU Int. 2006 Dec;98(6):1250-4. **Key Finding:** "These results show that aged garlic extract has a protective effect on WAS-induced degenerative changes in the urinary bladder."

Growth suppressing effect of garlic compound diallyl disulfide on **prostate cancer** *cell line (PC-3) in vitro.* Arunkumar A, Vijayababu MR, Kanagaraj P, Balasubramanian K, Aruldhas MM, Arunakaran J. Biol Pharm Bull. 2005 Apr;28(4):740-3. **Key Finding:** "It is concluded that diallyl disulfide, component of aged garlic extract, inhibits proliferation of prostate cancer cells through the induction of apoptosis."

Anticarcinogenic *properties of garlic: a review.* Khanum F, Anilakumar KR, Viswanathan KR. Crit Rev Food Sci Nutr. 2004;44(6):479-88. **Key Finding:** "This article focuses on the general chemistry, metabolism, anticarcinogenic properties, and mechanism of action behind the anticarcinogenic effects. Garlic has been thought to bring about its anticarcinogenic effect through a number of mechanisms, such as the scavenging of radicals, increasing glutathione levels, increasing the activities of enzymes, inhibition of cytochrome p4502E1, DNA repair mechanisms, prevention of chromosomal damage, etc."

Antimicrobial and chemo preventive properties of herbs and spices. Lai PK, Roy J. Curr Med Chem. 2004 Jun;11(11):1451-60. **Key Finding:** "A growing body of research has demonstrated that the commonly used herbs and spices such as garlic, black cumin, cloves, cinnamon, thyme, allspices, bay leaves, mustard and rosemary, possess antimicrobial properties that, in some cases, can be used therapeutically. Other spices, such as saffron, turmeric, green or black tea and flaxseed do contain potent phytochemicals, including carotenoids, curcumins, catechins, and lignin, which provide significant protection against **cancer.**"

Indian food ingredients and cancer prevention – an experimental evaluation of anticarcinogenic effects of garlic in rat colon. Sengupta A, Ghosh S, Bhattacharjee S, Das S. Asian Pac J Cancer Prev. 2004 Apr-Jun;5(2):126-32. **Key Finding:** "Following treatment, significant inhibition of cell proliferation and induction of apoptosis, as well as suppression of cyclooxygenase-2 activity were observed, associated with significant reduction in the incidence of aberrant crypt foci. The study points to combined protective effects of garlic components on **colon carcinogenesis**."

egetables, fruits and phytoestrogens in the prevention of diseases. Heber D. J Postgrad Med. 2004 Apr-Jun;50(2):145-9. **Key Finding:** "Consumers are advised to ingest one serving of each of the seven color groups daily. For instance, red foods contain lycopene which may be involved in maintaining **prostate** health and which has been linked to a decreased risk of **cardiovascular disease**. Green foods, including broccoli, Brussels sprouts and kale, have been associated with a decreased risk of cancer. White-green foods such as garlic may inhibit **cancer** cell growth. Grouping plants foods by color provides simplification, but it is also important as a method to help consumers make wise food choices and promote health."

Suppression of the nuclear factor-kappaB activation pathway by spice-derived phytochemicals: reasoning for seasoning. Aggarwal BB, Shishodia S. Ann N Y Acad Sci. 2004 Dec;1030:434-41. **Key Finding:** "The activation of nuclear transcription factor kappaB has now been linked with a variety of **inflammatory disease, including cancer, atherosclerosis, myocardial infarction, diabetes, allergy, asthma, arthritis, Crohn's disease, multiple sclerosis, Alzheimer's disease, osteoporosis, psoriasis, septic shock, and AIDS**. Extensive research in the last few years has shown that the pathway that activates this transcription factor can be interrupted by phytochemicals derived from spices such as turmeric (curcumin), red pepper (capsaicin), cloves (eugenol), ginger (gingerol), cumin, anise, and fennel (anethol), basil and rosemary (ursolic acid), garlic (diallyl sulfide, S-allylmercaptocysteine, ajoene), and pomegranate (ellagic acid). For the first time, therefore, research provides 'reasoning for seasoning.'"

*Ajoene (natural garlic compound): a new anti-**leukemia** agent for AML therapy.* Hassan HT. Leuk Res. 2004 Jul;28(7):667-71. **Key Finding:** "The recent findings of the potent enhancing activity of ajoene on chemotherapy-induced apoptosis in CD34-positive resistant human myeloid leukemia cells suggest a novel promising role for the treatment of refractory and/or relapsed AML (acute myeloid leukemia) patients as well as elderly AML patients."

Comparative effects of mono-, di-, tri-, and tetra sulfides derived from plants of the Allium family: redox cycling in vitro and hemolytic activity and Phase 2 enzyme induction in vivo. Munday R, Munday JS, Munday CM. Free Rad Biol Med. 2003 May 1;34(9):1200-1211. **Key Finding:** "Epidemiological evidence indicates that a high dietary intake of plants of the Allium family, such as garlic and onions, decreases the risk of **cancer** in humans. Allyl and propyl tri- and tetrasulfides, may contribute to the toxic effects of Allium vegetables, while only the allyl derivatives are effective in increasing tissue activities of cancer-protective enzymes."

*VBotanicals in **cancer** chemoprevention.* Park EJ, Pezzuto JM. Cancer Metastasis Rev. 2002;21(3-4):231-55. **Key Finding:** "In this review, we discuss the cancer chemo preventive activity of cruciferous vegetables such as cabbage and broccoli, Allium vegetables such as garlic and onion, green tea, citrus fruits, tomatoes, berries, ginger and ginseng. Phytochemicals of these types have great potential in the fight against human cancer, and a variety of delivery methods are available as a result of their occurrence in nature."

Inhibitory effect of whole strawberries, garlic juice or kale juice on endogenous formation of N-nitrosodimethylamine in humans. Chung MJ, Lee SH, Sung NJ. Cancer Lett. 2002 Aug 8;182(1):1-10. **Key Finding:** "When whole strawberries, garlic juice, or kale juice was provided immediately after an amine-rich diet with a nitrate, NDMA excretion was decreased by 70, 71, and 44% respectively, compared with NDMA excretion after ingestion of an amine-rich diet with a nitrate. These results suggest that consumption of whole strawberries, garlic juice, or kale juice can reduce endogenous NDMA formation."

*Garlic—A Natural Source of **Cancer** Preventive Compounds.* Das S. Asian Pac J Cancer Prev. 2002;3(4):305-311. **Key Finding:** "Garlic compounds have been found to block covalent binding of carcinogens to DNA, enhance degradation of carcinogens, have antioxidative and free radical scavenging properties and to regulate cell proliferation, apoptosis and immune responses. This has opened up a new avenue for researchers in the field of cancer chemoprevention."

*A historical perspective on garlic and **cancer**.* Milner JA. J Nutr. 2001 Mar;131(3s):1027S-31S. **Key Finding:** "Both water and lipid-soluble allyl sulfur compounds are effective in blocking a myriad of chemically induced tumors. Their ability to block experimentally induced tumors in a variety of sites including skin, mammary and colon, suggests a general mechanism of action. Some, but not all, allyl sulfur compounds can also effectively retard tumor proliferation and induce apoptosis."

Enhanced immune competence by garlic: role in **bladder cancer** *and other malignancies.* Lamm DL, Riggs DR. J Nutr. 2001 Mar;131(3s):1067S-70S. **Key Finding:** "Our previous animal studies demonstrated that aged garlic extract was highly effective for human bladder cancer. To elucidate the mechanism of this antitumor effect, the literature describing antitumor and immune enhancing effects of garlic is reviewed. Garlic can detoxify carcinogens by stimulation of cytochrome P(450) enzymes, antioxidant activity or sulfur compound binding. Studies demonstrate a direct toxic effect of garlic to s**arcoma** and **gastric colon**, bladder and **prostate cancer** cells in tissue culture. The most likely explanation of this effect is immune stimulation."

Mechanisms of inhibition of chemical toxicity and carcinogenesis by diallyl sulfide and related compounds from garlic. Yang CS, Chhabra SK, Hong JY, Smith TJ. Nutr. 2001 Mar;131(3s):1041S-5S. **Key Finding:** "The protective effect (of diallyl sulfide) was observed when the organosulfur compounds were given before, during or soon after chemical treatment. DAS and DASO(2) inhibited the bioactivation of 4-(methylnitrosamino)-1-(3-pyridyl)-1-butanone (NNK) and related **lung tumorigenesis** in A/J mice."

Garlic and **cancer***: a critical review of the epidemiologic literature.* Fleischauer AT, Arab L. Nutr. 2001 Mar;131(3s):1032S-40S. **Key Finding:** "Site-specific case-control studies of **stomach and colorectal cancer**, in which multiple reports were available, suggest a protective effect of high intake of raw and/or cooked garlic. Cohort studies confirm this inverse association for colorectal cancer. Few cohort and case-control studies for other sites of cancer exist."

Effects of diallyl disulfide and other donors of sulfane sulfur on the proliferation of human **hepatoma cell** *line (HepG2).* Iciek MB, Rokita HB, Wlodek LB. Neoplasma. 2001;48(4):307-12. **Key Finding:** "It may be concluded that these donors of reactive sulfane sulfur may be responsible for inhibition of the proliferation of HepG2 cells."

Effects of garlic oil on tumoragenecity and intercellular communication in human **gastric cancer** *cell line.* Li X, Xie J, Li W, Ji J, Zhao M, Sun M, Lu Y. Sci China C Life Sci. 2000 Feb;43(1):82-7. **Key Finding:** "Previous studies have demonstrated that garlic oil and its anti-tumor compound could inhibit DNA and RNA synthesis in human cancer cells. In order to explore the effects of garlic oil on carcinoma cells, a gastric carcinoma cell line BGC-823 was studied after garlic oil treatment. Data showed that the cell differentiation and suppression of tumorigenicity were significantly induced in tumor cells after garlic oil treatment."

The effects of garlic preparations against human **tumor cell** *proliferation.* Siegers CP, Steffen B, Robke A, Pentz R. Phytomedicine. 1999 Mar;6(1):7-11. **Key Finding:** "Our results suggest that the antiproliferative effects of garlic may be due to breakdown products of alliin, such as allicin or polysulfide, rather than alliin itself. Since the addition of an alliinase system (garlic powder) to an alliin enriched preparation without alliinase (garlic extract) potentiated the effects observed with the two preparations alone."

Protective effect of allium vegetables against both **esophageal and stomach cancer**: *a simultaneous case-referent study of a high-epidemic area in Jiangsu Province, China.* Gao CM, Takezaki T, Ding JH, Li MS, Tajima K. J Cancer Res. 1999 Jun;90(6):614-21. **Key Finding:** "The main results in the present study suggested that allium vegetables (such as garlic and onion), like raw vegetables, may have an important protecting effect against not only stomach cancer, but also esophageal cancer."

Low doses of diallyl disulfide, a compound derived from garlic, increase tissue activities of quinine reductase and glutathione transferase in the gastrointestinal tract of the rat. Munday R, Munday CM. Nutr Cancer. 1999;34(1):42-8. **Key Finding:** "In the present studies, increased activities of quinine reductase and glutathione transferase were recorded in the forestomach, glandular stomach, duodenum jejunum, ileum, cecum, colon, liver, kidneys, spleen, heart, lungs and urinary bladder of rats given diallyl disulfide over a wide range of dose levels. Such dose levels are close to that which may be achieved through human consumption of garlic, suggesting that induction of phase II enzymes may contribute to the protection that is afforded by this vegetable against **cancer of the gastrointestinal tract** in humans."

Heating garlic inhibits its ability to suppress 7, 12-dimethylbenz(a)anthracene-induced DNA adduct formation in rat **mammary tissue**. Song K, Milner JA. J Nutr. 1999 Mar;129(3):657-61. **Key Finding:** "These studies provide evidence that alliinase may be important for the formation of allyl sulfur compounds that contribute to a depression of DMBA metabolism and bio activation. Providing crushed garlic reduced by 64% the quantity of DMBA-induced DNA adducts present in mammary epithelial cells compared to controls. Microwave treatment decreased the protection provided by garlic resulting in a 90% loss of alliinase activity.

Heating in a convection oven also completely blocked the ability of uncrushed garlic to retard DMBA bio activation."

New pharmacological activities of garlic and its constituents. Sumiyoshi H. Nippon Yakurigaku Zasshi (Japan). 1997 Oct;110 Suppl 1;93P-97P. **Key Finding:** "Epidemiological studies in China, Italy and USA showed the inverse relationship between **stomach and colon cancer** incidences and dietary garlic intake. Anti-carcinogenic activities of garlic and its constituents including sulfides and S-allyl cysteine, have been demonstrated using several animal models. Garlic preparations has been also shown to lower serum cholesterol and triglyceride levels, which are major risk factors of **cardiovascular diseases**, through inhibition of their bio-synthesis in the liver, and to inhibit oxidation of low density lipoprotein. Furthermore, in vitro and in vivo studies have revealed that aged garlic extract stimulated immune functions, such as proliferation of lymphocyte, cytokine release, NK activity and phagocytosis. More recently, aged garlic extract has been demonstrated to **prolong life span** of senescence accelerated mice and prevent brain atrophy."

Garlic: its anticarcinogenic and antitumorigenic properties. Milner JA. Nutr Rev. 1996 Nov;54(11 Pt2):S82-6. **Key Finding:** "Several investigations indicate that garlic and its organic allyl sulfur components inhibit the cancer process. Furthermore, these studies reveal that the benefits of garlic are not limited to a specific species, a particular tissue, or a specific carcinogen. Although the evidence supports the benefits of garlic, additional evidence is needed to determine the quantity needed by humans to minimize **cancer** risk."

*Relation of vegetable, fruit, and grain consumption to **colorectal adenomatous polyps**.* Witte JS, Longnecker MP, Bird CL, Lee ER, Frankl HD, Haile RW. Am J Epidemiol. 1996 Dec 1;144(11):1015-25. **Key Finding:** "Frequent consumption of vegetables, fruits and grains was associated with decreased polyp prevalence. The authors also found inverse associations for high carotenoid vegetables such as garlic and cruciferous vegetables."

Therapeutic actions of garlic constituents. Agarwal KC. Med Res Rev. 1996 Jan;16(1):111-24. **Key Finding:** "In summary, the epidemiological, clinical, and laboratory data have proved that garlic contains many biologically and pharmacologically important compounds, which are beneficial to human health from **cardiovascular,** neoplastic, and several other diseases. Garlic contains several potentially important agents that possess **antitumor** and **anticarcinogenic properties**."

A prospective cohort study on the relationship between onion and leek consumption, garlic supplement use and the risk of **colorectal carcinoma** *in The Netherlands.* Dorant E, van den Brandt PA, Goldbohm RA. Carcinogenesis. 1996 Mar;17(3):477-84. **Key Finding:** "This study does not support an inverse association between the consumption of onions and leeks, or the use of garlic supplements and the incidence of male and female colon and rectum carcinoma."

Organosulfur compounds and **cancer.** Lea MA. Adv Exp Med Biol. 1996;401:147-54. **Key Finding:** "There is substantial evidence that constituents of garlic including diallyl sulfides can inhibit the induction of cancer in experimental animals. Effects on both tumor initiation and promotion have been documented. Some but not all epidemiological studies have also suggested that consumption of garlic can decrease cancer incidence."

Allium vegetable consumption, garlic supplement intake, and female **breast carcinoma** *incidence.* Dorant E, van den Brandt PA, Goldbohm RA. Breast Cancer Res Treat. 1995;33(2):163-70. **Key Finding:** "We found no association between the consumption of onions or leeks, or garlic supplement use, and the incidence of female breast carcinoma."

Chemo protective effects of capsaicin and diallyl sulfide against **mutagenesis** *or* **tumori-genesis** *by vinyl carbamate and N-nitrosodimethylamine.* Surh YJ, Lee RC, Park KK, Mayne ST, Liem A, Miller JA. Carcinogenesis. 1995 Oct;16(10):2467-71. **Key Finding:** "The results of this study suggest that capsaicin, a major ingredient of hot chili peppers, and diallyl sulfide from garlic suppress VC and NDMA-induced mutagenesis or tumorigenesis in part through inhibition of the cytochrome P-450 IIE1 isoform responsible for activation of these carcinogens."

Thioallyl compounds: potent inhibitors of cell proliferation. Lee ES, Steiner M, Lin R. Biochim Biophys Acta. 1994 Mar 10;1221(1):73-7. **Key Finding:** "We conclude that thioallyl compounds, natural constituents of garlic and known to inhibit **malignant cells,** can also reduce the proliferation of normal cells."

Highlights of the **cancer** *chemoprevention studies in China.* Han J. Prev Med. 1993 Sep;22(5):712-22. **Key Finding:** "Garlic has been used for thousands of years in Chinese cooking and folk medicine. Epidemiological studies show that the dietary intake of garlic is inversely related to gastric cancer incidence in Shandong Province. Field studies among a population at high risk for esophageal cancer in Linxian County, Henan Province, revealed that N-4-(ethoxycarbophenyl) retinamide decreased the incidence of this cancer."

Initiation and post-initiation chemo preventive effects of diallyl sulfide in **esophageal carcinogenesis***.* Wargovich MJ, Imada O, Stephens LC. Cancer Lett. 1992 May 30;64(1):39-42. **Key Finding:** "In this study, diallyl sulfide was examined for its chemo preventive effects in both the initiation and post-initiation phases of nitrosomethylbenzylamine-induced esophageal carcinogenesis in the Sprague-Dawley rat. Although highly inhibitory during initiation, DAS is ineffective when given after the carcinogen."

Protective effect of diallyl sulfide, a natural extract of garlic, on MNNG-induced damage of rat glandular stomach mucosa. Hu PJ. Zhonghua Zhong Liu Za Zhi (Chinese). 1990 Nov;12(6):429-31. **Key Finding:** "The results showed that nuclear aberration and ornithine decarboxylase activity were positively correlated to MNNG dose give. Oral or parenteral pretreatment with diallyl sulfide significantly and dose-dependently inhibited MNNG-induced NA and ODC. These data suggest that diallyl sulfide has the potential to inhibit **gastric cancer.**"

Inhibition of DMBA-induced mouse **skin tumorigenesis** *by garlic oil and inhibition of two tumor-promotion stages by garlic and onion oils.* Perchellet JP, Perchellet EM, Belman S. Nutr Cancer. 1990;14(3-4):183-93. **Key Finding:** "Onion and garlic oils inhibited the TPA-stimulated DNA synthesis when given as single doses of 5 mg one hour before TPA. The inhibition by garlic oil was most effective when given one hour before TPA but was evident when given from two hours before to two hours after TPA. These results indicate that onion and garlic oils inhibit all stages of mouse skin tumorigenesis."

Antitumor*-promoting activity of garlic extracts.* Nishino H, Iwashima A, Itakura Y, Matsuura H, Fuwa T. Oncology. 1989;46(4):277-80. **Key Finding:** "Garlic extract was proved to inhibit one of the earliest phenomena caused by 12-O-tetra-decanoyl-phorbol-13-acetate (TPA), a tumor promoter, in vitro; i.e., the enhancement of phospholipid metabolism. And also the first stage of tumor promotion in two-stage mouse skin carcinogenesis in vivo was suppressed by the treatment with garlic extract. Thus, garlic extract seems to be effective to inhibit initial events caused by TPA type tumor promoters in vitro and in vivo."

Inhibition of GSH-dependent PGH2 isomerase in **mammary adenocarcinoma** *cells by allicin.* Shalinsky DR, McNamara DB, Agrawal KC. Prostaglandins. 1989 Jan;37(1):135-48. **Key Finding:** "We studied the effect of allicin (from garlic) on PGE2 biosynthesis in a murine mammary adenocarcinoma cell line (No 4526). Allicin, over the range of 10-1000 microM, inhibited the formation of PGE2 in cells exposed to 2.0 microM 14C-AA for 20 min and in sonicated cells incubated with 20.0 microM 14C-PGH2 for 2 min."

Effects of organosulfur compounds from garlic and onions on benzo[a]pyrene-induced neoplasia and glutathione S-transferase activity in the mouse. Sparnins VL, Barany G, Wattenberg LW. Carcinogenesis. 1988 Jan;9(1):131-4. **Key Finding:** "All four allylic compounds (allyl methyl trisulfide, allyl methyl disulfide, diallyl trisulfide, and diallyl sulfide) from garlic and onions increased glutathione S-transferase activity in the forestomach, but varied in their capacity to induce GST in lung, liver and small bowel. In evaluating relationships between diet and **cancer**, it would be useful to consider the possible role of garlic and onion organosulfur compounds as protective agents."

*Onion and garlic oils inhibit **tumor** promotion.* Belman S. Carcinogenesis. 1983 Aug;4(8):1063-5. **Key Finding:** "The tumor yield and incidence of phorbol-myristate-acetate promotion were inhibited in a dose-dependent manner over the range of 10-10,000 micrograms onion oil, applied three times per week. Garlic oil was also inhibitor, but was less effective."

Candidiasis

*In vitro investigation of antifungal activity of allicin alone and in combination with azoles against **Candida species**.* Khodavandi A, Alizadeh F, Aala F, Et al. Mycopathologia. 2010 Apr;169(4):287-95. **Key Finding**: "Our results demonstrated the existing synergistic effect between allicin and azoles antifungals in some of the Candida spp. Such as C. albicans, C. glabrata and C. tropicalis, but synergy was not demonstrated in the majority of Candida spp. tested."

*Efficacy of niosomal formulation of diallyl sulfide against experimental **candidiasis** in Swiss albino mice.* Alam M, Dwivedi V, Khan AA, Mohammad O. Nanomed. 2009 Oct;4(7):713-24. **Key Finding:** "Incorporation of diallyl sulfide, a garlic oil component, in noisome enhances its antifungal efficacy."

*Potential of liposomal diallyl sulphide in treatment of experimental murine **candidiasis**.* Maroof A, Farazuddin M, Owais M. Biosci Rep. 2009 Jul 31. (Epub ahead of print). **Key Finding:** "The results of this study established that antifungal activity of diallyl sulphide, a poorly soluble compound, can be enhanced by incorporation into liposomes. Further studies and optimizations are needed to build upon the promising findings of the present study to enable development of an effective plant-derived antifungal formulation that can provide an alternative to the presently available antifungal drugs."

Synergistic Antiyeast Activity of Garlic Oil and Allyl Alcohol Derived from Alliin in Garlic. Chung I, Kwon SH, Shim ST, Kyung KH. Journal of Food Science. Vol. 72, Issue 9, pages M437-M440. Published online: 25 Oct 2007. **Key Finding:** "Combinations of AA and GO at 1 and 9 ppm, 5 and 5 ppm, and 6 and 3 ppm. Respectively, inhibited *C. utilis* **(Candida)** completely. The sum of the fractional inhibitory concentrations (FICs) in the 2-component (GO and AA) combination was as low as 0.37 for *C. utilis*, indicating strong synergism."

Cardiovascular disease

The effects of time-released garlic powder tablets on multifunctional cardiovascular risk in patients with coronary artery disease. Sobenin IA, Pryanishnikov W, Kunnova LM, Et al. Lipids Health Dis. 2010 Oct 19;9:119. **Key Finding**: "Allicin from garlic is safe with respect of adverse effects and allows even perpetual administration that may be crucial for the secondary prevention of atherosclerotic diseases in **coronary heart disease** patients."

Garlic (Allium sativum L.) and cardiovascular diseases. Ginter E, Simko V. Bratisl Lek Listy. 2010:111(8):452-6. **Key Finding**: "There are data on potential ability of garlic to inhibit the rate of progression of coronary calcification. Garlic as a dietary component appears to hold promise that it could reduce the risk of **cardiovascular disease**."

*Freshly crushed garlic is a superior **cardio protective** agent than processed garlic.* Mukherjee S, Lekli I, Goswami S, Das DK. J Agric Food Chem. 2009 Aug 12;57(15):7137-44. **Key Finding:** "The results thus show that although both freshly crushed garlic and processed garlic provide cardio protection, the former has additional cardio protective properties presumably due to the present of H2S. Freshly crushed garlic, but not the processed garlic, showed enhanced redox signaling as evident by increased level of p65 subunit of NFkappaB, Nrf2, and enhanced GLUT 4, PPARalpha, and PPARdelta."

Cardio protective *roles of aged garlic extract, grape seed proanthocyanidin, and hazelnut on doxorubicin-induced cardio toxicity.* Demirkaya E, Avci A, Kesik V, Karsliouglu Y, Oztas E, Kismet E, Gokcay E, Durak I, Koseoglu V. Can J Physiol Pharmacol. 2009 Aug;87(8):633-40. **Key Finding:** "The positive effects of natural antioxidant foods on the prevention of DXR-induced cardiac injury could not be clearly shown on the basis of antioxidant enzymes. However, the electron microscope changes clearly demonstrated the protective effects of aged garlic extract and grape seed proanthocyanidin. The supplementation of these antioxidant foods over longer periods may show more definitive results. Human studies with different doses are needed to evaluate the effects of these foods on the human heart."

Hydrogen sulfide mediates the vasoactivity of garlic. Benavides GA, Squadrito GL, Mills RW, Patel HD, Isbell TS, Patel RP, Darley-Usmar VM, Doeiler JE, Kraus DW. Proc Natl Acad Sci. 2007 Nov 13;104(46):17977-82. **Key Finding:** Garlic boosts the human body's own production of a compound which relaxes blood vessels, increases blood flow, and prevents blood clots and oxidative damage. When allicin and other compounds in garlic are metabolized, a chemical messenger, hydrogen sulphide, is produced which is responsible for the cellular signaling that is responsible for the **cardiovascular** benefits.

*Garlic reduces **dementia** and **heart-disease** risk.* Borek C. J Nutr. 2006 Mar;136(3 Suppl):810S-812S. **Key Finding:** "Although additional observations are warranted in humans, compelling evidence supports the beneficial health effects attributed to aged garlic extract in helping prevent **cardiovascular and cerebrovascular diseases** and lowering the risk of dementia and **Alzheimer's disease**."

Aged garlic extract maintains cardiovascular homeostasis in mice and rats. Morihara N, Sumioka I, Ide N, Moriguchi T, Uda N, Kyo E. J Nutr. 2006 Mar;136(3 Suppl):777S-781S. **Key Finding:** "Our data strongly suggest that aged garlic extract could be useful in preventing **cardiovascular diseases** associated with oxidative stress or dysfunctions of nitric oxide production."

*Garlic and **cardiovascular disease**: a critical review.* Rahman K, Lowe GM. J Nutr. 2006 Mar;136(3 Suppl):736S-740S. **Key Finding:** "This review analyzes in vitro and in vivo studies published since 1993 and concludes that although garlic appears to hold promise in reducing parameters associated with cardiovascular disease, more in-depth and appropriate studies are required."

*Homocysteine-lowering action is another potential **cardiovascular** protective factor of aged garlic extract.* Yeh YY, Yeh SM. J Nutr. 2006 Mar;136(3 Suppl):745S-749S. **Key Finding:** "The hypohomocysteinemic effect of aged garlic extract most likely stems from impaired remethylation of homocysteine to methionine and enhanced transsulfuration of homocysteine to cystathionine. More importantly, in addition to its cholesterol-lowering potential, blood pressure-lowering effect, and antioxidant property, a hypohomocysteinemic action may be another important cardiovascular protective factor of aged garlic extract."

Aged garlic extracts retards progression of coronary artery calcification. Budoff M. J Nutr. 2006 Mar;136(3 Suppl):741S-744S. **Key Finding:** "The role garlic might play in treating atherosclerotic **cardiovascular disease** has been postulated for many years, but until recently no studies on garlic's ability to inhibit the atherosclerotic process have been reported. A pilot study evaluating coronary artery calcification and the effect of garlic therapy in a group of patients who were also on statin therapy suggested incremental benefits."

Vegetables, fruits and phytoestrogens in the prevention of diseases. Heber D. J Postgrad Med. 2004 Apr-Jun;50(2):145-9. **Key Finding:** "Consumers are advised to ingest one serving of each of the seven color groups daily. For instance, red foods contain lycopene which may be involved in maintaining **prostate** health and which has been linked to a decreased risk of **cardiovascular disease**. Green foods, including broccoli, Brussels sprouts and kale, have been associated with a decreased risk of cancer. White-green foods such as garlic may inhibit **cancer** cell growth. Grouping plants foods by color provides simplification, but it is also important as a method to help consumers make wise food choices and promote health."

Cardiovascular *benefits of garlic.* Brace LD. J Cardiovasc Nurs. 2002 Jul;16(4):33-49. **Key Finding:** "The vast majority of recent randomized, placebo-controlled studies do not support a role for garlic in lowering blood lipids. There also is insufficient evidence to support a role in reducing blood pressure. While there have been indications of antiatherosclerotic effects associated with garlic consumption, there are insufficient data in humans. Investigation of antithrombotic effects of garlic consumption appears to hold promise."

Antioxidant health effects of aged garlic extract. Borek C. J Nutr. 2001 Mar;131(3s):1010S-5S. **Key Finding:** "Although additional observations are warranted in humans, compelling evidence supports the beneficial health effects attributed to aged garlic extract, i.e., reducing the risk of **cardiovascular disease, stroke, cancer and aging**, including the oxidant-mediated brain cell damage that is implicated in **Alzheimer's disease**."

Dietary Supplementation with Aged Garlic Extract Inhibits ADP-Induced Platelet Aggregation in Humans. Rahman K, Billington D. J Nutr. 2000;130:2662-2665. **Key Finding:** "We conclude that aged garlic extract, when taken as a dietary supplement by normolipidemic subjects, may be beneficial in protecting against **cardiovascular disease** as a result of inhibiting platelet aggregation."

*Garlic: its **cardio-protective** properties.* Neil A, Silagy C. Curr Opin Lipidol. 1994 Feb;5(1):6-10. **Key Finding:** "Evidence that garlic inhibits platelet aggregation, increases fibrinolysis, reduces blood pressure, enhances anti-oxidant activity, and reduces serum lipids suggests that it may have cardio-protective proper-ties. Quantitative pooling of data in meta-analyses of the primary trials strongly suggests that garlic is an effective **lipid-lowering** agent."

Cataracts

Prevention of selenite-induced **cataractogenesis** *in wistar albino rats by aqueous extract of garlic.* Javadzadeh A, Ghorbanjhaghjo A, Arami S, Rashtchizadeh N, Mesgari M, Rafeey M, Omidi Y. J Ocul Pharmacol Ther. 2009 Oct;25(5):395-400. **Key Finding:** "Intra peritoneal injection of the garlic in rat model appeared to effec-tively prevent Se-induced cataract, thus such herbal remedy may be considered for treatment of cataract."

Cerebrovascular disease

Garlic reduces **dementia** *and* **heart-disease** *risk.* Borek C. J Nutr. 2006 Mar;136(3 Suppl):810S-812S. **Key Finding:** "Although additional observations are warranted in humans, compelling evidence supports the beneficial health effects attributed to aged garlic extract in helping prevent **cardiovascular and cerebrovascular diseases** and lowering the risk of dementia and **Alzheimer's disease**."

Cholesterol

Effect of dietary **garlic** *and* **onion** *on biliary proteins and lipid peroxidation which influ-ence of cholesterol nucleation in bile.* Vidyashankar S, Sambaiah K, Srinivasan K. Steroids. 2010 Mar;75(3):272-81. **Key Finding**: "These data suggest that apart from the beneficial modulation of biliary cholesterol saturation index, Allium spices also influence cholesterol nucleating and antinucleating protein factors that contribute to their anti-lithogenic potential" preventing **cholesterol gall-stone** formation in the gallbladder.

Regression of pre-established **cholesterol gallstones** *by dietary* **garlic and onion** *in experimental mice.* Vidyashankar S, Sambaiah K, Srinivasan K. Metabolism. 2010 Oct;59(10):1402-12. **Key Finding:** "These results indicate that feeding garlic and onion effectively accelerates the regression of preformed cholesterol gall-stones by promoting cholesterol desaturation in bile."

The impact of garlic on lipid parameters: a systematic review and meta-analysis. Reinhart KM, Talati R, White CM, Coleman CI. Nutr Res Rev. 2009 Jun;22(1):39-48.

Key Finding: "Upon meta-analysis garlic was found to significantly reduce total **cholesterol,** but exhibited no significant effect on LDL or HDL."

Garlic supplementation and serum cholesterol: a meta-analysis. Khoo YS, Aziz Z. J Clin Pharm Ther. 2009 Apr;34(2):133-45. **Key Finding:** "Thirteen trials including 1056 subjects were eligible for the meta-analysis. Overall, administration of garlic did not show any significant difference in effects on all outcome measure examined when compared with placebo. Garlic therapy did not produce any statistically significant reduction in serum total **cholesterol** level."

*Dietary garlic and onion reduce the incidence of atherogenic diet-induced **cholesterol gall- stones** in experimental mice.* Vidyashankar S, Sambaiah K, Srinivasan K. Br J Nutr. 2009 Jun;101(11):1621-9. **Key Finding**: "Dietary garlic and onion reduce the cholesterol gallstones incidence by 15-39%. Dietary garlic and onion mark- edly reduced biliary cholesterol. Serum and liver cholesterol were decreased by feeding garlic or onion. Dietary Allium spices exerted antilithogenic influence by decreasing the cholesterol hyper-secretion into bile and increasing the bile acid output thus decreasing the formation of lithogenic bile in experimental mice."

*Effect of raw garlic vs. commercial garlic supplements on plasma lipid concentrations in adults with moderate **hypercholesterolemia**: a randomized clinical trial.* Gardner CD, Lawson LD, Block E, Chatteriee LM, Kiazand A, Balise RR, Kraemer HC. Arch Intern Med. 2007 Feb 26;167(4):346-53. **Key Finding:** "None of the forms of garlic used in this study, including raw garlic, when given at an approximate dose of a 4-g clove per day, 6 d/wk. for 6 months, had statistically or clinically significant effects on LDL-C or other plasma lipid concentrations in adults with moderate hypercholesterolemia."

*Comparison between swallowing and chewing of garlic on levels of **serum lipids**, cyclospo- rine, creatinine and lipid peroxidation in **renal transplant** recipients.* Jabbari A, Argani H, Ghorbanihaghjo A, Mahdavi R. Lipids Health Dis. 2005 May 19;4:11. **Key Finding:** "We conclude that undamaged garlic (swallowed) has no lowering effect on lipid level of serum. But crushed garlic (chewed) reduces cholesterol, triglyceride, MDA and blood pressure."

*Effects of garlic extract consumption on blood lipid and oxidant/antioxidant parameters in human with high blood **cholesterol**.* Durak I, Kavutcu M, Aytac B, Avci A, Ozbek H, Ozturk HS. J Nutr Biochem. 2004 Jun;15(6):373-7. **Key Finding:** "We conclude that garlic extract supplementation improves blood lipid profile, strengthens blood antioxidant potential, and causes significant reductions in systolic and diastolic **blood pressure**s. It also leads to a decrease in the level of oxidation product in the blood samples, which demonstrates reduced oxidation in the body."

Cholesterol-*lowering effect of organosulphur compounds from garlic: a possible mechanism of action.* Mathew BC, Prasad NV, Prabodh R. Kathmandu Univ Med J. 2004 Apr-Jun;2(2):100-2. **Key Finding:** "The antiatherogenic effects of these organosulphur compounds can be attributed to such reactions that inhibit HMG-CoA reductase and other lipgenic enzymes. The anticarcinogenic effects of these compounds may also be due to inhibitory reactions on enzymes that activate carcinogens."

Garlic attenuates **hypercholesterolemic** *risk factors in olive oil fed rats and high cholesterol fed rats.* Chetty KN, Calahan L, Harris KC, Dorsey W, Hill D, Chetty S, Jain SK. Pathophysiology. 2003 May;9(3):127-132. **Key Finding:** "The results suggest that the dietary olive oil regulated the levels of serum in cholesterol loaded rats. Garlic attenuated serum cholesterol in olive oil fed rats and decreased serum risk factors, both total cholesterol and LDL-C ration and LDL-Ch/HDL-Ch ratio."

Cholesterol-*Lowering Effect of Garlic Extracts and Organosulfur Compounds: Human and Animal Studies.* Yu-Yan Y, Lijuan L. J Nutr. 2001;131:989S-993S. **Key Finding:** "The results of our studies indicate that the cholesterol-lowering effects of garlic extract stem in part from inhibition of hepatic cholesterol synthesis by water-soluble sulfur compounds."

Garlic for treating **hypercholesterolemia**. *A meta-analysis of randomized clinical trials.* Stevinson C, Pittler MH, Ernst E. Ann Intern Med. 2000 Sep 19;133(6):420-9. **Key Finding:** "The available data suggest that garlic is superior to placebo in reducing total cholesterol levels. However, the size of the effect is modest."

Garlic powder and plasma lipids and lipoproteins: a multicenter, randomized, placebo-controlled trial. Isaacsohn JL, Moser M, Stein EA, Dudley K, Davey JA, Liskov E, Black HR. Arch Intern Med. 1998 Jun 8;158(11):1189-94. **Key Finding:** "Garlic powder (900 mg/d) treatment for 12 weeks was ineffective in lowering **cholesterol** levels in patients with hypercholesterolemia."

Garlic extract therapy in children with **hypercholesterolemia**. McCrindle BW, Helden E, Conner WT. Arch Pediatr Adolesc Med. 1998 Nov;152(11):1089-94. **Key Finding:** "Garlic extract therapy has no significant effect on cardiovascular risk factors in pediatric patients with familial hyperlipidemia."

Effect of a garlic oil preparation on serum lipoproteins and cholesterol metabolism: a random-ized controlled trial. Berthold HK, Sudhop T, von Bergmann K. JAMA. 1998 Jun 17;279(23):1900-2. **Key Finding:** "The commercial garlic oil preparation inves-tigated had no influence on serum lipoproteins, cholesterol absorption, or choles-terol synthesis. Garlic therapy for treatment of **hypercholesterolemia** cannot be recommended on the basis of this study."

*A double-blind crossover study in moderately **hypercholesterolemic** men that compared the effect of aged garlic extract and placebo administration on blood lipids.* Steiner M, Khan AH, Holbert D, Lin RI. Am J Clin Nutr. 1996;64:866-70. **Key Finding:** "We conclude that dietary supplementation with aged garlic extract has beneficial effects on the lipid profile and blood pressure of moderately hypercholesterol-emic subjects."

*Garlic powder in the treatment of moderate **hyperlipidemia**: a controlled trial and meta-analysis.* Neil HA, Silagy CA, Lancaster T, Hodgeman J, Vos K, Moore JW, Jones L, Cahill J, Fowler GH. J R Coll Physicians Lond. 1996 Jul-Aug;30(4):329-34. **Key Finding:** "In this trial, garlic was less effective in reducing total **cholesterol** than suggested by previous meta-analyses. Possible explanations are publication bias, overestimation of treatment effects in trials with inadequate concealment of treat-ment allocation, or type 2 errors. We conclude that meta-analyses should be inter-preted critically and with particular caution if the constituent trials are small."

*Alteration of lipid profile in **hyperlipidemic** rabbits by allicin, an active constituent of garlic.* Eilat S, Oestraicher Y, Rabinkov A, Ohad D, Mirelman D, Battler A, Eldar M, Vered Z. Coron Artery Dis. 1995 Dec;6(12):985-90. **Key Finding:** "Our results indicate that allicin has a beneficial effect on the serum lipid profile in hyperlipidemic rabbits, and should be further tested clinically."

Garlic (Allium sativum)—a potent medicinal plant. Resch KL, Ernst E. Fortschr Med (German). 1995 Jul 20;113(20-21):311-5. **Key Finding:** "A good deal of evidence suggests beneficial effects of the regular dietary intake of garlic, a traditional folk remedy, on mild **hypertension** and **hyperlipidemia**. Garlic seems to have **anti-microbial** and immunostimulating properties, enhance fibrinolytic activity, and exert favorable effects on **platelet aggregation** and adhesion."

Garlic as a lipid lowering agent—a meta-analysis. Silagy C, Neil A. J R Coll Physicians Lond. 1994 Jan-Feb;28(1):39-45. **Key Finding:** "Sixteen trials, with data from 952 subjects, were included in the analysis. The pooled mean difference in the absolute change (from baseline to final measurements in mmol/l) of total serum

cholesterol, triglycerides, and high-density lipoprotein (HDL)-cholesterol was compared between subjects treated with garlic therapy against those receiving placebo. The mean difference in reduction of total cholesterol was 12% with garlic therapy. The reduction was evident after one month of therapy and persisted for at least six months. Dried garlic powder preparations also significantly lowered serum triglycerides."

*Garlic: its **cardio-protective** properties.* Neil A, Silagy C. Curr Opin Lipidol. 1994 Feb;5(1):6-10. **Key Finding:** "Evidence that garlic inhibits platelet aggregation, increases fibrinolysis, reduces blood pressure, enhances anti-oxidant activity, and reduces serum lipids suggests that it may have cardio-protective properties. Quantitative pooling of data in meta-analyses of the primary trials strongly suggests that garlic is an effective **lipid-lowering** agent."

*Garlic reduces plasma lipids by inhibiting hepatic **cholesterol** and triacylglycerol synthesis.* Yeh YY, Yeh SM. Lipids. 1994 Mar;29(3):189-93. **Key Finding:** "When compared with the control group, cells treated with a high concentration of garlic extracts and water-extractable fractions from fresh garlic showed decreased rates of acetate incorporation into cholesterol (by 37-64%) and into fatty acids (by 28-64%). The results suggest that the hypocholesterolemic effect of garlic stems, in part, from decreased hepatic cholesterogenesis, whereas the triacylglycerol-lowering effect appears to be due to inhibition of fatty acid synthesis."

*Can garlic reduce levels of **serum lipids**? A controlled clinical study.* Jain AK, Vargas R, Gotzkowsky S, McMahon FG. Am J Med. 1993 Jun;94(6):632-5. **Key Finding:** "Forty-two healthy adults with a serum total cholesterol level of greater than or equal to 220 mg/dL received, in a randomized, double-blind fashion, either 300 mg three times a day of standardized garlic powder in tablet form, or placebo. Treatment with standardized garlic 900 mg/d produced a significantly greater reduction in serum total cholesterol and LDL-C than placebo. The garlic formulation was well tolerated without any odor problems."

*Effect of garlic on total serum **cholesterol**. A meta-analysis.* Warshafsky S, Kamer RS, Sivak SL. Ann Intern Med. 1993 Oct 1;119(7 Pt 1):599-605. **Key Finding:** "The best available evidence suggests that garlic, in an amount approximating one half to one clove per day, decreased total serum cholesterol levels by about 9% in the groups of patients studied."

*Inhibition of **cholesterol** synthesis in vitro by extracts and isolated compounds prepared from garlic and wild garlic.* Sendl A, Schliack M, Loser R, Stanislaus F, Wagner

H. Atherosclerosis. 1992 May;94(1):79-85. **Key Finding:** "The results demonstrate that garlic and wild garlic may reduce serum cholesterol levels primarily by inhibiting cholesterol synthesis if taken in sufficient amount and that this effect arises from a mixture of multiple compounds from the sulfur-containing class of thiosulfinates, ajoene and dithiines. Wild garlic extracts showed nearly identical efficiency to garlic extracts."

*Effect of ingestion of raw garlic on serum **cholesterol** level, clotting time and fibrinolytic activity in normal subjects.* Gadkari JV, Joshi VD. J Postgrad Med. 1991 Jul;37(3):128-31. **Key Finding**: "The effect of raw garlic was studied in 50 medical students. The subjects of the experimental group were given 10 gm of raw garlic after breakfast for two months. Fasting blood samples of all the subjects were investigated after two months. In the control group, there was no significant change in any of the parameters. In the experimental group, there was a significant decrease in serum cholesterol and an increase in clotting time and fibrinolytic activity. Hence, garlic may be a useful agent in prevent of thromboembolic phenomenon."

*Treatment of **hyperlipidemia** with garlic-powder tablets. Evidence from the German Association of general Practitioners' multicentric placebo-controlled double-blind study.* Mader FH. Arzneimittelforschung. 1990 Oct;40(10):1111-6. **Key Finding:** "Standardized garlic tablets were shown to be effective in the treatment of hyperlipidemia by lowering total cholesterol values by an average of 12% and triglyceride values by an average of 17%."

*Effect of dried garlic on blood coagulation, **fibrinolysis**, **and platelet aggregation** and serum **cholesterol** levels in patients with hyperlipoproteinemia.* Harenberg J, Giese C, Zimmermann R. Atherosclerosis. 1988 Dec;74(3):247-9. **Key Finding:** "The effects of dried garlic on blood coagulation, fibrinolysis, platelet aggregation, serum cholesterol levels, and blood pressure were studied in 20 patients with hyperlipoproteinemia over a period of four weeks. Fibrinogen and fibronopeptide A significantly decreased by 10%. Streptokinase activated plasminogen and fibrinopeptide B beta 15-42 significantly increased by about 10%. Serum cholesterol levels significantly decreased by 10%. Systolic and diastolic blood pressure decreased. ADP and collagen induced platelet aggregation were not influenced."

***Hypolipidemic** effect of garlic and thyroid function.* Chaudhuri BN, Mukherjee SK, Mongia SS, Chakravarty SK. Biomed Biocheim Acta. 1984;43(7):1045-7. **Key Finding:** "Male Sprague-Dawley rats were maintained on cholesterol and garlic oil for 12 weeks. Cholesterol induced hyperlipidemia was controlled by garlic feeding. Garlic treatment did not alter the concentrations of circulating thyroid hormones and thyroidal uptake of radioiodine. The results indicate that the hypolipidemic effect of garlic is probably not mediated through the thyroid."

*Effect of garlic oil in experimental **cholesterol atherosclerosis**.* Jain RC, Konar DB. Atherosclerosis. 1978 Feb;29(2):125-9. **Key Finding:** "Addition of cholesterol in the diet of male albino rabbits produced hypercholesterolemia, increased tissue cholesterol, and athermanous changes in the aorta. Supplementation of garlic oil along with cholesterol significantly inhibited the hypercholesterolemia, decreased tissue cholesterol and minimized the athermanous changes in the aorta. These results show that the active constituents in garlic responsible for its anti-atherogenic action are present in the oily fraction of garlic."

*Effects of essential oils of garlic and onion on alimentary **hyperlipemia**.* Bordia A, Bansal HC, Arora SK, Singh SV. Atherosclerosis. 1975 Jan-Feb;21(1):15-9. **Key Finding:** "The effect of garlic and onion on alimentary hyperlipemia, induced by feeding 100 g butter, has been studied in 10 healthy subjects. The freshly extracted juice of 50 g of garlic or onion, as well as an equivalent amount of their ether-extracted essential oils, was administered randomly on four different days during a one-week period. Garlic and onion have a significant protective action against fat-induced increases in serum cholesterol and plasma fibrinogen and decreases in coagulation time and fibrinolytic activity."

Colitis

*L-arginine augments the antioxidant effect of garlic against acetic acid-induced ulcerative **colitis** in rats.* Harisa GE, Abo-Salem OM, El-Sayed SM, El-Halawany N. Pak J Pharm Sci. 2009 Oct;22(4):373-80. **Key Finding:** "L-arginine can augment the protective effect of garlic against ulcerative colitis; an effect that might be mainly attributed to its NO precursor donating property resulting in enhancement of garlic antioxidant effects."

Common Cold

*Garlic for the **common cold**.* Lissiman E, Bhasale AL, Cohen M. Cochrane Database Syst Rev. 2009 Jul 8;(3):CD006206. **Key Finding:** "There is insufficient clinical trial evidence regarding the effects of garlic in preventing or treating the common cold. A single trial suggested that garlic may prevent occurrences of the common cold, but more studies are needed to validate this finding."

*Preventing the **common cold** with a garlic supplement: a double-blind, placebo-controlled survey.* Josling P. Adv Ther. 2001 Jul-Aug;18(4):189-93. **Key Finding:** "One hundred forty-six volunteers were randomized to receive a placebo or an allicin-containing garlic supplement, one capsule daily, over a 12-week period. The active treatment group had significantly fewer colds than the placebo group. The placebo group recorded significantly more days challenged virally (366 vs 111) and a significantly longer duration of symptoms (5.0 vs 1.5 days). An allicin-containing supplement can prevent attack by the common cold virus."

Crohn's disease

Suppression of the nuclear factor-kappaB activation pathway by spice-derived phytochemicals: reasoning for seasoning. Aggarwal BB, Shishodia S. Ann N Y Acad Sci. 2004 Dec;1030:434-41. **Key Finding:** "The activation of nuclear transcription factor kappaB has now been linked with a variety of **inflammatory disease, including cancer, atherosclerosis, myocardial infarction, diabetes, allergy, asthma, arthritis, Crohn's disease, multiple sclerosis, Alzheimer's disease, osteoporosis, psoriasis, septic shock, and AIDS**. Extensive research in the last few years has shown that the pathway that activates this transcription factor can be interrupted by phytochemicals derived from spices such as turmeric (curcumin), red pepper (capsaicin), cloves (eugenol), ginger (gingerol), cumin, anise, and fennel (anethol), basil and rosemary (ursolic acid), garlic (diallyl sulfide, S-allylmercaptocysteine, ajoene), and pomegranate (ellagic acid). For the first time, therefore, research provides 'reasoning for seasoning.'"

Dementia

*Garlic reduces **dementia** and **heart-disease** risk.* Borek C. J Nutr. 2006 Mar;136(3 Suppl):810S-812S. **Key Finding:** "Although additional observations are warranted in humans, compelling evidence supports the beneficial health effects attributed to aged garlic extract in helping prevent **cardiovascular and cerebrovascular diseases** and lowering the risk of dementia and **Alzheimer's disease**."

Diabetes

Cardiac contractile dysfunction and apoptosis in stretozotocin-induced diabetic rats are ameliorated by garlic oil supplementation. Ou HC, Tzang BS, Chang MH, Et al. J Agric Food Chem. 2010 Oct 13;58(19):10347-55. **Key Finding**: "Garlic oil possesses significant potential for protecting hearts from **diabetes**-induced cardiomyopathy."

*The **antidiabetic** effect of onion and garlic in experimental diabetic rats: meta-analysis.* Kook S, Kim GH, Choi K. J Med Food. 2009 Jun;12(3):552-60. **Key Finding:** "In the meta-analysis, the antidiabetic effects of onion extract and single components were significant for glucose concentration and body weight, but the effects of garlic extract were not significant. The results of the meta-analysis suggested that the single component intake and onion extract may be effective for lowering plasma glucose concentrations and body weight."

*Antioxidant effect of garlic and aged black garlic in animal model of **type 2 diabetes** mellitus.* Lee YM, Gweon OC, Seo YJ, Im J, Kang MJ, Kim MJ, Kim JI. Nutr Res Pract. 2009 Summer;3(2):156-61. **Key Finding:** "These results show that aged black garlic exerts stronger antioxidant activity than garlic in vitro and in vivo, suggesting that garlic and aged black garlic, to a greater extent, could be useful in preventing diabetic complications."

*Effect of fenugreek, onion and garlic on blood glucose and histopathology of pancreas of alloxan-induced **diabetic** rats.* Jelodar GA, Maleki M, Motadayen MH, Sirus S. Indian J Med Sci. 2005 Feb;59(2):64-9. **Key Finding**: "The results of this study indicate that only garlic was able to reduce blood glucose significantly compared with the control group."

Suppression of the nuclear factor-kappaB activation pathway by spice-derived phytochemicals: reasoning for seasoning. Aggarwal BB, Shishodia S. Ann N Y Acad Sci. 2004 Dec;1030:434-41. **Key Finding:** "The activation of nuclear transcription factor kappaB has now been linked with a variety of **inflammatory disease, including cancer, atherosclerosis, myocardial infarction, diabetes, allergy, asthma, arthritis, Crohn's disease, multiple sclerosis, Alzheimer's disease, osteoporosis, psoriasis, septic shock, and AIDS**. Extensive research in the last few years has shown that the pathway that activates this transcription factor can be interrupted by phytochemicals derived from spices such as turmeric (curcumin), red pepper (capsaicin), cloves (eugenol), ginger (gingerol), cumin, anise, and fennel (anethol), basil and rosemary (ursolic acid), garlic (diallyl sulfide, S-allylmercaptocysteine, ajoene), and pomegranate (ellagic acid). For the first time, therefore, research provides 'reasoning for seasoning.'"

*Reduced nociceptive responses in mice with alloxan induced **hyperglycemia** after garlic treatment.* Kumar GR, Reddy KP. Indian J Exp Biol. 1999 Jul;37(7):662-6. **Key Finding:** "The results suggest therapeutic potential of ethanol extract of garlic for anti-hyperglycemic and anti-nociceptive effects in **diabetes**."

Heart failure (myocardial infarction)

Suppression of the nuclear factor-kappaB activation pathway by spice-derived phytochemicals: reasoning for seasoning. Aggarwal BB, Shishodia S. Ann N Y Acad Sci. 2004 Dec;1030:434-41. **Key Finding:** "The activation of nuclear transcription factor kappaB has now been linked with a variety of **inflammatory disease, including cancer, atherosclerosis, myocardial infarction, diabetes, allergy, asthma, arthritis, Crohn's disease, multiple sclerosis, Alzheimer's disease, osteoporosis, psoriasis, septic shock, and AIDS**. Extensive research in the last few years has shown that the pathway that activates this transcription factor can be interrupted by phytochemicals derived from spices such as turmeric (curcumin), red pepper (capsaicin), cloves (eugenol), ginger (gingerol), cumin, anise, and fennel (anethol), basil and rosemary (ursolic acid), garlic (diallyl sulfide, S-allylmercaptocysteine, ajoene), and pomegranate (ellagic acid). For the first time, therefore, research provides 'reasoning for seasoning.'"

Hyperlipidemia (see cholesterol)

Hypertension

*Aged garlic extract lowers blood pressure in patients with treated but uncontrolled **hypertension**: a randomized controlled trial.* Ride K, Frank OR, Stocks NP. Maturitas. 2010 Oct;67(2):144-59. **Key Finding**: "Our trial suggests that aged garlic extract is superior to placebo in lowering systolic blood pressure similarly to current first line medications in patients with treated but uncontrolled hypertension."

Garlic components inhibit angiotensin II-induced cell-cycle progression and migration: Involvement of cell-cycle inhibitor p27(Kip1) and mitogen-activated protein kinase. Castro C, Lorenzo AG, Gonzalez A, Cruzado M. Mol Nutr Food Res. 2009 Nov 10. (Epub ahead of print). **Key Finding:** "We demonstrated that allyl methyl sulfide (AMS) and diallyl sulphide (DAS) inhibited aortic smooth muscle cell angiotensin II-stimulated cell-cycle progression and migration. Our findings show that AMS and DAS compounds derivate from garlic could be effective antioxidants targeted at the arterial remodeling seen in **hypertension**."

*A systematic review on the influence of trial quality on the effect of garlic on **blood pressure**.* Simons S, Wollersheim H, Thien T. Neth J Med. 2009 Jun;67(6):212-9. **Key Finding:** "The effect of garlic on blood pressure cannot be ascertained.

Previous meta-analyses have been based on trials with inadequate study designs, methodological deficiencies and with too little information about blood pressure measurement. In our view, use of garlic cannot be recommended as antihypertensive advice for hypertensive patients in daily practice."

Effect of garlic on **blood pressure**: *a systematic review and meta-analysis.* Ried K, Frank OR, Stocks NP, Fakler P, Sullivan T. BMC Cardiovasc Disord. 2008 Jun 16;8:13. **Key Finding:** "Eleven of 25 studies included in the systematic review were suitable for meta-analysis. Our meta-analysis suggests that garlic preparations are superior to placebo in reducing blood pressure in individuals with hypertension."

Garlic supplementation prevents oxidative DNA damage in essential **hypertension.** Dhawan V, Jain S. Mol Cell Biochem. 2005 Jul;275(1-2):85-94. **Key Finding:** "These findings point out the beneficial effects of **garlic** supplementation in reducing blood pressure and counteracting oxidative stress, and thereby, offering cardio protection in essential hypertensive."

Effects of garlic extract consumption on blood lipid and oxidant/antioxidant parameters in human with high blood **cholesterol.** Durak I, Kavutcu M, Aytac B, Avci A, Ozbek H, Ozturk HS. J Nutr Biochem. 2004 Jun;15(6):373-7. **Key Finding:** "We conclude that garlic extract supplementation improves blood lipid profile, strengthens blood antioxidant potential, and causes significant reductions in systolic and diastolic **blood pressure**s. It also leads to a decrease in the level of oxidation product in the blood samples, which demonstrates reduced oxidation in the body."

Garlic (Allium sativum)—a potent medicinal plant. Resch KL, Ernst E. Fortschr Med (German). 1995 Jul 20;113(20-21):311-5. **Key Finding:** "A good deal of evidence suggests beneficial effects of the regular dietary intake of garlic, a traditional folk remedy, on mild **hypertension** and **hyperlipidemia**. Garlic seems to have **anti-microbial** and immunostimulating properties, enhance fibrinolytic activity, and exert favorable effects on **platelet aggregation** and adhesion."

A meta-analysis of the effect of garlic on **blood pressure**. Silagy CA, Neil HA. J Hypertens. 1994 Apr;12(4):463-8. **Key Finding:** "The results suggest that this garlic powder preparation may be of some clinical use in subjects with mild hypertension."

Liver damage

Garlic extract prevents CCI(4)-induced liver fibrosis in rats: The role of tissue transfluta-minase. D'Argenio G, Amoruso DC, Massone G, Et al. Dig Liver Dis. 2010 Aug;42(8):571-7. **Key Finding:** "These findings concurrently suggest that trans-glutaminase may play a pivotal role in the pathogenesis of liver fibrosis and may identify garlic cystamine-like molecules as a potential therapeutic strategy in the treatment of **liver injury**."

Protective effects of garlic and silymarin on NDEA-induced rat's hepatoxicity. Shaarawy SM, Tohamy AA, Elgendy SM, Elmageed ZY, Bahnasy A, Mohamed MS, Kandil E, Matrougui K. Int J Biol Sci. 2009 Aug 11;5(6):549-57. **Key Finding:** "These novel findings suggest that silymarin and garlic have a synergistic effect, and could be used as hepatoprotective agents against **hepatotoxicity**."

Multiple sclerosis

Suppression of the nuclear factor-kappaB activation pathway by spice-derived phytochemi-cals: reasoning for seasoning. Aggarwal BB, Shishodia S. Ann N Y Acad Sci. 2004 Dec;1030:434-41. **Key Finding:** "The activation of nuclear transcription factor kappaB has now been linked with a variety of **inflammatory disease, including cancer, atherosclerosis, myocardial infarction, diabetes, allergy, asthma, arthritis, Crohn's disease, multiple sclerosis, Alzheimer's disease, osteoporosis, psoriasis, septic shock, and AIDS**. Extensive research in the last few years has shown that the pathway that acti-vates this transcription factor can be interrupted by phytochemicals derived from spices such as turmeric (curcumin), red pepper (capsaicin), cloves (eugenol), ginger (gingerol), cumin, anise, and fennel (anethol), basil and rosemary (ursolic acid), garlic (diallyl sulfide, S-allylmercaptocysteine, ajoene), and pomegranate (ellagic acid). For the first time, therefore, research provides 'reasoning for seasoning.'"

Neurodegeneration

*Nutraceutical antioxidants as novel **neuroprotective** agents.* Kelsey NA, Wilkins HM, Linseman DA. Molecules. 2010 Nov 3;15(11):7792-814. **Key Finding**: Thiosul-fonate allicin from garlic is an antioxidant that scavenges free radicals and has "potential therapeutic value in neurodegenerative diseases."

Protective effect of S-allyl-L-cysteine, a garlic compound, on amyloid beta-protein-induced cell death in nerve growth factor-differentiated PC12 cells. Ito Y, Kosuge Y, Sakikubo T, Horie K, Ishikawa N, Obokata N, Yokoyama E, Yamashina K, Yamamoto M, Saito H, Arakawa M, Ishige K. Neurosci Res. 2003 May;46(1):119-25. **Key Finding:** "Neuroactive compounds from aged garlic extract, S-allyl-L-cysteine, protected **neuronal cells** against Abeta-induced cell death in a concentration-dependent manner. It also protected them against tunicamycin-induced neuronal death."

*S-allyl-L-cysteine selectively protects cultured rat hippocampal neurons from amyloid beta-protein- and tunicamycin-induced **neuronal death**.* Kosuge Y, Koen Y, Ishige K, Minami K, Urasawa H, Saito H, Ito Y. Neuroscience. 2003;122(4):885-95. **Key Finding:** "These results suggest that S-allyl-L-cysteine found in aged garlic extract could protect against the neuronal cell death that is triggered by ER dysfunction in the hippocampus."

Obesity

1,2-vinyldithiin from garlic inhibits differentiation and inflammation of human preadipocytes. Keophyiphath M, Priem F, Jacquemond-Collet I, Clement K, Lacasa D. J Nutr. 2009 Nov;139(11):2055-60. **Key Finding:** "**Obesity** is a state of chronic low-grade inflammation. Limiting white adipose tissue expansion and therefore reducing inflammation could be effective in preventing the progression of obesity and the development of associated complications. We demonstrated that 1,2-DT, a garlic-derived organosulfur, has antiadipogenic and anti-inflammatory actions on human preadipocytes and may be a novel, antiobesity nutraceutical."

Osteoporosis

Suppression of the nuclear factor-kappaB activation pathway by spice-derived phytochemicals: reasoning for seasoning. Aggarwal BB, Shishodia S. Ann N Y Acad Sci. 2004 Dec;1030:434-41. **Key Finding:** "The activation of nuclear transcription factor kappaB has now been linked with a variety of **inflammatory disease, including cancer, atherosclerosis, myocardial infarction, diabetes, allergy, asthma, arthritis, Crohn's disease, multiple sclerosis, Alzheimer's disease, osteoporosis, psoriasis, septic shock, and AIDS**. Extensive research in the last few years has shown that the pathway that activates this transcription factor can be interrupted by phytochemicals derived from spices such as turmeric (curcumin), red pepper (capsaicin), cloves (eugenol), ginger (gingerol), cumin, anise, and fennel (anethol), basil and rosemary (ursolic acid), garlic (diallyl sulfide, S-allylmercaptocysteine, ajoene), and pomegranate (ellagic acid). For the first time, therefore, research provides 'reasoning for seasoning.'"

Rheumatoid arthritis

Garlic effectiveness in **rheumatoid arthritis**. Denisov LN, Andrianova IV, Timofeeva SS. Ter Arkh (Russian). 1999;71(8):55-8. **Key Finding:** "A garlic preparation (Alisate) can be recommended for treatment of rheumatoid arthritis patients in combined and monotherapy."

Septic shock

Suppression of the nuclear factor-kappaB activation pathway by spice-derived phytochemicals: reasoning for seasoning. Aggarwal BB, Shishodia S. Ann N Y Acad Sci. 2004 Dec;1030:434-41. **Key Finding:** "The activation of nuclear transcription factor kappaB has now been linked with a variety of **inflammatory disease, including cancer, atherosclerosis, myocardial infarction, diabetes, allergy, asthma, arthritis, Crohn's disease, multiple sclerosis, Alzheimer's disease, osteoporosis, psoriasis, septic shock, and AIDS**. Extensive research in the last few years has shown that the pathway that activates this transcription factor can be interrupted by phytochemicals derived from spices such as turmeric (curcumin), red pepper (capsaicin), cloves (eugenol), ginger (gingerol), cumin, anise, and fennel (anethol), basil and rosemary (ursolic acid), garlic (diallyl sulfide, S-allylmercaptocysteine, ajoene), and pomegranate (ellagic acid). For the first time, therefore, research provides 'reasoning for seasoning.'"

Sickle cell anemia

Sickle cell anemia*: a potential nutritional approach for a molecular disease.* Ohnishi ST, Ohnishi T, Ogunmola GB. Nutrition. 2000 May;16(5):330-8. **Key Finding:** "A certain population of red blood cells in patients with sickle cell anemia has an elevated density and possesses an abnormal membrane. These 'dense cells' have a tendency to adhere to neutrophils, platelets, and vascular endothelial cells, and, thus, they could trigger vasoocclusion and the subsequent painful crisis from which these patients suffer. We developed a laboratory method of preparing such dense cells and found that nutritional antioxidant supplements, hydroxyl radical scavengers, and iron-binding agents could inhibit the formation of dense cells in vitro. A cocktail consisting of daily doses of 6 g of aged garlic extract, 4-6 g of vitamin C, and 800 to 1200 IU of vitamin E may indeed be beneficial to the patients."

Stroke

*Aged garlic extract delays the appearance of infarct area in a cerebral **ischemia** model, an effect likely conditioned by the cellular antioxidant systems.* Aguilera P, Chanex-Cardenas ME, Ortiz-Plata A, Et al. Phytomedicine. 2010 Mar;17(3-4):241-7. **Key Finding**: "We conclude that the neuroprotective effect of aged garlic extract might be associated with control of the free-radical burst induced by perfusion, preservation of antioxidant enzyme activity, and the delay of other pathophysiological processes."

Antioxidant health effects of aged garlic extract. Borek C. J Nutr. 2001 Mar;131(3s):1010S-5S. **Key Finding:** "Although additional observations are warranted in humans, compelling evidence supports the beneficial health effects attributed to aged garlic extract, i.e., reducing the risk of **cardiovascular disease, stroke, cancer and aging**, including the oxidant-mediated brain cell damage that is implicated in **Alzheimer's disease**."

Thrombosis (blood clots)

*An evaluation of garlic and onion as **antithrombotic** agents.* Bordia T, Mohammed N, Thomason M, Ali M. Prostaglandins Leukot Essent Fatty Acids. 1996 Mar;54(3):183-6. **Key Finding:** "Garlic and onion should be consumed in a raw rather than cooked form in order to achieve a beneficial effect. Garlic was found to be more potent than onion in lowering the TXB2 (thromboxane) levels. These results show that garlic and onion can be taken frequently in low doses without any side effects, and can still produce a significant antithrombotic effect."

*Consumption of a garlic clove a day could be beneficial in preventing **thrombosis**.* Ali M, Thomson M. Prostaglandins Leukot Essent Fatty Acids. 1995 Sep;53(3):211-2. **Key Finding:** "A group of male volunteers in the age range 40-50 years participated in the study. Each volunteer consumed one clove of fresh garlic daily. After 26 weeks of garlic consumption, there was an approximately 20% reduction of serum cholesterol and about 80% reduction in serum thromboxane. No change in the level of serum glucose was observed. It appears that small amounts of fresh garlic consumed over a long period of time may be beneficial in the prevention of thrombosis."

Effects of a garlic-derived principle (ajoene) on aggregation and arachidonic acid metabolism in human blood platelets. Srivastava KC, Tyagi OD. Prostaglandins Leukot Essent Fatty Acids. 1993 Aug;49(2):587-95. **Key Finding:** "When garlic cloves are chopped or crushed several dialkyl thiosulfinates are rapidly formed by the action of the enzyme alliin lyase or alliinase (EC 4.4.1.4) on S(+)-alkyl-L-cysteine sulfoxides. One such compound identified recently is ajoene which has been reported to possess **antithrombotic** properties. We present here data on the antiplatelet properties of ajoene together with its effects on the metabolism of arachidonic acid in intact platelets. Thus, ajoene was found to inhibit platelet aggregation induced by AA, adrenaline, collagen, adenosine diphosphate and calcium ionophore; the nature of the inhibition was irreversible."

Aqueous extracts of onion, garlic and ginger inhibit platelet aggregation and alter arachidonic acid metabolism. Srivastava KC. Biomed Biochim Acta. 1984;43(8-9):S335-46. **Key Finding:** "Aqueous extracts of onion, garlic and ginger inhibited platelet aggregation induced by several aggregation agents, including arachidonate, in a dose-dependent manner. While onion and garlic extracts were found to be weak inhibitors of platelet thromboxane synthesis, ginger extract inhibited the platelet cyclooxygenase products and this effect correlated well with its inhibitory effects on the platelet aggregation induced by the above aggregation agents. The results indicate that if the same were happening in vivo, onion, garlic and ginger could be useful as natural **antithrombotic** materials."

Ulcers (peptic)

*Phytoceuticals: mighty but ignored weapons against **Helicobacter pylori** infection.* Lee SY, Shin YW, Hahm KB. J Dig Dis. 2008 Aug;9(3):129-39. **Key Finding:** "Helicobacter pylori infection causes peptic ulcer disease, mucosa-associated tissue lymphomas and gastric adenocarcinomas, for which the pathogenesis of chronic gastric inflammation prevails. Phytoceuticals such as Korean red ginseng, green tea, flavonoids, broccoli sprouts, garlic, and probiotics are known to inhibit H. pylori colonization, decrease gastric inflammation by inhibiting cytokine and chemokine release, and repress precancerous changes by inhibiting nuclear factor-kappa B DNA binding, inducing profuse levels of apoptosis and inhibiting mutagenesis."

Wound healing

*Effect of aged garlic extract on **wound healing**: a new frontier in wound management.* Ejaz S, Chekarova I, Cho JW, Lee SY, Ashraf S, Lim CW. Drug Chem Toxicol. 2009;32(3):191-203. **Key Finding:** "Successful wound healing depends upon angiogenesis, and impaired angiogenesis is a hallmark of the chronic wounds encountered with diabetes and venous or arterial insufficiency. Ninety chicks, aged 1 week and divided in 6 groups, were topically exposed to different concentrations of aged garlic extract (AGS) for 6 days. Different patterns, ranging from incomplete to almost complete wound closure, were observed with highly significant results in group E (the highest concentration of aged garlic extract.)These observations substantiate the beneficial use of AGS in the treatment of wounds."

Ginger

SOUTH ASIA IS CONSIDERED THE ANCIENT HOME of ginger cultivation and remains the primary source today. This plant is related to turmeric and like turmeric has been used for thousands of years as both a culinary spice and a therapeutic medicine. Fresh ginger is traditionally used as both a flavoring for many foods and drinks and as a key component in curries from India.

In recent studies, in the late twentieth century and early twenty-first century, gingerols, a primary chemical constituent of ginger, has been shown to be potent antidotes to certain cancers, such as ovarian and skin cancer. Its overall therapeutic effects are similar to those documented for onions and garlic.

Alzheimer's disease

Inhibition of acetyl cholinesterase activities and some pro-oxidant induced lipid peroxidation in rat brain by two varieties of ginger (Zingiber officinale). Oboh G, Ademilyui AO, Akinyemi AJ. Exp Toxicol Pathol. 2010 Oct 15. {Epub ahead of print}. **Key Finding:** "Some possible mechanism by which ginger extracts exert anti-**Alzheimer** properties could be through the inhibition of acetyl cholinesterase activities and prevention of lipid peroxidation in the brain."

Suppression of the nuclear factor-kappaB activation pathway by spice-derived phytochemicals: reasoning for seasoning. Aggarwal BB, Shishodia S. Ann N Y Acad Sci. 2004 Dec;1030:434-41. **Key Finding:** "The activation of nuclear transcription factor kappaB has now been linked with a variety of inflammatory disease, including **cancer, atherosclerosis, myocardial infarction, diabetes, allergy, asthma, arthritis, Crohn's disease, multiple sclerosis, Alzheimer's disease, osteoporosis, psoriasis, septic shock, and AIDS**. Extensive research in the last few years has shown that the pathway that activates this transcription factor can be interrupted by phytochemicals derived from spices such as turmeric (curcumin), red pepper (capsaicin), cloves (eugenol), ginger (gingerol), cumin, anise, and fennel (anethol), basil and rosemary (ursolic acid), garlic (diallyl sulfide, S-allylmercaptocysteine, ajoene), and pomegranate (ellagic acid). For the first time, therefore, research provides 'reasoning for seasoning.'"

Antioxidation

Herbal Antioxidants in Clinical Practice. Weiner MA. Journal of Orthomolecular Medicine. 1994; vol 9, no. 3:167-176. **Key Finding:** This paper present a discussion of herbs (ginger, ginkgo, licorice, schizandra, turmeric, quercetin) that may add to the optimization of **antioxidant** status and offer preventive values for overall human health.

Atherosclerosis

Suppression of the nuclear factor-kappaB activation pathway by spice-derived phytochemicals: reasoning for seasoning. Aggarwal BB, Shishodia S. Ann N Y Acad Sci. 2004 Dec;1030:434-41. **Key Finding:** "The activation of nuclear transcription factor kappaB has now been linked with a variety of inflammatory disease, including **cancer, atherosclerosis, myocardial infarction, diabetes, allergy, asthma, arthritis, Crohn's disease, multiple sclerosis, Alzheimer's disease, osteoporosis, psoriasis, septic shock, and AIDS**. Extensive research in the last few years has shown that the pathway that activates this transcription factor can be interrupted by phytochemicals derived from spices such as turmeric (curcumin), red pepper (capsaicin), cloves (eugenol), ginger (gingerol), cumin, anise, and fennel (anethol), basil and rosemary (ursolic acid), garlic (diallyl sulfide, S-allylmercaptocysteine, ajoene), and pomegranate (ellagic acid). For the first time, therefore, research provides 'reasoning for seasoning.'"

Ginger extract consumption reduces plasma **cholesterol,** *inhibits LDL oxidation and attenuates development of* **atherosclerosis** *in atherosclerotic, apolipoprotein E-deficient mice.* Fuhrman B, Rosenblat M; Hayek T, Coleman R, Aviram M. J Nutr. 2000 May;130(5):1124-31. Key Finding: "We conclude that dietary consumption of ginger extract by mice significantly attenuates the development of atherosclerotic lesions. This antiatherogenic effect is associated with a significant reduction in plasma and LDL cholesterol levels and a significant reduction in the LDL basal oxidative state."

Cancer (breast; colon; leukemia; lung; ovarian; skin)

6-Shogaol, an active constituent of ginger, inhibits **breast cancer** *cell invasion by reducing matrix metalloproteinase-9 expression via blockade of nuclear factor-kB activation.* Ling H, Yang H, Tan SH, Et al. Br J Pharmacol. 2010 Dec;161(8):1763-77. **Key**

Finding: "6-Shogaol from ginger is a potent inhibitor of MDA-MB-231 cell invasion, and the molecular mechanism involves at least in part the down-regulation of MMP-9 transcription by targeting the NF-kB activation cascade."

6-Dehydrogingerdione, an active constituent of dietary ginger, induces cell cycle arrest and apoptosis through reactive oxygen species/c-Jun N-terminal kinase pathways in human **breast cancer** *cells.* Hsu YL, Chen CY, Hou MF, Et al. Mol Nutr Food Res. 2010 Sep;54(9):1307-17. **Key Finding**: "6-dehydrogingerdione is an active constituent of dietary ginger. These findings suggest that a critical role for reactive oxygen species and c-Jun N-terminal kinase in 6-dehydrogingerdione-mediated apoptosis of human breast cancer."

Induction of apoptosis by {6}-gingerol associated with the modulation of p53 and involvement of mitochondrial signaling pathway in B{a{P-induced mouse **skin tumorigenesis**. Nigam N, George J, Srivastava S, Et al. Cancer Chemother Parmacol. 2010 Mar;65(4):687-96. **Key Finding**: "On the basis of the results we conclude that {6}-gingerol possesses apoptotic potential in mouse skin tumors as mechanism of chemoprevention hence deserves further investigation."

Induction of apoptosis by {8}-shogaol via reactive oxygen species generation, glutathione depletion, and caspase activation in human **leukemia** *cells.* Shieh PC, Chen YO, Kup DH, Et al. J Agric Food Chem. 2010 Mar 24;58(6):3847-54. **Key Finding**: "One of the pungent phenolic compounds in ginger, {8}-shogaol, was able to induce apoptosis in a time- and concentration-dependent manner. Taken together these results suggest for the first time that reactive oxygen species production and depletion of glutathione that contributed to {8}-shogaci-induced apoptosis in HL-60 human leukemia cells."

Ginger extract inhibits human telomerase reverse transcriptase and c-Myc expression in A549 **lung cancer** *cells.* Tuntiwechapikul W, Taka T, Songsomboon C, Et al. J Med Food. 2010 Dec;13(6):1347-54. **Key Finding**: "Ginger extract can inhibit the expression of the two prominent molecular targets of cancer, the human telomerase reverse transcriptase and c-Myc, in A549 lung cancer cells in a time- and concentration-dependent manner."

Increased growth inhibitory effects on human **cancer** *cells and anti-inflammatory potency of shogaols from Zingiber officinale relative to gingerols.* Sang S, Hong J, Wu H, Liu J, Yang CS, Pan MH, Badmaey V, Ho CT. J Agric Food Chem. 2009 Nov 25;57(22):10645-50. **Key Finding**: "Ginger has received extensive attention because of its antioxidant, anti-inflammatory and antitumor activities. Most researchers have considered gingerols as the active principles and have paid little attention to shogaols, the dehydration products of corresponding gingerols. In this study, we have purified and identified eight major components from ginger extract and compared their anticarcinogenic and anti-inflammatory activities. Our results showed that shogaols had much stronger growth inhibitory effects than gingerols on human **lung cancer** cells and human **colon cancer** cells."

{6}-Gingerol induces reactive oxygen species regulated mitochondrial cell death pathway in human epiermoid carcinoma A431 cells. Nigam N, Bhui K, Prasad S, George J, Shukla Y. Chem Biol Interact. 2009 Sep 14;181(1):77-84. **Key Finding**: "These results firmly suggest that {6}-gingerol can be effectively used for the treatment of **skin cancer**."

Potential of spice-derived phytochemicals for **cancer** *prevention.* Aggarwal BB, Kunnu-makkara AB, Harikumar KB, Tharakan ST, Sung B, Anand P. Planta Med. 2008 Oct;74(13):1560-9. **Key Finding:** "The potential of turmeric (curcumin), red chili (capsaicin), cloves (eugenol), ginger (zerumbone), fennel (anethole), kokum (gambogic acid), fenugreek (diosgenin), and black cumin (thymoquinone) in cancer prevention has been established. Additionally, the mechanism by which these agents mediate anticancer effects is also becoming increasingly evident. The current review describes the active components of some of the major spices, their mechanisms of action and their potential in cancer prevention."

Ginger inhibits cell growth and modulates angiogenic factors in **ovarian cancer** *cells.* Rhode J, Fogoros S, Zick S, Wahl H, Griffith KA, Huang J, Liu JR. BMC Complement Altern Med. 2007 Dec 20;7:44. **Key Finding:** "Ginger inhibits growth and modulates secretion of angiogenic factors in ovarian cancer cells. The use of dietary agents such as ginger may have potential in the treatment and prevention of ovarian cancer."

Role of chemo preventive agents in **cancer** *therapy.* Dorai T, Aggarwal BB. Cancer Lett. 2004 Nov 25;215(2):129-40. **Key Finding:** "Chemo preventive agents include genistein, resveratrol, diallyl sulfide, S-allyl cysteine, allicin, lycopene, capsaicin, curcumin, 6-gingerol, ellagic acid, ursolic acid, silymarin, anethol, catechins and eugenol. Because these agents have been shown to suppress cancer cell proliferation, inhibit growth factor signaling pathways, induce apoptosis, inhibit NF-kappaB, AP-1 and JAK-STAT activation pathways, inhibit angiogen-esis, suppress the expression of anti-apoptotic proteins, inhibit cyclooxygenase-2, they may have untapped therapeutic value. These chemo preventive agents also have very recently been found to reverse chemo resistance and radio resistance in patients undergoing cancer treatment."

Suppression of the nuclear factor-kappaB activation pathway by spice-derived phytochemicals: reasoning for seasoning. Aggarwal BB, Shishodia S. Ann N Y Acad Sci. 2004 Dec;1030:434-41. **Key Finding:** "The activation of nuclear transcription factor kappaB has now been linked with a variety of inflammatory disease, including **cancer, atherosclerosis, myocardial infarction, diabetes, allergy, asthma, arthritis, Crohn's disease, multiple sclerosis, Alzheimer's disease, osteoporosis, psoriasis, septic shock, and AIDS**. Extensive research in the last few years has shown that the pathway that activates this transcription factor can be interrupted by phytochemicals derived from spices such as turmeric (curcumin), red pepper (capsaicin), cloves (eugenol), ginger (gingerol), cumin, anise, and fennel (anethol), basil and rosemary (ursolic acid), garlic (diallyl sulfide, S-allylmercaptocysteine, ajoene), and pomegranate (ellagic acid). For the first time, therefore, research provides 'reasoning for seasoning.'"

Functional properties of spice extracts obtained via supercritical fluid extraction. Leal PF, Braga ME, Sato DN, Carvalho JE, Marques MO, Meireles MA. J Agric Food Chem. 2003 Apr 23;51(9):2520-5. **Key Finding:** "In the present study the antioxidant, **anticancer** and **antimicrobacterial** activities of extracts from ginger, rosemary and turmeric were evaluated. The rosemary extracts exhibited the strongest antioxidant and the lowest antimicrobacterial activities. Turmeric extracts showed the greatest antimicrobacterial activity. Ginger and turmeric extracts showed selected anticancer activities."

*Anti-**tumor** promoting potential of selected spice ingredients with antioxidative and anti-inflammatory activities: a short review.* Surh YJ. Food Chem Toxicol. 2002 Aug;40(8):1091-7. **Key Finding:** "This review summarizes the molecular mechanisms underlying chemo preventive effects of the spice ingredients curcumin, [6]-gingerol, and capsaicin, in terms of their effects on intracellular signaling cascades, particularly those involving NF-kappaB and mitogen-activated protein kinases."

*Botanicals in **cancer** chemoprevention.* Park EJ, Pezzuto JM. Cancer Metastasis Rev. 2002;21(3-4):231-55. **Key Finding:** "In this review, we discuss the cancer chemo preventive activity of cruciferous vegetables such as cabbage and broccoli, Allium vegetables such as garlic and onion, green tea, citrus fruits, tomatoes, berries, ginger and ginseng. Phytochemicals of these types have great potential in the fight against human cancer, and a variety of delivery methods are available as a result of their occurrence in nature."

*Anti-**tumor** promoting activities of selected pungent phenolic substances present in ginger.* Surh YJ, Park KK, Chun KS, Lee LJ, Lee E, Lee SS. J Environ Pathol Toxicol Oncol. 1999;18(2):131-9. **Key Finding:** "In our study, we found anti-tumor promoting properties of [6]-gingerol and [6]-paradol. These substances also significantly inhibited the tumor-promoter-stimulated inflammation, TNF-alpha production, and activation of epidermal ornithine decarboxylase in mice. In another study, [6]-gingerol and [6]-paradol suppressed the superoxide production stimulated by TPA in differentiated HL-60 cells. Taken together, these findings suggest that pungent vanilloids found in ginger possess potential chemo preventive activities."

Cholesterol

Antihypercholesterolaemic *effect of ginger rhizome (Zingiber officinale) in rats.* ElRokh el-SM, Yassin NA, Sl-Shenawy SM, Ibrahim BM. Inflammopharmachology. 2010 Dec;18(6):309-15. **Key Finding:** "The results revealed that the hypercholesterolemic rats treated with aqueous ginger infusion in the three doses used after 2 and 4 weeks of treatment induce significant decrease in all lipid profile parameters which were measured and improved the risk ratio."

*Ginger extract consumption reduces plasma **cholesterol,** inhibits LDL oxidation and attenuates development of **atherosclerosis** in atherosclerotic, apolipoprotein E-deficient mice.* Fuhrman B, Rosenblat M, Hayek T, Coleman R, Aviram M. J Nutr. 2000 May;130(5):1124-31. Key Finding: "We conclude that dietary consumption of ginger extract by mice significantly attenuates the development of atherosclerotic lesions. This antiatherogenic effect is associated with a significant reduction in plasma and LDL cholesterol levels and a significant reduction in the LDL basal oxidative state."

Colitis (and Crohn's disease)

*Suppression of dextran sodium sulfate-induced **colitis** in mice by zerumbone, a subtropical ginger sesquiterpene, and nimesulide, separately and in combination.* Murakami A, Hayashi R, Tanaka T, Kwon KH, Ohigashi H, Safitri R. Biochem Pharmacol. 2003 Oct 1;66(7):1253-61. **Key Finding:** "Ulcerative colitis and **Crohn's disease** are inflammatory disorders of unknown cause and difficult to treat. The present study was undertaken to explore the suppressive efficacy of zerumbone, a sesquiterpenoid used as a condiment in Southeast Asian countries. Our results suggest that zerumbone is a novel food factor for mitigating experimental ulcerative colitis and that use of a combination of agents, with different modes of action, may be an effective anti-inflammatory strategy."

Suppression of the nuclear factor-kappaB activation pathway by spice-derived phytochemicals: reasoning for seasoning. Aggarwal BB, Shishodia S. Ann N Y Acad Sci. 2004 Dec;1030:434-41. **Key Finding:** "The activation of nuclear transcription factor kappaB has now been linked with a variety of inflammatory disease, including **cancer, atherosclerosis, myocardial infarction, diabetes, allergy, asthma, arthritis, Crohn's disease, multiple sclerosis, Alzheimer's disease, osteoporosis, psoriasis, septic shock, and AIDS**. Extensive research in the last few years has shown that the pathway that activates this transcription factor can be interrupted by phytochemicals derived from spices such as turmeric (curcumin), red pepper (capsaicin), cloves (eugenol), ginger (gingerol), cumin, anise, and fennel (anethol), basil and rosemary (ursolic acid), garlic (diallyl sulfide, S-allylmercaptocysteine, ajoene), and pomegranate (ellagic acid). For the first time, therefore, research provides 'reasoning for seasoning.'"

Obesity

*Targeting inflammation-induced **obesity** and metabolic diseases by curcumin and other nutraceuticals.* Aggarwal BB. Annu Rev Nutr. 2010 Aug 21;30:173-99.
Key Finding: "Curcumin-induced alterations reverse insulin resistance, hyperglycemia, hyperlipidemia and other symptoms linked to obesity. Other structurally homologous nutraceuticals, derived from red **chili, cinnamon, cloves, black pepper and ginger**, also exhibit effects against obesity and insulin resistance."

Thrombosis (blood clots)

Aqueous extracts of onion, garlic and ginger inhibit platelet aggregation and alter arachidonic acid metabolism. Srivastava KC. Biomed Biochim Acta. 1984;43(8-9):S335-46.
Key Finding: "Aqueous extracts of onion, garlic and ginger inhibited platelet aggregation induced by several aggregation agents, including arachidonate, in a dose-dependent manner. While onion and garlic extracts were found to be weak inhibitors of platelet thromboxane synthesis, ginger extract inhibited the platelet cyclooxygenase products and this effect correlated well with its inhibitory effects on the platelet aggregation induced by the above aggregation agents. The results indicate that if the same were happening in vivo, onion, garlic and ginger could be useful as natural **antithrombotic** materials."

Grapefruit

ONLY IN THE EIGHTEENTH CENTURY, in Barbados, was the citrus hybrid known as grapefruit first bred, which makes it one of the newer therapeutic foods. After it was brought to Florida in the early nineteenth century, it became an increasingly popular cultivated crop. Today, the United States is the world's top producer, with most of the production occurring in Texas and Florida.

At least six types of cancer can be prevented or treated with grapefruit, according to medical studies. It has also been shown to be particularly beneficial in addressing health problems associated with diabetes.

Antioxidation

*Changes in **plasma lipid** and antioxidant activity in rats as a result of naringin and red grapefruit supplementation.* Gorinsetin S, Leontowicz H, Leontowicz M, Krzeminski R. Gralak M, Delgado-Licon E, Martinez-Avala AL, Katrich E, Trakhtenberg S. J Agric Food Chem. 2005 Apr 20;53(8):3223-8. **Key Finding**: "Naringin is a powerful plasma lipid lowering and plasma **antioxidant** activity increasing flavonone. However, fresh red grapefruit is preferable than naringin: it more effectively influences plasma lipid levels and plasma antioxidant activity and, therefore, could be used as a valuable supplement for disease-preventing diets."

***Antioxidant** and antiproliferative activities of common fruits.* Sun J, Chu YF, Wu X, Liu RH. J Agric Food Chem. 2002 Dec 4;50(25):7449-54. **Key Finding:** "This study was designed to investigate the profiles of total phenolic, including both soluble free and bound forms in common fruits, by applying solvent extraction, base digestion, and solid-phase extraction methods. Cranberry had the highest total phenolic content, followed by apple, red grape, strawberry, pineapple, banana peach, lemon, orange, pear, and grapefruit. Cranberry had the highest total antioxidant activity followed by apple, red grape, strawberry, peach, lemon, pear, banana, orange, grapefruit and pineapple. Cranberry showed the highest antiproliferation activity followed by lemon, apple, strawberry, red grape, banana, grapefruit, and peach."

Atherosclerosis

*Red grapefruit positively influences serum triglyceride level in patients suffering from **coronary atherosclerosis**: studies in vitro and in humans.* Gorinstein S, Caspi A, Libman I,

Lerner HT, Huang D, Leontowicz H, Leontowicz M, Tashma Z, Katrich E, Feng S, Trakhtenberg S. J Agric Food Chem. 2006 Mar 8;54(5):1887-92. **Key Finding**: "Diet supplemented with fresh red grapefruit positively influences serum lipid levels of all fractions, especially serum triglycerides and also serum antioxidant activity. The addition of fresh red grapefruit to generally accepted diets could be beneficial for hyperlipidemia, especially hypertriglyceridemia, patients suffering from coronary atherosclerosis."

Bone health

Grapefruit juice modulates bone quality in rats. Deyhim F, Mandadi K, Faraji B, Patil BS. J Med Food. 2008 Mar;11(1):99-104. **Key Finding**: "Drinking grapefruit juice positively affected **bone quality** by enhancing bone mineral deposition in ORX rats and by improving bone density in non-ORX rats via an undefined mechanism."

Cancer (breast; colon; lung; mouth; skin; stomach)

Quantification of 4'-geranyloxyferulic acid, a new natural colon cancer chemo preventive agent, by HPLC-DAD in **grapefruit skin** *extract.* Genovese S, Epifano F, Carlucci G, Et al. J Pharm Biomed Anal. 2010 Oct 10;53(2):212-4. **Key Finding**: "Many of the isolated oxyprenylated natural products from grapefruit have been shown to exert in vitro and in vivo remarkable anti-cancer and anti-inflammatory effects. 4'-geranyloxyferulic acid has been discovered as a valuable chemo preventive agent of **several types of cancer**."

Prospective study of the association between grapefruit intake and risk of **breast cancer** *in the European Prospective Investigation into Cancer and Nutrition (EPIC).* Spencer EA, Key TJ, Appleby PN, Et al. Cancer Causes Control. 2009 Aug;20(6):803-9. **Key Finding**: "There was no relationship between grapefruit intake and breast cancer risk among premenopausal women, all postmenopausal women, or post-menopausal women categorized by hormone replacement therapy use. In this study, we found no evidence of an association between grapefruit intake and risk of breast cancer."

Suppression of phorbol-12-myristate-13-acetate-induced tumor cell invasion by bergamottin via the inhibition of protein kinase Cdelta/p38 mitogen-activated protein kinase and JNK/ nuclear factor-kappB-dependent matrix metalloproteinase-9 expression. Hwang YP, Yun HJ,

Choi JH, Kang KW, Jeong HG. Mol Nutr Food Res. 2009 Nov 26 (Epub ahead of print). **Key Finding**: Bergamottin, a cytochrome P450 inhibitor from Citrus paradis (grapefruit), suppresses MMP and this expression contributes, at least in part, to the **antitumor** activity of bergamottin."

*Inhibition of **oral carcinogenesis** by citrus flavonoids.* Miller EG, Peacock JJ, Bourland TC, Taylor SE, Wright JM, Patil BS, Miller EG. Nutr Cancer. 2008;60(1):69-74. **Key Finding**: "The data suggest that naringin and naringenin, 2 flavonoids found in high concentrations in grapefruit, may be able to inhibit the development of **cancer**."

*Prospective study of grapefruit intake and risk of **breast cancer** in postmenopausal women: the Multiethnic Cohort Study.* Monroe KR, Murphy SP, Kolonel LN, Pike MC. Br J Cancer. 2007 Aug 6;97(3):440-5. **Key Finding**: "We investigated the association of grapefruit intake with breast cancer risk in 50,000 postmenopausal women from five racial/ethnic groups. Grapefruit intake was significantly associated with an increased risk of breast cancer for subjects in the highest category of intake, that is, one-quarter grapefruit or more per day compared to non-consumers. An increased risk of similar magnitude was seen in users of estrogen therapy, users of estrogen+progestin therapy, and among never users of hormone therapy."

*Lycopene and lutein inhibit proliferation in rat **prostate carcinoma** cells.* Gunasekera RS, Sewgobind K, Desai S, Dunn L, Black HS, McKeehan WL, Patil B. Nutr Cancer. 2007;58(2):171-7. **Key Finding**: "The effects of grapefruit-derived and commercial lycopene and lutein preparations on androgen independent cultured malignant type II tumor cells were compared to their benign parent type I tumor epithelial cells. Results demonstrated that both lycopene, in an alpha-Cyclodextrin water soluble carrier, and lutein inhibited malignant AT3 cells in a concentration and time-dependent manner."

Red Mexican grapefruit: a novel source for bioactive limonoids and their antioxidant activity. Mandadi KK, Jayaprakasha GK, Bhat NG, Patil BS. Z Naturforsch C. 2007 Mar-Apr;62(3-4):179-88. **Key Finding**: "Citrus limonoids have shown to inhibit the growth of **cancer in colon, lung, mouth, stomach and breast** in animal and cell culture studies. For the first time in the present study, an attempt has been made to isolate antioxidant fractions and five limonoids from red Mexican grapefruit seeds."

*Suppression of **colon carcinogenesis** by bioactive compounds in grapefruit.* Vanamala J, Leonardi T, Patil BS, Taddeo SS, Murphy ME, Pike LM, Chapkin RS, Lupton

JR, Turner ND. Carcinogenesis. 2006 Jun;27(6):1257-65. **Key Finding**: "These results suggest that consumption of grapefruit or limonin (an isolated citrus compound) may help to suppress colon cancer development."

*Naringenin inhibits glucose uptake in MCF-7 **breast cancer** cells: a mechanism for impaired cellular proliferation.* Harmon AW, Patel YM. Breast Cancer Res Treat. 2004 May;85(2):103-10. **Key Finding**: "We show that the grapefruit flavanone naringenin inhibited insulin-stimulated glucose uptake in proliferating and growth-arrested MCF-7 breast cancer cells. Naringenin may possess therapeutic potential as an anti-proliferative agent."

Effects of naringin on hydrogen peroxide-induced cytotoxicity and apoptosis in P388 cells. Kanno S, Shouji A, Asou K, Ishikawa M. Pharmacol Sci. 2003 Jun;92(2):166-70. **Key Finding**: "We examined the effects of naringin on H202-induced cytotoxicity and apoptosis in mouse **leukemia** P388 cells. These results indicate that naringin from grapefruit is a useful drug having antioxidant and anti-apoptopic properties."

*Intake of Flavonoids and **Lung Cancer**.* Marchand LL, Murphy SP, Hankin JH, Wilkens LR, Kolonel LN. J Natl Cancer Inst. 2000 Jan 19;92(2):154-60. **Key Finding:** "After adjusting for smoking and intakes of saturated fat and B-carotene, we found statistically significant inverse associations between lung cancer risk and the main food sources of the flavonoids quercetin (onions and apples) and naringin (white grapefruit.)"

*Citrus peel use is associated with reduced risk of squamous cell **carcinoma of the skin**.* Hakim IA, Harris RB. Ritenbaugh C. Nutr Cancer. 2000;37(2):161-8. Key Finding: "Limonene has demonstrated efficacy in preclinical models of breast and colon cancers. The principal sources of d-limonene are the oils of orange, grapefruit, and lemon. The present case-control study was designed to determine the usual citrus consumption patterns of an older Southwestern population and to then evaluate how this citrus consumption varied with history of squamous cell carcinoma of the skin. We found no association between the overall consumption of citrus fruits or citrus juices and skin squamous cell carcinoma. However, the most striking feature was the protection purported by citrus peel consumption. Moreover, there was a dose-response relationship between higher citrus peel in the diet and degree of risk lowering. This is the first study to explore the relationship between higher citrus peel consumption and human cancers."

*Inhibition of **mammary cancer** by citrus flavonoids.* Guthrie N, Carroll KK. Adv Exp Med Biol. 1998;439:227-36. **Key Finding**: "Double strength orange juice given to the rats in place of drinking water inhibited mammary tumorigenesis induced in female Sprague-Dawley rats by DMBA more effectively than double strength grapefruit juice. This may mean that hesperidin retains its effectiveness in vivo better than naringenin. It is also possible that orange juice contains other compounds that have anti-cancer activity and that may act synergistically with hesperidin."

Inhibition of human **breast cancer** *cell proliferation and delay of mammary tumorigenesis by flavonoids and citrus juices.* So FV, Guthrie N, Chamers AF, Moussa M, Carroll KK. Nutr Cancer. 1996;26(2):167-81. **Key Finding**: "Two citrus flavonoids, hesperidin and naringenin, found in oranges and grapefruit, respectively, and four noncitrus flavonoids, baicalein, galangin, genistein, and quercetin, were tested singly and in one-to-one combinations for their effects on proliferation and growth of a human breast carcinoma cell line, MDA-MB-435. Naringenin is present in grapefruit mainly as its glycosylated form, naringin. These compounds as well as grapefruit and orange juice concentrates were tested for their ability to inhibit development of mammary tumors in female Sprague-Dawley rats. Tumor development was delayed in the groups given orange juice or fed the naringin-supplemented diet. Rats given orange juice had a smaller tumor burden and grew better than any of the other groups. These experiments provide evidence that citrus flavonoids are effective inhibitors of human breast cancer cell proliferation in vitro, especially when paired with quercetin."

Inhibition of **carcinogenesis** *by some minor dietary constituents.* Wattenberg LW, Hanley AB, Barany G, Sparnins VL, Lam LK, Fenwick GR. Princess Takamatsu Symp. 1985;16:193-203. **Key Finding**: "Citrus fruit oil: orange, tangerine, lemon and grapefruit, induce glutathione S-transferase activity in tissues of the mouse. When fed in the diet prior to and during the course of administration of benzo(a)pyrene, the four citrus fruit oils inhibit formation of tumors of both the **forestomach and lungs** of mice."

Cardiovascular disease (and coronary artery disease)

The **grapefruit**: *an old wine in a new glass? Metabolic and cardiovascular perspectives.* Owira PM, Ojewole JA. Cardiovasc J Afr. 2010 Sep-Oct;21(5):280-5. **Key Finding**: "It has recently emerged that grapefruit, by virtue of its rich flavonoid content, is beneficial in the management of degenerative diseases such as **diabetes** and **cardiovascular disorders**."

Methanol seed extract of Citrus paradise Macfad lowers blood glucose, lipids and **cardiovascular disease** *risk indices in normal Wistar rats.* Adeneye AA. Nig Q J Hosp Med. 2008 Jan-Mar;18(1):16-20. **Key Finding**: "Citrus paradise (grapefruit) seed is traditionally used for the management of diabetes mellitus and obesity by the natives of South-West Nigeria. The present preliminary study was undertaken to evaluate blood glucose and lipid lowering effects as well as cardiovascular disease risk factor-reducing effect of Citrus paradise Macfad in male Wistar rats. Cardiovascular disease risk assessing factors such as **obesity** or body mass index, atherogenic index, coronary risk index were calculated. Results showed significant dose related lowering effects of the extract on FPG, cardiovascular disease risk and lipid parameters. These results lend support to the therapeutic potential of grapefruit seed in the management of suspected **type 2 diabetic** patients."

Effect of acute and chronic grapefruit, orange, and pineapple juice intake on blood lipid profile in normolipidemic rat. Daher CF, Abou-Khalil J, Baroody GM. Med Sci Monit. 2005 Dec;11(12):BR465-72. **Key Finding**: "High fruit intake is known to be associated with reduced risk of **coronary heart disease**. The card protective benefit of chronic juice intake in normolipidemic rat may be chiefly through mechanisms independent of a direct effect on blood lipid profile, although orange and pineapple, but not grapefruit, relatively improved the metabolism and clearance of blood lipoprotein particles. As a result of delayed gastric emptying, grapefruit and pineapple juices may moderate sharp increases in postprandial plasma TAG concentrations accompanying peak digestion and absorption."

Effects of tomato extract on human platelet aggregation in vitro. Dutta-Roy AK, Crosbie L, Gordon MJ. Platelets. 2001 Jun;12(4):218-27. **Key Finding:** "Among all fruits tested in vitro for their anti-platelet property, tomato had the highest activity followed by grapefruit, melon, and strawberry, whereas pear and apple had little or no activity. All these data indicate that tomato contains very potent anti-platelet components, and consuming tomatoes might be beneficial both as a preventive and therapeutic regime for **cardiovascular disease**."

Cholesterol

Changes in **plasma lipid** *and antioxidant activity in rats as a result of naringin and red grapefruit supplementation.* Gorinsetin S, Leontowicz H, Leontowicz M, Krzeminski R, Gralak M, Delgado-Licon E, Martinez-Avala AL, Katrich E, Trakhtenberg S. J Agric Food Chem. 2005 Apr 20;53(8):3223-8. **Key Finding**: "Naringin is a powerful plasma lipid lowering and plasma **antioxidant** activity increasing flavanone. However, fresh red grapefruit is preferable than naringin: it more effectively influences plasma lipid levels and plasma antioxidant activity and, therefore, could be used as a valuable supplement for disease-preventing diets."

Diabetes

The **grapefruit**: an old wine in a new glass? Metabolic and cardiovascular perspectives. Owira PM, Ojewole JA. Cardiovasc J Afr. 2010 Sep-Oct;21(5):280-5. **Key Finding**: "It has recently emerged that grapefruit, by virtue of its rich flavonoid content, is beneficial in the management of degenerative diseases such as **diabetes** and **cardiovascular disorders**."

Grapefruit juice improves glycemic control but exacerbates metformin-induced lactic acidosis in non-diabetic rats. Owira PM, Ojewole JA. Methods Find Exp Clin Pharmacol. 2009 Nov;31(9):563-70. **Key Finding**: "Recent clinical studies have indicated that grapefruit juice improves insulin resistance and reduces weight gain in humans. The effect of grapefruit juice on glucose tolerance and metformin-induced lactic acidosis in normal, non-diabetic rats is hereby investigated. Although grapefruit may be beneficial to diabetic patients, it may exacerbate lactic acidosis in **diabetic** patients taking metformin concurrently."

Hypoglycemic and hypolipidemic effects of methanol seed extract of Citrus paradise Macfad in alloxan-induced **diabetic** Wistar rats. Adeneye AA. Nig Q J Hosp Med. 2008 Oct-Dec;18(4):211-5. **Key Finding**: "Results of this study lend support to the traditional use of grapefruit seeds in the management of type 1 diabetic patients and may suggest a role in orthodox management of the disease."

Methanol seed extract of Citrus paradise Macfad lowers blood glucose, lipids and **cardiovascular disease** risk indices in normal Wistar rats. Adeneye AA. Nig Q J Hosp Med. 2008 Jan-Mar;18(1):16-20. **Key Finding**: "Citrus paradise (grapefruit) seed is traditionally used for the management of diabetes mellitus and obesity by the natives of South-West Nigeria. The present preliminary study was undertaken to evaluate blood glucose and lipid lowering effects as well as cardiovascular disease risk factor-reducing effect of Citrus paradise Macfad in male Wistar rats. Cardiovascular disease risk assessing factors such as **obesity** or body mass index, atherogenic index, coronary risk index were calculated. Results showed significant dose related lowering effects of the extract on FPG, cardiovascular disease risk and lipid parameters. These results lend support to the therapeutic potential of grapefruit seed in the management of suspected **type 2 diabetic** patients."

Epilepsy

*Effect of grapefruit juice on carbamazepine bioavailability in patients with **epilepsy.*** Garg SK, Kumar N, Bhargava VK, Prabhakar SK. Clin Pharmacol Thera. 1998;64:286-288. **Key Finding:** "Grapefruit juice increases the bioavailability of carbamazepine by inhibiting CYP3A4 enzymes in gut wall and in the liver."

Hepatitis C

*Apolipoprotein B-dependent **hepatitis C virus** secretion is inhibited by the grapefruit flavonoid naringenin.* Nahmias Y, Goldwasser J, Casali M, van Poll D, Wakita T, Chung RT, Yarmush ML. Hepatology. 2008 May;47(5):1437-45. **Key Finding:** "These results suggest a novel therapeutic approach for the treatment of Hepatitis C virus infection."

Hypertension

Effect of Citrus paradisi extract and juice on arterial pressure both in vitro and in vivo. Diaz-Juarez JA, Tenorio-Lopez FA, Zarco-Olvera G, Et al. Phytother Res. 2009 Jul;23(7):948-54. **Key Finding**: "Grapefruit consumption is considered as beneficial and it is popularly used for the treatment of a vast array of diseases, including **hypertension.** In the present study, the coronary vasodilator and hypotensive effects of Citrus paradise peel extract were assessed. It decreased coronary vascular resistance and mean arterial pressure when compared with control values."

*Antihypertensive effect of sweetie fruit in patients with stage I **hypertension.*** Reshef N, Hayari Y, Goren C, Boaz M, Madar Z, Knobler H. J Hypertens. 2005 Oct;18(10):1360-3. **Key Finding**: "Sweetie fruit, a hybrid between grapefruit and pummelo, was shown to have a significant beneficial effect in reducing diastolic blood pressure. These data suggest that the active ingredients associated with the antihypertensive effect of sweetie juice are the flavonoids naringin and narirutin."

Inflammatory bowel disease

*Dietary Factors in the Modulation of **Inflammatory Bowel Disease** Activity.* Shah S. MedGenMed. 2007;9(1):60. **Key Finding:** "Two studies have indicated that lycopene, an antioxidant, found in high quantities in foods that have a natural red color (e.g. tomato, watermelon, pink grapefruit) may play a role in attenuating the inflammatory process. Studies done using indoacetamide rat model of colitis showed that lycopene attenuated the inflammatory response."

Weight loss

Nootkatone, a characteristic constituent of grapefruit, stimulates energy metabolism and prevents diet-induced **obesity** *by activating AMPK.* Murase T, Misawa K, Haramizu S, Et al. Am J Physiol Endocrinal Metab. 2010 Aug;299(2):E266-75. **Key Finding**: "These findings indicate that long-term intake of nootkatone from grapefruit is beneficial toward preventing obesity and improving physical performance and that these effects are due, at least in part, to enhanced energy metabolism through AMPK activation in skeletal muscle and liver."

The effects of grapefruit on weight and insulin resistance: relationship to the **metabolic syndrome**. Fujioka K, Greenway F, Sheard J, Ying Y. J Med Food. 2006 Spring;9(1):49-54. **Key Finding**: "Half of a fresh grapefruit eaten before meals was associated with significant weight loss. In metabolic syndrome patients the effect was also seen with grapefruit products. Insulin resistance was improved with fresh grapefruit. Although the mechanism of this weight loss is unknown it would appear reasonable to include grapefruit in a **weight reduction** diet."

Grapes (see also Resveratrol)

DOMESTICATION OF GRAPES APPARENTLY BEGAN IN TURKEY at least five thousand years ago, though the first written records of purple grape use and cultivation appear in ancient Egyptian hieroglyphics. Later cultures, such as the ancient Greeks and Romans, introduced large-scale agricultural production of grapes for both eating and wine. In North America, wild purple grapes were part of the diet of Native tribes well before European colonists arrived.

Today, most of the world's grape production is concentrated in three countries—Spain, France and Italy—with the United States rapidly catching up. Both purple and green grapes have been intensively studied for their nutritional value. They naturally contain high levels of vitamin C, vitamin K, potassium, and phosphorus. These and other components help give grapes one of the best antioxidant profiles of any food, which helps explain their benefits in protecting the cardiovascular system.

Aging

Grape juice, berries, and walnuts affect **brain aging** *and behavior.* Joseph JA, Shukitt-Hale B, Willis LM. J Nutr. 2009 Sep;139(9):1813S-7S. **Key Finding:** "Research from our laboratory has suggested that dietary supplementation with fruit or vegetable extracts high in antioxidants (e.g. blueberries, strawberries, walnuts and Concord grape juice) can decrease the enhanced vulnerability to oxidative stress that occurs in aging and these reductions are expressed as improvements in behavior. Collaborative findings indicate that blueberry or Concord grape juice supplementation in humans with mild **cognitive impairment** increased verbal memory performance, thus translating our animal findings to humans."

Alzheimer's disease

Grape derived polyphenols attenuate tau neuropathology in a mouse model of **Alzheimer's disease.** Wang J, Santa-Maria I, Ho L, Et al. J Alzheimers Dis. 2010;22(2):653-61. **Key Finding**: "Oral administration of grape seed polyphenol extract significantly attenuated the development of Alzheimer's disease type tau neuropathology in the brain of TMHT mouse model through mechanisms associated with attenuation of extracellular signal-receptor kinase ½ signaling in the brain."

Antioxidation

Antioxidant and antigenotoxic activities of purple grape juice – organic and conventional – in adult rats. Dani C, Oliboni LS, Umezu FM, Pasquali MA, Salvador M, Moreira JC, Henriques JA. J Med Food. 2009 Oct;12(5):1111-8. **Key Finding:** "The aim of this study was to evaluate the protection of organic and conventional purple grape juices in brain, liver, and plasma from adult Wistar rats against the oxidative damage provoked by carbon tetrachloride. The chemical and analytical determination showed that the highest levels of total phenolic, resveratrol, and catechins were seen in organic purple grape juices. In all treatment groups it was observed that in all tissue and plasma, treatment increased the lipid peroxidation levels. Both grape juices were capable to reduce LP levels in cerebral cortex and hippocampus; however, in the striatum and substantia nigra on the organic grape juice reduced LP level."

Black grape and garlic extracts protect against cyclosporine a nephrotoxicity. Durak I, Cetin R, Candir O, Devrim E, Kilicoglu B, Avci A. Immunol Invest. 2007;36(1):105-14. **Key Finding:** "The results suggest that impaired oxidant/antioxidant balance may play part in the CsA-induced nephrotoxicity, and some foods with high **antioxidant** power may ameliorate this toxicity, in agreement with studies with antioxidant vitamins."

*Comparison of the **antioxidant** effects of Concord grape juice flavonoids alpha-tocopherol on markers of oxidative stress in healthy adults.* O'Byrne DJ, Devaraj S, Grundy SM, Jialal I. Am J Clin Nutr. 2002 Dec;76(6):1367-74. **Key Finding:** "Concord grape juice flavonoids are potent antioxidants that may protect against oxidative stress and reduce the risk of free radical damage and chronic diseases."

***Antioxidant** and antiproliferative activities of common fruits.* Sun J, Chu YF, Wu X, Liu RH. J Agric Food Chem. 2002 Dec 4;50(25):7449-54. **Key Finding:** "Phytochemicals, especially phenolics, in fruits and vegetables are suggested to be the major bioactive compound for the health benefits associated with reduced risk of chronic diseases such as **cardiovascular disease** and **cancer**. Cranberry had the highest total phenolic content, followed by apple, red grape, strawberry, pineapple, banana, peach, lemon, orange, pear, and grapefruit. Cranberry had the highest total antioxidant activity followed by apple, red grape, strawberry, peach, lemon, pear, banana, orange, grapefruit and pineapple. Antiproliferation activities were also studied in vitro using HepG(2) human liver-cancer cells, and cranberry showed the highest inhibitory effect followed by lemon, apple, strawberry, red grape, banana, grapefruit and peach."

Atherosclerosis

Effects of acute verjuice consumption with a high-cholesterol diet on some biochemical risk factors of atherosclerosis in rabbits. Setorki M, Asgary S, Eidi A, Et al. Med Sci Monit. 2010 Apr;16(4):BR124-130. **Key Finding**: "Verjuice is an acidic juice made from **unripe grape**. These results suggest that there might be an acute protective effect in the postprandial use of verjuice on some of the risk factors of **athero-sclerosis**, particularly as an antioxidant."

Cancer (colon; leukemia; prostate)

NFkappaB-dependent regulation of urokinase plasminogen activator by proanthocyanidin-rich **grape seed extract**: *effect on invasion by* **prostate cancer** *cells.* Uchino R, Madhy-astha R, Madhyastha H, Et al. Blood Coagul Fibrinolysis. 2010 Sep;21(6):528-33. **Key Finding**: "In-vitro experiments demonstrate the therapeutic property of grape seed extract as an antimetastatic agent by targeting uPA (urokinase plas-minogen activator system) in prostate cancer cells."

Apoptosis-inducing factor and caspase-dependent apoptotic pathways triggered by different **grape seed extracts** *on human* **colon cancer** *cell line Caco-2.* Dinicola S, Cucina A, Pasqualato A, Et al. Br J Nutr. 2010 Sep;104(6):824-32. **Key Finding**: "The focus of the present study is to determine the selective biological efficacy of grape seed extract obtained from three different sources on the human colon cancer cell line Caco-2. Irrespective of its source, high doses of grape seed extract induced a significant inhibition on Caco-2 cell growth."

Oligomer procyanidins from **grape seeds** *induce a paraptosis-like programmed cell death in human glioblastoma U-87 cells.* Zhang FJ, Yang JY, Mou YH, Et al. Pharm Biol. 2010 Aug;48(8):883-90. **Key Finding**: "We reported that F2, an oligomer procy-anidin fraction isolated from grape seeds, triggered an original form of cell death in U-87 human **glioblastoma cells**. We show that F2 induced a kind of cell death with a phenotype resembling morphological characteristics of paraptosis."

Intake of **grape-derived polyphenols** *reduces C26 tumor growth by inhibiting angio-genesis and inducing apoptosis.* Walter A, Etienne-Selloum N, Brasse D, Et al. FASEB J. 2010 Sep;24(9):3360-9. **Key Finding**: "Grape derived polyphenols effectively reduced the development of **colon carcinoma** tumors in vivo by blunting tumor vascularization and by inhibiting proliferation and promoting apoptosis of tumor cells subsequent to an up-regulation of tumor suppressor genes."

Anticancer and cancer chemo preventive potential of grape seed extract and other grape-based products. Kaur M, Agarwal C, Agarwal R. J Nutr. 2009 Sep;139(9):18065-125. **Key Finding:** "Completed studies from various scientific groups conclude that both grapes and grape-based products are excellent sources of various anti-cancer agents and their regular consumption should thus be beneficial to the general population."

Grape seed extract induces cell cycle arrest and apoptosis in human **colon carcinoma** *cells.* Kaur M, Mandair R, Agarwal R, Agarwal C. Nutr Cancer. 2008;60 (Suppl 1):2-11. **Key Finding:** "Our findings suggest that grape seed extract could be an effective CAM agent against colorectal cancer possibly due to its strong growth inhibitory and apoptosis-inducing effects."

Cranberry and Grape Seed Extracts Inhibit the Proliferative Phenotype of **Oral Squamous Cell Carcinomas**. Chatelain K, Phippen S, McCabe J, Teeters CA, O'Malley S, Kingsley K. Evid Based Complement Alternat Med. 2008 Jul 23. (Epub ahead of print). **Key Finding:** "This study represents one of the first comparative investigations of cranberry and grape seed extracts and their anti-proliferative effects on oral cancers. These observations provide evidence that cranberry and grape seed extracts not only inhibit oral cancer proliferation but also that the mechanism of this inhibition may function by triggering key apoptotic regulators in these cell lines."

Inhibition of **prostate cancer** *growth by muscadine grape skin extract and resveratrol through distinct mechanisms.* Hudson TS, Hartle DK, Hursting SD, Nunez NP, Wang TT, Young HA, Arany P, Green JE. Cancer Res. 2007 Sep 1;67(17):8396-405. **Key Finding:** "These results show that muscadine grape skin extract and resveratrol target distinct pathways to inhibit prostate cancer cell growth in this system and that the unique properties of MSKE suggest that it may be an important source for further development of chemo preventive or therapeutic agents against prostate cancer."

Purple grape juice inhibits 7,12-dimethylbenz[a]anthracene (DMBA)-induced rat **mammary tumorigenesis** *and in vivo DMBA-DNA adduct formation.* Jung KJ, Wallig MA, Singletary KW. Cancer Lett. 2006 Feb 28;233(2):279-88. **Key Finding:** "Grape juice constituents appear to have benefit in decreasing susceptibility of the rat mammary gland to the tumor-initiating action of DMBA."

Grape seed extract inhibits in vitro and in vivo growth of human **colorectal carcinoma** *cells.* Kaur M, Singh RP, Gu M, Agarwal R, Agarwal C. Clin Cancer Res.2006

Oct 15;12(20 Pt 1):6194-202. **Key Finding:** "Grape seed extract may be an effective chemo preventive agent against colorectal cancer, and that growth inhibitory and apoptotic effects of GSE against colorectal cancer could be mediated via an up-regulation of Cipl/p21."

Antioxidant *and antiproliferative activities of common fruits.* Sun J, Chu YF, Wu X, Liu RH. J Agric Food Chem. 2002 Dec 4;50(25):7449-54. **Key Finding:** "Phytochemicals, especially phenolics, in fruits and vegetables are suggested to be the major bioactive compound for the health benefits associated with reduced risk of chronic diseases such as **cardiovascular disease** and **cancer**. Cranberry had the highest total phenolic content, followed by apple, red grape, strawberry, pineapple, banana, peach, lemon, orange, pear, and grapefruit. Cranberry had the highest total antioxidant activity followed by apple, red grape, strawberry, peach, lemon, pear, banana, orange, grapefruit and pineapple. Antiproliferation activities were also studied in vitro using HepG(2) human liver-cancer cells, and cranberry showed the highest inhibitory effect followed by lemon, apple, strawberry, red grape, banana, grapefruit and peach."

Inhibition of rat ***mammary tumorigenesis*** *by concord grape juice constituents.* Singletary KW, Stansbury MJ, Giusti M, Van Breemen RB, Wallig M, Rimando A. J Agric Food Chem. 2003 Dec 3;51(25):7280-6. **Key Finding:** "These studies indicate that Concord grape juice constituents can inhibit the promotion stage of 7,12-dimethylbenz[a]anthracene (DMBA)-induced rat mammary tumorigenesis, in part by suppressing cell proliferation."

Cardiovascular Disease

eNOS activation induced by a polyphenol-rich grape skin extract in porcine ***coronary arteries***. Madeira SV, Auger C, Anselm E, Chataigneau M, Chataigneau T, Soares de Moura R, Schini-Kerth VB. J Vasc Res. 2009;46(5):406-16. **Key Finding:** "Grape skin extract causes endothelium-dependent NO-mediated relaxations of coronary arteries. This effect involves the intracellular formation of ROS in endothelial cells leading to the Src kinase/phosphinositide 3-kinase/Akt-dependent phosphorylation of eNOS."

Cardio protective *roles of aged garlic extract, grape seed proanthocyanidin, and hazelnut on doxorubicin-induced cardio toxicity.* Demirkaya E, Avci A, Kesik V, Karsliouglu Y, Oztas E, Kismet E, Gokcay E, Durak I, Koseoglu V. Can J Physiol Pharmacol. 2009 Aug;87(8):633-40. **Key Finding:** "The positive effects of natural antioxidant foods on the prevention of DXR-induced cardiac injury could not be clearly shown on the basis of antioxidant enzymes. However, the electron microscope changes clearly demonstrated the protective effects of aged garlic extract and grape seed proanthocyanidin. The supplementation of these antioxidant foods over longer periods may show more definitive results. Human studies with different doses are needed to evaluate the effects of these foods on the human heart."

Card protective actions of grape polyphenols. Leifert WR, Abeywardena MY. Nutr Res. 2008 Nov;28(11):729-37. **Key Finding**: "Consumption of grape and grape products may be beneficial in preventing the development of chronic degenerative diseases such as **cardiovascular disease**."

Grape juice causes endothelium-dependent relaxation via a redox-sensitive Src- and Akt-dependent activation of eNOS. Anselm E, Chataigneau M, Ndiaye M, Chataigneau T, Schini-Kerth VB. Cardiovasc Res. 2007 Jan 15;73(2):404-13. **Key Finding:** "Concord grape juice induces endothelium-dependent relaxations of **coronary arteries**, which involve a nitric oxide-mediated component and also, to a minor extent, an EDHF-mediated component."

Concentrated red grape juice exerts antioxidant, hypolipidemic, and anti-inflammatory effects in both hemodialysis patients and healthy subjects. Castilla P, Echarri R, Davalos A, Cerrato F, Ortega H, Teruel JL, Lucas MF, Gomez-Coronado D, Ortuno J, Lasuncion MA. Am J Clin Nutr. 2006 Jul;84(1):252-62. **Key Finding:** "Dietary supplementation with concentrated red grape juice improves the lipoprotein profile, reduces plasma concentrations of inflammatory biomarkers and oxidized LDL, and may favor a reduction in **cardiovascular disease** risk."

Antioxidant *and antiproliferative activities of common fruits.* Sun J, Chu YF, Wu X, Liu RH. J Agric Food Chem. 2002 Dec 4;50(25):7449-54. **Key Finding:** "Phytochemicals, especially phenolic, in fruits and vegetables are suggested to be the major bioactive compound for the health benefits associated with reduced risk of chronic diseases such as **cardiovascular disease** and **cancer**. Cranberry had the highest total phenolic content, followed by apple, red grape, strawberry, pineapple, banana, peach, lemon, orange, pear, and grapefruit. Cranberry had the highest total antioxidant activity followed by apple, red grape, strawberry, peach, lemon, pear, banana, orange, grapefruit and pineapple. Antiproliferation activities were also studied in vitro using HepG(2) human liver-cancer cells, and cranberry showed the highest inhibitory effect followed by lemon, apple, strawberry, red grape, banana, grapefruit and peach."

Grape polyphenols exert a cardio protective effect in pre- and postmenopausal women by lowering plasma lipids and reducing oxidative stress. Zern TL, Wood RJ, Greene C, West KL, Liu Y, Aggarwal D, Shachter NS, Fernandez ML. J Nutr. 2005 Aug;135(8):1911-7. **Key Finding:** "Through alterations in lipoprotein metabolism, oxidative stress, and inflammatory markers, lyophilized grape powder intake beneficially affected key risk factors for **coronary heart disease** in both pre- and postmenopausal women."

Select flavonoids and whole juice from purple grapes inhibit platelet function and enhance nitric oxide release. Freedman JE, Parker C, Li L, Perlman JA, Frei B, Ivanov V, Deak LR, Iafrati MD, Folts JD. Circulation. 2001 Jun 12;103(23):2792-8. **Key Finding:** "Both in vitro incubation and oral supplementation with purple grape juice decrease platelet aggregation, increase platelet-derived NO release, and decrease superoxide production. The suppression of platelet-mediated thrombosis represents a potential mechanism for the beneficial effects of purple grape products, independent of alcohol consumption, in **cardiovascular disease.**"

Purple Grape Juice Improves Endothelial Function and Reduces the Susceptibility of LDL Cholesterol to Oxidation in Patients with **Coronary Artery Disease**. Stein JH, Keevil JG, Wiebe DA, Aeschlimann S, Folts JD. Circulation. 1999;100:1050-1055. **Key Finding:** "Short-term ingestion of purple grape juice improves flow-mediated vasodilation and reduces LDL susceptibility to oxidation in coronary artery disease patients. Improved endothelium-dependent vasodilation and prevention of LDL oxidation are potential mechanisms by which flavonoids in purple grape products may prevent cardiovascular events, independent of alcohol content."

Cholesterol

Effects of grape pomace on the antioxidant defense system in diet-induced hypercholesterolemic rabbits. Choi CS, Chung HK, Choi MK, Kang MH. Nutr Res Pract. 2010 Apr;4(2):114-20. **Key Finding**: "**Grape pumice** (grape seed extract and grape peel powder) supplementation is considered to activate the antioxidant enzyme system and prevent damage with **hypercholesterolemia.**"

Red grape juice polyphenols alter **cholesterol** *homeostasis and increase LDL-receptor activity in human cells in vitro.* Davalos A, Fernandez-Hernando C, Cerrato F, Martinez-Botas J, Gomez-Coronado D, Gomez-Cordoves C, Lasuncion MA. J Nutr. 2006 Jul;136(7):1766-73. **Key Finding:** "These results indicate that red grape juice polyphenols disrupt or delay LDL trafficking through the endocytic pathway, thus preventing LDL cholesterol from exerting regulatory effects on intracellular lipid homeostasis."

Colitis

*Effects of proanthocyanidin from **grape seed** on treatment of recurrent ulcerative **colitis** in rats.* Wang YH, Yang XL, Wang L, Et al. Can J Physiol Pharmacol. 2010 Sep;88(9):888-98. **Key Finding**: "Grape seed proanthocyanidin exerted a protective effect on recurrent colitis in rats by modifying the inflammatory response, inhibiting inflammatory cell infiltration and antioxidation damage, promoting damaged tissue repair to improve colonic oxidative stress, and inhibiting colonic iNOS activity to reduce the production of nitric oxide."

Diabetes

*Antioxidant rich **grape pomace** extract suppresses postprandial hyperglycemia in diabetic mice by specifically inhibiting alpha-glucosidase.* Hogan S, Zhang L, Li J, Et al. Nutr Metab. 2010 Aug 27;7:71. **Key Finding**: "This is the first report that the grape pomace extracts selectively and significantly inhibits intestinal a-glucosidase and suppresses postprandial hyperglycemia in diabetic mice and therefore suggest a potential for utilizing grape pomace-derived bioactive compounds in management of **diabetes**."

***Type 2 diabetes** and glycemic response to grapes or grape products.* Zunino S. J Nutr. 2009 Sep;139(9):1794S-800S. **Key Finding:** "With a low mean glycemic index and glycemic load, grapes or grape products may provide health benefits to type 2 diabetics."

Hypertension

***Whole grape** intake impacts cardiac peroxisome proliferator-activator receptor and nuclear factor kappaB activity and cytokine expression in rats with diastolic dysfunction.* Seymour EM, Bennink MR, Watts SW, Bolling SF. Hypertension. 2010 May;55(5):1179-85. **Key Finding**: "Prolonged **hypertension** is the leading cause of heart failure. Grape-fed rats showed significantly reduced cardiac tumor necrosis factor-alpha and transforming growth factor-beta protein expression, increased inhibitor-kappaBalpha expression, and reduced cardiac fibrosis."

Inflammation

Grape seed and skin extracts inhibit platelet function and release of reactive oxygen intermediates. Vitseva O, Varghese S, Chakrabarti S, Folts JD, Freedman JE. J Cardiovasc Pharmacol. 2005 Oct;46(4):445-51. **Key Finding:** "The extracts from purple grape skins and seeds inhibit platelet function and platelet-dependent inflammatory responses at pharmacologically relevant concentrations. These findings suggest potentially beneficial platelet-dependent **antithrombotic** and **anti-inflammatory** properties of purple grape-derived flavonoids."

Obesity

*Effects of Grape Pomace Antioxidant Extract on Oxidative Stress and Inflammation in Diet Induced **Obese** Mice.* Hogan S, Canning C, Sun S, Et al. J Agric Food Chem. 2010 Oct 7 (Epub ahead of print.) **Key Finding**: "**Grape pomace extract** after 12-week treatment lowered plasma C-reactive protein levels by 15.5% in the high fat diet fed mice. The results showed that Norton grape pomace extract contained significant antioxidants and dietary grape pomace extract exerted an anti-inflammatory effect in diet induced obesity."

Oral health

*Grape products and **oral health**.* Wu CD. J Nutr. 2009 Sep;139(9):1818S-23S. **Key Finding:** "Grape seed extract, high in proanthocyanidin, positively affected the in vitro demineralization and/or remineralization processes of artificial root caries lesions, suggesting its potential as a promising natural agent for noninvasive root caries therapy. Raisins represent a healthy alternative to the commonly consumed sugary snack foods."

Thrombosis

Grape seed and skin extracts inhibit platelet function and release of reactive oxygen intermediates. Vitseva O, Varghese S, Chakrabarti S, Folts JD. Freedman JE. J Cardiovasc Pharmacol. 2005 Oct;46(4):445-51. **Key Finding:** "The extracts from purple grape skins and seeds inhibit platelet function and platelet-dependent inflammatory responses at pharmacologically relevant concentrations. These findings suggest potentially beneficial platelet-dependent **antithrombotic** and **anti-inflammatory** properties of purple grape-derived flavonoids."

Lemons and Limes

OF ALL THE CITRUS FRUITS, lemons and limes possess some of the strongest fragrance and flavors thanks to high levels of citric acid, flavonoids, and limonoids. This sharp flavor is an indicator that they're a great source of vitamin C and phytochemicals.

Agricultural experts believe that almost all varieties of cultivated citrus are hybrids derived from just four ancestral species. All lemons and most limes are considered to be hybrids. Some of the more promising experimental results with lemons and limes have found the limonoid content to be effective against at least six types of cancer.

Cancer (breast; colon; neuroblastoma; oral; pancreatic; skin)

Bioactive compounds from Mexican lime (Citrus aurantifolia) juice induce apoptosis in **human pancreatic** *cells.* Patil JR, Chidambara Murthy KN, Jayaprakasha GK, Chetti MG, Patil BS. J Agric Food Chem. 2009 Nov 25;57(22):10933-42. **Key Finding:** "All of the extracts of lime juice inhibited Panc-28 **cancer** cell growth. The inhibition of Panc-28 cells was in the range of 73-89% at 100 microg/ml. at 96 h. The results of the present study clearly indicate that antioxidant activity is proportionate to the content of flavonoids and proliferation inhibition ability is proportionate to the content of both flavonoids and limonoids (limonexic acid, isolimonexic acid and limonin)."

Antiproliferative effects of citrus limonoids against human **neuroblastoma and colonic adenocarcinoma** *cells.* Poulose SM, Harris ED, Patil BS. Nutr Cancer. 2006;56(1):103-12. **Key Finding**: Limonoids were tested against two human cancer cell lines, SH-SY5Y neuroblastoma and Caco-2 colonic adenocarcinoma. The results confirm that limonoids exert a strong multifaceted lethal action against cancer cells."

Citrus limonoids induce apoptosis in human **neuroblastoma** *cells and have radical scavenging activity.* Poulose SM, Harris ED, Patil BS. J Nutr. 2005 Apr;135(4):870-7. **Key Finding**: "We conclude that citrus limonoid glucosides are toxic to SH-SY5Y cancer cells. Cytotoxicity is exerted through apoptosis by an as yet unknown mechanism of induction."

Further studies on the anticancer activity of citrus limonoids. Miller EG, Porter JL, Binnie WH, Guo IY, Hasegawa S. J Agric Food Chem. 2004 Jul 28;52(15):4908-12. **Key Finding**: "Research in this laboratory has shown that some citrus limonoids can inhibit the development of 7,12-dimethylbenz{a}anthracene-induced **oral tumors**. In this experiment three limonoids (ichangensin, deoxylimonin, and obacunone) were tested for cancer chemo preventive activity. Obacunone reduced tumor number and burden by 25 to 40%; deoxylimonin reduced tumor number and burden by 30 to 50%."

Differential inhibition of human cancer cell proliferation by citrus limonoids. Tian Q, Miller EG, Ahmad H, Tang L, Patil BS. Nutr Cancer. 2001;40(2):180-4. **Key Finding:** "Limonoids have been shown to inhibit the growth of estrogen receptor-negative and –positive human **breast cancer** cells in culture. Four limonoids and a limonoid glucoside mixture had significant effects against MCF-7 breast cancer cells treated. All the limonoid samples could induce apoptosis in MCF-7 cells."

*Citrus peel use is associated with reduced risk of squamous cell **carcinoma of the skin**.* Hakim IA, Harris RB, Ritenbaugh C. Nutr Cancer. 2000;37(2):161-8. Key Finding: "Limonene has demonstrated efficacy in preclinical models of breast and colon cancers. The principal sources of d-limonene are the oils of orange, grapefruit, and lemon. The present case-control study was designed to determine the usual citrus consumption patterns of an older Southwestern population and to then evaluate how this citrus consumption varied with history of squamous cell carcinoma of the skin. We found no association between the overall consumption of citrus fruits or citrus juices and skin squamous cell carcinoma. However, the most striking feature was the protection purported by citrus peel consumption. Moreover, there was a dose-response relationship between higher citrus peel in the diet and degree of risk lowering. This is the first study to explore the relationship between higher citrus peel consumption and human cancers."

Cholesterol

Lime-treated maize husks lower plasma LDL-cholesterol levels in normal and hypercholesterolemic adult men from northern Mexico. Vidal-Quintanar RL, Mendivil RL, Pena M, Fernandez ML, Br J Nutr. 1999 Apr;81(4):281-8. **Key Finding**: Lime-treated maize husks, a by-product of tortilla manufacturing in Mexico, reduces plasma LDL-cholesterol levels in healthy and hypercholesterolemic subjects. LDL-cholesterol was reduced by 25% and improved the LDL:HDL value by 29-33%.

Diabetes

*Dietary sources of aldose reductase inhibitors: prospects for alleviating **diabetic** complications.* Sarawat M, Muthenna P, Suryanarayana P, Petrash JM, Reddy GB. Asia Pac J Clin Nutr. 2008;17(4):558-65. **Key Finding**: "Among 22 dietary sources tested for aldose reductase inhibitory potential to treat secondary complications of diabetes, 10 showed considerable inhibitory potential. These include spinach, black pepper, cumin, and **lemon**."

Immune system

Citrus pectin affects cytokine production by human peripheral blood mononuclear cells. Salman H, Bergman M, Djaldetti M, Orlin J, Bessler H. Biomed Pharmacother. 2008 Nov;62(9):579-82. **Key Finding**: "Pectin has anti-oxidative, hypocholesterolemic and anti-cancerous effects. The present study was undertaken to examine the effect of citrus pectin on the immune system via cytokine production by human peripheral blood cells. The findings indicate that citrus pectin possesses the capacity to exert an immunomodulatory response which may have a favorable effect on human health."

Obesity

*Lemon Polyphenols Suppress Diet-Induced **Obesity** by Up-Regulation of mRNA Levels of the Enzymes involved in beta-Oxidation in Mouse White Adipose Tissue.* Fukuchi Y, Hiramitsu M, Okada M, Hayashi S, Nabeno Y, Osawa T, Naito M. J Clin Biochem Nutr. 2008 Nov;43(3):201-9. **Key Finding**: "Feeding with lemon polyphenols suppressed body weight gain and body fat accumulation by increasing peroxisomal beta-oxidation through up-regulation of the mRNA level of ACO in the liver and white adipose tissue."

Oral thrush

*Treatment of **oral thrush** in HIV/AIDS patients with lemon juice and lemon grass (Cymbopogon citrates) and gentian violet.* Wright SC, Maree JE, Sibanyoni M. Phytomedicine. 2009 Mar;16(2-3):118-24. **Key Finding**: "The use of lemon juice and lemon grass for the treatment of oral candidiasis in an HIV population was validated by the randomized controlled trial."

Urinary stones

Lemonade therapy increases urinary citrate and urine volumes in patients with recurrent calcium oxalate stone formation. Penniston KL, Steele TH, Nakada SY. Urology. 2007 Nov;70(5):856-60. **Key Finding**: "Lemonade therapy resulted in favorable changes in urinary citrate and total urine volume."

Mushrooms (Maitake and Shiitake)

MUSHROOMS ARE THE SPORE-BEARING fruiting bodies of fungi, usually found aboveground. They have a long history among tribal cultures throughout the world for their medicinal properties and, secondarily, as a food source. Maitake and shiitake mushrooms, among the mushroom species most studied by contemporary medical science, have long been a fixture in traditional Chinese medicine.

These two mushrooms species have considerable documented benefits, alleviating at least sixteen health conditions, ranging from eleven types of cancer to diabetes and even malaria. Polysaccharides from these mushrooms are often identified as a key reason for the health-promoting effects observed in laboratory experiments.

Anti-Bacterial, Anti-Fungal

An examination of **antibacterial** *and* **antifungal** *properties of constituents of Shiitake (Lentinula edodes) and oyster (Pleurotus ostreatus) mushrooms.* Hearst R, Nelson D, McCollum G, Millar BC, Maeda Y, Goldsmith CE, Rooney PJ, Loughrey A, Rao JR, Moore JE. Complement Ther Clin Pract. 2009 Feb;15(1):5-7. **Key Finding**: "Aqueous extracts were tested against a panel of 29 bacterial and 10 fungal pathogens for the demonstration of microbial inhibition. Our data quantitatively showed that Shiitake mushroom extract had extensive antimicrobial activity against 85% of the organisms it was tested on."

Wild and commercial mushrooms as source of nutrients and nutraceuticals. Barros L, Cruz T, Baptista P, Estevinho LM, Ferreira IC. Food Chem Toxicol. 2008 Aug;46(8):2742-7. **Key Finding:** Experiments were performed in wild and commercial species of mushrooms to analyze nutrient and phytochemical levels. Commercial species seemed to have higher concentrations of sugars, while wild species had higher contents of alpha-Tocopherol. Wild also had a higher content of phenols but a lower content of ascorbic acid than commercial species. There was no difference found in the **antimicrobial** properties of wild and commercial species.

Antibiotic *properties of the strains of the basidiomycete Lentinus edodes.* Soboleva A, Krasnopolskaia LM, Fedorova GB, Katrukha GS. Antibiot Khimioter (Russian). 2006;51(7):3-8. **Key Finding**: "Antibiotic properties of the extracts from the fermentation broth and mycelium of 15 strains of the edible and medicinal basidomycete L. edodes were studied and it was shown that the extracts were active against gram-positive and gram-negative bacteria, yeasts and mycelia fungi, including dermatophytes and phytopathogens."

Atherosclerosis

The bioactive agent ergothioneine, a key component of dietary mushrooms, inhibits monocyte binding to endothelial cells characteristic of early cardiovascular disease. Martin KR. J Med Food. 2010 Dec;13(6):1340-6. **Key Finding**: "These data provide evidence that ergothioneine found in commonly consumed dietary mushrooms can protect against events observed in **atherogenesis,** suggesting increased dietary intake of edible mushrooms would be a prudent medicinal means of reducing cardiovascular disease risk."

Antiatherosclerotic effect of the edible mushrooms Pleurotus eryngii (Eringi), Grifola frondosa (Maitake), and Hypsizygus marmoreus (Bunashimeji) in apolipoptortin E-deficient mice. Mori K, Kobayashi C, Tomita T, Inatomi S, Ikeda M. Nutr Res. 2008 May;28(5):335-42. **Key Finding**: "Supplementation of the 3 edible mushrooms prevents the development of **atherosclerosis.** Antiatherosclerotic effect is partly via lowering of serum TC concentrations."

Cancer (bladder; brain; breast; colon; esophageal; gastric; liver; lung; prostate; rectum; skin)

*Synergistic potentiation of interferon activity with **maitake** mushroom d-fraction on **bladder cancer** cells.* Louie B, Rajamahanty S, Won J, Et al. BJU Int. 2010 Apr;105(7):1011-5. **Key Finding**: "The combination of interferon-alpha and maitake mushroom D-fraction reduced growth by approximately 75% in T24 bladder cancer cells. This appears to be due to a synergistic potentiation of these two agents inducing a G9!) arrest with DNA-PK activation."

*Commonly consumed and specialty dietary mushrooms reduce cellular proliferation in MCF-7 human **breast cancer** cells.* Martin KR, Brophy SK. Exp Biol Med. 2010 Nov;235(11):1306-14. **Key Finding**: "Overall, all test mushrooms significantly suppressed cellular proliferation with **maitake** further significantly inducing apoptosis and cytotoxicity in human breast cancer cells. This suggests that both common and specialty mushrooms may be chemo protective against breast cancer."

Novel medicinal mushroom blend suppresses growth and invasiveness of human **breast cancer** *cells.* Jiang J, Silva D. Int J Oncol. 2010 Dec;37(6):1529-36. **Key Finding:** "MycoPhyto Complex (MC) is a novel medicinal mushroom blend which consists of mushroom mycelia from the species Agaricus blazei, Codryceps sinensis, Coriolus versicolor, Ganoderma lucidum, Grifola frondosa and Polyporus umbellaturs. Here we shot that MC demonstrates cytostatic effects through the inhibition of cell proliferation and cell cycle arrest at the G2/M phase of highly invasive human breast cancer cells MDA-MB-231."

Effect of the culture extract of Lentinus edodes mycelia on splenic sympathetic activity and cancer cell proliferation. Shen J, Tanida M, Fujisaki Y, Horii Y, Hashimoto K, Nagai K. Uton Neurosci. 2009 Jan 28;145(1-2):50-4. **Key Finding**: "These findings suggest that shiitake mushroom has tumor-inhibitory effects in the tumor volume of human **colon and breast cancer** cells implanted in athymic nude mice."

Possible disease remission in patient with invasive **bladder cancer** *with D-fraction regimen.* Rajamahanty S, Louie B, O'Neill C, Choudhury M, Konno S. Int J Gen Med. 2009 Jul 30;2:15-7. **Key Finding**: "D-fraction, the bioactive extract of Maitake mushroom, is a natural agent that may have clinical implications in patients with superficial bladder tumors."

Synergistic potentiation of D-fraction with vitamin C as possible alternative approach for **cancer** *therapy.* Konno S. Int J Gen Med. 2009 Jul 30;2:91-108. **Key Finding**: "Maitake mushroom D-fraction in numerous studies performed in vitro and in vivo or in clinical settings showed that it was capable of modulating immunologic and hematologic parameters, inhibiting or regressing the cancer cell growth. Synergistic potentiation of Maitake D-fraction with vitamin C demonstrated in vitro may have clinical implication because such combination therapy appears to help improve the efficacy of currently ongoing cancer therapies."

A phase I/II trial of polysaccharide extract from Grifola frondose (Maitake mushroom) in **breast cancer** *patients: immunological effects.* Deng G, Lin H, Seidman A, Fornier M, D'Andrea G, Wesa K, Yeung S, Cunningham-Rundles S, Vickers AJ, Cassileth B. J Cancer Res Clin Oncol. 2009 Sep;135(9):1215-21. **Key Finding**: "Oral administration of a polysaccharide extract from Maitake mushroom is associated with both immunologically stimulatory and inhibitory measurable effects in peripheral blood. Cancer patients should be made aware of the fact that botanical agents produce more complex effects than assumed, and may depress as well as enhance immune function."

*Antitumor effects of a water-soluble extract from Maitake (Grifola frondosa) on human **gastric cancer** cell lines.* Shomori K, Yamamoto M, Arifuku I, Teramachi K, Ito H. Oncol Rep. 2009 Sep;22(3):615-20. **Key Finding**: "These results suggest that Maitake extract induces apoptosis of TMK-1 human gastric cancer cells by caspase-3-dependent and independent pathways, resulting in potential antitumor effects on gastric cancer."

Maitake beta-glucan enhances therapeutic effect and reduces myelosupression and nephrotoxicity of cisplatin in mice. Masuda Y, Inoue M, Miyata A, Mizuno S, Nanba H. Int Immunopharmacol. 2009 May;9(5):620-6. **Key Finding**: "These results suggest that MD-Fraction from maitake in combination with cisplatin, an anticancer drug, cannot only enhance **antitumor** and antimetastatic activity, but also reduce cisplatin-induced myelotoxicity and nephrotoxicity."

*Pleurotus ostreatus inhibits proliferation of human **breast and colon cancer** cells through p53-dependent as well as p53-independent pathway.* Jedinak A, Silva D. Int J Oncol. 2008 Dec;33(6):1307-13. **Key Finding**: "In the present study we evaluated whether extracts from edible mushrooms Agaricus bisporus (portabella), Flammulina velutipes (enoki), Lentinula edodes (shiitake) and Pleurotus ostreatus (oyster) affect the growth of breast and colon cancer cells. Here, we identified was the most potent, P. ostreatus (oyster mushroom) which suppressed proliferation of breast cancer (MCF-7, MDA-MB-231) and colon cancer (HT-29, HCT-116) cells, without affecting proliferation of epithelial mammary MCF-10A and normal colon FHC cells. Our results indicated that the edible oyster mushroom has potential therapeutic/preventive effects on breast and colon cancer."

*Inhibitory effect of MD-Fraction on tumor metastasis: involvement of NK cell activation and suppression of intercellular adhesion molecule (ICAM)-1 expression in **lung vascular** endothelial cells.* Masuda Y, Murata Y, Hayashi M, Nanba H. Biol Pharm Bull. 2008 Jun;31(6):1104-8. **Key Finding**: "These results suggest that MD-Fraction from the maitake mushroom inhibits tumor metastasis by activating NK cells and APCs, and by suppressing of ICAM-1 leading to the inhibition of tumor cell adhesion to vascular endothelial cells."

A polysaccharide extracted from rice bran fermented with Lentinus edodes enhances natural killer cell activity and exhibits anticancer effects. Kim HY, Kim JH, Yang SB, Hong SG, Lee SA, Hwang SJ, Shin KS, Suh HJ, Park MH. J Med Food. 2007 Mar;10(1):25-31. **Key Finding**: "We suggest that the administration of rice bran cultured with Lentinus edodes may be effective for preventing and/or treating **cancer** through NK cell activation."

Induction of apoptosis in SGC-7901 cells by polysaccharide-peptide GFPS1b from the cultured mycelia of Grifola frondosa GF9801. Cui FJ, Li Y, Xu YY, Liu ZQ, Huang DM, Zhang ZC, Tao WY. Toxicol In Vitro. 2007 Apr;21(3):417-27. **Key Finding:** "GFPPS1b, a novel polysaccharide-peptide isolated from Grifola frondosa, has **anti-tumor** activity and can significantly inhibit the proliferation of SGC-7901 cells, whereas slightly influences the growth of human normal liver cell line L-02."

*Effect of various natural products on growth of **bladder cancer** cells: two promising mushroom extracts.* Konno S. Altern Med Rev. 2007 Mar;12(1):63-8. **Key Finding**: "The present study indicates that GD- and PL-fractions mushroom extracts demonstrated a significant (>90 percent) growth reduction in 72 hours in human bladder cancer T24 cells. Vitamin C appears to act synergistically with these fractions to potentiate their bioactivity."

Antitumor activities of O-sulfonated derivatives of (1>3)-alpha-D-glucan from different Lentinus edodes. Unursaikhan S, Xu X, Zeng F, Zhang L. Biosci Biotechnol Biochem. 2006 Jan;70(1):38-46. **Key Finding:** "The in vivo and in vitro antitumor activities of the native alpha-D-glucans and their O-sulfonated derivatives (from four kinds of fruiting bodies of Lentinus edodes) against solid **tumor Sarcoma** 180 cells were evaluated. All of the O-sulfonated derivatives exhibited higher antitumor activities than those of the native glucans."

Inhibition of growth and induction of apoptosis in human cancer cell lines by an ethyl acetate fraction from shiitake mushrooms. Fang N, Li Q, Yu S, Zhang J, He L, Ronis MJ, Badger TM. J Altern Complement Med. 2006 Mar;12(2):125-32. **Key Finding**: "These data suggest that inhibition of growth in tumor cells (two human **breast carcinoma** cells lines, MDA-MB-453 and MCF-7) by 'mycochemicals' in shiitake mushrooms may result from induction of apoptosis."

Protection against D-galactosamine-induced acute liver injury by oral administration of extracts from Lentinus edodes mycelia. Watanabe A, Kobayashi M, Hayashi S, Kodama D, Isoda K, Kondoh M, Kawase M, Tamesada M, Yagi K.

Biol Pharm Bull. 2006 Aug;29(8):1651-4. **Key Finding**: "Our findings indicate that an extract of Lentinus edodes administration is a promising treatment for protecting the **liver** from acute injury."

*Anti-tumor activities of lentinan and micellapist in **tumor**-bearing mice.* Maruyama S, Sukekawa Y, Kaneko Y, Fujimoto S. Gan To Kagaku Ryoho (Japanese). 2006 Nov;33(12):1726-9. **Key Finding**: "In the mice treated with Lentinan (isolated from shiitake mushroom) CD8-positive cells appeared to have suppressed tumor cell proliferation."

o-Orsellinaldehyde from the submerged culture of the edible mushroom Grifola frondosa exhibits selective cytotoxic effects against Hep 3B cells through apoptosis. Lin JT, Liu WH. J Agric Food Chem. 2006 Oct 4;54(20):7564-9. **Key Finding:** "Grifola frondosa extract showed a selective cytotoxic effect against Hep 3B cells (human **carcinoma**) and MRC-5, normal human lung fibroblast."

Characterization and immunomodulating activities of polysaccharide from Lentinus edodes. Zheng R, Jie S, Hanchuan D, Moucheng W. Int Immunopharmacol. 2005 May;5(5):811-20. **Key Finding**: "We evaluated the effects of the polysaccharide L-II (from the fruiting body of Lentinus edodes) on the cellular immune response of **Sarcoma** 180-bearing mice. Results of these studies demonstrated the antitumor activity of the polysaccharide L-II on mice-transplanted sarcoma 180 was mediated by **immunomodulation** in inducing T-cells and macrophage-dependent immune system responses."

Maitake D-Fraction enhances antitumor effects and reduces immunosuppression by mitomycin-C in tumor-bearing mice. Kodama N, Murata Y, Asakawa A, Inui A, Hayashi M, Sakai N, Nanba H. Nutrition. 2005 May;21(5):624-9. **Key Finding**: "These results suggest that D-Fraction can decrease the effective dosage in tumor-bearing mice by increasing the proliferation, differentiation, and activation of immunocompetent cells and thus provide a potential clinical benefit for patients with **cancer.**"

Selective induction of apoptosis in murine skin carcinoma cells (CH72) by an ethanol extract of Lentinula edodes. Gu YH, Belury MA. Cancer Lett. 2005 Mar 18;220(1):21-8. **Key Finding**: "Cell cycle analysis demonstrated that L. edodes extract induced a transient G(1) arrest in **skin carcinoma** cells with no changes observed in the non-tumorigenic cells."

Lentinan from shiitake mushroom (Lentinus edodes) suppresses expression of cytochrome P450 1A subfamily in the mouse liver. Okamoto T, Kodoi R, Nonaka

Y, Fukuda I, Hashimoto T, Kanazawa K, Misuno M, Ashida H. Bio factors. 2004;21(1-4):407-9. **Key Finding**: "Our studies have demonstrated that lentinan suppresses hepatic CYP1As expression in the both constitutive and inducible levels through the production of **tumor necrosis** factor-alpha and an increase in the DNA-binding activity of nuclear factor-kappaB."

*Maitake beta-glucan MD-fraction enhances **bone marrow** colony formation and reduces doxorubicin toxicity in vitro.* Lin H, She YH, Cassileth BR, Sirotnak F, Cunningham RS. Int Immunopharmacol. 2004 Jan;4(1):91-9. **Key Finding**: "These studies provided the first evidence that MD-fraction from maitake acts directly in a dose dependent manner on hematopoietic BMC and enhances bone marrow cells growth and differentiation into colony forming cells."

*Lentin, a novel and potent antifungal protein from shitake mushroom with inhibitory effects on activity of human immunodeficiency virus-1 reverse transcriptase and proliferation of **leukemia** cells.* Ngai PH, Ng TB. Life Sci. 2003 Nov 14;73(26):3363-74. **Key Finding**: "From the fruiting bodies of the edible mushroom Lentinus edodes, a novel protein designated lentin with potent antifungal activity was isolated. Lentin exerted an inhibitory activity on HIV-1 reverse transcriptase and proliferation of leukemia cells."

*Effect of Maitake (Grifola frondosa) D-Fraction on the activation of NK cells in **cancer** patients.* Kodama N, Komuta K, Nanba H. Med Food. 2003 Winter;6(4):371-7. **Key Finding**: "In the present study, we administered maitake D-Fraction to cancer patients without anticancer drugs, and at the same time NK cell activity was monitored. Maitake D-Fraction hindered metastatic progress, lessened the expression of tumor markers, and increased NK cell activity in all patients examined. Maitake D-Fraction appears to repress cancer progression and primarily exerts its effect through stimulation of NK activity."

*White button mushroom phytochemicals inhibit aromatase activity and **breast cancer** cell proliferation.* Grube BJ, Eng ET, Kao YC, Kwon A, Chen S. J Nutr. 2001 Dec;131(12):3288-93. **Key Finding:** "Phytochemicals in the mushroom aqueous extract inhibited aromatase activity and proliferation of MCF-7aro cells. These results suggest that diets high in mushrooms may modulate the aromatase activity and function in chemoprevention in postmenopausal women by reducing the in situ production of estrogen."

*Dietary intakes of mushrooms and green tea combine to reduce the risk of **breast cancer** in Chinese women.* Zhang M, Huang J, Xie X, Holman CD. Int J Cancer.

2009 Mar 15;124(6):1404-8. **Key Finding:** "We conclude that higher dietary intake of mushrooms decreased breast cancer risk in pre and postmenopausal Chinese women and an additional decreased risk of breast cancer from joint effect of mushrooms and green tea was observed."

Inhibition of human **colon carcinoma** *development by lentinan from shiitake mushrooms (Lentinus edodes).* Ng ML, Yap AT. J Altern Complement Med. 2002 Oct;8(5):581-9. **Key Finding**: "This study showed that the antitumor property of lentinan was maintained with oral administration. In addition, 'primed' lymphocytes, when given passively to immunodeficient mice, were able to retard the development of tumors in these mice."

Can maitake MD-fraction aid cancer patients? Kodama N, Komuta K, Nanba H. Altern Med Rev. 2002 Jun;7(3):236-9. **Key Finding**: "In this non-random case series, a combination of MD-fraction and whole maitake powder was investigated to determine its effectiveness for 22- to 57-year old cancer patients in stages II-IV. Cancer regression or significant symptom improvement was observed in 58.3 percent of **liver cancer** patients, 68.8 percent of **breast cancer** patients, and 62.5 percent of **lung cancer** patients. The trial found a less than 10-20 percent improvement for **leukemia, stomach cancer, and brain cancer** patients."

Chemo sensitization of carmustine with maitake beta-glucan on androgen-independent prostatic cancer cells: involvement of glyoxalase I. Finkelstein MP, Aynehchi S, Samadi AA, Drinis S, Choudhury MS, Taxaki H, Konno S. J Altern Complement Med. 2002 Oct;8(5):573-80. **Key Finding**: "This study demonstrates a sensitized cytotoxic effect of the anticancer agent carmustine with beta-glucan in PC-3 cells, which was associated with a drastic (approximately 80%) inactivation of Gly-I, which appears to be critically involved in **prostate cancer** viability."

Effects of maitake (Grifola frondosa) D-Fraction on the carcinoma angiogenesis. Matsui K, Kodama N, Nanba H. Cancer Lett. 2001 Oct 30;172(2):193-8. **Key Finding:** "These results suggest that the anti-tumor activity of the D-Fraction is not only associated with the activation of the immune-competent cells but also possibly related to the **carcinoma** angiogenesis induction."

Maitake extracts and their therapeutic potential. Mayell M. Altern Med Rev. 2001 Feb;6(1):48-60. **Key Finding**: "The D-fraction, the MD-fraction, and other extracts of maitake, often in combination with whole maitake powder, have shown particular promise as immunomodulating agents, and as an adjunct to **cancer** and **HIV** therapy. They may also provide some benefit in the treatment of **hyperlipidemia**, **hypertension**, and **hepatitis**."

The use of mushroom glucans and proteoglycans in cancer treatment. Kidd PM. Altern Med Rev. 2000 Feb;5(1):4-27. **Key Finding**: "More than 50 mushroom species have yielded potential immunoceuticals that exhibit anticancer activity in vitro or in animal models and of these, six have been investigated in human cancers. All are non-toxic and very well tolerated. Two proteoglycans from Coriolus versicolor have demonstrated the most promise. In Japanese trials since 1970, PSK (Polysaccharide-K) significantly extended survival at five years or beyond in cancers of the **stomach, colon-rectum, esophagus, nasopharynx, and lung** and in a HLA B40-positive **breast cancer** subset."

*Induction of apoptosis in human **prostatic cancer** cells with beta-glucan (maitake mushroom polysaccharide).* Fullerton SA, Samadi AA, Tortorelis DG, Choudhury MS, Malouh C, Tazaki H, Konno S. Mol Urol. 2000 Spring;4(1):7-13. **Key Finding**: "A bioactive beta-glucan from the Maitake mushroom has a cytotoxic effect, presumably through oxidative stress, on prostatic cancer cells in vitro, leading to apoptosis."

*Mushrooms, **tumors**, and immunity.* Borchers AT, Stern JS, Hackman RM, Keen CL, Gershwin ME. Proc Soc Exp Biol Med. 1999 Sep;221(4):281-93. **Key Finding**: "In this paper, we review existing data on the mechanism of whole mushrooms and isolated mushroom compounds, in particular (1->3)-beta-D-glucans and the means by which they modulate the immune system and potentially exert tumor-inhibitory effects. We believe that the antitumor mechanisms of several species of whole mushrooms as well as of polysaccharides isolated from Lentinus edodes, Schizophyllium commune, Grifola frondosa, and Sclerotinia sclerotiorum are mediated largely by T cells and macrophages."

*Effects of Lentinus edodes, Grifola frondosa and Pleurotus ostreatus administration on **cancer** outbreak, and activities of macrophages and lymphocytes in mice treated with a carcinogen, N-butyl-N-butanonitrosoamine.* Kurashige S, Akuzawa Y, Endo F. Immunopharmacol Immunotoxicol. 1997 May;19(2):175-83. **Key Finding**: "Significantly higher cytotoxic activity against P-815 cells was observed in lymphocytes from mice treated with BBN plus each mushroom than that in lymphocytes from normal mice or mice treated with BBN alone."

*Inhibitory effect of Chinese herb medicine zhuling on urinary **bladder cancer**: An experimental and clinical study.* Yang DA. Zhonghua Wai Ke Za Zhi (Chinese). 1991 Jun;29(6):393-5. **Key Finding**: "Inhibitory effect of Zhuling (Grifola umbellate pilat) on urinary bladder cancer was determined. The experimental results showed that zhuling inhibited significantly the induction of bladder cancer in rats. Zhuling was given to 22 clinical patients with recurrent bladder cancer. The patients were followed up for 12 to 38 months. Bladder cancer recurred in seven of the patients with a longer recurrence interval (19.2 months) after medication than before medication. The remaining 15 patients had no recurrence."

Host-mediated **antitumor** *effect of grifolan NMF-5N, a polysaccharide obtained from Grifola frondosa.* Takeyama T, Suzuki I, Ohno N, Oikawa S, Sato K, Ohsawa M, Yadomae T. J Pharmacobiodyn. 1987 Nov;10(11):644-51. **Key Finding**: "these results suggested that grifolan NMF-5N shows antitumor activity via host-mediated mechanisms and both macrophages and T cells play important roles in this mechanism."

Antitumor *effect of polysaccharide grifolan NMF-5N on syngeneic tumor in mice.* Suzuki I, Takeyama T, Ohno N, Oikawa S, Sato K, Suzuki Y, Yadomae T. J Pharmacobiodyn. 1987 Feb;10(2):72-7. **Key Finding**: "These results suggest that antitumor activities of grifolan NMF-5N in murine syngeneic tumor systems depend on not only dosage but also injection routes and timing."

Antitumor *activity of a beta-1,3-glucan obtained from liquid cultured mycelium of Grifola frondosa.* Ohno N, Adachi Y, Suzuki I, Oikawa S, Sato K, Ohsawa M, Yadomae T. J Pharmacobiodyn. 1986 Oct;9(10):861-4. **Key Finding**: "The mice cured from the solid form of sarcoma 180 by administration of grifolan LE had the ability to reject the same tumor cell. From these results, it is suggested that the antitumor activity of grifolan LE occurred by modification of biological responses."

Cholesterol

Beta-glucans in higher fungi and their health benefits. Rop O, Micek J, Jurikova T. Nutr Rev. 2009 Nov;67(11):624-31. **Key Finding**: "A number of beta-glucans, such as lentinan from Shiitake, have shown marked anticarcinogenic activity. In addition to having an immunity-stimulating effect, beta-glucans may participate in physiological processes related to the metabolism of fats in the human body. Their application results in a decrease in the total **cholesterol** content in blood and may also contribute to reductions in **body weight**."

Cholesterol-*lowering effects of maitake (Grifola frondosa) fiber, shiitake (Lentinus edodes) fiber, and enokitake (Flammulina velutipes) fiber in rats.* Fukushima M, Ohashi T, Fujiwara Y, Sonoyama K, Nakano M. Exp Biol Med (Maywood). 2001 Sep;226(8):758-65. **Key Finding**: "The results of this study demonstrate that maitake and enokitake lowered the serum total cholesterol level by enhancement of fecal cholesterol excretion, and in particular, by enhancement of hepatic LDL receptor mRNA in EF group."

Diabetes

Phytochemical characteristics and hypoglycemic activity of fraction from mushroom Inonotus oblique. Lu X, Chen H, Dong P, Fu L, Zhang X. J Sci Food Agric. 2010 Jna 30;90(2):276-80. **Key Finding**: "Inonotus obliquus is a medicinal mushroom that has been used as an effective agent to treat various diseases such as diabetes, tuberculosis and cancer. The effects on hyperglycemia were investigated and the main constituents were isolated. Inonotus obliquus showed significant **antihyperglycemic** and **antilipidperoxidative** effects in alloxan-induced diabetic mice."

Activity and toxicity of Cr(lll)-enriched Grifola frondosa in insulin-resistant mice. Xu Q, Guo J. Biol Trace Elem Res. 2009 Dec;131(3):271-7. **Key Finding**: "These results indicate that chromium-enriched Grifola frondosa may have potential beneficial effects in insulin-resistant **prediabetic** conditions."

*Submerged culture mycelium and broth of Grifola frondosa improve glycemic responses in **diabetic** rats.* Lo HC, Hsu TH, Chen CY. Am J Clin Med. 2008;36(2):265-85. **Key Finding**: "Our results revealed that submerged-culture mycelia and broth of Grifola frondosa have bioactivities for improving glycemic responses."

***Anti-diabetic** effect of an alpha-glucan from fruit body of maitake (Grifola frondosa) on KK-Ay mice.* Hong L, Xun M, Wutong W. J Pharm Pharmacol. 2007 Apr;59(4):575-82. **Key Finding**: "These data suggest that MT-alpha-glucan from the fruit body of maitake mushrooms has an anti-diabetic effect which might be related to its effect on insulin receptors."

Enhanced insulin-hypoglycemic activity in rats consuming a specific glycoprotein extracted from maitake mushroom. Preuss HG, Echard B, Bagchi D, Perricone NV, Zhuang C. Mol Cell Biochem. 2007 Dec;306(1-2):105-13. **Key Finding**: "A glycoprotein extract from Maitake mushroom (SX-fraction) should be considered as an alternative method for improving **insulin sensitivity**."

***Antihypertensive** and metabolic effects of whole Maitake mushroom powder and its fractions in two rat strains.* Talpur NA, Echard BW, Fan AY, Jaffari O, Bagchi D, Preuss HG. Mol Cell Biochem. 2002 Aug;237(1-2):129-36. **Key Finding:** "We conclude that the examined forms of Maitake mushrooms have antihypertensive and **antidiabetic** potential which differ among rat strains. The soluble fraction may decrease systolic **blood pressure** in hypertensive rats via alteration in the rennin-angiotensin system."

Anti-diabetic activity present in the fruit body of Grifola Frondosa (Maitake). Kubo K, Aoki H, Nanba H. Biol Pharm Bull. 1994 Aug;17(8):1106-10. **Key Finding**: "The fruit body of Grifola frondosa (maitake) was confirmed to contain substances with anti-diabetic activity. Moreover, levels of insulin and triglyceride in plasma demonstrated a change similar to blood glucose with feeding of maitake."

Hepatitis

Maitake extracts and their therapeutic potential. Mayell M. Altern Med Rev. 2001 Feb;6(1):48-60. **Key Finding**: "The D-fraction, the MD-fraction, and other extracts of maitake, often in combination with whole maitake powder, have shown particular promise as immunomodulating agents, and as an adjunct to **cancer** and **HIV** therapy. They may also provide some benefit in the treatment of **hyperlipidemia**, **hypertension**, and **hepatitis**."

HIV

Maitake extracts and their therapeutic potential. Mayell M. Altern Med Rev. 2001 Feb;6(1):48-60. **Key Finding**: "The D-fraction, the MD-fraction, and other extracts of maitake, often in combination with whole maitake powder, have shown particular promise as immunomodulating agents, and as an adjunct to **cancer** and **HIV** therapy. They may also provide some benefit in the treatment of **hyperlipidemia**, **hypertension**, and **hepatitis**."

Hyperglycemia

Hypoglycemic activity of Grifola frondosa rich in vanadium. Cui B, Han L, Qu J, Lv Y. Biol Trace Elem Res. 2009 Nov;131(2):186-91. **Key Finding**; "In the fermented mushroom of G. frondosa, vanadium at lower doses in combination with G. frondosa induced significant decreases of the blood glucose and HbA1c levels in **hyperglycemic** mice."

A comparison of hypoglycemic activity of three species of basidiomycetes rich in vanadium. Han C, Liu T. Biol Trace Elem Res. 2009 Feb;127(2):177-82. **Key Finding**: "The hypoglycemic activity of fermented mushroom of three fungi of basidiomycetes rich in vanadium was studied. Compared with Ganoderma rich in vanadium and Grifola frondosa rich in vanadium, the hypoglycemic effects of Coprinus comatus rich in vanadium on hyperglycemic animals are significant; it may be used as a hypoglycemic food or medicine for **hyperglycemic** people."

Hyperlipidemia

Maitake extracts and their therapeutic potential. Mayell M. Altern Med Rev. 2001 Feb;6(1):48-60. **Key Finding**: "The D-fraction, the MD-fraction, and other extracts of maitake, often in combination with whole maitake powder, have shown particular promise as immunomodulating agents, and as an adjunct to **cancer** and **HIV** therapy. They may also provide some benefit in the treatment of **hyperlipidemia**, **hypertension**, and **hepatitis**."

Hypertension

Maitake *mushroom extracts ameliorate progressive hypertension and other chronic metabolic perturbations in aging female rats.* Preuss HG, Echard B, Bagchi D, Perricone NV. Int J Med Sci. 2010 Jun 7;7(4):169-80. **Key Finding**: "we believe our data suggest that maitake mushroom fractions lessen age-related **hypertension,** at least in part, via effects on the rennin-angiotensin system, enhance insulin sensitivity, and reduce some aspects of inflammation, actions that should lead to a longer, healthier life span."

Antihypertensive *and metabolic effects of whole Maitake mushroom powder and its fractions in two rat strains.* Talpur NA, Echard BW, Fan AY, Jaffari O, Bagchi D, Preuss HG. Mol Cell Biochem. 2002 Aug;237(1-2):129-36. **Key Finding:** "We conclude that the examined forms of Maitake mushrooms have antihypertensive and **antidiabetic** potential which differ among rat strains. The soluble fraction may decrease systolic **blood pressure** in hypertensive rats via alteration in the rennin-angiotensin system."

Maitake extracts and their therapeutic potential. Mayell M. Altern Med Rev. 2001 Feb;6(1):48-60. **Key Finding**: "The D-fraction, the MD-fraction, and other extracts of maitake, often in combination with whole maitake powder, have shown particular promise as immunomodulating agents, and as an adjunct to **cancer** and **HIV** therapy. They may also provide some benefit in the treatment of **hyperlipidemia**, **hypertension**, and **hepatitis**."

Immune system

Lentinula edodes (Shiitake) mushroom extract protects against hydrogen peroxide induced cytotoxicity in peripheral blood mononuclear cells. Kuppusamy UR, Chong YL, Mahmood AA, Indran M, Abdullah N, Vikineswary S. Indian J Biochem Biophys. 2009 Apr;46(2):161-5. **Key Finding**: "Lentinula edodes, commonly known as Shiitake mushroom, has been used as medicinal food in Asian countries and is believed to possess strong **immunomodulatory** property. In the present study, the methanolic extract of the fruit bodies of L. edodes was investigated for cytoprotection effect against H2O2-induced cytotoxicity in human peripheral blood mononuclear cells. The extract improved PBMC viability and exerted a dose-dependent protection against H2O2-induced cytotoxicity."

*The effects of whole mushrooms during **inflammation**.* Yu S, Weaver V, Martin K, Cantorna MT. BMC Immunol. 2009 Feb 20;10-12. **Key Finding**: "The data support a model whereby edible mushrooms (such as maitake and shiitake) regulate **immunity** in vitro. There are modest effects of in vivo consumption of edible mushrooms on induced inflammatory responses."

Oral administration of submerged cultivated Grifola frondosa enhances phagocytic activity in normal mice. Wang L, Ha CL, Cheng TL, Cheng SY, Lian TW, Wu MJ. Pharm Pharmacol. 2008 Feb;60(2):237-43. **Key Finding**: "These results suggested that oral administration of submerged cultivated G. frondosa mixture may enhance host innate **immunity** against foreign pathogens without eliciting adverse inflammatory response."

The immune effects of edible fungus polysaccharides compounds in mice. Yin Y, Fu W, Fu M, He G, Traore L. Asia Pac J Clin Nutr. 2007;16 Suppl 1:258-60. **Key Finding:** "The main objective of this study was to evaluate mice's immune effects of the mixed polysaccharides extracted from Lentinus edodes, Ganoderma lucidium and Grifola frondosa. Polysaccharides compounds significantly increased the thymus and NK cells activities as well as the ability of macrophages to phagocyte latex particles and the activity of macrophages. The results indicated that the mixed polysaccharides compounds could enhance the **cell immune** of mice."

Immunomodulatory properties of Grifola frondosa in submerged culture. Wu MJ, Cheng TL, Cheng SY, Lian TW, Wang L, Chiou SY. Agric Food Chem. 2006 Apr 19;54(8):2906-14. **Key Finding**: "These results imply that the relatively low molecular mass polysaccharides isolated from mycelia of G. frondosa can enhance innate **immunity** in vitro and therefore may serve as biological response modifiers."

Characterization and immunomodulating activities of polysaccharide from Lentinus edodes. Zheng R, Jie S, Hanchuan D, Moucheng W. Int Immunopharmacol. 2005 May;5(5):811-20. **Key Finding**: "We evaluated the effects of the polysaccharide L-II (from the fruiting body of Lentinus edodes) on the cellular immune response of **Sarcoma** 180-bearing mice. Results of these studies demonstrated the anti-tumor activity of the polysaccharide L-II on mice-transplanted sarcoma 180 was mediated by **immunomodulation** in inducing T-cells and macrophage-dependent immune system responses."

*Administration of a polysaccharide from Grifola frondosa stimulates **immune func-tion** of normal mice.* Kodama N, Murata Y, Nanba H. J Med Food. 2004 Summer;7(2):141-5. **Key Finding**: "These results indicate that D-Fraction from maitake enhances both the innate and adaptive arms of the immune response in normal mice. Its administration may enhance host defense against foreign pathogens and protect healthy individuals from infectious diseases."

Inflammation

*The effects of whole mushrooms during **inflammation**.* Yu S, Weaver V, Martin K, Cantorna MT. BMC Immunol. 2009 Feb 20;10-12. **Key Finding**: "The data support a model whereby edible mushrooms (such as maitake and shiitake) regulate **immunity** in vitro. There are modest effects of in vivo consumption of edible mushrooms on induced inflammatory responses."

Irritable Bowel Syndrome

Grifola frondosa water extract alleviates intestinal inflammation by suppressing TNF-alpha production and its signaling. Lee JS, Park SY, Thapa D, Et al. Exp Mol Med. 2010 Feb 28;42(2):143-54. **Key Finding:** "Taken together, the results strongly suggest **Grifola frondosa** is a valuable medicinal food for **irritable bowel syndrome** treatment and thus may be used as an alternative medicine."

Malaria

The shiitake mushroom-derived immune-stimulant lentinan protects against murine malaria blood-stage infection by evoking adaptive immune-responses. Zhou LD, Zhang QH, Zhang Y, Liu J, Cao YM. Int Immunopharmacol. 2009 Apr;9(4):455-62. **Key Finding**: "Our findings suggest that lentinan from Lentinus edodes has prophylactic potential for the treatment of **malaria**."

Weight loss

Beta-glucans in higher fungi and their health benefits. Rop O, Micek J, Jurikova T. Nutr Rev. 2009 Nov;67(11):624-31. **Key Finding**: "A number of beta-glucans, such as lentinan from Shiitake, have shown marked anticarcinogenic activity. In addition to having an immunity-stimulating effect, beta-glucans may participate in physiological processes related to the metabolism of fats in the human body. Their application results in a decrease in the total **cholesterol** content in blood and may also contribute to reductions in **body weight**."

Nuts

(Almonds, Macadamias, Peanuts, Pistachios, Walnuts)

ALMOND TREES MAY HAVE BEEN THE FIRST DOMESTICATED NUT in human history. Almond nuts, which are the tree's cultivated seeds, were found in the Egyptian Pharaoh Tutankhamnun's tomb when it was opened by archaeologists about 3,250 years after his birth. Cultivation of almonds spread from the Middle East and India into southern Europe, and finally to California during the nineteenth century.

When scientists began to measure the nutrient content of almonds, it was discovered that they contain a remarkably wide variety, from the minerals zinc, potassium, iron, and magnesium, to most of the B vitamins along with vitamins C and E. Vitamin E concentrations alone, in a 3.5 ounce serving of almonds, have been measured at 175% of the USDA recommended daily consumption of that vitamin for adults.

Aging

Grape juice berries, and walnuts affect **brain aging** *and behavior.* Joseph JA, Shukitt-Hale B, Willis LM. J Nutr. 2009 Sep;139(9):1813S-7S. **Key Finding:** "Research from our laboratory has suggested that dietary supplementation with fruit or vegetable extracts high in antioxidants (e.g. blueberries, strawberries, **walnuts** and Concord grape juice) can decrease the enhanced vulnerability to oxidative stress that occurs in aging and these reductions are expressed as improvements in behavior. Collaborative findings indicate that blueberry or Concord grape juice supplementation in humans with mild **cognitive impairment** increased verbal memory performance, thus translating our animal findings to humans."

Antioxidation

The phytochemical composition and antioxidant actions of tree nuts. Bolling BW, McKay DL, Blumberg JB. Asia Pac j Clin Nutr. 2010;19(1):117-23. **Key Finding**: "Most tree nuts provide an array of phytochemicals that may contribute to the health benefits attributed to this whole food. A limited number of human studies indicate these nut phytochemicals are bio accessible and bioavailable and have **antioxidant** actions in vivo."

Acute effect of nut consumption on plasma total polyphenols, **antioxidant capacity and lipid peroxidation.** Torabian S, Haddad E, Rajaram S, Banta J, Sabate J. Hum Nutr Diet. 2009 Feb;22(1):64-71. **Key Finding:** "Consumption of walnuts and almonds increased plasma polyphenol concentrations increased the total antioxidant capacity and reduced plasma lipid peroxidation."

Comparative flavan-3-ol profile and antioxidant capacity of roasted **peanut, hazelnut, and almond** *skins.* Monagas M, Garrido I, Lebron-Aguilar R, Gomez-Cordoves MC, Rybarczyk A, Amarowicz R, Bartolome B. J Agric Food Chem. 2009 Nov 25;57(22):10590-9. **Key Finding:** "The **antioxidant** capacity as determined by various methods was higher for whole extracts from roasted hazelnut and peanut skins than for almond skins; however, the antioxidant capacities of the high molecular weight fraction of the three types of nut skins were equivalent."

Flavonoids from almond skins are bioavailable and act synergistically with vitamins C and E to enhance hamster and human **LDL resistance to oxidation.** Hen CY, Milbury PE, Lapsley K, Blumberg JB. J Nutr. 2005 Jun;135(6):1366-73. **Key Finding:** "**Almond** skin flavonoids possess antioxidant capacity in vitro; they are bioavailable and act in synergy with vitamins C and E to protect LDL against oxidation in hamsters."

Melatonin in walnuts: influence on levels of melatonin and total antioxidant capacity of blood. Reiter RJ, Manchester LC, Tan DX. Nutrition. 2005 Sep;21(9):920-4. **Key Finding:** "Melatonin is present in walnuts and, when eaten, increase blood melatonin concentrations. The increase in blood melatonin levels correlates with an increased **antioxidative** capacity."

Antioxidative *phenolic compounds isolated from* **almond** *skins (Prunus amygdalus Batsch).* Sang S, Lapsley K, Jeong WS, Lachance PA, Ho CT, Rosen RT. J Agric Food Chem. 2002 Apr 10;50(8):2459-63. **Key Finding:** "Nine phenolic compounds were isolated from the ethyl acetate and n-butanol fractions of almond skins. Compounds 6 and 7 show very strong DPPH radical scavenging activity. Compounds 1-3,5,8 and 9 show strong activity, whereas compound 4 has very weak activity."

Cancer (breast; colon; leukemia; lung; ovarian)

Intake of fiber and nuts during adolescence and incidence of proliferative benign breast disease. Su X, Tamimi RM, Collins LC, Et al. Cancer Causes Control. 2010 Jul;21(7):1033-46. **Key Finding:** "These findings from among 29,480 women who completed a high school diet questionnaire in 1998 support the hypothesis that dietary intake of fiber and nuts during adolescence influences subsequent risk of breast disease and may suggest a viable means for **breast cancer** prevention."

Human cancer cell antiproliferative and antioxidant activities of Juglans regia L. Carvalho M, Ferreira PJ, Mendes VS, Et al. Food Chem Toxicol. 2010 Jan;48(1):441-7. **Key Finding**: "**Walnut** methanolic extracts were assayed for their antiproliferative effectiveness using human **renal cancer** cell lines A-498 and 769-P and the **colon cancer** cells. All extracts exhibited similar growth inhibition activity. The results obtained strongly indicate that walnut tree constitutes an excellent source of effective chemo preventive agents."

*Arachidin-1, a **Peanut** Stillbenoid, Induces Programmed Cell Death in Human **Leukemia** HL-60 Cells.* Huang CP, Au LC, Chiou RY, Et al. J Agric Food Chem. 2010 Nov 10 {Epub ahead of print}. **Key Finding**: "**Resveratrol**, a stilbenoid isolated from germinating peanut kernels, possesses anticancer activity and studies have indicated that it induces programmed cell death in human leukemia HL-60 cells. In this study, the anticancer activity of these stilbenoids was determined in HL-60 cells."

*Suppression of implanted MDA-MB 231 human **breast cancer** growth in nude mice by dietary **walnut**.* Hardman WE, Ion G. Nutr Cancer. 2008;60(5):666-74. **Key Finding:** Mice eating a diet with walnuts (equivalent to two ounces a day for humans) were compared to mice eating a similar diet without walnuts. The walnut consuming mice were less likely to develop breast tumors. After 145 days, 100 percent of the mice engineered to develop cancer had developed cancer, whereas only 50 percent of the cancer-engineered mice that ate walnuts had cancer.

*Inhibition of the phosphatidy linositol 3-kinase/Akt pathway by inositol pentakisphosphate results in **antiangiogenic** and **antitumor** effects.* Maffucci T, Piccolo E, Cumashi A, Iezzi M, Riley AM, Saiardi A, Godage HY, Rossi C, Broggini M, Iacobelli S, Potter BV, Innocenti P, Falasca M. Cancer Res. 2005 Spe 15;65(18):8339-49. **Key Finding:** A natural compound found in many legumes and nuts blocks a key enzyme involved in tumor growth. When this compound was tested on mice with **ovarian** and **lung cancers**, it sabotaged tumor growth and was also non-toxic, unlike conventional chemotherapy drugs.

*Whole **almonds** and almond fractions reduce aberrant crypt foci in a rat model of **colon carcinogenesis**.* Davis PA, Iwahashi CK. Cancer Lett. 2001 Apr 10;165(1):27-33. **Key Finding:** "These results suggest that almond consumption may reduce colon cancer risk and does so via at least one almond lipid-associated component."

Cardiovascular disease

Nuts, blood lipids and **cardiovascular disease**. Sabate J, Wien M. Asia Pac J Clin Nutr. 2010;19(1):131-6. **Key Finding**: "Over 40 dietary intervention studies have been conducted evaluating the effect of nut containing diets on blood lipids. These studies have demonstrated that intake of different kinds of nuts lower total and LDL **cholesterol a**nd the LDL: HDL ratio in healthy subjects or patients with moderate hypercholesterolemia even in the context of healthy diets. Additional cardio protective nutrients found in nuts include phytochemicals."

Peanut *consumption and* **cardiovascular** *risk*. Ghadimi NM, Kimiagar M, Abadi A, Et al. Public Health Nutr. 2010 Oct;13(10):1581-5. **Key Finding**: "Short-term peanut consumption might improve lipid profiles, the atherogenic index of plasma and coronary heart disease risk in hypercholesterolemic men."

Peanuts, peanut oil, and fat free peanut flour reduced cardiovascular disease risk factors and the development of **atherosclerosis** *in Syrian golden hamsters*. Stephens AM, Dean LL, Davis JP, Et al. J Food Sci. 2010 May;75(4):H116-22. **Key Finding**: "Peanut and peanut component diets retarded an increase in total **cholesterol** and cholesteryl ester. Because cholesteryl ester is an indicator of the development of atherosclerosis this study demonstrated that peanuts, peanut oil, and peanut components retarded the development of atherosclerosis in animals consuming an atherosclerosis inducing diet."

Nuts, blood lipis and **cardiovascular disease**. Sabate J, Wien M. Asia Pac J Clin Nutr. 2010;19(1):131-6. **Key Finding**: "Nuts have a unique fatty acid profile and feature a high unsaturated to saturated fatty acid ratio, an important contributing factor to the beneficial health effects of nut consumption. Additional cardio protective nutrients found in nuts include vegetable protein, fiber, alpha-tocopherol, folic acid, magnesium, copper, phytosterols and other phytochemicals."

Effects of **walnut** *consumption on blood lipids and other* **cardiovascular risk** *factors: a meta-analysis and systematic review*. Banel DK, Hu FB. Am J Clin Nutr. 2009 July;90(1):56-63. **Key Finding:** "Thirteen studies representing 365 participants were included in the analysis. Overall, high-walnut-enriched diets significantly decreased total and LDL **cholesterol** for the duration of the short-term trials. Larger and longer-term trials are needed to address the effects of walnut consumption on cardiovascular risk and body weight."

Effects of **pistachios** *on* **cardiovascular disease** *risk factors and potential mechanisms of action: a dose-response study*. Gebauer SK, West SG, Kay CD, Alaupovic

P, Bagshaw D, Kris-Etherton PM. Am J Clin Nutr. 2008 Sep;88(3):651-9. **Key Finding:** "Inclusion of pistachios in a healthy diet beneficially affects cardiovascular disease risk factors in a dose-dependent manner."

*A **macadamia** nut-rich diet reduces total and LDL-**cholesterol** in mildly hypercholesterolemic men and women.* Griel AE, Cao Y, Bagshaw DD, Cifelli AM, Holub B, Kris-Etherton PM. J Nutr. 2008 Apr;138(4):761-7. **Key Finding:** "Macadamia nuts can be included in a heart-healthy dietary pattern that reduces lipid/lipoprotein **cardiovascular disease** risk factors. Nuts as an isocaloric substitute for high SFA foods increase the proportion of unsaturated fatty acids and decrease SFA, thereby lowering CVD risk."

*Dietary omega-3 fatty acid intake and **cardiovascular disease**.* Psota TL, Gebauer SK, Kris-Etherton P. Am J Cardiol. 2006 Aug 21;98(4A): 3i-18i. **Key Finding:** "Sources of plant-derived omega-3 fatty acids include **walnuts,** flaxseed and soybean oil. Because of the remarkable cardio protective effects of omega-3 fatty acids, consumption of food sources that provide them should be increased in the diet."

A diet rich in walnuts favorably influences plasma fatty acid profile in moderately hyperlipidemia subjects. Chisholm A, Mann J, Skeaff M, Frampton C, Sutherland W, Duncan A, Tiszavari S. Eur J Clin Nutr. 1998 Jan;52(1):12-6. **Key Finding:** "Despite an unintended increase in the total fat intake on the **walnut** diet, fatty acid profile of the major lipid fractions showed changes which might be expected to reduce risk of **cardiovascular disease**."

Cholesterol

*Nut consumption and **blood lipid levels***: *a pooled analysis of 25 intervention trials.* Sabate J, Oda K, Ros E. Arch Intern Med. 2010 May 10;170(9):821-7. **Key Finding**: "We pooled individual primary data from 25 nut consumption trials conducted in 7 countries among 583 men and women with normolipidemia and hypercholesterolemia. Nut consumption improves blood lipid levels in a dose-related manner, particularly among subjects with higher LDL-C or with lower body mass index."

Nuts and berries for heart health. Ros E, Tapsell LC, Sabate J. Curr Atheroscler Rep. 2010 Nov;12(6):397-406. **Key Finding**: "Nuts are likely to beneficially impact heart health. Epidemiologic studies have associated nut consumption with a reduced incidence of **coronary heart disease** in both genders and **diabetes** in women. Limited evidence also suggests beneficial effects on hypertension and inflammation. Intervention studies consistently show that nut intake has a **cholesterol-lowering effect** and there is emerging evidence of beneficial effects on oxidative stress, **inflammation**, and vascular reactivity. **Blood pressure**, visceral adiposity, and glycemic control also appear to be positively influenced by frequent nut consumption without evidence of undue weight gain. Berries are another plant food rich in bioactive phytochemicals, particularly flavonoids, for which there is increasing evidence of benefits on cardio metabolic risk that are linked to their potent antioxidant power."

*Peanuts, peanut oil, and fat free **peanut** flour reduced cardiovascular disease risk factors and the development of **atherosclerosis** in Syrian golden hamsters.* Stephens AM, Dean LL, Davis JP, Et al. J Food Sci. 2010 May;75(4):H116-22. **Key Finding**: "Peanut and peanut component diets retarded an increase in total **cholesterol** and cholesteryl ester. Because cholesteryl ester is an indicator of the development of atherosclerosis this study demonstrated that peanuts, peanut oil, and peanut components retarded the development of atherosclerosis in animals consuming an atherosclerosis inducing diet."

*Long-term **walnut** supplementation without dietary advice induces favorable serum lipid changes in free-living individuals.* Torabian S, Haddah E, Cordero-MacIntyre Z, Et al. Eur J Clin Nutr. 2010 Mar;64(3):274-9. **Key Finding**: "Including walnuts as part of a habitual diet favorably altered the plasma lipid profile. The **lipid-lowering** effects of walnuts were more evident among subjects with higher lipid baseline values, precisely those people with greater need of reducing plasma total and LDL-cholesterol."

*Effects of **almond** dietary supplementation on **coronary heart disease** lipid risk factors and serum lipid oxidation parameters in men with mild hyperlipidemia.* Jalali-Khanabadi BA, Mozaffari-Khosravi H, Parsaeyan N. J Altern Complement Med. 2010 Dec;16(12):1279-83. **Key Finding**: "After 4 weeks, almond supplementation significantly decreased low-density lipoprotein **cholesterol,** total cholesterol, and apolipoprotein in 30 healthy volunteer men with mild hyperlipidemia."

***Pistachios** increase serum antioxidants and lower serum oxidized-LDL in hypercholesterolemic adults.* Kay CD, Gebauer SK, West SG. J Nutr. 2010 Jun;140(6):1093-8. **Key Finding**: "A heart-healthy diet including pistachios contributes to the decrease in the serum oxidized-LDL concentration through **cholesterol**-lowering and may provide an added benefit as a result of the antioxidants the pistachios contain."

*Effects of **walnut** consumption on blood lipids and other **cardiovascular risk** factors: a meta-analysis and systematic review.* Banel DK, Hu FB. Am J Clin Nutr. 2009 July;90(1):56-63. **Key Finding:** "Thirteen studies representing 365 participants were included in the analysis. Overall, high-walnut-enriched diets significantly decreased total and LDL **cholesterol** for the duration of the short-term trials. Larger and longer-term trials are needed to address the effects of walnut consumption on cardiovascular risk and body weight."

*A macadamia nut-rich diet reduces total and LDL-**cholesterol** in mildly hypercholesterolemic men and women.* Griel AE, Cao Y, Bagshaw DD, Cifelli AM, Holub B, Kris-Etherton PM. J Nutr. 2008 Apr;138(4):761-7. **Key Finding: "Macadamia** nuts can be included in a heart-healthy dietary pattern that reduces lipid/lipoprotein **cardiovascular disease** risk factors. Nuts as an isocaloric substitute for high SFA foods increase the proportion of unsaturated fatty acids and decrease SFA, thereby lowering CVD risk."

The energetics of nut consumption. Mattes RD. Asia Pac J Clin Nutr. 2008;17 Suppl 1:337-9. **Key Finding:** "Nuts are a nutrient-rich food group. Depending on the type, they may provide substantive concentrations of Vitamin E, magnesium, folate, essential fatty acids, fiber and protein to the diet. They also contain potentially important phytochemicals. By mechanisms yet to be identified, they are reported to improve postprandial **lipid profiles** and may hold other health benefits. However, they are also energy dense so a theoretical contributor to positive energy balance and **weight gain**. Epidemiological studies have consistently revealed an inverse association between the frequency of nut consumption and body mass index. Intervention trials demonstrate less than predicted weight gain following inclusion of nuts in the diet."

***Pistachio** Nut Consumption and Serum Lipid Levels.* Sheridan MJ, Cooper JN, Erario M, Cheifetz CE. J Am Coll Nutr. 2007;26(2):141-148. **Key Finding:** "A diet consisting of 15% of calories as pistachio nuts (about 2-3 ounces per day) over a four week period can favorably improve some lipid profiles in subjects with moderate **hypercholesterolemia** and may reduce risk of **coronary disease**."

*Effects of **pistachio** nuts consumption on plasma lipid profile and oxidative status in healthy volunteers.* Kocyigit A, Koylu AA, Keles H. J Nutr Meta Cardio Dis. 2006 April;16(3):202-209. **Key Finding:** "These results indicated that consumption of pistachio nuts decreased oxidative stress, and improved total **cholesterol** and HDL levels in healthy volunteers."

A Systematic Review of the Effects of Nuts on **Blood Lipid Profiles** *in Humans.* Mukuddem-Petersen J, Oosthuizen W, Jerling JC. J Nutr. 2005 Sep;135:2082-2089. **Key Finding:** "From the literature search, 415 publications were screened and 23 studies were included. The results of 3 almond, 2 peanut, 1 pecan nut, and 4 walnut studies showed decreases in total cholesterol between 2 and 16% and LDL cholesterol between 2 and 19% compared with subjects consuming control diets. Consumption of macadamia nuts produced less convincing results."

Flavonoids from almond skins are bioavailable and act synergistically with vitamins C and E to enhance hamster and human **LDL resistance to oxidation.** Chen CY, Milbury PE, Lapsley K, Blumberg JB. J Nutr. 2005 Jun;135(6):1366-73. **Key Finding:** "**Almond** skin flavonoids possess antioxidant capacity in vitro; they are bioavailable and act in synergy with vitamins C and E to protect LDL against oxidation in hamsters."

Serum lipid response to the graduated enrichment of a Step I diet with **almonds**: *a randomized feeding trial.* Sabate J, Haddad E, Tanzman JS, Jambazian P, Rajaram S. Am J Clin Nutr. 2003 Jun;77(6):1379-84. **Key Finding:** "Isoenergetic incorporation of approximately 68 g of almonds into a Step I diet markedly improved the serum lipid profile of healthy and mildly hypercholesterolemic adults. Total and **LDL-cholesterol** concentrations declined with progressively higher intakes of almonds."

Effects of plant-based diets high in raw or roasted **almonds** *or roasted almond butter on serum lipoproteins in humans.* Spiller GA, Miller A, Olivera K, Reynolds J, Miller B, Morse SJ, Dewell A, Farquhar JW. J Am Coll Nutr. 2003 Jun;22(3):195-200. **Key Finding:** "These results suggest that unblanched almonds –whether raw, dry roasted, or in roasted butter form—can play an effective role in **cholesterol-lowering** plant-based diets."

Antihypertriglyceridemic *effect of* **walnut** *oil.* Zibaeenezhad MJ, Rezaiezadeh M, Mowla A, Ayatollahi SM, Panjehshahin MR. Angiology. 2003 Jul-Aug;54(4):411-4. **Key Finding:** "This randomized, double blind case-control study was conducted to evaluate the lipid-lowering effect of Persian walnut oil. Sixty hyperlipidemia subjects were randomized into two groups. Plasma TG concentrations decreased by 19% to 33% in the walnut oil group. It was concluded that walnut oil is a good antihypertriglyceridemic natural remedy and should be further explored in more detail."

Almonds *and almond oil have similar effects on* **plasma lipids** *and LDl oxidation in healthy men and women.* Hyson DA, Schneeman BO, Davis PA. J Nutr. 2002

Apr;132(4):703-7. **Key Finding:** "22 normolipemic men and women replaced half of their habitual fat with either whole almonds (WA) or almond oil (AO) for 6-wk periods. Fat replacement with either WA or AO resulted in a 54% increase in percentage of energy as MUFA with declines in both saturated fat and cholesterol intake. Total and LDL cholesterol significantly decreased, whereas HDL cholesterol increased."

*A Monosaturated Fatty Acid-Rich **Pecan**-Enriched Diet Favorably Alters the **Serum Lipid Profile** of Healthy Men and Women.* Rajaram S, Burke K, Connell B, Myint T, Sabate J. J Nutr. 2001;131:2275-2279. **Key Finding:** "Nuts such as pecans that are rich in monosaturated fat may be recommended as part of prescribed cholesterol-lowering diet of patients or habitual diet of healthy individuals."

*Nut consumption, lipids, and risk of a **coronary** event.* Fraser GE. Asia Pac J Clin Nutr. 2000;9(Suppl):S28-S32. **Key Finding:** "Human feeding studies have demonstrated reductions of 8-12% in low-density lipoprotein (LDL) **cholesterol** when **almonds and walnuts** are substituted for more traditional fats."

***Pecans** Lower Low Density Lipoprotein **Cholesterol** in People with Normal Lipid Levels.* Morgan WA, Clayshulte BJ. J Am Dietetic Asso. 2000 Mar;100(3):312-318. **Key Finding:** "LDL-C was lowered in the pecan treatment group from 2.61+0.49 mmol/L at baseline to 2.35+0.49 at week 4. At week 8, total cholesterol and HDL-C in the pecan treatment group were significantly lower than in the control group."

*Effect of **Pistachio** Nuts on Serum Lipid Levels in Patients with Moderate **Hypercholesterolemia**.* Edwards K, Kwaw I, Matud J, Kurtz I. J Am Coll Nutr. 1999;18(3):229-232. **Key Finding:** "After three weeks, there was a decrease in total cholesterol, an increase in HDL, a decrease in the total cholesterol/HDL ratio and a decrease in the LDL/HDL ratio."

*Nuts and plasma lipids: an **almond**-based diet lowers LDL-C while preserving HDL-C.* Spiller GA. Jenkins DA, Bosello O, Gates JE, Cragen LN, Bruce B. J Am Coll Nutr. 1998 Jun;17(3):285-90. **Key Finding:** "Results suggest that the more favorable **lipid-altering** effects induced by the almond group (against an olive oil-based diet and a cheese and butter-based control diet) may be due to interactive or additive effects of the numerous bioactive constituents found in almonds."

*Effects of walnuts on **serum lipid** levels and **blood pressure** in normal men.* Sabate J, Fraser GE, Burke K, Knutsen SF, Bennett H, Lindsted KD. N Eng J Med. 1993 Mar 4;328(9):603-7. **Key Finding:** "Incorporating moderate quantities of walnuts into the recommended cholesterol-lowering diet while maintaining the intake of total dietary fat and calories decreases serum levels of total cholesterol and favorably modifies the lipoprotein profile in normal men."

*Effect of a diet high in monounsaturated fat from **almonds** on plasma **cholesterol** and lipoproteins.* Spiller GA, Jenkins DJ, Cragen LN, Gates JE, Bosello O, Berra K, Rudd C, Stevenson M, Superko R. J Am Coll Nutr. 1992 Apr;11(2):126-30. **Key Finding:** "The effect of almonds (raw) as part of a low saturated fat, low cholesterol, and high-fiber diet was studied in 26 adults. There was a rapid and sustained reduction in low-density lipoprotein cholesterol without changes in high-density lipoprotein cholesterol."

Cognition

*Grape juice, berries, and **walnuts** affect **brain aging** and behavior.* Joseph JA, Shukitt-Hale B, Willism LM. J Nutr. 2009 Sep;139(9):1813S-7S. **Key Finding:** "Research from our laboratory has suggested that dietary supplementation with fruit or vegetable extracts high in antioxidants (e.g. blueberries, strawberries, walnuts and Concord grape juice) can decrease the enhanced vulnerability to oxidative stress that occurs in aging and these reductions are expressed as improvements in behavior. Collaborative findings indicate that blueberry or Concord grape juice supplementation in humans with mild **cognitive impairment** increased verbal memory performance, thus translating our animal findings to humans."

Coronary artery disease

*Effects of **almond** dietary supplementation on **coronary heart disease** lipid risk factors and serum lipid oxidation parameters in men with mild hyperlipidemia.* Jalali-Khanabadi BA, Mozaffari-Khosravi H, Parsaeyan N. J Altern Complement Med. 2010 Dec;16(12):1279-83. **Key Finding**: "After 4 weeks, almond supplementation significantly decreased low-density lipoprotein **cholesterol,** total cholesterol, and apolipoprotein in 30 healthy volunteer men with mild hyperlipidemia."

The Traditional and Emerging Role of Nuts in Healthful Diets. Dreher ML, Maher CV, Kearney P. Nutr Rev. 2009 Apr;54(8):241-245. **Key Finding:** "Nuts have been a staple food providing energy, protein, essential fatty acids, vitamins and minerals. Research suggests there may be a connection between frequent nut consumption and a reduced incidence of **coronary heart disease**."

*The Effects of Nuts on **Coronary Heart Disease** Risk.* Kris-Etherton PM, Zhao G, Binkoski AE, Coval SM, Etherton TD. Nutr Rev. 2009 Apr;59(4):103-111. **Key Finding:** "Epidemiological studies have consistently demonstrated beneficial effects of nut consumption on coronary heart disease morbidity and mortality in different population groups. Clinical studies have reported total and low-density lipoprotein cholesterol-lowering effects of heart-healthy diets that contain various nuts or legume peanuts. It is evidenced that the favorable fatty acid profile of nuts (high in unsaturated fatty acids and low in saturated fatty acids) contributes to cholesterol lowering and, hence, CHD risk reduction. Dietary fiber and other bioactive constituents in nuts may confer additional cardio protective effects."

Nuts and health outcomes: new epidemiologic evidence. Sabate J, Ang Y. Am J Clin Nutr. 2009 May;89(5):1643S-1648S. **Key Finding:** "Epidemiologic studies have been remarkably consistent in showing an association between nut consumption and a reduced risk of **coronary heart disease**. Frequent nut intake probably reduces risk of **diabetes** mellitus among women, but its effects on men are unknown. Evidence on the **anticarcinogenic** effects of nuts is somewhat limited because studies in the past 2 decades have examined only 3 tumor sites and the benefits appear to be manifested only in women. However, the protective benefits of frequent nut consumption on **gallstone diseases** are observed in both sexes. Long-term nut consumption is linked with lower body weight and lower risk of **obesity** and weight gain."

*The role of tree nuts and peanuts in the prevention of **coronary heart disease**: multiple potential mechanisms.* Kris-Etherton PM, Hu FB, Ros E, Sabate J. J Nutr. 2008 Sep;138(9):1746S-1751S. **Key Finding:** "Nuts and peanuts are food sources that are a composite of numerous cardio protective nutrients and if routinely incorporated in a healthy diet, population risk of coronary heart disease would therefore be expected to decrease markedly."

***Almonds** reduce biomarkers of lipid peroxidation in older **hyperlipidemia** subjects.* Jenkins DJ, Kendall CW, Marchie A, Josse AR, Nguyen TH, Faulkner DA, Lapsley KG, Blumberg J. J Nutr. 2008 May;138(5):908-13. **Key Finding:** "Almond antioxidant activity was demonstrated by their effect on 2 biomarkers of lipid peroxidation, serum MDA and urinary isoprostanes, and supports the previous finding that almonds reduced oxidation of LDL-C. Antioxidant activity provides an additional possible mechanism, in addition to lowering cholesterol, which may account for the reduction in **coronary heart disease** risk with nut consumption."

Pistachio Nut Consumption and Serum Lipid Levels. Sheridan MJ, Cooper JN, Erario M, Cheifetz CE. J Am Coll Nutr. 2007;26(2):141-148. **Key Finding:** "A diet consisting of 15% of calories as pistachio nuts (about 2-3 ounces per day) over a four week period can favorably improve some lipid profiles in subjects with moderate **hypercholesterolemia** and may reduce risk of **coronary disease**."

*Dose Response of **Almonds** on Coronary Heart Disease Risk Factors: Blood Lipids, Oxidized Low-Density Lipoproteins, Lipoprotein (a), Homocysteine, and Pulmonary Nitric Oxide.* Jenkins DJA, Kendall CWC, Marchie A, Parker TL, Connelly PW, Qian W, Haight JS, Faulkner D, Vidgen E, Lapsley KG, Spiller GA. Circulation. 2002;106:1327-1332. **Key Finding:** "Almonds used as snacks in the diets of hyperlipidemia subjects significantly reduce **coronary heart disease** risk factors, probably in part because of the nonfat (protein and fiber) and monosaturated fatty acid components of the nut."

*The scientific evidence for a beneficial health relationship between walnuts and **coronary heart disease**.* Feldman EB. J Nutr. 2002 May;132(5):10625-11015. **Key Finding:** "Five controlled, peer-reviewed human clinical walnut intervention trials, involving approximately 200 subjects at risk of coronary heart disease were reviewed. The intervention trials consistently demonstrated **walnuts** as part of a heart-healthy diet, lower blood cholesterol concentrations. These results were supported by several large prospective observational studies in humans, all demonstrating a dose response-related inverse association of the relative risk of coronary heart disease with the frequent daily consumption of small amounts of nuts, including walnuts."

*Frequent nut intake and risk of death from **coronary heart disease** and all causes in postmenopausal women: the Iowa Women's Health Study.* Ellsworth JL, Kushi LH, Folsom AR. Nutr Metab Cardiovasc Dis. 2001 Dec;11(6):372-7. **Key Finding:** "Frequent nut consumption may offer postmenopausal women modest protection against the risk of death from all causes and coronary heart disease."

*Nut consumption and risk of **coronary heart disease**: a review of epidemiologic evidence.* Hu FB, Stampfer MJ. Curr Atheroscler Rep. 1999 Nov;1(3):204-9. **Key Finding:** "Based on the data from the Nurses' Health Study, we estimated that substitution of the fat from 1 ounce of nuts for equivalent energy from carbohydrate in an average diet was associated with a 30% reduction in coronary heart disease risk and the substitution of nut fat for saturated fat was associated with 45% reduction in risk."

Nut consumption, lipids, and risk of a coronary event. Fraser GE. Clin Cardiol. 1999 Jul;22(7 Suppl):11-5. **Key Finding:** "Nuts are nutrient-dense and perhaps the best natural source of vitamin E and are relatively concentrated repositories of dietary fiber, magnesium, potassium, and arginine, the dietary precursor of nitric oxide. Human feeding studies have demonstrated reductions of 8-12% in low-density lipoprotein (LDL) cholesterol when **almonds and walnuts** are substituted for more traditional fats. Four of the best and largest cohort studies in nutritional epidemiology have now reported that eating nuts frequently is associated with a decreased risk of **coronary heart disease** of the order of 30-50%."

Nuts: a new protective food against **coronary heart disease**. Sabate J, Fraser GE. Curr Opin Lipidol. 1994 Feb;5(1):11-6. **Key Finding:** "Recent epidemiological findings indicate that frequent nut consumption offers protection from fatal and non-fatal coronary heart disease events. Although human nutrition studies seem to indicate that nut consumption lowers total and LDL cholesterol, the unique nutrient composition of nuts invites speculation on other mechanisms of protection."

Diabetes

Nuts and berries for heart health. Ros E, Tapsell LC, Sabate J. Curr Atheroscler Rep. 2010 Nov;12(6):397-406. **Key Finding**: "Nuts are likely to beneficially impact heart health. Epidemiologic studies have associated nut consumption with a reduced incidence of **coronary heart disease** in both genders and **diabetes** in women. Limited evidence also suggests beneficial effects on hypertension and inflammation. Intervention studies consistently show that nut intake has a **cholesterol-lowering effect** and there is emerging evidence of beneficial effects on oxidative stress, **inflammation**, and vascular reactivity. **Blood pressure**, visceral adiposity, and glycemic control also appear to be positively influenced by frequent nut consumption without evidence of undue weight gain. Berries are another plant food rich in bioactive phytochemicals, particularly flavonoids, for which there is increasing evidence of benefits on cardio metabolic risk that are linked to their potent antioxidant power."

Health benefits of nuts in prevention and management of **diabetes.** Kendall CW, Esfahani A, Truan J, Et al. Asia Pac J Clin Nutr. 2010;19(1):110-6. **Key Finding**: "Overall, there are good reasons to justify further exploration of the use of nuts in the prevention of diabetes and its micro- and macro vascular complications."

Almond consumption and cardiovascular risk factors in adults with prediabetes. Wien M, Bleich D, Raghuwanshi M, Et al. J Am Coll Nutr. 2010 Jun;29(3):189-97. **Key Finding**: "An almond-enriched American Diabetes Association diet consisting of 20% of calories as almonds over a 16-week period is effective in improving markers of insulin sensitivity and yields clinically significant improvement in LDL-C in adults with prediabetes."

Long-term effects of increased dietary polyunsaturated fat from **walnuts** *on metabolic parameters in* **type II diabetes**. Tapsell LC, Batterham MJ, Teuss G, Tan SY, Dalton S, Quick CJ, Gillen LJ, Charlton KE. Eur J Clin Nutr. 2009 Aug;63(8):1008-15. **Key Finding:** "The walnut group produced significantly greater reductions in fasting insulin levels, an effect seen largely in the first 3 months."

Possible Benefit of Nuts in **Type 2 Diabetes**. Jenkins DJA, Hu FB, Tapsell LC, Josse AR, Kendall CWC. J Nutr. 2008 Sep;138(9):1752S-1756S. **Key Finding:** "We conclude that there is justification to consider the inclusion of nuts in the diets of individuals with diabetes in view of their potential to reduce cardiovascular disease risk, even though their ability to influence overall glycemic control remains to be established."

Effect of diets enriched in **almonds** *on insulin action and serum lipids in adults with normal glucose tolerance or* **type 2 diabetes**. Lovejoy JC, Most MM, Lefevre M, Greenway FL, Rood JC. Am J Clin Nutr. 2002 Nov;76(5):1000-6. **Key Finding:** "Almond-enriched diets do not alter insulin sensitivity in healthy adults or glycaemia in patients with diabetes. Almonds had beneficial effects on serum lipids in healthy adults and produced changes similar to high monounsaturated fat oils in diabetic patients."

Heart failure (myocardial infarction)

Effect of antioxidant-rich foods on plasma ascorbic acid, cardiac enzyme, and lipid peroxide levels in patients hospitalized with **acute myocardial infarction**. Singh RB, Niaz MA, Agarwal P, Begom R, Rastogi SS. J Am Diet Assoc. 1995 Jul;95(7):775-80. **Key Finding:** "Consumption of an antioxidant-rich diet (which includes crushed **almonds and walnuts**) may reduce the plasma levels of lipid peroxide and cardiac enzyme and increase the plasma level of ascorbic acid. Antioxidant-rich foods may reduce myocardial necrosis and reperfusion injury induced by oxygen free radicals."

Hyperlipidemia

*Almonds reduce biomarkers of lipid peroxidation in older **hyperlipidemia** subjects.* Jenkins DJ, Kendall CW, Marchie A, Josse AR, Nguyen TH, Faulkner DA, Lapsley KG, Blumberg J. J Nutr. 2008 May;138(5):908-13. **Key Finding:** "Almond antioxidant activity was demonstrated by their effect on 2 biomarkers of lipid peroxidation, serum MDA and urinary isoprostanes, and supports the previous finding that almonds reduced oxidation of LDL-C. Antioxidant activity provides an additional possible mechanism, in addition to lowering cholesterol, which may account for the reduction in **coronary heart disease** risk with nut consumption."

Inflammation

Nuts and berries for heart health. Ros E, Tapsell LC, Sabate J. Curr Atheroscler Rep. 2010 Nov;12(6):397-406. **Key Finding**: "Nuts are likely to beneficially impact heart health. Epidemiologic studies have associated nut consumption with a reduced incidence of **coronary heart disease** in both genders and **diabetes** in women. Limited evidence also suggests beneficial effects on hypertension and inflammation. Intervention studies consistently show that nut intake has a **cholesterol-lowering effect** and there is emerging evidence of beneficial effects on oxidative stress, **inflammation**, and vascular reactivity. **Blood pressure**, visceral adiposity, and glycemic control also appear to be positively influenced by frequent nut consumption without evidence of undue weight gain. Berries are another plant food rich in bioactive phytochemicals, particularly flavonoids, for which there is increasing evidence of benefits on cardio metabolic risk that are linked to their potent antioxidant power."

*Effect of **almond**-enriched high-monounsaturated fat diet on selected markers of **inflammation**: a randomized, controlled, crossover study.* Rajaram S, Connell KM, Sabate J. Br J Nutr. 2009 Oct 29:1-6. **Key Finding:** "Consumption of almonds influenced a few but not all of the markers of **inflammation** and hemostasis."

Metabolic syndrome

*Lifestyle counseling and supplementation with flaxseed or **walnuts** influence the management of metabolic syndrome.* Wu H, Pan A, Yu Z, Et al. J Nutr. 2010 Nov;140(11):1937-42. **Key Finding**: "Our results suggest that flaxseed and walnut supplementation may ameliorate central obesity. Further studies with larger sample sizes and of longer duration are needed to examine the role of these foods in the prevention and management of metabolic syndrome."

*Effects of one serving of mixed nuts on serum lipids, insulin resistance and inflammatory markers in patients with the **metabolic syndrome**.* Casas-Agustench P, Lopez-Uriarte P, Bullo M, Ros E, Cabre-Vila JJ, Salas-Salvado J. Nutr Metab Cardiovasc Dis. 2009 Dec 21. (Epub ahead of print). **Key Finding:** "In a randomized, parallel-group, 12-week feeding trial, 50 patients with metabolic syndrome were given recommendations for a healthy diet with or without supplementation with 30g/day of raw nuts (15g walnuts, 7.5g almonds and 7.5g hazelnuts.) Patients with metabolic syndrome show decreased lipid responsiveness but improved insulin sensitivity after daily intake of 30g of mixed nuts."

Obesity

***Pistachio** nuts reduce triglycerides and body weight by comparison to refined carbohydrate snack in obese subjects on a 12-week weight loss program.* Li Z. Song P, Nguyen C, Et al. J Am Coll Nutr. 2010 Jun;29(3):198-203. **Key Finding**: "Pistachios can be consumed as a portion-controlled snack for individuals restricting calories to lose weight without concern that pistachios will cause weight gain. By comparison to refined carbohydrate snacks such as pretzels, pistachios may have beneficial effects on triglycerides as well."

The energetics of nut consumption. Mattes RD. Asia Pac J Clin Nutr. 2008;17 Suppl 1:337-9. **Key Finding:** "Nuts are a nutrient-rich food group. Depending on the type, they may provide substantive concentrations of Vitamin E, magnesium, folate, essential fatty acids, fiber and protein to the diet. They also contain potentially important phytochemicals. By mechanisms yet to be identified, they are reported to improve postprandial **lipid profiles** and may hold other health benefits. However, they are also energy dense so a theoretical contributor to positive energy balance and **weight gain**. Epidemiological studies have consistently revealed an inverse association between the frequency of nut consumption and body mass index. Intervention trials demonstrate less than predicted weight gain following inclusion of nuts in the diet."

Prostate health

*The effect of **walnut** intake on factors related to **prostate and vascular health** in older men.* Spaccarotella KJ, Kris-Etherton PM, Stone WL, Bagshaw DM, Fishell VK, West SG, Lawrence FR, Harman TJ. Nutr J. 2008 May 2;7:13. **Key Finding:** "The significant decrease in the alpha-T gamma-T ratio with an increase in serum gamma-T and a trend towards an increase in the ratio of free PSA: total PSA following the 8-week supplement study suggest that walnuts may improve biomarkers of prostate and vascular status."

Olive and Olive Oil

SINCE PREHISTORIC TIMES, olives have been an important crop in the Middle East. Records from about four thousand years ago in ancient Mesopotamia show that the olive oil was a valuable export. However, much of the oil produced during this period was apparently used for grooming rather than as a food source.

With the advent of ancient Greece and Rome, olives and their oil became a standard fixture in cooking and as a food crop, with up to fifteen varieties being cultivated at the height of the Roman Empire's power. Today, Spain, Italy, and Greece produce about three-fourths of all the world's olives. Thanks to publicity about the health benefits of the Mediterranean diet, in which olives and olive oil are a primary food, much medical research looked into the connections between olives' high levels of monounsaturated fat, vitamin E, and phenols and their positive effects against cholesterol, cardiovascular disease, and other ailments.

Aging

Dietary **extra-virgin olive oil** *rich in phenolic antioxidants and the* **aging process***: long-term effects in the rat.* Jacomelli M, Pitozzi V, Zaid M, Et al. J Nutr Biochem. 2010 Apr;21(4):290-6. **Key Finding**: "We did detect a protective effect of olive oil on some age-related pathology and on blood pressure, of which the former was associated with the antioxidant content."

Olive oil and **cognition***: results from the three-city study.* Berr C, Portet F, Carriere I, Akbaraly TN, Feart C, Gourlet V, Combe N, Barberger-Gateau P, Richie K. Dement Geriatr Cogn Disord. 2009;28(4):357-64. **Key Finding**: "Our objective was to examine the association between olive oil use, cognitive deficit and cognitive decline in a large elderly population. We followed 6,947 subjects. Participants with moderate or intensive use of olive oil compared to those who never used olive oil showed lower odds of cognitive deficit for verbal fluency and visual memory."

Olive-oil consumption and health: the possible role of antioxidants. Owen RW, Giacosa A, Hull WE, Haubner R, Wurtele G, Spiegelhalder B, Bartsch H. Lancet Oncol. 2000 Oct;1:107-12. **Key Finding**: "High consumption of extra-virgin olive oils, which are particularly rich in phenolic antioxidants (as well as squalene and oleic acid), should afford considerable protection against **cancer (colon, breast, skin) coronary heart disease**, and **aging** by inhibiting oxidative stress."

Antioxidation

*A 3 years follow-up of a Mediterranean diet rich in virgin olive oil is associated with high plasma **antioxidant** capacity and reduced body **weight gain**.* Razquin C, Martinez JA, Martinez-Gonzalez MA, Mitjavila MT, Estruch R, Marti A. Eur J Clin Nutr. 2009 Dec;63(12):1387-93. **Key Finding**: "Mediterranean diet, especially rich in virgin olive oil, is associated with higher levels of plasma antioxidant capacity. Plasma total antioxidant capacity is related to a reduction in body weight after 3 years of intervention in a high cardiovascular risk population with a Mediterranean-style diet rich in virgin olive oil."

*Olive-oil consumption and health: the possible role of **antioxidants**.* Owen RW, Giacosa A, Hull WE, Haubner R, Wurtele G, Spiegelhalder B, Bartsch H. Lancet Oncol. 2000 Oct;1:107-12. **Key Finding**: "High consumption of extra-virgin olive oils, which are particularly rich in phenolic antioxidants (as well as squalene and oleic acid), should afford considerable protection against **cancer (colon, breast, skin) coronary heart disease**, and **aging** by inhibiting oxidative stress."

Cancer (bladder; breast; colon; esophageal; leukemia; oral; larynx; prostate)

***Olive oil** and health: summary of the II international conference on olive oil and health consensus report, Jaen and Cordoba (Spain) 2008.* Lopez-Miranda J, Perez-Jimenez F, Ros E, Et al. Nutr Metab Cardiovasc Dis. 2010 May;20(4):284-94. **Key Finding**: "Experimental and human cellular studies have provided new evidence on the potential protective effect of olive oil on cancer. Furthermore, results of case-control and cohort studies suggest that monounsaturated fatty acids intake including olive oil is associated with a reduction in cancer risk (mainly **breast, colorectal and prostate** cancers.)"

***Extra-virgin olive oil**-enriched diet modulates DSS-colitis-associated colon carcinogenesis in mice.* Sanchez-Fidalgo S, Villegas I, Cardeno A, Et al. Clin Nutr. 2010 Oct;29(5):663-73. **Key Finding**: "These results confirm that extra virgin olive oil diet has protective/preventive effect in the ulcerative colitis associated **colorectal cancer**."

***Mediterranean diet** and upper **aero digestive tract cancer**: the Greek segment of the Alcohol-Related Cancers and Genetic Susceptibility in Europe study.* Samoli E, Lagiou A, Nikolopoulos E, Et al. Br J Nutr. 2010 Nov;104(9):1369-74. **Key Finding**:

"Adherence to the traditional Mediterranean diet is associated with reduced risk of upper aero digestive tract cancers (oral, larynx and esophagus) and may explain the lower incidence of these cancers in Greece, in spite of the smoking and drinking habits of this population."

Oleuropein and hydroxytyrosol inhibit **MCF-7 breast cancer** *cell proliferation interfering with ERK1/2 activation.* Sirianni R, Chimento A, De Luca A, Et al. Mol Nutr Food Res. 2010 Jun;54(6):833-40. **Key Finding:** "Our study demonstrated that hydroxytyrosol and oleuropein, two polyphenols contained in **extra virgin olive oil**, can have a chemo-preventive role in breast cancer cell proliferation through the inhibition of estrogen-dependent rapid signals involved in uncontrolled tumor cell growth."

Phytochemicals in olive-leaf extracts and their antiproliferative activity against **cancer** *and endothelial cells.* Goulas V, Exarchou V, Troganis AN, Psomiadou E, Fotsis T, Briasoulis E, Gerothanassis IP. Mol Nutr Food Res. 2009 May;53(5):600-8. **Key Finding:** "The dominant compound of the extracts was oleuropein; phenols and flavonoids were also identified. These phytochemicals demonstrated strong antioxidant potency and inhibited cancer and endothelial cell proliferation at low micro molar concentrations, which is significant considering their high abundance in fruits and vegetables. The antiproliferative activity of crude extracts and phytochemicals against the cell lines used in this study is demonstrated for the first time."

Postmenopausal **breast cancer** *risk and dietary patterns in the E3N-EPIC prospective cohort study.* Cottet V, Touvier M, Fournier A, Touillaud MS, Lafay L, Clavel-Chapelon F, Boutron-Ruault MC. Am J Epidemiol. 2009 Nov 15;170(10):1257-67. **Key Finding**: "The analyses in this French cohort study included 2,381 postmenopausal invasive breast cancer cases diagnosed during a median 9.7 year follow-up period among 65,374 women. Two dietary patterns were identified: "alcohol/Western" (essentially meat products, French fries, appetizers, rice/pasta, potatoes, pulses, pizza/pies, canned fish, eggs, alcoholic beverages, cakes, mayonnaise, and butter/cream; and "healthy/Mediterranean" (essentially vegetables, fruits, seafood, olive oil and sunflower oil.) The first pattern was positively associated with breast cancer risk. The healthy/Mediterranean pattern was negatively associated with breast cancer risk."

Phytochemicals in olive-leaf extracts and their antiproliferative activity against **cancer** *and endothelial cells.* Goulas V, Exarchou V, Troganis AN, Psomiadou E, Fotsis T, Briasoulis E, Gerothanassis IP. Mol Nutr Food Res. 2009 May;53(5):600-8. **Key Finding:** "We investigated the antioxidant potency and antiproliferative activity against cancer and endothelial cells of water and methanol olive leaves extracts and analyzed their content in phytochemicals. Olive-leaf crude extracts were found to inhibit cell proliferation of human **breast adenocarcinoma** (MCF-7) human **urinary bladder carcinoma** (T-24). The dominant compound of the extracts was oleuropein; phenols and flavonoids were also identified. These phytochemicals demonstrated strong antioxidant potency and inhibited cancer and endothelial cell proliferation at low micro molar concentrations."

*Lupeol, a novel anti-inflammatory and **anti-cancer** dietary triterpene.* Saleem M. Cancer Lett. 2009 Nov 28;285(2):109-15. **Key Finding**: "Lupeol, a triterpene found in green pepper, white cabbage, olive, strawberry, mangoes and grapes, was reported to possess beneficial effects as a therapeutic and preventive agent for a range of disorders. Lupeol at its effective therapeutic doses exhibit no toxicity to normal cells and tissues. This mini review provides detailed account of preclinical studies conducted to determine the utility of lupeol as a therapeutic and chemo preventive agent for the treatment of inflammation and cancer."

Oleanolic acid, a pentacyclic triterpenoid, induces rabbit platelet aggregation through a phospholipase C-calcium dependent signaling pathway. Lee JJ, Jin YR, Lim Y, Yu JY, Kim TJ, Yoo HS, Shin HS, Yun YP. Arch Pharm Res. 2007 Feb;30(2):210-4. **Key Finding**: "Oleanolic acid has a wide variety of pharmacologic effects such **as antitumor, antifungal, insecticidal, hepatoprotective and anti-HIV activities.** This paper reports that oleanolic acid induces the aggregation of rabbit platelets."

*Olive Fruit Extracts Inhibit Proliferation and Induce Apoptosis in HT-29 Human **Colon Cancer** Cells.* Juan ME, Wenzel U, Ruiz-Gutierrez V, Daniel H, Planas JM. J Nutr. 2006 Oct;136:2553-2557. **Key Finding:** "Our results report for the first time, to our knowledge, the inhibition of cell proliferation without cytotoxicity and the restoration of apoptosis in colon cancer cells by maslinic and oleanolic acids present in olive fruit extracts."

*Virgin Olive Oil Phenols Inhibit Proliferation of Human Promyelocytic **Leukemia** Cells (HL60) by Inducing Apoptosis and Differentiation.* Fabiani R, De Bartolomeo A, Rosignoli P, Servili M., Selvaggini R, Montedoro GF, Di Saverio C, Morozzi G. J Nutr. 2006 Mar;136:614-619. **Key Finding:** "These results support the hypothesis that polyphenols play a critical role in the anticancer activity of olive oil."

Olives and olive oil in **cancer** *prevention.* Owen RW, Haubner R, Wurtele G, Hull E, Spiegelhalder B, Bartsch H. Eur J Cancer Prev. 2004 Aug;13(4):319-26. **Key Finding:** "Both olives and olive oil contain substantial amounts of compounds deemed to be anticancer agents (e.g. squalene and terpenoids) as well as the peroxidation-resistant lipid oleic acid. It seems probably that olive and olive oil consumption in southern Europe represents an important contribution to the beneficial effects on health of the Mediterranean diet."

Cancer *chemoprevention by hydroxytyrosol isolated from virgin olive oil through G1 cell cycle arrest and apoptosis.* Fabiani R, De Bartolomeo A, Rosignoli P, Servili M, Montedoro G, Morozzi G. Eur J Cancer Prev. 2002 Aug;11(4):351-358. **Key Finding:** "Hydroxytyrosol inhibited proliferation of both human promyelocytic **leukemia** cells and **colon adenocarcinoma** cells. These results support the hypothesis that hydroxytyrosol may exert a protective activity against cancer by arresting the cell cycle and inducing apoptosis in tumor cells, and suggest that hydroxytyrosol, an important component of virgin olive oil, may be responsible for its anticancer activity."

*The antioxidant/***anticancer** *potential of phenolic compounds isolated from olive oil.* Owen RW, Giacosa A, Hull WE, Haubner R, Spiegelhalder B, Bartsch H. Eur J Cancer. 2000 Jun;36(10):1235-1247. **Key Finding:** "Using the newly developed methodology we can demonstrate that the antioxidant phenolic compounds present in olive oil are potent inhibitors of free radical generation by the faucal matrix. This indicates that the study of the inter-relation between reactive oxygen species and dietary antioxidants is an area of great promise for elucidating mechanisms of colorectal carcinogenesis and possible future chemo preventive strategies."

Olive-oil consumption and health: the possible role of antioxidants. Owen RW, Giacosa A, Hull WE, Haubner R, Wurtele G, Spiegelhalder B, Bartsch H, Lancet Oncol. 2000 Oct;1:107-12. **Key Finding**: "High consumption of extra-virgin olive oils, which are particularly rich in phenolic antioxidants (as well as squalene and oleic acid), should afford considerable protection against **cancer (colon, breast, skin) coronary heart disease**, and **aging** by inhibiting oxidative stress."

Tumor-promoting and tumor-protective effects of high-fat diets on chemically induced **mammary cancer** *in rats.* Zusman I, Gurevich P, Madar Z, Nyska A, Korol D, Timar B, Zuckerman A. Anticancer Res. 1997 Jan-Feb;17(1A):349-56. **Key Finding**: "We studied the effects of different dietary fats on experimental rat mammary tumorigenesis induced by DMBA. The olive diet was associated with a significant reduction in the tumorigenic effect of DMBA: tumor incidence decreased to 30% as compared to 44%-55% in the other dietary groups studied. The protective antitumor effect of the olive diet was found to be connected to its dietary content of monounsaturated fatty acids such as oleic and palmitic acids and with serum concentrations of stearic acid."

Cardiovascular disease

Gene expression changes in mononuclear cells in patients with metabolic syndrome after acute intake of phenol-rich **virgin olive oil**. Camargo A, Ruano J, Fernandez JM, Et al. BMC Genomics. 2010 Apr 20;11:253. **Key Finding**: "This study shows that intake of virgin olive oil based breakfast, which is rich in phenol compounds, is able to repress in vivo expression of several pro-inflammatory genes, thereby switching activity of peripheral blood mononuclear cells to a less deleterious inflammatory profile. These results provide at least a partial molecular basis for reduced risk of **cardiovascular disease** observed in Mediterranean countries where virgin olive oil represents a main source of dietary fat."

*Reduction in systemic and VDL triacylglycerol concentration after a 3-month Mediterranean-style diet in high-***cardiovascular-risk*** subjects.* Perona JS, Covas MI, Fito M, Et al. J Nutr Biochem. 2010 Sep;21(9):892-8. **Key Finding**: "We conclude that the reduction in systemic triacylglycerol concentrations observed after consumption of the Mediterranean Diet supplemented with **virgin olive oil** may be explained by reduction of the lipid core of very low-density lipoprotein and a selective modification of the molecular species composition in the particle."

Effect of Mediterranean diet on the expression of pro-atherogenic genes in a population at high **cardiovascular risk**. Llorente-Cortes V, Estruck R, Mena MP, Et al. Atherosclerosis. 2010 Feb;208(2):442-50. **Key Finding**: "Our findings showed that the Mediterranean diet supplemented with **virgin olive oil** influences expression of key genes involved in vascular inflammation, foam cell formation and thrombosis. Dietary intervention can thus actively modulate the expression of pro-atherothrombotic genes even in a high-risk population."

Olive oil and **cardiovascular health**. Covas Ml, Konstantinidou V, Fito M. Cardiovasc Pharmacol. 2009 Dec;54(6):477-82. **Key Finding**: "The wide range of benefits associated with olive oil consumption could contribute to explaining the low rate of cardiovascular mortality found in southern European-Mediterranean countries in comparison to other westernized countries."

*Effects of a Mediterranean-style diet on **cardiovascular risk** factors: a randomized trial.* Estruch R, Martinez-Gonzalez MA, Corella D, Et al. Ann Intern Med. 2006 Jul 4;145(1):1-11. **Key Finding:** "Compared with a low-fat diet, Mediterranean diets supplemented with olive oil or nuts have beneficial effects on cardiovascular risk factors."

Olive oil and modulation of cell signaling in disease prevention. Wahle KW, Caruso D, Ochoa JJ, Quiles JL. Lipids. 2004 Dec;39(12):1223-31. **Key Finding**: "Increased olive oil consumption is implicated in a reduction in **cardiovascular risk, rheumatoid arthritis**, and, to a lesser extent, a variety of **cancers**. Olive oil intake also has been shown to modulate immune function, particularly the inflammatory processes associated with the immune system."

Cholesterol

*Garlic attenuates **hypercholesterolemic** risk factors in olive oil fed rats and high cholesterol fed rats.* Chetty KN, Calahan L, Harris KC, Dorsey W, Hill D, Chetty S, Jain SK. Pathophysiology. 2003 May;9(3):127-132. **Key Finding:** "The results suggest that the dietary **olive oil** regulated the levels of serum in cholesterol loaded rats. Garlic attenuated serum cholesterol in olive oil fed rats and decreased serum risk factors, both total cholesterol and LDL-C ration and LDL-Ch/HDL-Ch ratio."

Cognition

*Olive oil and **cognition**: results from the three-city study.* Berr C, Portet F, Carriere I, Akbaraly TN, Feart C, Gourlet V, Combe N, Barberger-Gateau P, Richie K. Dement Geriatr Cogn Disord. 2009;28(4):357-64. **Key Finding**: "Our objective was to examine the association between olive oil use, cognitive deficit and cognitive decline in a large elderly population. We followed 6,947 subjects. Participants with moderate or intensive use of olive oil compared to those who never used olive oil showed lower odds of cognitive deficit for verbal fluency and visual memory."

Coronary artery disease

*Anti-inflammatory effect of virgin olive oil in stable **coronary disease** patients: a randomized, crossover, controlled trial.* Alcantara M, Covas MI, Fito M, Marrugat J, Schroder H, Weinbrenner T, ALcantara M, Munoz D, Guxens M, de la Torre R, Farre M,

Menoyo E, Pujadas-Bastardes M, Closas N, Khymenets O, de la Torre-Boronat C, Gimeno E, Lamuela R, Lopez MC. Eur J Clin Nutr. 2008 Apr;62(4):570-4. **Key Finding**: "Consumption of virgin olive oil could provide beneficial effects in stable coronary heart disease patients as an additional intervention to the pharmacological treatment."

Olive-oil consumption and health: the possible role of **antioxidants**. Owen RW, Giacosa A, Hull WE, Haubner R, Wurtele G, Spiegelhalder B, Bartsch H. Lancet Oncol. 2000 Oct;1:107-12. **Key Finding**: "High consumption of extra-virgin olive oils, which are particularly rich in phenolic antioxidants (as well as squalene and oleic acid), should afford considerable protection against **cancer (colon, breast, skin) coronary heart disease**, and **aging** by inhibiting oxidative stress."

Diabetes

Effect of **virgin olive oil** *plus acetylsalicylic acid on brain slices damage after hypoxia-reoxygenation in rats with* **type 1-like diabetes** *mellitus.* De La Cruz JP, Del Rio S, Arrebola MM, Et al. Neurosci Lett. 2010 Mar 3;471(2):89-93. **Key Finding**: "The main conclusion of our study is that daily oral administration of virgin olive oil to diabetic rats may be a natural way to increase the neuroprotection of aspirin in diabetic animals."

Renal effects of plant-derived oleanolic acid in streptozotocin-induced diabetic rats. Mapanga RF, Tufts MA, Shode FO, Musabayane CT. Ren Fail. 2009;31(6):481-91. **Key Finding**: "These findings suggest that oleanolic acid may have beneficial effects on some processes associated with renal derangement of STZ-induced diabetic rats. This bioactive compound has potential in **diabetes** management."

HIV

Oleanolic acid, a pentacyclic triterpenoid, induces rabbit platelet aggregation through a phospholipase C-calcium dependent signaling pathway. Lee JJ, Jin YR, Lim Y, Yu JY, Kim TJ, Yoo HS, Shin HS, Yun YP. Arch Pharm Res. 2007 Feb;30(2):210-4. **Key Finding**: "Oleanolic acid has a wide variety of pharmacologic effects such **as antitumor, antifungal, insecticidal, hepatoprotective and anti-HIV activities.** This paper reports that oleanolic acid induces the aggregation of rabbit platelets."

Hypertension

Mediterranean-style diet effect on the structural properties of the erythrocyte cell membrane of **hypertensive** *patients: the Prevencion con Dieta Mediterranea Study.* Barcelo R, Perona JS, Prades J, Funari SS, Gomez-Gracia E, Conde M, Estruch R, Ruiz-Gutierrez V. Hypertension. 2009 Nov;54(5):1143-50. **Key Finding**: "A currently ongoing randomized trial has revealed that the Mediterranean diet, rich in virgin olive oil or nuts, reduces systolic blood pressure in high-risk cardiovascular patients. Here, we present a structural sub study to assess the effect of a Mediterranean-style diet supplemented with nuts or virgin olive oil on erythrocyte membrane properties in 36 hypertensive participants after 1 year of intervention. These data suggest that the diet affects the lipid metabolism that is altered in hypertensive patients, influencing the structural membrane properties."

Immunity

Olive oil, immune system *and infection.* Puertollano MA, Puertollano E, Alvarez de Cienfuegos G, Et al. Nutr Hosp. 2010 Jan-Feb;25(1):1-8. **Key Finding**: "This review contributes to clarify the interaction between the administration of diet containing olive oil and immune system, as well as to determine the effect promoted by this essential component in the Mediterranean diet in the immunomodulation against an infectious agent."

Inflammation

Phytochemistry: Ibuprofen-like activity in extra-virgin olive oil. Beauchamp GK, Keast RSJ, Morel D, Lin J, Pika J, Han Q, Lee CH, Smith AB, Breslin PAS. Nature. 2005 Sep;437:45-46. **Key Finding**: "Newly pressed extra-virgin olive oil contains oleocanthal—a compound whose pungency induces a strong stinging sensation in the throat, not unlike that caused by solutions of the non-steroidal anti-inflammatory drug ibuprofen. We show there that this similar perception seems to be an indicator of a shared pharmacological activity, with oleocanthal acting as a natural **anti-inflammatory** compound that has a potency and profile strikingly similar to that of ibuprofen."

Osteoarthritis

Effect of oleocanthal and its derivatives on inflammatory response induced by Lipopolysaccharide in a murine chondrocyte cell line. Iacono A, Gomez R, Sperry J, Et al. Arthritis

Rheum. 2010 Jun;62(6):1675-82. **Key Finding**: "This class of molecules from olecanthal isolated from **extra virgin olive oil** was found to display nonsteroidal anti-inflammatory drug activity similar to that of ibuprofen and thus shows potential as a therapeutic weapon for the treatment of inflammatory degenerative joint diseases such as **osteoarthritis.**"

Hydrolyzed Olive Vegetation Water in Mice Has Anti-Inflammatory Activity. Bitler CM, Viale TM, Damaj B, Crea R. J. Nutr. 2005 June;135:1475-1479. **Key Finding:** Olive vegetation water when combined with glucosamine "acted synergistically to reduce serum TNF levels in LPS-treated mice," which means this combination "may be an effective therapy for a variety of inflammatory processes, including **rheumatoid** and **osteoarthritis.**"

Peripheral vascular disease

*Extra-Virgin Olive Oil Increases the Resistance of LDL to Oxidation More than Refined Olive Oil in Free-living Men with **Peripheral Vascular Disease**.* Ramirez-Tortosa MC, Urbano G, Lopez-Jurado M, Nestares T, Gomez MC, Mir A, Ros E, Mataix J, Gil A. Journal of Nutrition. 1999;129:2177-2183. **Key Finding:** "We suggest that antioxidants present in extra-virgin olive oil may protect LDL against oxidation more than does refined olive oil in men with peripheral vascular disease."

Rheumatoid arthritis

Hydrolyzed Olive Vegetation Water in Mice Has Anti-Inflammatory Activity. Bitler CM, Viale TM, Damaj B, Crea R. J. Nutr. 2005 June;135:1475-1479. **Key Finding:** Olive vegetation water when combined with glucosamine "acted synergistically to reduce serum TNF levels in LPS-treated mice," which means this combination "may be an effective therapy for a variety of inflammatory processes, including **rheumatoid** and **osteoarthritis.**"

Olive oil and modulation of cell signaling in disease prevention. Wahle KW, Caruso D, Ochoa JJ, Quiles JL. Lipids. 2004 Dec;39(12):1223-31. **Key Finding**: "Increased olive oil consumption is implicated in a reduction in **cardiovascular risk, rheumatoid arthritis**, and, to a lesser extent, a variety of **cancers**. Olive oil intake also has been shown to modulate immune function, particularly the inflammatory processes associated with the immune system."

Stroke

*Dietary **virgin olive oil** reduces blood brain barrier permeability, brain edema, and brain injury in rats subjected to **ischemia**-reperfusion.* Mohagheghi R, Bigdeli MR, Rasoulian B, Et al. ScientificWorldJournal. 2010 Jun 29;10:1180-91. **Key Finding:** "Oral administration of virgin olive oil reduce infarct volume, brain edema, blood brain barrier permeability, and improves neurologic deficit scores after transient middle cerebral artery occlusion in rats."

Weight loss

*A 3 year follow-up of a Mediterranean diet rich in virgin olive oil is associated with high plasma **antioxidant** capacity and reduced body **weight gain**.* Razquin C, Martinez JA, Martinez-Gonzalez MA, Mitjavila MT, Estruch R, Marti A. Eur J Clin Nutr. 2009 Dec;63(12):1387-93. **Key Finding**: "Mediterranean diet, especially rich in virgin olive oil, is associated with higher levels of plasma antioxidant capacity. Plasma total antioxidant capacity is related to a reduction in body weight after 3 years of intervention in a high cardiovascular risk population with a Mediterranean-style diet rich in virgin olive oil."

Onions

BULBS OF THE ONION FAMILY from the genus *Allium* have been found by archaeologists in seven-thousand-year-old Bronze Age settlements, so we know it was one of the earliest foods cultivated. Ancient Egyptians consumed large quantities of onions, as did the ancient Greeks and Romans, who also prized their medicinal qualities. It is said that Christopher Columbus first brought onions to the Americas on his inaugural voyage of discovery.

As with garlic, onions contain phytochemicals with a variety of anti-inflammatory and antioxidant health benefits. At least twenty health conditions may be ameliorated by onion consumption, according to in vitro and laboratory studies and epidemiological analyses of populations who consume high quantities of onions. Besides quercetin and related phytochemicals, onions are high in B vitamins, vitamin C, phosphorus, potassium, and zinc.

Aging

*Onion flesh and onion peel enhance antioxidant status in **aged** rats.* Park J, Kim J, Kim MK. J Nutr Sci Vitaminol (Tokyo). 2007 Feb;53(1):21-9. **Key Finding**: "This study was designed to investigate the effects of dietary onion flesh or onion peel on lipid peroxides and DNA damage in aged rats. Onion flesh or onion peel enhanced antioxidant status in aged rats and may be beneficial for the elderly as a means of lowering lipid peroxide levels."

Antioxidation

Flavonoid quercetin protects against swimming stress-induced changes in oxidative biomarkers in the hypothalamus of rats. Haleagrahara N, Radhakrishnan A, Lee N, Kumar P. Eur J Pharmacol. 2009 Oct 25;621(1-3):46-52. **Key Finding**: "These data demonstrate that forced swimming stress produced a severe oxidative damage in the hypothalamus and treatment with quercetin markedly attenuated these stress-induced changes. Antioxidant action of quercetin may be beneficial for the prevention and treatment of stress-induced **oxidative damage in the brain**."

*Alleviative effects of quercetin and onion on male **reproductive toxicity** induced by diesel exhaust particles.* Izawa H, Kohara M, Aizawa K, Suganuma H, Inakuma T, Watanabe G, Taya K, Sagai M. Biosci Biotechnol Biochem. 2008 May;72(5):1235-41.

Key Finding: "These results clearly indicate alleviative effects of quercetin and onion against the male reproductive toxicity induced by diesel exhaust particles."

Protective roles of onion and garlic extracts on cadmium-induced changes in sperm characteristics and testicular oxidative damage in rats. Ola-Mudathir KF, Suru SM, Fafunso MA, Obioha UE, Faremi TV. Food Chem Toxicol. 2008 Dec;46(12):3604-11. **Key Finding**: "Our study demonstrated that aqueous extracts of onion and garlic could proffer a measure of protection against Cd-induced **testicular oxidative damage and spermiotoxicity** by possibly reducing lipid peroxidation and increasing the antioxidant defense mechanism in rats."

Antioxidative activity and ameliorative effects of **memory impairment** *of sulfur-containing compounds in Allium species.* Nishimura H, Higuchi O, Tateshita K, Tomobe K, Okuma Y, Nomura Y. Biofactors. 2006;26(2):135-46. **Key Finding**: "These results suggest that di-n-propyl trisulfide contained in onion ameliorates memory impairment in SAMPS mouse by its antioxidant effect."

Antioxidative and antihypertensive effects of Welsh onion on rats fed with a high-fat high-sucrose diet. Yamamoto Y, Aoyama S, Hamaguchi N, Rhi GS. Biosci Biotechnol Biochem. 2005 Jul;69(7):1311-7. **Key Finding**: "These results suggest that the green-leafy Welsh onion, but not the white type, reduced superoxide generation by suppressing the angiotensin II production and then the NADH/NADPH oxidase activity, increasing the NO availability in the aorta, and consequently lowering the blood pressure in the rats fed with the high-fat high-sucrose diet. The radical scavenging and reducing antioxidative activities of green Welsh onion may also be effective in decreasing superoxide."

Varietal differences in phenolic content and **antioxidant** *and* **antiproliferative** *activities of onions.* Yang J, Meyers KJ, Van der Heide J, Liu RH. J Agric Food Chem. 2004 Nov 3;52(22):6787-93. **Key Finding:** "The proliferation of HepG(2) and Caco-2 cells was significantly inhibited in a dose-dependent fashion after exposure to the Western Yellow, shallots, New York Bold, and Northern Red extracts of onion. Western Yellow, shallots, and New York Bold exhibited the highest antiproliferative activity against HepG(2) cells and New York Bold and Western Yellow exhibited the highest antiproliferative activity against Caco-2 cells. However, the varieties of Western White, Peruvian Sweet, Empire Sweet, Mexico, Texas 1015, Imperial Valley Sweet, and Vidalia demonstrated weak antiproliferative activity against both HepG(2) and Caco-2 cells. These results may influence consumers toward purchasing onion varieties exhibiting greater potential health benefits."

Antimutagenic, antioxidant and free radical scavenging activity of ethyl acetate extracts from white, yellow and red onions. Shon MY, Choi SD, Kahng GG, Nam SH, Sung NJ. Food Chem Toxicol. 2004 Apr;42(4):659-66. **Key Finding:** "Yellow onion extracts had more organic acid and free sugar than those detected in the white and red onion extract. After ingested, extracts showed antimutagenic activities. This study demonstrated that the antimutagenicity and antioxidant properties of ethyl acetate extract against mutagens were related to their phenols and flavonoids."

Arthritis

*Natural products as a gold mine for **arthritis** treatment.* Khanna D, Sethi G, Ahn KS, Pandey MK, Kunnumakkara AB, Sung B, Aggarwal A, Aggarwal BB. Curr Opin Pharmacol. 2007 Jun;7(3):344-51. **Key Finding:** "The large numbers of inexpensive natural products that can modulate inflammatory responses, but lack side effects, constitute 'goldmines' for the treatment of arthritis. Numerous agents derived from plants can suppress cell signaling intermediates, including curcumin, resveratrol, cranberries and peanuts, tea polyphenols, genistein, quercetin from onions, silymarin from artichoke."

Bone density

*The association between onion consumption and **bone density** in perimenopausal and postmenopausal non-Hispanic white women 50 years and older.* Matheson EM, Mainous AG, Carnemolla MA. Menopause. 2009 Jul-Aug;16(4):756-9. **Key Finding**: "Onion consumption seems to have a beneficial effect on bone density in perimenopausal and postmenopausal non-Hispanic white women 50 years and older. Furthermore, older women who consume onions most frequently may decrease their risk of **hip fracture** by more than 20% versus those who never consume onions."

*Dietary quercetin inhibits **bone loss** without effect on the uterus in ovarietomized mice.* Tsuji M, Yamamoto H, Sato T, Mizuha Y, Kawai Y, Taketani Y, Kato S, Terao J, Inakuma T, Takeda E. J Bone Miner Metab. 2009;27(6):673-81. **Key Finding**: "These results suggest that dietary quercetin inhibits bone loss without effect on the uterus in OVX mice and does not act as a potent inhibitor of osteoclastogenesis or as a selective estrogen receptor modulator in vivo."

*Effect of quercetin on **bone formation.*** Wong RW, Rabie AB. J Orthop Res. 2008 Aug;26(8):1061-6. **Key Finding**: "Quercetin in a collagen matrix has the effect of increasing new bone formation locally, and can be used as a bone graft material."

Cancer (colon; endometrial; esophageal; leukemia; lung; stomach)

Quercetin inhibited murine **leukemia** *WEHI-3 cells in vivo and promoted immune response.* Yu CS, Lai KC, Yang JS, Et al. Phytother Res. 2010 Feb;24(2):163-8. **Key Finding**: "Based on pathological examination of injected mice, an effect of quercetin isolated from onion was observed in the spleen of mice. Apparently, quercetin affects WEHI-3 cells in vivo."

Luteolin inhibits protein kinase C(epsilon) and c-Src activities and UVB-induced **skin cancer**. Byun S, Lee KW, Jung SK, Et al. Cancer Res. 2010 Mar 15;70(6):2415-23. **Key Finding**: "Luteolin, a flavonoid present in **onion and broccoli**, exerts potent chemo preventive activity against UVB-induced skin cancer mainly by targeting PKC(epsilon) and Src."

Allium vegetables intake and **endometrial cancer** *risk.* Galeone C, Pelucchi C, Dal Maso L, Negri E, Montella M, Zucchetto A, Talamini R, La Vecchia C. Public Health Nutr. 2009 Sep;12(9):1576-9. **Key Finding**: "We analyzed data from a multi-center case-control study of 454 endometrial cancer cases and 908 controls. Our study found a moderate protective role of allium vegetables (onions and garlic) on the risk of endometrial cancer."

Quercetin-induced apoptotic cascade in **cancer** *cells: antioxidant versus estrogen receptor alpha-dependent mechanisms.* Galluzzo P, Martini C, Bulzomi P, Leone S, Bolli A, Pallottini V, Marino M. Mol Nutr Food Res. 2009 Jun;53(6):699-708. **Key Finding**: "These findings suggest that quercetin results in HeLa cell death through an ERalpha-dependent mechanism involving caspase- and p38 kinase activation. These findings indicate new potential chemo preventive actions of flavonoids on cancer growth."

Food intake and the occurrence of squamous cell carcinoma in different sections of the esophagus in Taiwanese men. Chen YK, Lee CH, Wu IC, Liu JS, Wu DC, Lee JM, Goan YG, Chou SH, Huang CT, Lee CY, Hung HC, Yang JF, Wu MT. Nutrition. 2009 Jul-Aug;25(7-8):753-61. **Key Finding**: "We found that intake of vegetables, raw onions and raw garlic, and fruits significantly protective against **esophageal squamous cell carcinoma** risk."

Dietary flavonoids and **colorectal adenoma** *recurrence in the Polyp Prevention Trial.* Bobe G, Sansbury LB, Albert PS, Cross AJ, Kahle L, Ashby J, Slattery ML, Caan B, Paskett E, Iber F, Kikendall JW, Lance P, Daston C, Marshall JR, Schatzkin

A, Lanza E. Cancer Edpiemiol Biomarkers Prev. 2008 Jun;17(6):1344-53. **Key Finding**: "Total flavonoid intake was not associated with any or advanced adenoma recurrence. However, high intake of flavonols, which are at greater concentrations in beans, onions, apples and tea, was associated with decreased risk of advanced adenoma recurrence. Similar inverse associations were observed to a smaller extent for isoflavonoids, the flavonol kaempferol, and the isoflavonoids genistein and formononetin."

Chemoprevention of aberrant crypt foci in the colon of rats by dietary onion. Tache S, Ladam A, Corpet DE. Eur J Cancer. 2007 Jan;43(2):454-8. **Key Finding**: "Onion intake might reduce the risk of **colorectal cancer**, according to epidemiology. We tested 60 rats given a 5% dried onion diet. Data show that a 5% onion diet reduced carcinogenesis during initiation and promotion stages, and suggest this chemoprevention is due to known phytochemicals."

*Dietary quercetin inhibits proliferation of **lung carcinoma** cells.* Hung H. Forum Nutr. 2007;60:146-57. **Key Finding**: "Quercetin and other related flavonoids have been shown to inhibit carcinogen-induced tumors in rodents. In humans, the total average intake of quercetin and kaempferol is estimated at 20 mg/day and consumption of quercetin from onions and apples was inversely correlated with lung cancer risk. In this study, we report that quercetin-inhibited A549 lung carcinoma cells proliferation."

*Fruit and vegetable intake and prevalence of **colorectal adenoma** in a cancer screening trial.* Millen AE, Subar AF, Graubard BI, Peters U, Hayes RB, Weissfeld JL, Yokochi LA, Ziegler RG. Am J Clin Nutr. 2007 Dec;86(6):1754-64. **Key Finding:** "Diets rich in fruit and deep-yellow vegetables, dark-green vegetables, and onions and garlic are modestly associated with reduced risk of colorectal adenoma, a precursor of colorectal cancer."

*Anti-proliferative and pro-apoptotic effects of 2, 3-dihydro-3, 5-dihydroxy-6-methyl-4H-pyranone (DDMP) through inactivation of NF-kappaB in human **colon cancer** cells.* Ban JO, Hwang IG, Kim TM, Hwang BY, Lee US, Jeong HS, Yoon YW, Kimz DJ, Hong JT. Arch Pharm Res. 2007 Nov; 30(11):1455-63. **Key Finding**: "These results suggest that DDMP from onions inhibit **colon cancer** cell growth by inducing apoptotic cell death through the inhibition of NF-kappaB."

The production of reactive oxygen species and the mitochondrial membrane potential are modulated during onion oil-induced cell cycle arrest and apoptosis in A549 cells. Wu XJ, Stahl T, Hu Y, Kassie F, Mersch-Sundermann V. J Nutr. 2006 Mar;136(3):608-13. **Key**

Finding: "Protective effects of Allium vegetables against cancers have been shown extensively in experimental animals and epidemiologic studies. We investigated cell proliferation and the induction of apoptosis by onion oil extracted from Allium cepa, a widely consumed Allium vegetable, in human **lung cancer** A549 cells. These results suggest that onion oil may exert chemo preventive action by inducing cell cycle arrest and apoptosis in tumor cells."

*Growth inhibitory effect of alk(en)yl thiosulfates derived from onion and garlic in human immortalized and **tumor cell** lines.* Chang HS, Yamato O, Yamasaki M, Ko M, Maede Y. Cancer Lett. 2005 Jun 1;223(1):47-55. **Key Finding**: "Natural constituents of onion and garlic were shown to inhibit the in vitro proliferation of three human tumorigenic cell lines, WiDr, 293 and HL-60, in a dose-dependent manner. These results suggest that the alk(en)yl thiosulfates have an antitumor effect through the induction of apoptosis initiated by oxidative stress."

*Allium vegetables and **stomach cancer** risk in China.* Setiawan VW, Yu GP, Lu QY, Lu ML, Yu SZ, Mu L, Zhang JG, Kurtz RC, Cai L, Hsieh CC, Zhang ZF. Asian Pac J Cancer Prev. 2005 Jul-Sep;6(3):387-95. **Key Finding**: An epidemiological study in Shanghai (750 cases and 750 age- and gender- matched controls) and in Qingdao (201 cases and 201 age- and gender- matched controls) was conducted by a standard questionnaire. "Our results confirm protective effects of allium vegetables (especially onions and garlic) against stomach cancer."

*Varietal differences in phenolic content and **antioxidant** and **antiproliferative** activities of onions.* Yang J, Meyers KJ, Van der Heide J, Liu RH. J Agric Food Chem. 2004 Nov 3;52(22):6787-93. **Key Finding:** "The proliferation of HepG(2) and Caco-2 cells was significantly inhibited in a dose-dependent fashion after exposure to the Western Yellow, shallots, New York Bold, and Northern Red extracts of onion. Western Yellow, shallots, and New York Bold exhibited the highest antiproliferative activity against HepG(2) cells and New York Bold and Western Yellow exhibited the highest antiproliferative activity against Caco-2 cells. However, the varieties of Western White, Peruvian Sweet, Empire Sweet, Mexico, Texas 1015, Imperial Valley Sweet, and Vidalia demonstrated weak antiproliferative activity against both HepG(2) and Caco-2 cells. These results may influence consumers toward purchasing onion varieties exhibiting greater potential health benefits."

Comparative effects of mono-, di-, tri-, and tetrasulfides derived from plants of the Allium family: redox cycling in vitro and hemolytic activity and Phase 2 enzyme induction in vivo. Munday R, Munday JS, Munday CM. Free Rad Biol Med. 2003 May 1;34(9):1200-1211.

Key Finding: "Epidemiological evidence indicates that a high dietary intake of plants of the Allium family, such as garlic and onions, decreases the risk of **cancer** in humans. Allyl and propyl tri- and tetrasulfides, may contribute to the toxic effects of Allium vegetables, while only the allyl derivatives are effective in increasing tissue activities of cancer-protective enzymes."

*Botanicals in **cancer** chemoprevention.* Park EJ, Pezzuto JM. Cancer Metastasis Rev. 2002;21(3-4):231-55. **Key Finding:** "In this review, we discuss the cancer chemo preventive activity of cruciferous vegetables such as cabbage and broccoli, Allium vegetables such as garlic and onion, green tea, citrus fruits, tomatoes, berries, ginger and ginseng. Phytochemicals of these types have great potential in the fight against human cancer, and a variety of delivery methods are available as a result of their occurrence in nature."

*Intake of Flavonoids and **Lung Cancer**.* Marchand LL, Murphy SP, Hankin JH, Wilkens LR, Kolonel LN. J Natl Cancer Inst. 2000 Jan 19;92(2):154-60. **Key Finding:** "After adjusting for smoking and intakes of saturated fat and B-carotene, we found statistically significant inverse associations between lung cancer risk and the main food sources of the flavonoids quercetin (onions and apples) and naringin (white grapefruit.)"

*Protective effect of allium vegetables against both **esophageal and stomach cancer**: a simultaneous case-referent study of a high-epidemic area in Jiangsu Province, China.* Gao CM, Takezaki T, Ding JH, Li MS, Tajima K. J Cancer Res. 1999 Jun;90(6):614-21. **Key Finding:** "The main results in the present study suggested that allium vegetables (such as garlic and onion), like raw vegetables, may have an important protecting effect against not only stomach cancer, but also esophageal cancer."

*Consumption of onions and a reduced risk of **stomach carcinoma**.* Dorant E, van den Brandt PA, Goldbohm RA, Sturmans F. Gastroenterology. 1996 Jan;110(1):12-20. **Key Finding**: "The association between onion and leek consumption, garlic supplement use, and the incidence of stomach carcinoma was investigated in the Netherlands Cohort Study on diet and cancer, which started in 1986 with 120,852 men and women ranging in age from 55 to 69 years. The Netherlands Cohort Study provides evidence for a strong inverse association between onion consumption and stomach carcinoma incidence. The consumption of leeks and use of garlic supplements were not associated with stomach carcinoma risk."

*A prospective cohort study on the relationship between onion and leek consumption, garlic supplement use and the risk of **colorectal carcinoma** in The Netherlands.* Dorant E, van den Brandt PA, Goldbohm RA. Carcinogenesis. 1996 Mar;17(3):477-84.

Key Finding: "This study does not support an inverse association between the consumption of onions and leeks, or the use of garlic supplements and the incidence of male and female colon and rectum carcinoma."

Allium vegetable consumption, garlic supplement intake, and female **breast carcinoma** *incidence.* Dorant E, van den Brandt PA, Goldbohm RA. Breast Cancer Res Treat. 1995;33(2):163-70. **Key Finding:** "We found no association between the consumption of onions or leeks, or garlic supplement use, and the incidence of female breast carcinoma."

Inhibition of DMBA-induced mouse **skin tumorigenesis** *by garlic oil and inhibition of two tumor-promotion stages by garlic and onion oils.* Perchellet JP, Perchellet EM, Belman S. Nutr Cancer. 1990;14(3-4):183-93. **Key Finding:** "Onion and garlic oils inhibited the TPA-stimulated DNA synthesis when given as single doses of 5 mg one hour before TPA. The inhibition by garlic oil was most effective when given one hour before TPA but was evident when given from two hours before to two hours after TPA. These results indicate that onion and garlic oils inhibit all stages of mouse skin tumorigenesis."

Effects of organosulfur compounds from garlic and onions on benzo[a]pyrene-induced neoplasia and glutathione S-transferase activity in the mouse. Sparnins VL, Barany G, Wattenberg LW. Carcinogenesis. 1988 Jan;9(1):131-4. **Key Finding:** "All four allylic compounds (allyl methyl trisulfide, allyl methyl disulfide, diallyl trisulfide, and diallyl sulfide) from garlic and onions increased glutathione S-transferase activity in the forestomach, but varied in their capacity to induce GST in lung, liver and small bowel. In evaluating relationships between diet and **cancer**, it would be useful to consider the possible role of garlic and onion organosulfur compounds as protective agents."

Onion and garlic oils inhibit **tumor** *promotion.* Belman S. Carcinogenesis. 1983 Aug;4(8):1063-5. **Key Finding:** "The tumor yield and incidence of phorbol-myristate-acetate promotion were inhibited in a dose-dependent manner over the range of 10-10,000 micrograms onion oil, applied three times per week. Garlic oil was also inhibitor, but was less effective."

Cardiovascular disease

An **onion byproduct** *affects plasma lipids in healthy rats.* Roldan-Marlin E, Jensen RI, Krath BN, Et al. J Agric Food Chem. 2010 May 12;58(9):5308-14. **Key Finding:** "The aim of this study is to elucidate the safety and potential role of onion byproducts in affecting risk markers of **cardiovascular disease.** The effects of an onion byproduct, Allium cepa L. cepa 'Recas' (OBP) and its two derived fractions were measured. Onion byproduct contains factors with the ability to modulate plasma lipids and lipoprotein levels, but did not present significant beneficial effects on individual markers related to plasma lipid transport in the rat model."

Methanolic extract of onion (allium cepa) attenuates ischemia/hypoxia-induced apoptosis in cardiomyocytes via antioxidant effect. Park S, Kim MY, Lee DH, Lee SH, Baik EJ, Moon CH, Park SW, Ko EY, Oh SR, Jung YS. Eur J Nutr. 2009 Jun;48(4):235-42. **Key Finding**: "Although there is growing awareness of the beneficial potential of onion intake to lower the risk of **cardiovascular disease**, there is little information about the effect of onion on ischemic heart injury, one of the most common cardiovascular diseases. This study investigates the effect of the methanol-soluble extract of onion on ischemic injury in heart-derived H9c2 cells in vitro and in rat hearts in vivo. The results of this study suggest that the methanolic extract of onion attenuates ischemia/hypoxia-induced apoptosis in heart-derived H9c2 cells in vitro and in rat hearts in vivo, though, at least in part, an antioxidant effect."

Pure dietary flavonoids quercetin and (1)-epicatechin augment nitric oxide products and reduce endothelin-1 acutely in healthy men. Loke WM, Hodgson JM, Proudfoot JM, McKinley AJ, Puddey IB, Croft KD. Am J Clin Nutr. 2008 Oct;88(4):1018-25. **Key Finding**: "Dietary flavonoids may improve endothelial function and ultimately lead to beneficial **cardiovascular** effects. A randomized, placebo-controlled, crossover trial in 12 healthy men was conducted. It was found that dietary flavonoids such as quercetin and (a)-epicatechin can augment nitric oxide status and reduce endothelin-1 concentrations and may thereby improve endothelial function."

*Vegetable flavonoids and **cardiovascular disease**.* Terao J, Kawai Y, Murota K. Asia Pac J Clin Nutr. 2008;17 Suppl 1:291-3. **Key Finding**: "We focused on quercetin, a major flavonoid in onion, and its anti-atherosclerotic effect was examined from the aspect of the bioavailability and translocation to the target site. We discovered that quercetin metabolites accumulate in the aorta tissue and exerted their antioxidant activity. Furthermore, quercetin metabolites were detected in human atherosclerotic aorta exclusively. These imply that quercetin metabolites are incorporated into the atherosclerotic region and act as complementary antioxidants, when oxidative stress is loaded in the vascular system."

Ingestion of onion soup high in quercetin inhibits platelet aggregation and essential components of the collagen-stimulated platelet activation pathway in man: a pilot study. Hubbard GP, Wolffram S, de Vos R, Bovy A, Gibbons JM, Lovegrove JA. Br J Nutr. 2006 Sep;96(3):482-8. **Key Finding**: "The ingestion of quercetin from a dietary source of onion soup could inhibit some aspects of collagen-stimulated platelet aggregation and signaling ex vivo. This further substantiates the epidemiological data suggesting that those who preferentially consume high amounts of quercetin-containing foods have a reduced risk of thrombosis and potential **cardiovascular disease** risk."

*Dietary onion intake as part of a typical high fat diet improves indices of **cardiovascular** health using the mixed sex pig model.* Gabler NK, Ostrowska E, Imsic M, Eagling DR, Jois M, Tatham BG, Dunshea FR. Plant Foods Hum Nutr. 2006 Dec;61(4):179-85. **Key Finding**: "These data demonstrate that consumption of onions can have positive health effects in both male and female pigs consuming a high fat diet."

Consumption of foods rich in flavonoids is related to a decreased cardiovascular risk in apparently healthy French women. Menngen LI, Sapinho D, de Bree A, Arnault N, Bertrais S, Galan P, Hercberg S. J Nutr. 2004 Apr;134(4):923-6. **Key Finding:** "A cross-sectional analysis was performed in 1286 women and 1005 men. Dietary intakes were estimated using six 24-h dietary records. In women, flavonoid rich (such as onions) food consumption was inversely related to systolic blood pressure. Women in the highest tertile of flavonoid-rich food consumption were at lower risk for **cardiovascular disease**, whereas a positive tendency was seen in men."

Cataracts

*Preventive effect of onion juice on selenite-induced experimental **cataract**.* Javadzadeh A, Ghorbanihaghjo A, Bonyadi S, Rashidi MR, Mesgari M, Rashtchizadeh N, Argani H. Indian J Ophthalmol. 2009 May-Jun;57(3):185-9. **Key Finding:** "Instillation of onion juice into the rat eyes effectively prevents selenite-induced cataract formation. This effect was associated with increased TA level, SOD and GPX activities in the lens."

Cerebral ischemia

Neuroprotective effects of onion extract and quercetin against ischemic neuronal damage in the gerbil hippocampus. Hwang IK, Lee CH, Yoo KY, Choi JH, Park OK, Lim SS, Kang IJ, Kwon DY, Park J, Yi JS, Bae YS, Won MH. J Med Food. 2009

Oct;12(5):990-5. **Key Finding**: "We suggest that repeated administration of onion extract and quercetin can protect against neuronal damage from transient **cerebral ischemia**."

Neuroprotective effect of methanolic extracts of Allium cepa on ischemia and reperfusion-induced cerebral injury. Shri R, Singh BK. Fitoterapia. 2008 Feb;79(2):86-96. **Key Finding**: "The present study investigated the effect of methanol extract of outer scales and edible portions of Allium cepa bulb on ischemia and reperfusion-dinced cerebral injury. A. cepa bulb markedly reduced cerebral infarct size and attenuated impairment in short-term memory and motor coordination."

Cholesterol

*Effect of dietary **garlic** and **onion** on biliary proteins and lipid peroxidation which influence of cholesterol nucleation in bile.* Vidyashankar S, Sambaiah K, Srinivasan K. Steroids. 2010 Mar;75(3):272-81. **Key Finding**: "These data suggest that apart from the beneficial modulation of biliary cholesterol saturation index, Allium spices also influence cholesterol nucleating and antinucleating protein factors that contribute to their anti-lithogenic potential" preventing **cholesterol gallstone** formation in the gallbladder.

Welsh onion *attenuates **hyperlipidemia** in rats fed on high-fat high-sucrose diet.* Yamamoto Y, Yasouka A. Biosci Biotechnol Biochem. 2010;74(2):402-4. **Key Finding**: "The results suggest that the green Welsh onion might be effective in attenuating hyperlipidemia in a manner other than affecting fatty acid metabolism in the liver. Kaempferol seemed to be one of the components in green Welsh onion acting to lower lipid deposition."

*Regression of pre-established **cholesterol gallstones** by dietary **garlic and onion** in experimental mice.* Vidyashankar S, Sambaiah K, Srinivasan K. Metabolism. 2010 Oct;59(10):1402-12. **Key Finding:** "These results indicate that feeding garlic and onion effectively accelerates the regression of preformed cholesterol gallstones by promoting cholesterol desaturation in bile."

*Dietary garlic and onion reduce the incidence of atherogenic diet-induced **cholesterol gallstones** in experimental mice.* Vidyashankar S, Sambaiah K, Srinivasan K. Br J Nutr. 2009 Jun;101(11):1621-9. **Key Finding**: "Dietary garlic and onion reduce the cholesterol gallstones incidence by 15-39%. Dietary garlic and onion markedly reduced biliary cholesterol. Serum and liver cholesterol were decreased by feeding garlic or onion. Dietary Allium spices exerted antilithogenic influence by decreasing the cholesterol hyper-secretion into bile and increasing the bile acid output thus decreasing the formation of lithogenic bile in experimental mice."

Consumption of brown onions (Allium cepa var. cavalier and var. destiny) moderately modulates **blood lipids**, *hematological and hemostatic variables in healthy pigs.* Ostrowska E, Gabler NK, Sterling SJ, Tatham BG, Jones RB, Eagling DR, Jois M, Dunshea FR. Br J Nutr. 2004 Feb;91(2):211-8. **Key Finding**: "Onion supplementation, regardless of the variety, resulted in dose-dependent reductions in erythrocyte counts and Hb levels, while the white blood cell concentrations, particularly lymphocytes, were increased in pigs that consumed onions. Dietary supplementation with raw brown onions has moderate lipid-modulating and immunostimulatory properties."

Effects of essential oils of garlic and onion on alimentary **hyperlipemia**. Bordia A, Bansal HC, Arora SK, Singh SV. Atherosclerosis. 1975 Jan-Feb;21(1):15-9. **Key Finding:** "The effect of garlic and onion on alimentary hyperlipemia, induced by feeding 100 g butter, has been studied in 10 healthy subjects. The freshly extracted juice of 50 g of garlic or onion, as well as an equivalent amount of their ether-extracted essential oils, was administered randomly on four different days during a one-week period. Garlic and onion have a significant protective action against fat-induced increases in serum cholesterol and plasma fibrinogen and decreases in coagulation time and fibrinolysis activity."

Coronary artery disease

Dietary intakes of flavonols, flavones and isoflavones by Japanese women and the inverse correlation between quercetin intake and plasma LDL cholesterol concentration. Arai Y, Watanabe S, Kimira M, Shimoi K, Mochizuki R, Kinae N. J Nutr. 2000 Sep;130(9):2243-50. **Key Finding:** Subjects were 115 women volunteers. The major source of flavonoids was onions and that of isoflavones was tofu. "These results suggest that a high consumption of both flavonoids and isoflavones by Japanese women may contribute to their low incidence of **coronary heart disease** compared with women in other countries."

Dietary antioxidant flavonoids and risk of **coronary heart disease**: *the Zutphen Elderly Study.* Hertog MG, Feskens EJ, Hollman PC, Katan MB, Kromhout D. Lancet. 1993 Oct 23;342(8878):1007-11. **Key Finding:** The flavonoid intake of 805 men aged 65-84 years was measured. The major sources of intake were tea, onions and apples. "Flavonoid intake was significantly inversely associated with mortality from coronary heart disease. Flavonoids in regularly consumed foods may reduce the risk of death from coronary heart disease in elderly men."

Diabetes

*The **antidiabetic** effect of onion and garlic in experimental diabetic rats: meta-analysis.* Kook S, Kim GH, Choi K. J Med Food. 2009 Jun;12(3):552-60. Key Finding: "In the meta-analysis, the antidiabetic effects of onion extract and single components were significant for glucose concentration and body weight, but the effects of garlic extract were not significant. The results of the meta-analysis suggested that the single component intake and onion extract intake may be effective for lowering plasma glucose concentrations and body weight."

Depression

*Antidepressant-like effect of onion (Allium cepa L.) powder in a rat behavioral model of **depression**.* Sakakibara H, Yoshino S, Kawai Y, Terao J. Biosci Biotechnol Biochem. 2008 Jan;72(1):94-100. **Key Finding:** "The results of the present study suggest that onion exerted antidepressant-like activity in a behavioral model that acted independently of the hypothalamic-pituitary-adrenal axis."

Gallstones

*Dietary garlic and onion reduce the incidence of atherogenic diet-induced **cholesterol gallstones** in experimental mice.* Vidyashankar S, Sambaiah K, Srinivasan K. Br J Nutr. 2009 Jun;101(11):1621-9. **Key Finding**: "Dietary garlic and onion reduce the cholesterol gallstones incidence by 15-39%. Dietary garlic and onion markedly reduced biliary cholesterol. Serum and liver cholesterol were decreased by feeding garlic or onion. Dietary Allium spices exerted antilithogenic influence by decreasing the cholesterol hyper-secretion into bile and increasing the bile acid output thus decreasing the formation of lithogenic bile in experimental mice."

Heart failure (myocardial infarction)

*Allium vegetable intake and risk of **acute myocardial infarction** in Italy.* Galeone C, Tavani A, Pelucchi C, Negri E, La Vecchia C. Eur J Nutr. 2009 Mar;48(2):120-3. **Key Finding**: "The current study, the first from Mediterranean countries, suggests that a diet rich in onions may have a favorable effect on the risk of myocardial infarction."

Hip fractures

*The association between onion consumption and **bone density** in perimenopausal and post-menopausal non-Hispanic white women 50 years and older.* Matheson EM, Mainous AG, Carnemolla MA. Menopause. 2009 Jul-Aug;16(4):756-9. **Key Finding**: "Onion consumption seems to have a beneficial effect on bone density in perimenopausal and postmenopausal non-Hispanic white women 50 years and older. Further-more, older women who consume onions most frequently may decrease their risk of **hip fracture** by more than 20% versus those who never consume onions."

Hypertension

*Quercetin reduces **blood pressure** in hypertensive subjects.* Edwards RL, Lyon T, Litwin SE, Rabovsky A, Symons JD, Jalili T. J Nutr. 2007 Nov;137(11):2405-11. **Key Finding**: "Men and women with prehypertension and stage 1 hypertension were enrolled in a randomized, double-blind, placebo-controlled crossover study to test the efficacy of 730 mg quercetin a day for 28 days vs. placebo. These data are the first to our knowledge to show that quercetin supplementation reduces blood pressure in hypertensive subjects."

*Quercetin-supplemented diets lower **blood pressure** and attenuate cardiac hypertrophy in rats with aortic constriction.* Jalili T, Carlstrom J, Kim S, Freeman D, Jin H, Wu TC, Litwin SE, Symons J. J Cardiovasc Pharmacol. 2006 Apr;47(4):531-41. **Key Finding**: "Our data supports an antihypertensive and antihypertrophic effect of quercetin (from onions) in vivo in the absence of changes concerning vascular and myocardial function."

Antioxidative and antihypertensive *effects of Welsh onion on rats fed with a high-fat high-sucrose diet.* Yamamoto Y, Aoyama S, Hamaguchi N, Rhi GS. Biosci Biotechnol Biochem. 2005 Jul;69(7):1311-7. **Key Finding**: "These results suggest that the green-leafy Welsh onion, but not the white type, reduced super-oxide generation by suppressing the angiotensin II production and then the NADH/NADPH oxidase activity, increasing the NO availability in the aorta, and consequently lowering the blood pressure in the rats fed with the high-fat high-sucrose diet. The radical scavenging and reducing antioxidative activities of green Welsh onion may also be effective in decreasing superoxide."

Memory impairment

Neuroprotective effect of methanolic extracts of Allium cepa on ischemia and reperfusion-induced cerebral injury. Shri R, Singh BK. Fitoterapia. 2008 Feb;79(2):86-96. **Key Finding**: "The present study investigated the effect of methanolic extract of outer scales and edible portions of Allium cepa bulb on ischemia and reperfusion-dinced cerebral injury. A. cepa bulb markedly reduced cerebral infarct size and attenuated impairment in short-term memory and motor coordination."

*Antioxidative activity and ameliorative effects of **memory impairment** of sulfur-containing compounds in Allium species.* Nishimura H. Higuchi O, Tateshita K, Tomobe K, Okuma Y, Nomura Y. Bio factors. 2006;26(2):135-46. **Key Finding**: "These results suggest that di-n-propyl trisulfide contained in onion ameliorates memory impairment in SAMP8 mouse by its antioxidant effect."

Periodontal disease

*Inhibitory effect of quercetin on **periodontal pathogens** in vitro.* Geoghegan F, Wong RW, Rabie AB. Phytother Res. 2010 Jun;24(6):817-20. **Key Finding:** "The results suggest that quercetin possesses significant antimicrobial properties on periodontal pathogens in vitro."

Prostate Hyperplasia (benign)

*Onion and garlic intake and the odds of **benign prostatic hyperplasia**.* Galeone C, Pelucchi C, Talamini R, Negri E, Dal Maso L, Montella M, Ramazzotti V, Franceschi S, La Vecchia C. Urology. 2007 Oct;70(4):672-6. **Key Finding**: "This uniquely large data set from European populations (1369 patients and 1451 controls) showed an inverse association between allium vegetable consumption and benign prostatic hyperplasia."

Thrombosis (blood clots)

*An evaluation of garlic and onion as **antithrombotic** agents.* Bordia T, Mohammed N, Thomason M, Ali M. Prostaglandins Leukot Essent Fatty Acids. 1996 Mar;54(3):183-6. **Key Finding:** "Garlic and onion should be consumed in a raw rather than cooked form in order to achieve a beneficial effect. Garlic was found to be more potent than onion in lowering the TXB2 (thromboxane) levels.

These results show that garlic and onion can be taken frequently in low doses without any side effects, and can still produce a significant antithrombotic effect."

Onion exerts antiaggregatory effects by altering arachidonic acid metabolism in platelets. Srivastava KC. Prostaglandins Leukot Med. 1986 Sep;24(1):43-50. **Key Finding:** "In vitro effects of an oily extract of onion were examined on the metabolism of arachidonic acid in human platelets. Onion was found to reduce the formation of thromboxane and lipoxygenase products from exogenous arachidonic acid in platelets."

Aqueous extracts of onion, garlic and ginger inhibit platelet aggregation and alter arachidonic acid metabolism. Srivastava KC. Biomed Biochim Acta. 1984;43(8-9):S335-46. **Key Finding:** "Aqueous extracts of onion, garlic and ginger inhibited platelet aggregation induced by several aggregation agents, including arachidonate, in a dose-dependent manner. While onion and garlic extracts were found to be weak inhibitors of platelet thromboxane synthesis, ginger extract inhibited the platelet cyclooxygenase products and this effect correlated well with its inhibitory effects on the platelet aggregation induced by the above aggregation agents. The results indicate that if the same were happening in vivo, onion, garlic and ginger could be useful as natural antithrombotic materials."

Oranges

BOTANISTS BELIEVE THAT ORANGES probably originated in Southeast Asia and that, over the generations, a series of mutations created the variety of oranges we see today. The original hybrid may have been a cross between the pummelo and the mandarin orange, while the navel orange might have been resulted from a mutation in a Selecta orange tree sometime in the early nineteenth century. Oranges were introduced to the Americas shortly after the first Columbus expedition, with Florida being one of the first sites where they were cultivated.

Of all the vitamins and minerals present in the typical Florida orange, levels of vitamin C are by far the highest. Because they could prevent scurvy among sailors, oranges became a staple food along eighteenth-century trade routes. Six of the B vitamins are also present, along with calcium, magnesium, and potassium, among other minerals. Science experiments have found that the most nutritious and health beneficial part of the orange is its peel.

Alzheimer's

Effects of banana, orange, and apple on oxidative stress-induced neurotoxicity in PC12 cells. Heo HJ, Choi SJ, CHoi SG, Shin DH, Lee JM, Lee CY. J Food Sci. 2008 Mar;73(2):H28-32. **Key Finding:** "These results suggest that fresh apples, banana, and orange in our daily diet along with other fruits may protect neuron cells against oxidative-stress-induced neurotoxicity and may play an important role in reducing the risk of neurodegenerative disorders such as **Alzheimer's** disease."

Antioxidation

Antioxidant effectiveness of organically and non-organically grown red oranges in cell culture systems. Tarozzi A, Hrelia S, Angeloni C, Morroni F, Biagi P, Guardigli M, Cantelli-Forti G, Hrelia P. Eur J Nutr. 2006 Mar;45(3):152-8. **Key Finding:** "Our results clearly show that organic red oranges have a higher phytochemical content (i.e., phenolic, anthocyanin and ascorbic acid), total **antioxidant** activity and bioactivity than integrated nonorganic red oranges."

Bladder ischemia

Antioxidant levels of common fruits, vegetables, and juices versus protective activity against in vitro **ischemia/***reperfusion.* Bean H, Schuler C, Leggett RE, Levin RM. Int Urol Nephrol. 2009 Sep 19. (Epub ahead of print). **Key Finding:** "An assay was utilized to determine the antioxidant reactivity of a series of fruits, vegetables, and juices, and the results were compared to the protective ability of selected juices in an established in vitro rabbit bladder model of ischemia/reperfusion. The results showed that cranberry juice had the highest level of antioxidant reactivity, blueberry juice had an intermediate activity, and orange juice had the lowest. It was determined, however, that contrary to the hypothesis, the orange juice was significantly more potent in protecting the bladder against ischemia/reperfusion damage than either blueberry or cranberry juice."

Cancer (breast; colon; leukemia; lung; prostate; urinary; skin)

Bioactive compounds from **sour orange** *inhibit* **colon cancer** *cell proliferation and induce cell cycle arrest.* Jayaprakasha GK, Jadegoud Y, Nagana Gowda GA, Patil BS. J Agric Food Chem. 2010 Jan 13;58(1):180-6. **Key Finding:** "These findings support the hypothesis that limonoids and phytosterols are effective apoptosis-promoting agents and incorporation of enriched fractions of these compounds in the diet may serve to prevent colon cancer."

Monodemethylated polymethoxyflavones from sweet orange (Citrus sinensis) peel inhibit growth of human **lung cancer** *cells by apoptosis.* Xiao H, Yang CS, Li S, Jin H, Ho CT, Patel T. Mol Nutr Food Res. 2009 Mar;53(3):398-406. **Key Finding:** "Our results provide rationale to develop orange peel extract enriched with monode-methylated PMFs into value-added nutraceutical products for cancer prevention."

Chemo preventive effects of orange peel extract (OPE). I: OPE inhibits intestinal tumor growth in ApcMin/+ mice. Fan K, Kurihara N, Abe S, Ho CT, Ghai G, Yang K. J Med Food. 2007 Mar;10(1):11-7. **Key Finding:** "Findings indicated that orange peel inhibited tumorigenesis in this preclinical mouse model for human familial adenomatous polyposis, an intestinal **tumor growth**."

Chemo preventive effects of orange peel extract (OPE). II: OPE inhibits atypical hyperplastic lesions in rodent **mammary gland***.* Abe S, Fan K, Ho CT, Ghai G, Yang K. J

Med Food. 2007 Mar;10(1):18-24. **Key Finding**: "A standardized preparation of orange peel extract with 30% polymethoxyflavones decreased development of an atypical hyperplastic lesion and increased apoptosis in ductal epithelial cells of mouse mammary gland."

*Apoptosis-inducing activity of hydroxylase polymethoxyflavones and polymethoxyflavones from orange peel in human **breast cancer** cells.* Sergeev IN, Ho CT, Li S, Colby J, Dushenkov S. Mol Nutr Food Res. 2007 Dec;51(12):1478-84. **Key Finding**: "Our results strongly imply that bioactive polymethoxyflavones from sweet orange peel exert proapoptotic activity in human breast cancer cells, which depends on their ability to induce an increase in intracellular Ca(2+) and thus activate Ca(2+)-dependent apoptotic proteases."

Protective effects of a red orange extract on UVB-induced damage in human keratinocytes. Cimino F, Cristani M, Saija A, Bonina FP, Virgili F. Biofactors. 2007;30(2):129-38. **Key Finding**: "We can propose extract from red orange as a useful natural standardized extract in **skin photoprotection** with promising applications in the field of dermatology."

*Dietary beta-cryptoxanthin inhibits N-butyl-N-(4-hydroxybutyl) nitrosamine-induced **urinary bladder carcinogenesis** in male ICR mice.* Miyazawa K, Miyamoto S, Suzuki R, Yasui Y, Ikeda R, Kohno H, Yano M, Tanaka T, Hata K, Suzuki K. Oncol Rep. 2007 Feb;17(2):297-304. **Key Finding**: "These findings suggest that beta-cryptoxanthin extracted from Citrus unshiu oranges is able to prevent OH-BBN induced bladder carcinogenesis in mice."

*Apigenin and **cancer** chemoprevention: progress, potential and promise (review).* Patel D, Shukla S, Gupta S. Int J Oncol. 2007 Jan;30(1):233-45. **Key Finding**: "Apigenin is a flavones present in oranges, parsley and onions, and has been shown to possess remarkable anti-inflammatory, antioxidant and anti-carcinogenic properties. This review examines the cancer chemo preventive effects of apigenin."

*Plymethoxylated flavones induce Ca(2+)-mediated apoptosis in **breast cancer** cells.* Sergeev IN, Li S, Colby J, Ho CT, Dushenkov S. Life Sci. 2006 Dec 23;80(3):245-53. **Key Finding**: "We report that polymethoxyflavones derived from sweet orange inhibit growth of human breast cancer cells. Our results strongly suggest that the cellular Ca(2+) modulating activity of flavonoids underlies their apoptotic mechanism and that hydroxylation of PMFs (from sweet orange, Citrus sinensis L) is critical for their ability to induce an increase in {Ca(2+)}(i) and, thus, activate Ca(2+)-dependent apoptotic proteases."

*Zanthoxyli Fructus induces growth arrest and apoptosis of LNCaP human **prostate cancer** cells in vitro and in vivo in association with blockade of the AKT and AR signal pathways.* Yang Y, Ikezoe T, Takeuchi T, Adachi Y, Ohtsuki Y, Koeffler HP, Taguchi H. Oncol Rep. 2006 Jun;15(6):1581-90. **Key Finding**: "Zanthoxyli Fructus belong to the family of oranges and might be useful as an adjunctive therapeutic agent for the treatment of individuals with a variety of cancer types."

Biological activity of carotenoids in red paprika, Valencia orange and golden delicious apple. Molnar P, Kawase M, Satoh K, Sohara Y, Tanaka T, Tani S, Sakagami H, Nakashima H, Motohashi N, Gyemant N, Molnar J. Phytother Res. 2005 Aug;19(8):700-7. **Key Finding:** "Carotenoid fractions were extracted from red paprika, Valencia orange peel and the peel of Golden delicious apple. Apple showed potent anti-H. Pylori activity. The extracts were inactive against HIV. Apple and orange showed slightly higher cytotoxic activity against three human tumor cells lines (**squamous cell carcinoma HSC-2, HSC-3, submandibular gland carcinoma HSG, and human promyelocytic leukemic HL-60 cells**. Paprika scavenged efficiently. The data suggest the potential importance of carotenoids as possible anti-H. Pylori and multidrug resistance reversal agents."

*Food consumption by children and the risk of childhood acute **leukemia**.* Kwan ML, Block G, Selvin S, Month S, Buffler PA. Am J Epidemiol. 2004 Dec 1;160(11):1098-107. **Key Finding**: "Regular consumption of oranges and orange juice during the first 2 years of life was associated with a reduction in risk of childhood leukemia diagnosed between the ages of 2 and 14 years. Restricting the analysis to leukemia diagnosed between the ages of 2 and 5 years reflected a similar pattern of reduced risk."

*Influence of the diet on the development of **colorectal cancer** in a population of Madrid.* Juarranz Sanz M, Soriano Llora T, Et al. Rev Clin Esp. (Spanish). 2004 Jul;204(7):355-61. **Key Finding**: "The objective of this study is to evaluate the relationship between daily consumption of specific food groups and development of colorectal carcinoma. A modest inverse association was found with consumption of oranges, grapefruits, strawberries and cherries."

*Effects of commonly consumed fruit juices and carbohydrates on redox status and **anticancer** biomarkers in female rats.* Breinholt VM, Nielsen SE, Knuthsen P, Lauridsen ST, Daneshvar B, Sorensen A. Nutr Cancer. 2003;45(1):46-52. **Key Finding:** "The results of the present study suggest that commonly consumed fruit juices {apple juice, orange juice, black currant juice} can alter lipid and protein oxidation biomarkers in the blood as well as hepatic quinine reductase activity and that quercetin may not be the major active principle."

Carotenoids and **colon cancer**. Slattery ML, Benson J, Curtin K, Ma KN, Schaeffer D, Potter JD. Am J Clin Nutr. 2000 Feb;71(2):575-82. **Key Finding:** "Lutein was inversely associated with colon cancer in both men and women studied. The major dietary sources of lutein in subjects with colon cancer and in control subjects were spinach, broccoli, lettuce, tomatoes, oranges and orange juice, carrots, celery, and greens. These data suggest that incorporating these foods into the diet may help reduce the risk of developing colon cancer."

Citrus peel use is associated with reduced risk of squamous cell **carcinoma of the skin.** Hakim IA, Harris RB, Ritenbaugh C. Nutr Cancer. 2000;37(2):161-8. Key Finding: "Limonene has demonstrated efficacy in preclinical models of breast and colon cancers. The principal sources of d-limonene are the oils of orange, grapefruit, and lemon. The present case-control study was designed to determine the usual citrus consumption patterns of an older Southwestern population and to then evaluate how this citrus consumption varied with history of squamous cell carcinoma of the skin. We found no association between the overall consumption of citrus fruits or citrus juices and skin squamous cell carcinoma. However, the most striking feature was the protection purported by citrus peel consumption. Moreover, there was a dose-response relationship between higher citrus peel in the diet and degree of risk lowering. This is the first study to explore the relationship between higher citrus peel consumption and human cancers."

Inhibition of **mammary cancer** *by citrus flavonoids.* Guthrie N, Carroll KK. Adv Exp Med Biol. 1998;439:227-36. **Key Finding**: "Double strength orange juice given to the rats in place of drinking water inhibited mammary tumorigenesis induced in female Sprague-Dawley rats by DMBA more effectively than double strength grapefruit juice. This may mean that hesperidin retains its effectiveness in vivo better than naringenin. It is also possible that orange juice contains other compounds that have anti-cancer activity and that may act synergistically with hesperidin."

Inhibition of human **breast cancer** *cell proliferation and delay of mammary tumorigenesis by flavonoids and citrus juices.* So FV, Guthrie N, Chamers AF, Moussa M, Carroll KK. Nutr Cancer. 1996;26(2):167-81. **Key Finding**: "Two citrus flavonoids, hesperidin and naringenin, found in oranges and grapefruit, respectively, and four noncitrus flavonoids, baicalein, galangin, genistein, and quercetin, were tested singly and in one-to-one combinations for their effects on proliferation and growth of a human breast carcinoma cell line, MDA-MB-435. Naringenin is present in grapefruit mainly as its glycosylated form, naringin. These compounds as well as grapefruit and orange juice concentrates were tested for their ability to inhibit development of mammary tumors in female Sprague-Dawley rats. Tumor development was delayed in the groups given orange juice or fed the naringin-supplemented diet. Rats given orange juice had a smaller tumor burden and grew better than any of the other groups. These experiments provide evidence that citrus flavonoids are effective inhibitors of human breast cancer cell proliferation in vitro, especially when paired with quercetin."

Cholesterol

*Orange juice decreases low-density lipoprotein **cholesterol** in hypercholesterolemic subjects and improve lipid transfer to high-density lipoprotein in normal and hypercholesterolemic subjects.* Cesar TB, Aptekmann NP, Araujo MP, Et al. Nutr Res. 2010 Oct;30(10):689-94. **Key Finding**: "Orange juice may be beneficial as free-cholesterol transfer to HDL is crucial for cholesterol esterification and reverse cholesterol transport. Orange juice consumption decreased low-density lipoprotein cholesterol."

Coronary artery disease

Effect of acute and chronic grapefruit, orange, and pineapple juice intake on blood lipid profile in normolipidemic rat. Daher CF, Abou-Khalil J, Baroody GM. Med Sci Monit. 2005 Dec;11(12):BR465-72. **Key Finding**: "High fruit intake is known to be associated with reduced risk of **coronary heart disease**. The card protective benefit of chronic juice intake in normolipidemic rat may be chiefly through mechanisms independent of a direct effect on blood lipid profile, although orange and pineapple, but not grapefruit, relatively improved the metabolism and clearance of blood lipoprotein particles. As a result of delayed gastric emptying, grapefruit and pineapple juices may moderate sharp increases in postprandial plasma TAG concentrations accompanying peak digestion and absorption."

Obesity

Blood orange juice inhibits fat accumulation in mice. Titta L, Trinei M, Stendardo M, Et al. Int J Obes (London). 2010 Mar;34(3):578-88. **Key Finding**: "Dietary supplementation of Moro juice (a blood orange), but not Navelina juice (a blond orange), significantly reduced body **weight gain** and fat accumulation regardless of the increased energy intake because of sugar content. Furthermore, mice drinking Moro juice were resistant to HFD-induced **obesity** with no alterations in food intake."

Pecans (see Nuts)

Peppers (Chile, Bell, and Black)

CAPSICUM IS A GENUS OF FLOWERING PLANTS native to the Americas, where they have been cultivated as a food, spice, and medicine for thousands of years by the native peoples of what are now the United States, Mexico, and Central and South America. The fruit of *Capsicum* plants include chile peppers and bell peppers. Cayenne powder and paprika powder, made by grinding dried peppers, are used for seasoning in many cuisines.

About forty species of *Capsicum* are known to exist, five of which have been domesticated for agricultural production. Each species includes many varieties; for example, bell peppers and jalapenos are both varieties of *Capsicum annuum*. Capsaicin is the primary flavonoid in most *Capsicum* peppers and is what endows them with their varying degrees of hot, pungent flavors and aromas. In addition to creating a strong burning sensation in the mouth, capsaicin is an antioxidant with cancer-fighting powers and one of the primary sources of many of the health benefits of peppers.

Antioxidation

Antioxidant *and* ***antiproliferative*** *activities of common vegetables.* Chu YF, Sun J, WuX, Liu RH. J Agric Food Chem. 2002 Nov 6;50(23):6910-6. **Key Finding:** "In this study, 10 common vegetables were selected on the basis of consumption per capita data in the U.S. Broccoli possessed the highest total phenolic content, followed by spinach, yellow onion, red pepper, carrot, cabbage, potato, lettuce, celery, and cucumber. Red pepper had the highest total antioxidant activity, followed by broccoli, carrot, spinach, cabbage, yellow onion, celery, potato, lettuce and cucumber. Antiproliferative activities were also studied in vitro using human liver cancer cells. Spinach showed the highest inhibitory effect, followed by cabbage, red pepper, onion, and broccoli."

Cancer (bladder; breast; colon; esophageal; leukemia; melanoma; oral; pancreatic; prostate; tongue)

Capsaicin *induces apoptosis through ubiquitin-proteasome system dysfunction.* Maity R, Sharma J, Jana NR. J Cell Biochem. 2010 Apr 1;109(5):933-42. **Key Finding:** "Capsaicin is an active component of red pepper having an antiproliferative effect in a **variety of cancer cells** due to its ability to induce apoptosis. Treatment of capsaicin to mouse neuro 2a cells results in the inhibition of proteasome activity in a dose- and time-dependent manner that seems to correlate with its effect on cell death. Our results strongly support the use of capsaicin as an anticancer drug."

In vitro investigation of the potential immunomodulatory and anti-cancer activities of **black pepper** *(Piper Nigrum) and cardamom (Elettaria cardamomum).* Majdalawieh AF, Carr RI. J Med Food. 2010 Apr;13(2):371-81. **Key Finding**: "Our findings strongly suggest that black pepper and cardamom exert immunomodulatory roles and **antitumor** activities and hence they manifest themselves as natural agents that can promote the maintenance of a healthy immune system."

Capsaicin *induces apoptosis in SCC-4 human* **tongue cancer** *cells through mitochondria-dependent and –independent pathways.* Ip SW, Lan SH, Huang AC, Et al. Environ Toxicol. 2010 Oct 5 (Epub ahead of print). **Key Finding**: "Herein, we investigated whether capsaicin induces apoptosis in human tongue cancer SCC-4 cells. Capsaicin decreased the percentage of viable cells in a dose-dependent manner and produced DNA fragmentation and GO/G1 phase arrest in SCC-4 cells."

Apoptosis induced by capsaicin and resveratrol in **colon carcinoma** *cells requires nitric oxide production and caspase activation.* Kim MY, Trudel LJ, Wogan GN. Anticancer Res. 2009 Oct;29(10):3733-40. **Key Finding:** "We examined the role of nitric oxide and influence of p53 status during apoptosis induced by these agents in two isogenic HCT116 human colon carcinomas, wild-type p53 and complete knockout of p53 cells. Capsaicin and resveratrol, alone or in combination, inhibited cell growth and promoted apoptosis by the elevation of nitric oxide; combined treatment in p53-WT cells was most effective. These findings offer exciting opportunities to improve the effectiveness of colon cancer treatment."

Capsaicin-induced apoptosis in human **hepatoma** *HepG2 cells.* Huang SP, Chen JC, Wu CC, Chen CT, Tang NY, Ho YT, Lin JP, Chung JG, Lin JG. Anticancer Res. 2009 Jan;29(1):165-74. **Key Finding**: "Our results indicated that the capsaicin-induced apoptosis in HepG2 cells may result from the elevation of intracellular Ca2+ production, ROS, disruption of alpha psi(m), regulation of Bcl-2 family protein expression and caspase-3 activity."

Suppression of cFLIP by lupeol, a dietary triterpene, is sufficient to overcome resistance to TRAIL-mediated apoptosis in chemo resistant human **pancreatic cancer** *cells.* Murtaza I, Saleem M, Adhami VM, Hafeez BB, Mukhtar H. Cancer Res. 2009 Feb

1;69(3):1156-65. **Key Finding**: "Our findings showed the anticancer efficacy of lupeol with mechanistic rationale against highly chemo resistant human PaC cells. We suggest that lupeol, alone or as an adjuvant to current therapies, could be useful for the management of human PaC."

Lupeol triterpene, a novel diet-based microtubule targeting agent: disrupts surviving/cFLIP activation in **prostate cancer** *cells.* Saleem M, Murtaza I, Witkowsky O, Kohl AM, Maddodi N. Biochem Biophys Res Commun. 2009 Oct 23;388(3):576-82. **Key Finding**: "We conclude that the Lupeol-induced growth inhibition of CaP cells is a net outcome of simultaneous effects on stathmin, cFLIP, and surviving which results in the disruption of microtubule assembly. We suggest that Lupeol alone or as an adjuvant to other microtubule agents could be developed as a potential agent for the treatment of human CaP."

Lupeol, a novel anti-inflammatory and **anti-cancer** *dietary triterpene.* Saleem M. Cancer Lett. 2009 Nov 28;285(2):109-15. **Key Finding**: "Lupeol, a triterpene found in green pepper, white cabbage, olive, strawberry, mangoes and grapes, was reported to possess beneficial effects as a therapeutic and preventive agent for a range of disorders. Lupeol at its effective therapeutic doses exhibit no toxicity to normal cells and tissues. This mini review provides detailed account of preclinical studies conducted to determine the utility of lupeol as a therapeutic and chemo preventive agent for the treatment of inflammation and cancer."

Capsaicin, a component of red peppers, induces expression of androgen receptor via PI3K and MAPK pathways in **prostate** *LNCaP cells.* Malagarie-Cazenave S, Olea-Herrero N, Vara D, Diaz-Laviada I. FEBS Lett. 2009 Jan 5;583(1):141-7. **Key Finding**: "In this study, capsaicin induced an increase in the cell viability of the androgen-responsive prostate cancer LNCaP cells."

Capsaicin induces apoptosis by generating reactive oxygen species and disrupting mitochondrial transmembrane potential in human **colon cancer** *cell lines.* Yang KM, Pyo JO, Kim GY, Yu R, Han IS, Ju SA, Kim WH, Kim BS. Cell Mol Biol Lett. 2009;14(3):497-510. **Key Finding**: "Our results clearly showed that capsaicin induced apoptosis in colon cancer cells. Although the actual mechanisms of capsaicin-induced apoptosis remain uncertain, it may be a beneficial agent for colon cancer treatment and chemoprevention."

Capsaicin-induced apoptosis in human **breast cancer** *MCF-7 cells through caspase-independent pathway.* Chou CC, Wu YC, Wang YF, Chou MJ, Kuo SJ, Chen DR. Oncol Rep. 2009 Mar;21(3):665-71. **Key Finding**: "Our results suggest that capsaicin induces cellular apoptosis (in MCF-7 breast cancer cells) through a caspase-independent pathway and that reactive oxygen species and intracellular calcium ion fluctuation has a minimal role in the process."

A case-control study of **gallbladder cancer** *in Hungary.* Nakadaira H, Lang I, Szentirmay Z, Hitre E, Kaster M, Yamamoto M. Asian Pac J Cancer Prev. 2009;10(5):833-6. **Key Finding**: "Our previous study indicated an association of chili pepper consumption with gallbladder cancer in the presence of gall-stones in Chile. We investigated whether or not a similar association was present in Hungary, where mortality from gallbladder cancer is high and chili peppers are frequently consumed. Hungarian hot pepper consumption was identified as a risk factor for gallbladder cancer by multivariate logistic regression analysis."

Lupeol inhibits growth of highly aggressive human metastatic melanoma cells in vitro and in vivo by inducing apoptosis. Saleem M, Maddodi N, Abu Zaid M, Khan N, bin Hafeez B, Asim M, Suh Y, Yun JM, Setaluri V, Mukhtar H. Clin Cancer Res. 2008 Apr 1;14(7):2119-27. **Key Finding**: "Our findings showed the anticancer efficacy of lupeol, a triterpene, with mechanistic rationale against metastatic human **mela-noma** cells. We suggest that lupeol, alone or as an adjuvant to current therapies, could be useful for the management of human melanoma."

Growth inhibition of human **colon cancer** *cells by plant compounds.* Duessel S, Heuertz RM, Ezekiel UR. Clin Lab Sci. 2008 Summer;21(3):151-7. **Key Finding**: "The purpose of this study was to determine if resveratrol from red grapes, cinnam-aldehyde from cinnamon, and piperine from black pepper has anti-proliferative effects on colon cancer. All phytochemicals displayed anti-proliferative effects on DLD-1 colon cancer cells in culture. These results taken together with everyday dietary availability of concentrations used in this study strongly suggest that regular intake of low doses of these phytochemicals offer preventive effects against colon cancer."

Fruits, vegetables, soy foods and **breast cancer** *in pre- and postmenopausal Korean women: a case-control study.* Do MH, Lee SS, Kim JY, Jung PJ, Lee MH. Int J Vitam Nutr Res. 2007 Mar;77(2):130-41. **Key Finding**: "High tomato intake was associated with reduced breast cancer risk in premenopausal women. In postmenopausal women, green pepper intake showed an inverse association of breast cancer risk."

Immunotherapy of **tumors** *with neuroimmune ligand capsaicin.* Beltran J, Ghosh AK, Basu S. J Immunol. 2007 Mar 1;178(5):3260-4. **Key Finding**: "In this study, we demonstrate that intratumoral administration of capsaicin into a preexisting tumor results in retarded progression of the injected tumor regardless of whether the tumor is at its early or late stage. Furthermore, it leads to significant inhibition of growth of other, uninjected tumors in the same animal. Capsaicin-elicited immunity is shown to be T cell-mediated and tumor-specific."

Capsaicin induced apoptosis of B16-F10 **melanoma** *cells through down-regulation of Bci-2.* Jun HS, Park T, Lee CK, Kang MK, Park MS, Kang H, Surh YJ, Kim OH. Food Chem Toxicol. 2007 May;45(5):708-15. **Key Finding**: "These findings indicate that capsaicin from hot chili peppers induces apoptosis of B16-F10 melanoma cells via down-regulation the Bci-2."

Apoptosis induced by capsaicin in prostate PC-3 cells involves ceramide accumulation, neutral sphingomyelinase, and JNK activation. Sanchez AM, Malagarie-Cazenave S, Olea N, Vara D, Chiloeches A, Diaz-Laviada I. Apoptosis. 2007 Nov;12(11):2013-24. **Key Finding**: "Numerous studies have recently focused on the anticarcinogenic, antimutagenic, or chemo preventive activities of the main pungent component of red pepper, capsaicin. We have previously shown that, in the androgen-independent **prostate cancer** PC-3 cells, capsaicin inhibits cell growth and induces apoptosis through reactive oxygen species generation. In the present study, we investigated the signaling pathways involved in the antiproliferative effect of capsaicin."

Catechin-vanilloid synergies with potential clinical applications in **cancer**. Morre DM, Morre DJ. Rejuvenation Res. 2006 Spring;9(1):45-55. **Key Finding**: "A cancer-specific cell surface protein, tNOX, has been identified as a target for low-dose cell killing (apoptosis) of cancer cells by green tea catechins and Capsicum vanilloid combinations. This protein is uniquely associated with all forms of cancer and is absent from normal cells and tissues. Its activity is correlated with cancer growth. When blocked, cancer cells fail to enlarge after division and eventually die."

Capsaicin induced cell cycle arrest and apoptosis in human esophagus epidermoid carcinoma CE 81T/VGH cells through the elevation of intracellular reactive oxygen species and Ca2+ productions and caspase-3 activation. Wu CC, Lin JP, Yang JS, Chou ST, Chen SC, Lin YT, Lin HL, Chung JG. Mutat Res. 2006 Oct 10;601(1-2):71-82. **Key Finding**: "These results suggest that the capsaicin-induced apoptosis in the CE 81T/VGH cells may result from the activation of caspase-3 and intracellular Ca2+ release pathway and it is further suggested that capsaicin has potential as a novel therapeutic agent for the treatment of **esophagus epidermoid carcinoma** cells."

Biological activity of carotenoids in red paprika, Valencia orange and golden delicious apple. Molnar P, Kawase M, Satoh K, Sohara Y, Tanaka T, Tani S, Sakagami

H, Nakashima H, Motohashi N, Gyemant N, Molnar J. Phytother Res. 2005 Aug;19(8):700-7. **Key Finding:** "Carotenoid fractions were extracted from red paprika, Valencia orange peel and the peel of Golden delicious apple. Apple showed potent anti-H. Pylori activity. The extracts were inactive against HIV. Apple and orange showed slightly higher cytotoxic activity against three human **tumor cells lines (squamous cell carcinoma HSC-2, HSC-3, submandibular gland carcinoma HSG, and human promyelocytic leukemic HL-60 cells.** Paprika scavenged efficiently. The data suggest the potential importance of carotenoids as possible anti-H. Pylori and multidrug resistance reversal agents."

Bioactivities of Anastasia black (Russian sweet pepper). Shirataki Y, Kawase M, Sakagami H, Nakashima H, Tani S, Tanaka T, Sohara Y, Schelz Z, Molnar J, Motohashi N. Anticancer Res. 2005 May-Jun;25(38):1991-9. **Key Finding**: "Some fractions of hexane and acetone extracts of Russian sweet pepper showed higher cytotoxic activity against **three human oral tumor cell lines (squamous cell carcinoma HSC-2, HSC-3, submandibular gland carcinoma HSG)** than against three normal human oral cells. No fractions displayed anti-HIV activity, but some hydrophobic fractions showed higher anti-H. Pylori activity."

Capsaicin-induced apoptosis and reduced release of reactive oxygen species in MBT-2 murine **bladder tumor** *cells.* Lee JS, Chang JS, Lee JY, Kim JA. Arch Pharm Res. 2004 Nov;27(11):1147-53. Key Finding: "These results suggest that capsaicin may be a valuable intravesical chemotherapeutic agent for bladder cancers."

Induction of apoptosis in **leukemic** *cells by homovanillic acid derivative, capsaicin, through oxidative stress: implication of phosphorylation of p53 at Ser-15 residue by reactive oxygen species.* Ito K, Nakazato T, Yamato K, Miyakawa Y, Yamada T, Hozumi N, Segawa K, Ikeda Y, Kizaki M. Cancer Res. 2004 Feb 1;64(3):1071-8. **Key Finding**: "Capsaicin effectively inhibited tumor growth and induced apoptosis in vivo using NOD/SCID mice with no toxic effects. We conclude that capsaicin has potential as a novel therapeutic agent for the treatment of leukemia."

Capsaicin, a spicy component of hot pepper, induces apoptosis by activation of the peroxisome proliferator-activated receptor gamma in HT-29 human **colon cancer** *cells.* Kim CS, Park WH, Park JY, Kang JH, Kim MO, Kawada T, Yoo H, Han IS, Yu R. J Med Food. 2004 Fall;7(3):267-73. **Key Finding**: "Our data suggest that capsaicin-induced apoptotic cell death in HT-29 human colon cancer cells could be associated with the PPARgamma pathway without the involvement of the vanilloid receptor. Capsaicin may have a beneficial effect for the treatment of colon cancer."

Non-pungent capsaicinoids from sweet pepper synthesis and evaluation of the chemo preventive and anticancer potential. Macho A, Lucena C, Sancho R, Daddario N, Minassi A, Munoz E, Appendino G. Eur J Nutr. 2003 Jan;42(1):2-9. **Key Finding:** "These results (from tumoral cells) suggest that capsiates target a variety of pathways involved in **cancer** development and inflammation, and have considerable potential for dietary health benefits."

*Capsaicin inhibits growth of adult T-cell **leukemia** cells.* Zhang J, Nagasaki M, Tanaka Y, Morikawa S. Leuk Res. 2003 Mar;27(3):275-83. **Key Finding**: "Capsaicin treatment inhibited the growth of ATL cells both in dose and time-dependent manner. The inhibitory effect was mainly due to the induction of cell cycle arrest and apoptosis. Based on these findings, capsaicin may be considered for chemo-prevention of adult T-cell leukemia."

*Synergistic Capsicum-tea mixtures with **anticancer** activity.* Morre DJ, Morre DM. J Pharm Pharmacol. 2003 Jul;55(7):987-94. **Key Finding**: "We have demon-strated a synergy between a decaffeinated green tea concentrate and a vanilloid-containing Capsicum preparation. At a ratio of 25 parts green tea concentrate to 1 part Capsicum preparation, the resultant product exhibited efficacy in the killing of cancer cells in culture 100-times that of green tea on a weight basis."

Cytotoxic and multidrug resistance reversal activity of a vegetable, 'Anastasia Red', a variety of sweet pepper. Motohashi N, Wakabayashi H, Kurihara T, Takada Y, Maruyama S, Sakagami H, Nakashima H, Tani S, Shirataki Y, Kawase M, Wolfard K, Molnar J. Phytother Res. 2003 Apr;17(4):348-52. **Key Finding**: "These extracts showed relatively higher cytotoxic activity against two human **oral tumors** cell lines (HSC-2, HSG) than against normal human gingival fibroblasts, suggesting a tumor-specific cytotoxic activity."

Antioxidant and **antiproliferative** *activities of common vegetables.* Chu YF, Sun J, Wu X, Liu RH. J Agric Food Chem. 2002 Nov 6;50(23):6910-6. **Key Finding:** "In this study, 10 common vegetables were selected on the basis of consumption per capita data in the U.S. Broccoli possessed the highest total phenolic content, followed by spinach, yellow onion, red pepper, carrot, cabbage, potato, lettuce, celery, and cucumber. Red pepper had the highest total antioxidant activity, followed by broccoli, carrot, spinach, cabbage, yellow onion, celery, potato, lettuce and cucumber. Antiproliferative activities were also studied in vitro using human liver cancer cells. Spinach showed the highest inhibitory effect, followed by cabbage, red pepper, onion, and broccoli."

Antimutagenic activity of carotenoids in green peppers against some nitroarenes. Gonzalez de Mejia E, Quintanar-Hernandez A, Loarca-Pina G. Mutat Res. 1998 Aug 7;416(1-2):11-9. **Key Finding**: "These results suggest that each one of the pepper extracts have more than one **antimutagenic** compound (e.g., beta-carotene and xanthophyll) and those functional nutrients apparently have a synergistic effect."

*Chemo protective effects of capsaicin and diallyl sulfide against **mutagenesis** or **tumori-genesis** by vinyl carbamate and N-nitrosodimethylamine.* Surh YJ, Lee RC, Park KK, Mayne ST, Liem A, Miller JA. Carcinogenesis. 1995 Oct;16(10):2467-71. **Key Finding:** "The results of this study suggest that capsaicin, a major ingredient of hot chili peppers, and diallyl sulfide from garlic suppress VC and NDMA-induced mutagenesis or tumorigenesis in part through inhibition of the cyto-chrome P-450 IIE1 isoform responsible for activation of these carcinogens."

Cholesterol

*Hypoxanthine levels in human urine serve as a screening indicator for the plasma total **choles-terol** and low-density lipoprotein modulation activities of **fermented red pepper paste**.* Kim Y, Park YJ, Yang SO, Et al. Nutr Res. 2010 Jul;30(7):455-61. **Key Finding**: "Marked cholesterol modulation was observed in the fermented red pepper paste treated group compared with the placebo group."

Administration of tomato and paprika beverages modifies hepatic glucose and lipid metabolism in mice: a DNA microarray analysis. Aizawa K, Matsumoto T, Inakuma T, Ishijima T, Nakai Y, Abe K, Amano F. J Agric Food Chem. 2009 Nov 25;57(22):10964-71. **Key Finding**: "To examine whether the expression of hepatic genes, including biomarkers, is affected by the ingestion of tomato or paprika, mice were given tomato beverage, paprika beverage, or water control for 6 weeks. The ingestion of tomato or paprika un-regulated the expression of 687 and 1045 genes and down-regulated the expression of 841 and 653 genes respectively. These changes in gene expression suggest that tomato ingestion promotes flycogen accumulation and stimulates some specific steps in fatty acid oxidation. Paprika ingestion promoted the entire glucose and fatty acid metabolic pathways to improve lipid profiles."

Effects of daily ingestion of chili on serum lipoprotein oxidation in adult men and women. Ahuja KD, Ball MJ. Br J Nutr. 2006 Aug;96(2):239-42. **Key Finding**: "Regular consumption of chili for 4 weeks increases the resistance of serum lipoproteins to oxidation. Laboratory studies had shown that the resistance of isolated LDL-

cholesterol or linoleic acid to oxidation is increased in incubations with chili extracts or capsaicin, the active ingredient of chili."

Diabetes

*Kochujang, a Korean fermented red pepper plus soybean paste, improves glucose homeostasis in 90% pancreatectomized **diabetic** rats.* Kwon DY, Hong SM, Ahn IS, Kim YS, Shin DW, Park S. Nutrition. 2009 Jul-Aug;25(7-8):790-9. **Key Finding:** Kochujuan, the fermented product of red pepper, and soybeans have been reported to modulate energy and glucose metabolism. "The combination of red pepper and fermented soybeans in kochujang improves glucose homeostasis by reducing insulin resistance."

Inflammation

Immunosuppressive activity of capsaicinoids: capsiate derived from sweet peppers inhibits NF-kappaB activation and is a potent anti-inflammatory compound in vivo. Sancho R, Lucena C, Macho A, Calzado MA, Blanco-Molina M, Minassi A, Appendino G, Munoz E. Eur J Immunol. 2002 Jun;32(6):1753-63. **Key Finding**: "These results suggest that capsaicin target specific pathways involved in **inflammation,** and hold considerable potential for dietary health benefits as well as for pharmaceutical development."

Obesity/Weight loss

*Targeting inflammation-induced **obesity** and metabolic diseases by curcumin and other nutraceuticals.* Aggarwal BB. Annu Rev Nutr. 2010 Aug 21;30:173-99. **Key Finding**: "Curcumin-induced alterations reverse insulin resistance, hyperglycemia, hyperlipidemia and other symptoms linked to obesity. Other structurally homologous nutraceuticals, derived from red **chili, cinnamon, cloves, black pepper and ginger**, also exhibit effects against obesity and insulin resistance."

*Maximum tolerable dose of red pepper decreases **fat intake** independently of spicy sensation in the mouth.* Yoshioka M, Imanaga M, Ueyama H, Yamane M, Kubo Y, Boivin A, St-Amand J, Tanaka H, Kiyonaga A. Br J Nutr. 2004 Jun;91(6):991-5. **Key Finding**: "The present results indicate that the maximum tolerable dose is necessary to have a suppressive effect of red pepper on fat intake."

*Effects of red pepper on **appetite** and **energy intake**.* Yoshioka M, St-Pierre S, Drapeau V, Dionne I, Doucet E, Suzuki M, Tremblay A. Br J Nutr. 1999 Aug;82(2):115-23. **Key Finding**: "These results indicate that the ingestion of red pepper decreases appetite and subsequent protein and fat intakes in Japanese females and energy intake in Caucasian males."

Pineapple (see Fruit)

Pomegranates

POMEGRANATES ARE NATIVE TO IRAN AND IRAQ and have been cultivated throughout the Mediterranean since ancient times. They are mentioned by the Greek writer Homer in his epic poems, archaeologists have found Mesopotamian cuneiform tablets from at least four thousand years ago describing pomegranates. They have long been valued both as a food and as a source for remedies in the Ayurvedic system of medicine in India, where they are used to treat diarrhea, intestinal parasites, bleeding, and cataracts.

During the twentieth century, Western science began to extensively study the health benefits of pomegranate consumption. Pomegranates are high in vitamin C and polyphenols, the most common being ellagitannins and punicalagins, both of which are antioxidants. Its other phytochemicals include catechins, gallocatechins, and anthocyanins. Laboratory research and preliminary human trials have shown pomegranates to be effective in reducing the risk of atherosclerosis and cardiovascular disease, along with a variety of other maladies.

Aging

Extract of Punica granatum inhibits **skin photo aging** *induced by UVB irradiation.* Park HM. Moon E, Kim AJ, Et al. Int J Dermatol. 2010 Mar;49(3):276-82. **Key Finding**: "The major polyphenols in **pomegranate**, particularly catechin, play a significant role in its photoprotective effects on UVB-induced skin damage."

Dietary compound ellagic acid alleviates **skin wrinkle** *and inflammation induced by UV-B irradiation.* Bae JY, Choi JS, Kang SW, Et al. Exp Dermatol. 2010 Aug;19(8):e182-90. **Key Finding:** "These results demonstrate that ellagic acid present in **berries and pomegranate** prevented collagen destruction and inflammatory responses caused by UV-B. Dietary and pharmacological interventions with ellagic acid may be promising treatment strategies interrupting skin wrinkle and inflammation associated with chronic UV exposure leading to photo aging."

Pomegranate juice is potentially better than apple juice in improving antioxidant function in **elderly** *subjects.* Guo C, Wei J, Yang J, Xu J, Pang W, Jiang Y. Nutr Res. 2008 Feb;28(2):72-7. **Key Finding:** "26 elderly subjects were divided into two groups, an apple and pomegranate, consumed daily for 4 weeks. Changes in plasma antioxidant capacity, activity of antioxidant enzymes, contents of ascorbic acid, vitamin E, reduced glutathione, oxidized low density lipoprotein and carbonyls, and the degree of DNA damage in mononuclear blood cells were measured. It is concluded that daily consumption of pomegranate juice is potentially better than apple juice in improving antioxidant function in the elderly. Phenolic may be the functional components contained in pomegranate juice that accounted for the observations."

Antioxidation

Consumption of polyphenol-rich beverages (mostly **pomegranate and black currant juices***) by healthy subjects for a short term increased serum antioxidant status, and the serum's ability to attenuate macrophage cholesterol accumulation.* Rosenblat M, Volkova N, Attias J, Et al. Food Funct. 2010 Oct;1(1):99-109. **Key Finding:** "100% Wonderful-variety pomegranate and 100% black currant juices were the most potent **antioxidative** effects of 35 beverages studies."

Comparison of **antioxidant** *potency of commonly consumed polyphenol-rich beverages in the United States.* Seeram NP, Aviram M, Zhang Y, Henning SM, Feng L, Dreher M, Heber D. J Agric Food Chem. 2008 Feb 27;56(4):1415-22. **Key Finding:** "The present study applied four tests of antioxidant potency. The beverages included several different brands as follows: apple juice, acai juice, black cherry juice, blueberry juice, cranberry juice, Concord grape juice, orange juice, red wines, iced tea beverages, black tea, green tea, white tea, and a major pomegranate juice available in the U.S. market. Pomegranate juice had the greatest antioxidant potency composite index among the beverages tested and was at least 20% greater than any of the other beverages tested."

Intervention of antioxidant system function of aged rats by giving fruit juices with different antioxidant capacities. Xu J, Guo CJ, Yang JJ, Wei JY, Li YF, Pang W, Jiang YG, Cheng S. Zhonghua Yu Fang Yi Xue Za Zhi (in Chinese). 2005 Mar;39(2):80-3. **Key Finding**: "The pomegranate juice should possess higher antioxidant capacity and might improve the antioxidant system function of aged rats, while the apple juice is relatively lower in antioxidant capacity and not very effective."

Atherosclerosis

Effects of a pomegranate fruit extract rich in punicalagin on oxidation-sensitive genes and eNOS activity at sites of perturbed shear stress and **atherogenesis***.*de Nigris F, Williams-Ignarro S, Sica V, Lerman LO, D'Armiento FP, Byrns RE, Casamassimi A,

Carpentiero D, Schiano C, Sumi D, Fiorito C, Ignarro LJ, Napoli C. Cardiovasc Res. 2007 Jan 15;73(2):414-23. **Key Finding:** "This study indicates that the proatherogenic effects induced by perturbed shear stress can be also reversed by chronic administration of pomegranate fruit extract."

Beneficial effects of pomegranate juice on oxidation-sensitive genes and endothelial nitric oxide synthase activity at sites of perturbed shear stress. De Nigris F, Williams-Ignarro S, Lerman LO, Crimi E, Botti C, Mansueto G, D'Armiento FP, De Rosa G, Sica V, Ignarro LJ, Napoli C. Proc Natl Acad Sci. 2005 Mar 29;102(13):4896-901. **Key Finding:** "Oral administration of pomegranate juice to hypercholesterolemic mice at various stages of disease reduced significantly the progression of **atherosclerosis.** This experimental study indicates that the proatherogenic effects induced by perturbed shear stress can be reversed by chronic administration of PJ. This approach may have implications for the prevention or treatment of atherosclerosis and its clinical manifestations."

*Pomegranate juice supplementation to atherosclerotic mice reduces macrophage lipid peroxidation, cellular **cholesterol** accumulation and development of **atherosclerosis.*** Kaplan M, Hayek T, Raz A, Coleman R, Dornfeld L, Vaya J, Aviram M. J Nutr. 2001 Aug;131(8):2082-9. **Key Finding:** "Pomegranate juice supplementation to mice with advanced atherosclerosis reduced the lesion size by 17% compared with placebo-treated mice. In a separate study, supplementation of young (2-mo-old) mice for 2 mo. with a tannin fraction isolated from PJ reduced their atherosclerotic lesion size, paralleled by reduced plasma lipid peroxidation and decreased Ox-LDL MPM uptake. PJ supplementation to mice with advanced atherosclerosis reduced their macrophage oxidative stress, their macrophage cholesterol flux and even attenuated the development of atherosclerosis."

Pomegranate juice consumption inhibits serum angiotensin converting enzyme activity and reduces systolic blood pressure. Aviram M, Dornfeld L. Atherosclerosis. 2001 Sep;158(1):195-8. **Key Finding**: "Consumption of pomegranate juice which is rich in tannins, possess anti-atherosclerotic properties which could be related to its potent anti-oxidative characteristics. A 36% decrement in serum ACE activity and a 5% reduction in systolic **blood pressure** were noted in hypertensive patients. As reduction in serum ACE activity, even with no decrement in blood pressure, was previously shown to attenuate **atherosclerosis,** pomegranate juice can offer a wide protection against cardiovascular diseases."

Pomegranate juice consumption reduces oxidative stress, atherogenic modifications to LDL, and platelet aggregation: studies in humans and in atherosclerotic apolipoprotein E-deficient mice. Aviram M, Dornfeld L, Rosenblat M, Volkova N, Kaplan M, Coleman R, Hayek T, Presser D, Fuhrman B. Am J Clin Nutr. 2000 May;71(5):1062-76. **Key Finding:** "Pomegranate juice had potent antiatherogenic effects in healthy humans and in **atherosclerotic** mice that may be attributable to its antioxidative properties."

Cancer (breast; colon; lung; prostate; skin)

Pomegranate extract inhibits the proliferation and viability of MMTV-Wnt-1 mouse mammary cancer stem cells in vitro. Dai Z, Nair V, Khan M, Ciolino HP. Oncol Rep. 2010 Oct;24(4):1087-91. **Key Finding**: "These data suggest that pomegranate extract, which is a proven and safe dietary supplement, has promise as a treatment against **breast cancer** by preventing proliferation of cancer stem cells."

Pomegranate *ellagitannins-derived compounds exhibit antiproliferative and antiaromatase activity in **breast cancer** cells in vitro.* Adams LS, Zhang Y, Seeram NP, Et al. Cancer Prev Res. 2010 Jan;3(1):108-13. **Key Finding**: "These studies suggest that pomegranate ellagitannins-derived compounds have potential for the prevention of estrogen-responsive breast cancers."

*Occurrence of urolithins, gut microbiota ellagic acid metabolites and proliferation markers expression response in the human **prostate** gland upon consumption of walnuts and **pomegranate** juice.* Gonzalez-Sarrias A, Gimenez-Bastida JA, Garcia-Conesa MT, Et al. Mol Nutr Food Res. 2010 Mar;54(3):311-22. **Key Finding**: "Pomegranate juice exerts protective effects against prostate cancer, mainly attributed to ellagitannins. Our results suggest that urolithin glucuronides and dimethyl ellagic acid may be the molecules responsible for the beneficial effects of pomegranate juice against prostate cancer."

Effects of fruit ellagitannins extracts, ellagic acid, and their colonic metabolite, urolithin A, on Wnt signaling. Sharma M, Li L, Celver J, Et al. J Agric Food Chem. 2010 Apr 14;58(7):3965-9. **Key Finding**: "Ellagitannin rich-foods such as **pomegranate** have potential against **colon carcinogenesis** and that urolithins are relevant bioactive constituents in the colon."

Colon cancer *chemo preventive activities of **pomegranate** ellagitannins and urolithins.* Kasimsetty SG, Bialonskia D, Reddy MK, Et al. J Agric Food Chem. 2010 Feb 24;58(4):2180-7. **Key Finding**: "These results indicate that the ellagitannins and urolithins released in the colon upon consumption of pomegranate juice in considerable amounts could potentially curtail the risk of colon cancer development by inhibiting cell proliferation and inducing apoptosis."

*Oral feeding of **pomegranate fruit extract** inhibits early biomarkers of UVB radiation-induced **carcinogenesis** in SKH-1 hairless mouse **epidermis**.* Afaq F, Khan N, Syed DN, Mukhtar H, Et al. Photochem Photobiol. 2010 Nov-Dec;86(6):1316-26. **Key Finding**: "We provide evidence that oral feeding of pomegranate fruit extract to mice affords substantial protection from the adverse effects of UVB radiation via modulation in early biomarkers of photo carcinogenesis."

*Pomegranate fruit extract impairs invasion and motility in human **breast cancer**.* Khan GN, Gorin MA, Rosenthal D, Pan Q, Bao LW, Wu ZF, Newman RA, Pawlus AD, Yang P, Lansky EP, Merajver SD. Integr Cancer Ther. 2009 Sep;8(3):242-53. **Key Finding: "**Pomegranate fruit extracts (PFE) possess polyphenol and other compounds with antiproliferative, pro-apoptotic and anti-inflammatory effects in prostate, lung, and other cancers. The authors investigated the effect of a novel, defined PFE consisting of both fermented juice and seed oil on the NF-kB pathway, which is constitutively active in aggressive breast cancer cell lines. Inhibition of motility and invasion by PFEs, coincident with suppressed RhoC and RhoA protein expression, suggests a role for these defined extracts in lowering the metastatic potential of aggressive breast cancer species."

Cellular antioxidant activity of common fruits. Wolfe KL, Kang X, He X, Dong M, Zhang Q, Liu RH. J Agric Food Chem. 2008 Sep 24;56(18):8418-26. **Key Finding:** "The objective of this study was to determine the cellular antioxidant activity, total phenolic contents, and oxygen radical absorbance capacity values of 25 fruits commonly consumed in the United States. Pomegranate and berries (wild blueberry, blackberry, raspberry, and blueberry) had the highest cellular antioxidant activity, whereas banana and melons had the lowest. Apple and strawberries were the biggest suppliers of cellular antioxidant activity to the American diet. Increasing fruit consumption is a logical strategy to increase antioxidant intake and decrease oxidative stress and may lead to reduced risk of **cancer.**"

*Pomegranate juice inhibits sulfoconjugation in Caco-2 human **colon carcinoma** cells.* Saruwatari A, Okamura S, Nakajima Y, Narukawa Y, Takeda T, Tamura H. J Med Food. 2008 Dec;11(4):623-8. **Key Finding**: "These data suggest that punicalagin (pomegranate's most abundant antioxidant polyphenol) is mainly responsible for the inhibition of sufloconjugation by pomegranate juice."

Pomegranate fruit extract inhibits pro survival pathways in human A549 lung carcinoma cells and tumor growth in athymic nude mice. Khan N, Hadi N, Afaq F, Syed DN, Kweon

MH, Mukhtar H. Carcinogenesis. 2007 Jan;28(1):163-73. **Key Finding:** "Our results provide a suggestion that pomegranate fruit extract can be a useful chemo preventive/chemotherapeutic agent against human **lung cancer**."

*Phase II study of pomegranate juice for men with rising prostate-specific antigen following surgery or radiation for **prostate cancer**.* Pantuck AJ, Leppert JT, Zomorodian N, Aronson W, Hong J, Barnard RJ, Seeram N, Liker H, Wang H, Elashoff R, Heber D, Aviram M, Ignarro L, Belldegrun A. Clin Cancer Res. 2006 Jul 1;12(13):4018-26. **Key Finding:** "We report the first clinical trial of pomegranate juice in patients with prostate cancer. The statistically significant prolongation of PSA doubling time, coupled with corresponding laboratory effects on **prostate cancer** in vitro cell proliferation and apoptosis as well as oxidative stress, warrant further testing in a placebo-controlled study."

*Pomegranate juice, total pomegranate ellagitannins, and punicalagin suppress inflammatory cell signaling in **colon cancer** cells.* Adams LS, Seeram NP, Aggarwal BB, Takada Y, Sand D, Heber D. J Agric Food Chem. 2006 Feb 8;54(3):980-5. **Key Finding:** "The polyphenol phytochemicals in the pomegranate can play an important role in the modulation of inflammatory cell signaling in colon cancer cells."

In vitro antiproliferative, apoptotic and antioxidant activities of punicalagin, ellagic acid and a total pomegranate tannin extract are enhanced in combination with other polyphenols as found in pomegranate juice. Seeram NP, Adams LS, Henning SM, Niu Y, Zhang Y, Nair MG, Heber D. J Nutr Biochem. 2005 Jun;16(6):360-7. **Key Finding:** "Pomegranate juice showed greatest antiproliferative activity against all **colon cancer** cell lines by inhibiting proliferation from 30% to 100%. The superior bioactivity of **pomegranate juice** compared to its purified polyphenols illustrated the multifactorial effects and chemical synergy of the action of multiple compounds compared to single purified active ingredients."

*Pomegranate fruit juice for chemoprevention and chemotherapy of **prostate cancer**.* Malik A, Afaq F, Sarfaraz S, Adhami VM, Syed DN, Mukhtar H. Proc Natl Acad Sci. 2005 Oct 11;102(41):14813-8. **Key Finding:** "Pomegranate from the tree Punica granatum possesses strong antioxidant and anti-inflammatory properties. We recently showed that pomegranate fruit extract possesses remarkable antitumor-promoting effects in mouse skin. In this study, employing human prostate cancer cells, we evaluated the antiproliferative and proapoptotic properties of pomegranate. We suggest that pomegranate juice may have cancer-chemo preventive as well as cancer-chemotherapeutic effects against prostate cancer in humans."

Chemo preventive and adjuvant therapeutic potential of pomegranate (Punica granatum) for human **breast cancer**. Kim ND, Mehta R, Yu W, Neeman I, Livney T, Michay A, Et al. Breast Cancer Res Treat. 2002 Feb;71(3):203-17. **Key Finding:** "The ability to affect a blockade of endogenous active estrogen biosynthesis was shown by polyphenols from fermented organically grown pomegranate juice. The findings suggest that clinical trials to further assess chemo preventive and adjuvant therapeutic applications of pomegranate in human breast cancer may be warranted."

Cardiovascular disease

Pomegranate *(Punica granatum L.) juice supplementation attenuates isoproterenol-induced cardiac necrosis in rats.* Jadeja RN, Thounaojam MC, Patel DK, Et al. Cardiovasc Toxicol. 2010 Sep;10(3):174-80. **Key Finding**: "Present study provides first scientific report on protect effect of supplementation of pomegranate juice against isoproterenol-induced cardiac necrosis in rats."

Pomegranate juice flavonoids inhibit low-density lipoprotein oxidation and **cardiovascular diseases***: studies in atherosclerotic mice and in humans.* Aviram M, Dornfeld L, Kaplan M, Coleman R, Gaitini D, Nitecki S, Hofman A, Rosenblat M, Volkova N, Presser D, Attias J, Hayek T, Fuhrman B. Drugs Exp Clin Res. 2002;28(2-3):49-62. **Key Finding:** "Dietary supplementation of polyphenol-rich pomegranate juice to atherosclerotic mice significantly inhibited the development of atherosclerotic lesions and this may be attributed to the protection of LDL against oxidation."

Cholesterol

Cholesterol*-lowering effect of concentrated pomegranate juice consumption in* **type II diabetic** *patients with hyperlipidemia.* Esmaillzadeh A, Tahbaz F, Gaieni I, Alavi-Majd H, Azadbakht L. Int J Vit Nutr Res. 2006;76(3):147-151. **Key Finding:** "It is concluded that concentrated pomegranate juice consumption could modify heart disease risk factors in hyperlipidemia patients."

Pomegranate juice inhibits oxidized LDL uptake and **cholesterol** *biosynthesis in macrophages.* Fuhrman B, Volkova N, Aviram M. J Nutr Biochem. 2005 Sep;16(9):570-6. **Key Finding:** "We conclude that pomegranate juice-mediated suppression of Ox-LDL degradation and of cholesterol biosynthesis in macrophages can lead to reduced cellular cholesterol accumulation and foam cell formation."

*Pomegranate juice supplementation to atherosclerotic mice reduces macrophage lipid peroxidation, cellular **cholesterol** accumulation and development of **atherosclerosis**.* Kaplan M, Hayek T, Raz A, Coleman R, Dornfeld L, Vaya J, Aviram M. J Nutr. 2001 Aug;131(8):2082-9. **Key Finding:** "Pomegranate juice supplementation to mice with advanced atherosclerosis reduced the lesion size by 17% compared with placebo-treated mice. In a separate study, supplementation of young (2-mo-old) mice for 2 months with a tannin fraction isolated from PJ reduced their atherosclerotic lesion size, paralleled by reduced plasma lipid peroxidation and decreased Ox-LDL MPM uptake. PJ supplementation to mice with advanced atherosclerosis reduced their macrophage oxidative stress, their macrophage cholesterol flux and even attenuated the development of atherosclerosis."

Coronary artery disease

Vascular action of polyphenols. Ghosh D, Scheepens A. Mol Nutr Food Res. 2009 Mar;53(3):322-31. **Key Finding**: "Several epidemiological studies suggest that the regular consumption of foods and beverages rich in flavonoids is associated with a reduction in the risk of several pathological conditions ranging from **hypertension to coronary heart disease, stroke and dementia**. The major polyphenols shown to have some of these effects in humans are primarily from tomatoes (polyphenols and nonpolyphenol), soy, pomegranate, grape seed and berries."

Dementia

Vascular action of polyphenols. Ghosh D, Scheepens A. Mol Nutr Food Res. 2009 Mar;53(3):322-31. **Key Finding**: "Several epidemiological studies suggest that the regular consumption of foods and beverages rich in flavonoids is associated with a reduction in the risk of several pathological conditions ranging from **hypertension to coronary heart disease, stroke and dementia**. The major polyphenols shown to have some of these effects in humans are primarily from tomatoes (polyphenols and nonpolyphenol), soy, pomegranate, grape seed and berries."

Dental plaque

Punica granatum (pomegranate) extract is active against dental plaque. Menezes SM, Cordeiro LN, Viana GS. J Herb Pharmacother. 2006;6(2):79-92. **Key Finding**: Extract from pomegranate was studied on 60 healthy patients using fixed orthodontic appliances. Those in the pomegranate mouth wash group were very effective against dental plaque microorganisms. Pomegranate juice may be a possible alternative for the treatment of dental plaque bacteria.

Diabetes

Effect of **pomegranate seed oil** *on hyperlipidemia subjects: a double-blind placebo-controlled clinical trial.* Mirmiran P, Fazeli MR, Asghari G, Et al. Br J Nutr. 2010 Aug;104(3):402-6. **Key Finding**: "It is concluded that administration of pomegranate seed oil for 4 weeks in **hyperlipidemia** subjects had favorable effects on lipid profiles including TAG and TAG:HDL-C ratio."

The effects of polyphenol-containing antioxidants on oxidative stress and lipid peroxidation in **Type 2 diabetes** *mellitus without complications.* Fenercioglu AK, Saler T, Genc E, Et al. J Endocrinol Invest. 2010 Feb;33(2):118-24. **Key Finding**: "These observations indicated that the polyphenol-rich antioxidant supplement containing **pomegranate extract**, green tea extract, and ascorbic acid has important antagonizing effects on oxidative stress and lipid peroxidation in patients with Type 2 diabetes mellitus and might be beneficial in preventing cardiovascular complications."

Effect of **pomegranate juice** *on Angiotensin II-induced* **hypertension** *in* **diabetic** *Wistar rats.* Mohan M, Waghulde H, Kasture S. Phytother Res. 2010 Jun;24 Suppl 2:S196-203. **Key Finding:** "The results suggest that the pomegranate juice extract could prevent the development of high blood pressure induced by Ang II in diabetic rats probably by combating the oxidative stress induced by diabetes and Ang II and by inhibiting ACE activity."

Cholesterol-*lowering effect of concentrated pomegranate juice consumption in* **type II diabetic** *patients with hyperlipidemia.* Esmaillzadeh A, Tahbaz F, Gaieni I, Alavi-Majd H, Azadbakht L. Int J Vit Nutr Res. 2006;76(3):147-151. **Key Finding:** "It is concluded that concentrated pomegranate juice consumption could modify heart disease risk factors in hyperlipidemia patients."

Concentrated pomegranate juice improves lipid profiles in diabetic patients with hyperlipidemia. Esmaillzadeh A, Tahbaz F, Gaieni I, Alavi-Majid H, Azadbakht L. J Med Food. 2004 Fall;7(3):305-8. **Key Finding**: "It is concluded that concentrated pomegranate juice consumption may modify **heart disease** risk factors in hyperlipidemia patients, and its inclusion therefore in their diets may be beneficial."

Heart Disease

Concentrated pomegranate juice improves lipid profiles in diabetic patients with hyperlipidemia. Esmaillzadeh A, Tahbaz F, Gaieni I, Alavi-Majid H, Azadbakht L. J Med Food. 2004 Fall;7(3):305-8. **Key Finding**: "It is concluded that concentrated pomegranate juice consumption may modify **heart disease** risk factors in hyperlipidemia patients, and its inclusion therefore in their diets may be beneficial."

HIV

Punica granatum (Pomegranate) juice provides an HIV-1 entry inhibitor and candidate topical microbicide. Neurath AR, Strick N, Li YY, Debnath AK. BMC Infect Dis. 2004 Oct 14;4:41. **Key Finding**: "HIV-1 entry inhibitors from pomegranate juice absorb onto corn starch. The resulting complex blocks virus binding to CD4 and CXCR4/CCRS and inhibits infection by primary virus clades A to G and group O. These results suggest the possibility of producing an anti-HIV-1 microbicide from inexpensive, widely available sources whose safety has been established throughout centuries."

Hypertension

Effect of **pomegranate juice** *on Angiotensin II-induced* **hypertension** *in* **diabetic** *Wistar rats.* Mohan M, Waghulde H, Kasture S. Phytother Res. 2010 Jun;24 Suppl 2:S196-203. **Key Finding:** "The results suggest that the pomegranate juice extract could prevent the development of high blood pressure induced by Ang II in diabetic rats probably by combating the oxidative stress induced by diabetes and Ang II and by inhibiting ACE activity."

Vascular action of polyphenols. Ghosh D, Scheepens A. Mol Nutr Food Res. 2009 Mar;53(3):322-31. **Key Finding**: "Several epidemiological studies suggest that the regular consumption of foods and beverages rich in flavonoids is associated with a reduction in the risk of several pathological conditions ranging from **hypertension to coronary heart disease, stroke and dementia**. The major polyphenols shown to have some of these effects in humans are primarily from tomatoes (polyphenols and nonpolyphenol), soy, pomegranate, grape seed and berries."

Pomegranate juice consumption for 3 years by patients with **carotid artery stenosis** *reduces common carotid intima-media thickness, blood pressure and LDL oxidation.* Aviram

M, Rosenblat M, Gaitini D, Nitecki S, Hoffman A, Dornfeld L, Volkova N, Presser D, Attias J, Liker H, Hayek T. 2004 Clin Nutr. 2004 Jun;23(3):423-33. **Key Finding:** "The results of the present study thus suggest that pomegranate juice consumption by patients with carotid artery stenosis decreases carotid IMT and systolic **blood pressure** and these effects could be related to the potent antioxidant characteristics of pomegranate juice polyphenols."

Pomegranate juice consumption inhibits serum angiotensin converting enzyme activity and reduces systolic blood pressure. Aviram M, Dornfeld L. Atherosclerosis. 2001 Sep;158(1):195-8. **Key Finding**: "Consumption of pomegranate juice which is rich in tannins, possess anti-atherosclerotic properties which could be related to its potent anti-oxidative characteristics. A 36% decrement in serum ACE activity and a 5% reduction in systolic **blood pressure** were noted in hypertensive patients. As reduction in serum ACE activity, even with no decrement in blood pressure, was previously shown to attenuate **atherosclerosis,** pomegranate juice can offer a wide protection against cardiovascular diseases."

Inflammatory diseases

Suppression of the nuclear factor-kappaB activation pathway by spice-derived phytochemicals: reasoning for seasoning. Aggarwal BB, Shishodia S. Ann N Y Acad Sci. 2004 Dec;1030:434-41. **Key Finding:** "The activation of nuclear transcription factor kappaB has now been linked with a variety of inflammatory disease, including **cancer, atherosclerosis, myocardial infarction, diabetes, allergy, asthma, arthritis, Crohn's disease, multiple sclerosis, Alzheimer's disease, osteoporosis, psoriasis, septic shock, and AIDS**. Extensive research in the last few years has shown that the pathway that activates this transcription factor can be interrupted by phytochemicals derived from spices such as turmeric (curcumin), red pepper (capsaicin), cloves (eugenol), ginger (gingerol), cumin, anise, and fennel (anethol), basil and rosemary (ursolic acid), garlic (diallyl sulfide, S-allylmercaptocysteine, ajoene), and pomegranate (ellagic acid). For the first time, therefore, research provides 'reasoning for seasoning.'"

Influenza

Influenza virus *variation in susceptibility to inactivation by* **pomegranate** *polyphenols is determined by envelope glycoproteins.* Sundararajan A, Ganapathy R, Huan L, Et al. Antiviral Res. 2010 Oct;88(1):1-9. **Key Finding:** "Our findings demonstrate that the direct anti-influenza activity of pomegranate polyphenols is substantially modulated by small changes in envelope glycoproteins."

Pomegranate (Punica granatum) purified polyphenol extract inhibits **influenza** *virus and has a synergistic effect with oseltamivir.* Haidariab M, Muzammil A, Illab SW, Madjidab M. Phytomedicine. 2009 Dec;16(12):1127-1136. **Key Finding:** "Pomegranate polyphenol extract inhibited the replication of human influenza A/Hong Kong (H3N2) in vitro. Pomegranate extracts should be further studied in therapeutic and prophylactic potential especially for influenza epidemics and pandemics."

Skin damage

Extract of Punica granatum inhibits **skin photoaging** *induced by UVB irradiation.* Park HM, Moon E, Kim AJ, Et al. Int J Dermatol. 2010 Mar;49(3):276-82. **Key Finding**: "The major polyphenols in **pomegranate**, particularly catechin, play a significant role in its photo protective effects on UVB-induced skin damage."

Dietary compound ellagic acid alleviates **skin wrinkle** *and inflammation induced by UV-B irradiation.* Bae JY, Choi JS, Kang SW, Et al. Exp Dermatol. 2010 Aug;19(8):e182-90. **Key Finding:** "These results demonstrate that ellagic acid present in **berries and pomegranate** prevented collagen destruction and inflammatory responses caused by UV-B. Dietary and pharmacological interventions with ellagic acid may be promising treatment strategies interrupting skin wrinkle and inflammation associated with chronic UV exposure leading to photo aging."

Stroke

Vascular action of polyphenols. Ghosh D, Scheepens A. Mol Nutr Food Res. 2009 Mar;53(3):322-31. **Key Finding**: "Several epidemiological studies suggest that the regular consumption of foods and beverages rich in flavonoids is associated with a reduction in the risk of several pathological conditions ranging from **hypertension to coronary heart disease, stroke and dementia**. The major polyphenols shown to have some of these effects in humans are primarily from tomatoes (polyphenols and nonpolyphenol), soy, pomegranate, grape seed and berries."

Pumpkins

THE GOURD-LIKE SQUASH WE CALL PUMPKIN (a variety of winter squash) may have originated in North America, since the oldest pumpkin seeds ever found, about seven thousand to nine thousand years in age, were discovered at an archaeological dig in Mexico. Today, pumpkins are grown on all the continents except Antarctica, with the US state of Illinois being one of the primary producers.

Nutritionally, pumpkin contains high levels of vitamin A, vitamin E, riboflavin, potassium, iron, and phytosterols. Medical studies show that these chemical compounds can help prevent and alleviate diabetes. Pumpkin seeds and pumpkin seed oil, with their high fatty acid content, are also beneficial in lowering cholesterol, treating prostate problems, and maintaining healthy blood vessels.

Cancer (breast; colon; gastric; lung; melanoma; prostate)

*Medicinal and biological potential of **pumpkin**: an updated review.* Yaday M, Jain S, Tomar R, Et al. Nutr Res Rev. 2010 Dec;23(2):184-90. **Key Finding**: "Various important medicinal properties of pumpkin and its phyto-constituents include anti-diabetic, antioxidant, **anti-carcinogenic**, anti-inflammatory and other well documented properties."

*Do dietary lycopene and other carotenoids protect against **prostate cancer**?* Jian L, Du CJ, Lee AH, Binns CW. Int J Cancer. 2005 Mar 1;113(6):1010-4. **Key Finding:** "Intake of pumpkin rich in carotenoids was inversely associated with prostate cancer risk.

*Comparison of lifestyle risk factors by family history for **gastric, breast, lung and colorectal cancer**.* Huang XE, Hirose K, Wakai K, Matsuo K, Ito H, Xiang J, Takezaki T, Tajima K. Asian Pac J Cancer Prev. 2004 Oct-Dec;5(4):419-27. **Key Finding**: "Frequent intake of pumpkin, cabbage, lettuce and fruits and raw vegetables were associated with decreased risk for all four sites of cancer— gastric, breast, lung and colon."

Anticancer and anti-inflammatory activities of cucurbitacins from Cucurbita andreana. Jayaprakasam B, Seeram NP, Nair MG. Cancer Lett. 2003 Jan 10;189(1):11-6. **Key Finding**: "Cucurbitacins from Cucurbita andreana were evaluated for their inhibitory effects on the growth of human **colon, breast, lung**, and central nervous system cancer cell lines. All cell lines were inhibited dose-dependent; colon from 65 to 81.5%; breast from 12 to 87%; lung from 2 to 96%."

Purification and characterization of Moschatin, a novel type I ribosome-inactivating protein from the mature seeds of pumpkin (Curcurbita moschata), and preparation of its immuno- toxin against human melanoma cells. Xia HC, Li F, Li Z, Zhang ZC. Cell Res. 2003 Oct;13(5):369-74. **Key Finding**: "The results implied that Moschatin from the mature seeds of pumpkin can be used as a new potential anticancer agent against **melanoma**."

Diabetes

*Flax and **Pumpkin seeds** mixture ameliorates **diabetic** nephropathy in rats.* Makni M, Sefi M, Fetoui H, Et al. Food Chem Toxicol. 2010 Aug-Sep;48(8-9):2407- 12. **Key Finding**: "Our results suggest that Flax and Pumpkin seeds mixture supplemented in diet of diabetic rats may be helpful to prevent diabetes and its complications."

***Anti-diabetic** effects of pumpkin and its components, trigonelline and nicotinic acid, on Goto-Kakizaki rats.* Yoshinari D, Sato H, Igarashi K. Biosci Biotechnol Biochem. 2009 May;73(5):1033-41. **Key Finding**: "The compounds considered to be effective in improving glucose tolerance and contained in the methanol extract of the pumpkin in relatively abundant amounts were isolated and identified as trigonelline and nicotinic acid."

*Effects of protein-bound polysaccharide isolated from pumpkin on insulin in **diabetic** rats.* Quanhong L, Caili F, Yukui R, Guanghui H, Tongyi C. Plant Foods Hum Nutr. 2005 Mar;60(1):13-6. **Key Finding**: "The results suggest that the hypoglycemic effect of polysaccharide from pumpkin depends on the dose and it possesses the possibility of being developed as a new antidiabetic agent."

Hyperglycemia

*Health benefits of traditional corn, beans, and pumpkin: in vitro studies for **hyperglycemia** and **hypertension** management.* Kwon YI, Apostolidis E, Kim YC, Shetty K. J Med Food. 2007 Jun;10(2):266-75. **Key Finding:** "In this study antidiabetic and antihypertension relevant potentials of phenolic phytochemicals were confirmed in select important traditional plant foods of indigenous communities such as pumpkin, beans and maize. Pumpkin showed the best overall potential."

Hypertension

*Health benefits of traditional corn, beans, and pumpkin: in vitro studies for **hyperglycemia** and **hypertension** management.* Kwon YI. Apostolidis E, Kim YC, Shetty K. J Med Food. 2007 Jun;10(2):266-75. **Key Finding:** "In this study antidiabetic and antihypertension relevant potentials of phenolic phytochemicals were confirmed in select important traditional plant foods of indigenous communities such as pumpkin, beans and maize. Pumpkin showed the best overall potential."

Prostate hyperplasia

Effects of pumpkin seed oil and saw palmetto oil in Korean men with symptomatic benign prostatic hyperplasia. Hong H, Kim CS, Maeng S. Nutr Res. Pract. 2009 Winter;3(4):323-7. **Key Finding**: "From these results, it is suggested that administration of pumpkin seed oil and saw palmetto oil are clinically safe and may be effective as treatments for **benign prostatic hyperplasia**."

Inhibition of Testosterone-Induced Hyperplasia of the Prostate of Sprague-Dawley Rats by Pumpkin Seed Oil. Gossell-Williams M, Davis A, O'Connor N. J Med Food. 2006 Summer;9(2):284-286. **Key Finding:** "We conclude pumpkin seed oil can inhibit testosterone-induced hyperplasia of the prostate and therefore may be beneficial in the management of **benign prostatic hyperplasia**."

*Pumpkin Seed Oil and Phytosterol-F Can Block Testosterone/Prazosin-Induced **Prostate Growth** in Rats.* Tsai YS, Tong YC, Cheng JT, Less CH, Yang FS, Lee HY. Urologia Int. 2006;77(3):269-74. **Key Finding:** ""Pumpkin seed oil alone or combined with Phytosterol-F can block the T-P-induced increases in prostatic weight-to-body weight ratio and protein synthesis."

Raspberries

IT MAY COME AS A SURPRISE that more raspberries are grown in Russia than anywhere else, with an output more than twice that of the United States. Although red raspberries are most common, red and black raspberries have been crossbred to produce purple raspberries and various hybrids, including loganberries and boysenberries.

Thanks to their high levels of anthocyanins and phenolic compounds, raspberries have powerful antioxidant properties. Medical studies have found both red and black raspberries to be beneficial in preventing or treating at least eight types of cancer.

Antibacterial

Antibacterial *activity of berry fruits used for culinary purposes.* Cavanagh HM, Hipwell M, Wilkinson JM. J Med Food. 2003 Spring;6(1):57-61. **Key Finding:** "Commercial raspberry, black current, cranberry, and blackberry cordials (100% fruit) as well as fresh berries were assessed for their ability to inhibit the growth of various bacteria and the yeast Candida albicans. Three of the six raspberry cordials and the blackcurrant cordial inhibited all 12 bacteria and C. albicans. Bacteria showed varying susceptibilities to the remaining cordials. All cordials inhibited the growth of Mycobacterium phlei. Of the fresh berries, mulberries and boysenberries did not inhibit any bacteria, and the remaining berries inhibited the growth of varying numbers of bacteria."

Antibacterial *activity of raspberry cordial in vitro.* Ryan T, Wilkinson JM, Cavanaugh HM. Res Vet Sci. 2001 Dec;71(3):155-9. **Key Finding:** "Raspberry juice cordial has a long anecdotal use in Australia for the prophylaxis and treatment of gastroenteritis in livestock, cage birds and humans. The antimicrobial properties of raspberry juice cordial, raspberry juice, raspberry leaf extract and commercial brand of raspberry leaf tea were investigated against five human pathogenic bacteria and two fungi. Raspberry cordial and juice were found to significantly reduce the growth of several species of bacteria, including Salmonella, Shigella and E. coli, but demonstrated no antifungal activity. No antimicrobial activity was detected in the leaf extract or tea."

Antioxidation

Antioxidant properties of raspberry seed extracts on micronucleus distribution in peripheral blood lymphocytes. Godevac D, Tesevic V, Vajs V, Milosavljevic S, Stankovic M. Food Chem Toxicol. 2009 Nov;47(11):2853-9. **Key Finding:** "These results demonstrate that the constituents of raspberry seed extracts may be important in the prevention of oxidative lymphocyte damage by reactive oxygen species and may also reduce the level of DNA damage."

*Prevention of **oxidative DNA damage** by bioactive berry components.* Aiyer HS, Kichambare S, Gupta RC. Nutr Cancer. 2008;60 Suppl 1:36-42. **Key Finding:** "The hormone 17ss-estradiol (E(2)) causes oxidative DNA damage via redox cycling of its metabolites. In this study, ACI rats were fed either AIN-93M diet or diets supplemented with 0.5% each of mixed berries (strawberry, blueberry, blackberry, and red and black raspberry), blueberry along or ellagic acid. Ellagic acid (EA) diet significantly reduced E(2)-induced levels of 8-oxodG. Blueberry alone also significantly reduced the levels. Mixed berries were ineffective. In addition, aqueous extracts of berries (2%) and EA (100 microM) were tested for their efficacy in diminishing oxidative DNA adducts induced by redox cycling of 4E(2) catalyzed by copper chloride in vitro. EA was the most efficacious (90%) followed by extracts of red raspberry (70%), blueberry and strawberry (50% each; P<0.001)."

*Cellular **antioxidant** activity of common fruits.* Wolfe KL, Kang X, He X, Dong M, Zhang Q, Liu RH. J Agric Food Chem. 2008 Sep 24;56(18):8418-26. **Key Finding:** "The objective of this study was to determine the cellular antioxidant activity, total phenolic contents, and oxygen radical absorbance capacity values of 25 fruits commonly consumed in the United States. Pomegranate and berries (wild blueberry, blackberry, raspberry, and blueberry) had the highest cellular antioxidant activity, whereas banana and melons had the lowest. Apple and strawberries were the biggest suppliers of cellular antioxidant activity to the American diet. Increasing fruit consumption is a logical strategy to increase antioxidant intake and decrease oxidative stress and may lead to reduced risk of **cancer.**"

*The effects of dietary phenolic compounds on cytokine and **antioxidant** production by A549 cells.* Gauliard B, Grieve D, Wilson R, Crozier A, Jenkins C, Mullen WD, Lean M. J Med Food. 2008 Jun;11(2):382-4. **Key Finding:** "A commercially available raspberry juice (Bouvrage) was purified by high-performance liquid chromatography and gave three fractions: Fraction 1 contained phenolic acid and vitamin

C; Fraction 2 contained flavonoids and ellagic acid; Fraction 3 contained anthocyanins and ellagitannins. None of the compounds tested had any significant effect on glutathione. However, the phenolic compounds can significantly alter cytokine and antioxidant production."

*Safety and whole-body **antioxidant** potential of a novel anthocyanin-rich formulation of edible berries.* Bagchi D, Roy S, Patel V, He G, Khanna S, Ojha N, Phillips C, Ghosh S, Bagchi M, Sen CK. Mol Cell Biochem. 2006 Jan;281(1-2):197-209. **Key Finding:** "Six berry extracts (wild blueberry, bilberry, cranberry, elderberry, raspberry seeds and strawberry) singly and in combinations, were studied in our laboratories for antioxidant efficacy, cytotoxic potential, cellular uptake and anti-angiogenic properties. Combinations of edible berry extracts were evaluated to develop a synergistic formula, OptiBerry, which exhibited high oxygen radical absorbance capacity (ORAC) value, low cytotoxicity and superior **anti-angiogenic** properties compared to the other combinations tested."

The effects of an antioxidant-supplemented beverage on exercise-induced oxidative stress: results from a placebo-controlled double-blind study in cyclists. Morillas-Ruiz J, Zafrilla P, Almar M, Cuevas MJ, Lopez FJ, Abellan P, Villegas JA, Gonzalez-Gallego J. Eur J Appl Physiol. 2005 Dec;95(5-6):543-9. **Key Finding:** "These results suggest that in moderately trained cyclists, **antioxidant** supplementation (with black grape, raspberry and red currant) counters oxidative stress induced by a 90 min exercise at 70% VO2max."

Inhibition of protein and lipid oxidation in liposomes by berry phenolic. Viljanen K, Kylli P, Kivikari R, Heinonen M. J Agric Food Chem. 2004 Dec 1;52(24):7419-24. **Key Finding:** "Bilberry and raspberry phenolic exhibited the best overall **antioxidant** activity toward protein oxidation. In raspberries, ellagitannins were responsible for the antioxidant activity. While the antioxidant effect of berry proanthocyanidin and anthocyanin was dose-dependent, ellagitannins appeared to be equally active at all concentrations."

***Antioxidant** and **antiproliferative** activities of raspberries.* Liu M, Li XQ, Weber C, Lee CY, Brown J, Liu RH. J Agric Food Chem. 2002 May 8;50(10):2926-30. **Key Finding:** "To study the health benefits of raspberries, four fresh raspberry varieties (Heritage, Kiwigold, Goldie and Anne) were evaluated for total antioxidant and antiproliferative activities. The total amount of phenolic and flavonoids for each of the four raspberry varieties was determined. The Heritage raspberry had the highest total phenolic content (512.7 +/-4.7 mg/100 g of raspberry) of the varieties measured followed by Kiwigold (451.1 +/-4.5 mg/100 g of raspberry), followed by Goldie and Anne. Similarly, the Heritage raspberry variety contained the highest total flavonoids (103.4 +/- 2.0 mg/100g of raspberry) of the varieties tested, followed by Kiwigold (87.3 +/- 1.8mg/100 g of raspberry), followed by Goldie and Anne. The color of the raspberry juice correlated well to the total phenolic, flavonoid and anthocyanin contents of the raspberry. Heritage had the highest a/b ratio and the darkest colored juice. Heritage variety had the highest total antioxidant activity followed by Kiwigold. The antioxidant activity of the raspberry was directly related to the total amount of phenolic and flavonoids."

Cyclooxygenase inhibitory and **antioxidant** *cyaniding glycosides in cherries and berries.* Seeram NP, Momin RA, Nair MG, Bourquin LD. Phytomedicine. 2001 Sep;8(5):362-9. **Key Finding:** "Anthocyanins from raspberries and sweet cherries demonstrated 45% and 47% cyclooxygenase-I and cyclooxygenase-II inhibitory activities, respectively, when assayed at 125 microg/ml. Anthocyanins 1 and 2 are present in both cherries and raspberry. Fresh blackberries and strawberries contained only anthocyanin 2 in yields of 24 and 22.5 mg/100 g, respectively. Anthocyanins 1 and 2 were not found in bilberries, blueberries, cranberries or elderberries."

Cancer (breast; cervical; colon; esophageal; leukemia; prostate; skin; stomach)

Effect of **black raspberry** *extract in inhibiting NFkappa B dependent radioprotection in human* **breast cancer** *cells.* Madhusoodhanan R, Natarajan M, Singh JV, Et al. Nutr Cancer. 2010;62(1):93-104. **Key Finding**: "These results suggest that black raspberry extracts may act as a potent radio sensitizer by overcoming the effects of NFkappa B mediated radioprotection in human breast cancer cells."

Black raspberries *inhibit intestinal tumorigenesis in apc1638+/- and Muc2-/- mouse models of* **colorectal cancer**. Bi X, Fang W, Wang LS, Et al. Cancer Prev Res. 2010 Nov;3(11):1443-50. **Key Finding**: "Collectively, our data suggest that freeze-dried black raspberries are highly effective in preventing intestinal tumor development in both mouse models of colorectal cancer through targeting multiple signaling pathways."

Red raspberries *have antioxidant effects that play a minor role in the killing of* **stomach and colon cancer** *cells.* God J, Tate PL, Larcom LL. Nutr Res. 2010 Nov;30(11):777-82. **Key Finding**: "We conclude that the antioxidant effect plays a minor role in the killing of 2 gastrointestinal cell types, but its role in inactivating a breast cancer cell line is much more significant."

Topical treatment with **black raspberry** *extract reduces cutaneous UVB-induced carcinogenesis and inflammation.* Duncan FJ, Martin JR, Wulff BC, Stoner GD, Tober KL, Oberyszyn TM, Kusewitt DF, Van Buskirk AM. Cancer Prev Res. 2009 Jul;2(7):665-72. **Key Finding:** "The ability of black raspberry extract to reduce acute UVB-induced inflammation and to decrease tumor development in a long-term model provides compelling evidence to explore the clinical efficacy of black raspberry extract in the prevention of human **skin cancers**."

Carcinogen-altered genes in rat esophagus positively modulated to normal levels of expression by both **black raspberries** *and phenyl ethyl isothiocyanate.* Stoner GD, Dombkowski AA, Reen RK, Cukovic D, Salagrama S, Wang LS, Lechner JF. Cancer Res. 2008 Aug 1;68(15):6460-7. **Key Finding:** "Herein, we report our results with companion animals that were fed a diet containing 5% freeze-dried black raspberries (BRB) instead of PEITC. We found that 462 of the 2,261 NMBA-dysregulated genes in rat esophagus were restored to near-normal levels of expression by BRB. Further, we have identified 53 NMBA-dysregulated genes that are positively modulated by both PEITC and BRB. Their dysregulation during the early phase of NMBA-induced **esophageal cancer** may be especially important in the genesis of the disease."

Differential effects of black raspberry and strawberry extracts on BaPDE-induced activation of transcription factors and their target genes. Li J, Zhang D, Stoner GD, Huang C. Mol Carcinog. 2008 Apr;47(4):286-94. **Key Finding:** "These results suggest that black raspberry and strawberry components may target different signaling pathways in exerting their **anti-carcinogenic** effects." For example, tumor necrosis factor-alpha (TNF-alpha) induction by BaPDE was blocked by extract fractions of both black raspberries and strawberries, whereas vascular endothelial growth factor (VEGF) expression, which depends on AP-1 activation, was suppressed by black raspberry fractions but not strawberry fractions.

Berry extracts exert different antiproliferative effects against **cervical** *and* **colon cancer** *cells grown in vitro.* McDougall GJ, Ross HA, Ikeji M, Stewart D. J Agric Food Chem. 2008 May 14;56(9):3016-23. **Key Finding:** "Polyphenol-rich berry extracts were screened for their antiproliferative effectiveness using human cervical cancer (HeLa) cells grown in micro titer plates. Rowan berry, raspberry, lingonberry, cloudberry, arctic bramble, and strawberry extracts were effective, but blueberry, sea buckthorn and pomegranate extracts were considerably less effective. The most effective extracts (strawberry>arctic bramble>cloudberry>lingonberry) gave EC 50 values in the range of 25-40 microg/(mL of phenols). These extracts were also effective against human colon cancer (CaCo-2) cells, which were generally more sensitive at low concentrations but conversely less sensitive at higher concentrations. The strawberry, cloudberry, arctic bramble and the raspberry extracts share common polyphenol constituents, especially the ellagitannins, which have been shown to be effective antiproliferative agents."

Dietary berries and ellagic acid prevent oxidative DNA damage and modulate expression of DNA repair genes. Aiyer HS, Vadhanam MV, Stoyanova R, Caprio GD, Clapper ML, Gupta RC. Int J Mol Sci. 2008 Mar;9(3):327-41. **Key Finding:** "DNA damage is a pre-requisite for the initiation of cancer and agents that reduce this damage are useful in **cancer** prevention. In this study, results suggest that red raspberry and ellagic acid reduce endogenous oxidative DNA damage by mechanisms which may involve increase in DNA repair. "

Dietary berries and ellagic acid diminish estrogen-mediated **mammary tumorigenesis** *in ACI rats.* Aiyer HS, Srinivasan C, Gupta RC. Nutr Cancer. 2008;60(2):227-34. **Key Finding:** "We investigated the efficacy of dietary berries and ellagic acid to reduce estrogen-mediated mammary tumorigenesis. Compared with the control group, ellagic acid reduced the tumor volume by 75% and tumor multiplicity by 44%. Black raspberry followed closely with tumor volume diminished by >69% and tumor multiplicity by 37%. Blueberry showed a reduction (40%) only in tumor volume. This is the first report showing the significant efficacy of both ellagic acid and berries in the prevention of solely estrogen-induced mammary tumors."

Cellular **antioxidant** *activity of common fruits.* Wolfe KL, Kang X, He X, Dong M, Zhang Q, Liu RH. J Agric Food Chem. 2008 Sep 24;56(18):8418-26. **Key Finding:** "The objective of this study was to determine the cellular antioxidant activity, total phenolic contents, and oxygen radical absorbance capacity values of 25 fruits commonly consumed in the United States. Pomegranate and berries (wild blueberry, blackberry, raspberry, and blueberry) had the highest cellular antioxidant activity, whereas banana and melons had the lowest. Apple and strawberries were the biggest suppliers of cellular antioxidant activity to the American diet. Increasing fruit consumption is a logical strategy to increase antioxidant intake and decrease oxidative stress and may lead to reduced risk of **cancer.**"

Effects of a black raspberry diet on gene expression in the rat esophagus. Lechner JF, Reen RK, Dombkowski AA, Cukovic D, Salagrama S, Wang LS, Stoner GD. Nutr Cancer. 2008;60 Suppl 1:61-9. **Key Finding:** "Histological and molecular studies indicate that a 5% freeze-dried black raspberry diet produces only modest effects on the **esophagus**, the target tissue for NMBA **carcinogenesis** in the rat."

*Effects of a topically applied bio adhesive berry gel on loss of heterozygosis indices in **premalignant oral lesions**.* Shumway BS, Kresty LA, Larsen PE, Zwick JC, Lu B, Fields HW, Mumper RJ, Stoner GD, Mallery SR. Clin Cancer Res. 2008 Apr 15;14(8):2421-30. **Key Finding:** "Confirming earlier phase I data, none of the 27 participants developed freeze-dried black raspberry gel-associated toxicities. Furthermore, our results show histologic regression in a subset of patients as well as statistically significant reduction in loss of heterozygosity at tumor suppressor gene-associated loci. These preliminary data suggest that further evaluation of berry gels for oral intraepithelial neoplasia chemoprevention is warranted."

*Cyanidin-3-rutinoside, a natural polyphenol antioxidant, selectively kills **leukemic cells** by induction of oxidative stress.* Feng R, Ni HM, Wang SY, Tourkova IL, Shurin MR, Harada H, Yin XM. J Biol Chem. 2007 May 4;282(18):13468-76. **Key Finding:** "We found that cyaniding-3-rutinoside extracted and purified from the black raspberry cultivar Jewel induced apoptosis in HL-60 cells in a dose- and time-dependent manner (causing about 50% of human leukemia programmed cell death within 18 hours of treatment). These results indicate that cyaniding-3-rutinoside has the potential to be used in leukemia therapy with the advantages of being widely available and selective against tumors."

*Inhibition of **cancer** cell proliferation and suppression of TNF-induced activation of NFkappaB by edible berry juice.* Boivin D, Blanchette M, Barrette S, Moghrabi A, Beliveau R. Anticancer Res. 2007 Mar-Apr;27(2):937-48. **Key Finding:** "These results illustrate that berry juices have striking differences in their potential chemo preventive activity and that the inclusion of a variety of berries in the diet might be useful for preventing the development of tumors. The growth of various cancer cell lines, including those of **stomach, prostate, intestine and breast**, was strongly inhibited by raspberry, black currant, white currant, gooseberry, velvet leaf blueberry, low-bush blueberry, sea buckthorn and cranberry juice, but not (or only slightly) by strawberry, high-bush blueberry, serviceberry, red currant, or blackberry juice. "

Differential inhibition of UV-induced activation of NF kappaB and AP-1 by extracts from black raspberries, strawberries, and blueberries. Huang C, Zhang D, Li J, Tong Q, Stoner GD. Nutr Cancer. 2007;58(2):205-12. **Key Finding:** "Our results showed that black raspberries inhibited UVB-induced activation of NF kappaB in mouse epidermal cells (**skin carcinogenesis**) in a time- and dose- dependent manner; however, the methanol fractions from strawberries and blueberries were ineffective. Cycandin-3-rutinoside, an anthocyanin found in abundance in black raspberries and not in strawberries or high-bush blueberries, was found to contribute to the inhibition of UVG-induced activation of NF kappB."

Colon-available raspberry polyphenols exhibit anti-cancer effects on in vitro models of **colon cancer**. Coates EM, Popa G, Gill CI, McCann MJ, McDougall GJ, Stewart D, Roswland I. J Carcinog. 2007 Apr 18;6:4. **Key Finding:** "The results indicate that raspberry phytochemicals likely to reach the colon are capable of inhibiting several important stages in colon carcinogenesis in vitro."

Antiproliferative activity is predominantly associated with ellagitannins in raspberry extracts. Ross HA, McDougall GJ, Stewart D. Phytochemistry. 2007 Jan;68(2):218-28. **Key Finding:** "Raspberry extracts enriched in polyphenols, but devoid of organic acids, sugars and vitamin C, were prepared by sorption to C18 solid phase extraction matrices and tested for their ability to inhibit the proliferation of human **cervical cancer** (HeLa) cells in vitro. The raspberry extract reduced proliferation in a dose-dependent manner whether this was judged by cell number or measurements of cell viability. The ellagitannins-rich bound fraction had the highest antioxidant capacity."

Berry phenolic extracts modulate the expression of p21(WAF1) and Bax but not Bcl-2 in HT-29 **colon cancer** *cells.* Wu QK, Koponen JM, Mykkanen HM, Torronen AR. J Agric Food Chem. 2007 Feb 21;55(4):1156-63. **Key Finding:** "Colon cancer cells were exposed to 0-60 mg/ml of extracts and the cell growth inhibition was determined after 24 h. The degree of cell growth inhibition was as follows: bilberry>black currant>cloudberry>lingonberry>raspberry>strawberry. A 14-fold increase in the expression of p21WAF1, an inhibitors of cell proliferation and a member of the cyclin kinase inhibitors, was seen in cells exposed to cloudberry extract compared to other berry treatments. The pro-apoptosis marker, Bax, was increased 1.3-fold only in cloudberry and bilberry-treated cells. Cloudberry, despite its very low anthocyanin content, was a potent inhibitor of cell proliferation. Therefore, it is concluded that, in addition to anthocyanin, also other phenolic or nonphenolic phytochemicals are responsible for the antiproliferative activity of berries."

Blackberry, black raspberry, blueberry, cranberry, red raspberry, and strawberry extracts inhibit growth and stimulate apoptosis of human **cancer** *cells in vitro.* Seeram NP, Adams LS, Zhang Y, Lee R, Sand D, Scheuller HS, Heber D. J Agric Food Chem. 2006 Dec 13;54(25):9329-39. **Key Finding:** "The berry extracts were evaluated for their ability to inhibit the growth of human **oral, breast, colon and prostate tumor cell** lines at concentrations ranging from 25 to 200 micro g/ml. With increasing concentration of berry extract, increasing inhibition of cell proliferation in all of the cancer cell lines was observed, with different degrees of potency between cell lines. The berry extracts were also evaluated for their ability to stimulate apoptosis of the COX-2 expressing **colon cancer** cell line, HT-29. Black raspberry and strawberry extracts showed the most significant pro-apoptotic effects against this cell line."

In vitro **antileukaemic** *activity of extracts from berry plant leaves against sensitive and multidrug resistant HL60 cells.* Skupien K, Oszmianski J, Kostrzewa-Kowak D, Tarasiuk J. Cancer Lett. 2006 May 18;236(2):282-91. **Key Finding:** "It was found that the blueberry extract was the most efficient against sensitive HL60 cell line (about 2-fold more active than strawberry and raspberry extracts) but presented much lower activity towards resistant cells. In contrast, strawberry and raspberry extracts exhibited the high cytotoxic activity against sensitive leukemia HL60 cell line as well as its MDR sublines."

Protection against **esophageal cancer** *in rodents with lyophilized berries: potential mechanisms.* Stoner GD, Chen T, Kresty LA, Aziz RM, Reinemann T, Nines R. Nutr Cancer. 2006;54(1):33-46. **Key Finding:** "Our laboratory has been evaluating the ability of lyophilized (freeze-dried) black raspberries, blackberries and strawberries to inhibit carcinogen-induced cancer in the rodent esophagus. At 25 wks. of the bioassay, all three berry types were found to inhibit the number of esophageal tumors in NMBA-treated animals by 24-56% relative to NMBA controls. Black raspberries and strawberries were also tested in a post initiation scheme and were found to inhibit NMBA-induced esophageal tumorigenesis by 31-64% when administered in the diet following treatment of the animals with NMBA. Berries, therefore, inhibit tumor promotion and progression events as well as tumor initiation."

Black raspberry extracts inhibit benzo(a)pyrene diol-epoxide-induced activator protein 1 activation and VEGF transcription by targeting the phosphatidylinositol 3-kinase/Akt pathway. Huang C, Li J, Song L, Zhang D, Tong Q, Ding M, Bowman L, Aziz R, Stoner GD. Cancer Res. 2006 Jan 1;66(1):581-7. **Key Finding:** "In view of the important roles of AP-1 and VEGF in **tumor** development, one mechanism for the chemo preventive activity of black raspberries may be inhibition of the PI-3K/Akt/AP-1/VEGF pathway."

Molecular mechanisms involved in chemoprevention of black raspberry extracts: from transcription factors to their target genes. Lu H, Li J, Zhang D, Stoner GD, Huang C. Nutr Cancer. 2006;54(1):69-78. **Key Finding:** "We anticipate that the ability of black raspberries to inhibit **tumor** development may be mediated by impairing signal transduction pathways leading to activation of AP-1 and NFkappaB, subsequently resulting in down-regulation of VEGF and COX-2 expression. The RO-ME fraction appears to be the major fraction responsible for the inhibitory activity of black raspberries."

Black raspberries inhibit N-nitrosomethylbenzylamine (NMBA)-induced ***angiogenesis*** *in rat esophagus parallel to the suppression of COX-2 and iNOS.* Chen T, Rose ME, Hwang H, Nines RG, Stoner GD. Carcinogenesis. 2006 Nov;27(11):2301-7. **Key Finding:** "Angiogenesis, the formation of new blood vessels, is critical to **tumor** growth and metastasis. Vascular endothelial growth factor (VEGF), an important angiogenic activator, is essential for angiogenesis. We report that dietary black raspberry powder inhibits N-nitromethylbenzylamine-induced tumor development in the rat esophagus by inhibiting the formation of DNA adducts and reducing the proliferation rate of preneoplastic cells."

Suppression of the tumorigenic phenotype in human ***oral squamous cell carcinoma*** *cells by an ethanol extract derived from freeze-dried black raspberries.* Rodrigo KA, Rawal Y, Renner RJ, Schwartz SJ, Tian Q, Larsen PE, Mallery SR. Nutr Cancer. 2006;54(1):58-68. **Key Finding:** "Our results demonstrate that freeze-dried black raspberry ethanol extract suppresses cell proliferation without perturbing viability, inhibits translation of the complete angiogenic cytokine vascular endothelial growth factor, suppresses nitric oxide synthase activity, and induces both apoptosis and terminal differentiation. These data imply that freeze-dried black raspberry is a promising candidate for use as a chemo preventive agent in persons with **oral epithelial dysplasia**."

Inhibition of the growth of premalignant and malignant human oral cell lines by extracts and components of black raspberries. Han C, Ding H, Casto B, Stoner GD, D'Ambrosio SM. Nutr Cancer. 2005;51(2):207-17. **Key Finding:** "These results show for the first time that the growth inhibitory effects of black raspberries on premalignant and **malignant human oral cells** may reside in specific components (ferulic acid and beta-sitosterol) that target aberrant signaling pathways regulating cell cycle progression."

Black raspberry extract and fractions contain angiogenesis inhibitors. Liu Z, Schwimer J, Liu D, Greenway FL, Anthony CT, Woltering EA. J Agric Food Chem. 2005 May 18;53(10):3909-15. **Key Finding:** "These findings suggest that an active black raspberry fraction may be a promising complementary **cancer** therapy. It is natural and potent enough for manageable dosing regimens. These extracts contain multiple active ingredients that may be additive or synergistic in their antiangiogenic effects. These observations warrant further investigations in animals and human trials."

Antimutagenic activity of berry extracts. Hope Smith S, Tate PL, Huang G, Magee JB, Meepagala KM, Wedge DE, Larcom LL. J Med Food. 2004 Winter;7(4):450-5. **Key Finding:** "Identification of phytochemicals useful in dietary prevention and intervention of **cancer** is of paramount important. Juice from strawberry, blueberry, and raspberry fruit significantly inhibited **mutagenesis** caused by both carcinogens tested (methyl methanesulfonate and benzo{a}pyrene). Ethanol extracts from freeze-dried fruits of strawberry cultivars (Sweet Charlie and Carlsbad) and blueberry cultivars (Tifblue and Premier) were also tested. Of these, the hydrolysable tannin-containing fraction from Sweet Charlie strawberries was most effective at inhibiting mutations."

Inhibition of benzo(a)pyrene diol-epoxide-induced transactivation of activated protein 1 and nuclear factor kappaB by black raspberry extracts. Huang C, Huang Y, Li J, Hu W, Aziz R, Tang MS, Sun N, Cassidy J, Stoner GD. Cancer Res. 2002 Dec 1;62(23):6857-63. **Key Finding:** "Freeze-dried black raspberries have been shown to inhibit the development of chemically induced **esophageal and colon cancer** in rodents. The molecular mechanisms through which black raspberries inhibit **carcinogenesis** remain unclear. We investigated the effects of black raspberry extracts on transactivation of activate protein 1 (AP-1) and nuclear factor kappaB (NFkappaB) induced by BaP diol-epoxide (BPDE), the ultimate carcinogen of BaP in mouse epidermal JB6 CI 41 (CI 41) cells. In view of the important roles of Ap-1 and NFkappaB in **tumor** promotion/progression, these results suggest that the ability of black raspberries to inhibit tumor development may be mediated by impairing signal transduction pathways leading to activation of Ap-1 and NFkappaB. The RU-ME fraction appears to be the major fraction responsible for the inhibitory activity of black raspberries."

*Anticarcinogenic Activity of Strawberry, Blueberry, and Raspberry Extracts to **Breast and Cervical Cancer** Cells.* Wedge DE, Meepagala KM, Magee JB, Smith SH, Huang G, Larcom LL. J Med Food. 2001 Spring;4(1):49-51. **Key Finding:** "Freeze-dried fruits of two strawberry cultivators, Sweet Charlie and Carlsbad, and two blueberry cultivars, Tifblue and Premier, were sequentially extracted and tested separately for in vitro anticancer activity on cervical and breast cancer cell lines. Ethanol extracts from all four fruits strongly inhibited CaSki and SiHa cervical cancer cell lines and MCF-7 and T47-D breast cancer cell lines. An unfractionated aqueous extract of raspberry and the ethanol extract of Premier blueberry significantly inhibited mutagenesis by both direct-acting and metabolically active carcinogens."

Hypercholesteremia

Efficiency of pharmacologically-active antioxidant phytomedicine Radical Fruits in treatment **hypercholesteremia** *in men.* Abidov M, Jimenez Del Rio M, Ramazanov A, Kalyuzhin O, Chkhikvishvili I. Georgian Med News. 2006 Nov;(140):78-83. **Key Finding:** "Radical Fruits is a dietary supplement that contains standardized extracts and concentrates of prune, pomegranate, apple, grape, raspberry, blueberry, white cherry and strawberry. Forty-four non-obese, non-smoking, non-diabetic hypercholesteremic male volunteers took part in a 4 week double-blind, randomized, placebo-controlled clinical trial. Administration of pharmacologically active antioxidant supplement Radical Fruit in hypercholesteremic men significantly increased plasma HDL and reduced total cholesterol and LDL, and urinary oxidative and inflammatory isoprostanes and thromboxane."

Intestinal pathogens

Berry phenolics selectively inhibit the growth of **intestinal pathogens**. Puupponen-Pimia R, Nohynek L, Hartmann-Schmidlin S, Kahkonen M, Heinonen M, Maatta-Riihinen K, Oksman-Caldentey KM. J Appl Microbiol. 2005;98(4):991-1000. **Key Finding:** "Berries and their phenolic selectively inhibit the growth of human pathogenic bacteria. Cloudberry and raspberry were the best inhibitors, and Staphylococcus and Salmonella the most sensitive bacteria."

The action of berry phenolic against human **intestinal pathogens**. Puupponen-Pimia R, Nohynek L, Alakomi HL, Oksman-Caldentey KM. Biofactors. 2005;23(4):243-51. **Key Finding:** "Phenolic compounds present in berries selectively inhibit the growth of human gastrointestinal pathogens. Especially cranberry, cloudberry, raspberry, strawberry and bilberry possess clear antimicrobial effects against e.g. salmonella and staphylococcus."

Resveratrol
(in Grapes and Berries)

WHEN STRESSED OR UNDER ATTACK BY PATHOGENS, several species of plants, including grapes, produce resveratrol to counteract the effects of these stresses. Although this phytochemical wasn't discovered until the late 1930s, subsequent research has placed it high in the pantheon of natural plant compounds that benefit human health in multiple ways.

Using yeast, then worms, and finally a species of short-lived fish, researchers have found resveratrol to be an effective life-extension agent. In the case of the fish, which usually live only nine weeks, a diet rich in resveratrol extended their natural life by 56 percent compared to a control group. In studies with mice, resveratrol has also counteracted the effects of high-fat diets and prevented the development of skin cancer. As you will see below, lab studies have found resveratrol to be beneficial for at least twenty-three medical conditions, including ten types of cancer.

Aging (and life expectancy)

*Life span extension by resveratrol, rapamycin, and metformin: The promise of dietary restriction mimetics for a **healthy aging**.* Mouchiroud L, Molin L, Dalliere N, Solari F. Biofactors. 2010 Sep;36(5):377-82. **Key Finding**: "We will report evidences supporting resveratrol as a molecule that acts by mimicking the beneficial effects of dietary restriction. Although this molecule does not reveal all the secrets of the fountain of youth, it may help us maintain the quality of life in old age."

Protective action of resveratrol in human skin: possible involvement of specific receptor binding sites. Bastianetto S, Dumont Y, Duranton A, Et al. PLoS One. 2010 Sep 23;5(9):12935. **Key Finding**: "Taken together, these findings suggest that resveratrol, by acting on specific polyphenol binding sites in epidermis, may be useful to prevent **skin disorders associated with aging**."

Ageing *and neurodegenerative diseases.* Hung CW, Chen YC, Hsieh WL, Et al. Ageing Res Rev. 2010 Nov;9 Suppl 1:S36-46. **Key Finding**: "The beneficial effects of resveratrol are believed to be associated with the activation of a longevity gene, SirT1. In this review, we discuss the pathogenesis of age-related neurodegenerative diseases including **Alzheimer's disease, Parkinson's disease and**

cerebrovascular disease. The therapeutic potential of resveratrol, diet and the roles of stem cell therapy are discussed to provide a better understanding of the ageing mystery."

Polyphenols and aging. Queen BL, Tollefsbol TO. Curr Aging Sci. 2010 Feb;3(1):34-42. **Key Finding**: "Increasingly well-documented results have begun to provide a basis for considering the use of polyphenols such as resveratrol in the development of novel therapies for certain **age-associated diseases**."

Cellular mechanisms of **cardio protection** *by calorie restriction: state of the science and future perspectives.* Marzetti E, Wohlgemuth SE, Anton SD, Bernabei R, Carter CS, Leeuwenburgh C. Clin Geriatr Med. 2009 Nov;25(4):715-32. **Key Finding:** "Preclinical studies indicate that specific compounds, such as **resveratrol,** may mimic many of the effects of calorie restriction, thus potentially obviating the need for drastic food intake reductions. Results from ongoing clinical trials will reveal whether the intriguing alternative of calorie restriction represents a safe and effective strategy to promote cardiovascular health and delay cardiac **aging** in humans."

Curcumin, resveratrol and flavonoids as **anti-inflammatory**, *cyto- and DNA-protective dietary compounds.* Bisht K, Wagner KH, Bulmer AC. Toxicology. 2009 Nov 10. (Epub ahead of print). **Key Finding:** "The polyphenols afford protection against various stress-induced toxicities through modulating intercellular cascades which inhibit inflammatory molecule synthesis, the formation of free radicals, nuclear damage and induce antioxidant enzyme expressions. These responses have the potential to increase **life expectancy**."

Induction of a reversible, non-cytotoxic S-phase delay by resveratrol: implications for a mechanism of **lifespan** *prolongation and* **cancer** *protection.* Zhou R, Fukui M, CHoi HJ, Zhu BT. Br J Pharmacol. 2009 Sep;158(2):462-74. **Key Finding:** "Resveratrol has been shown to prolong lifespan and prevent cancer formation. At present, the precise cellular mechanisms of resveratrol's action are still not clearly understood, and this is the focus of this study. It is hypothesized that the induction of a non-cytotoxic S-phase delay may represent a useful mechanistic strategy for lifespan prolongation and cancer prevention."

Metabolic effects of resveratrol in mammals—a link between improved insulin action and **aging**. Frojdo S, Durand C, Pirola L. Curr Aging Sci. 2008 Dec;1(3):145-51. **Key Finding:** "Resveratrol, a polyphenol, has been shown to possess lifespan-promoting properties in yeast and metazoans, including small mammals. The action of resveratrol has been linked to its capability to i) prolong lifespan following chronic administration to mice and ii) protect from the development of diet-induced obesity and obesity-dependent metabolic disorders. Here we summarize the current understanding on how resveratrol displays its remarkable properties by acting on the control of insulin secretion and by modulation of insulin action in peripheral insulin-responsive tissues. Resveratrol has the potential to prevent the establishment of insulin-resistance and thus postpone or even prevent the onset of **type 2 diabetes**."

Alzheimer's disease

*Oxidative stress and **Alzheimer's disease**: dietary polyphenols as potential therapeutic agents.* Darvesh AS, Carroll RT, Bishayee A, Geldenhuys WJ, Van der Schyf CJ. Expert Rev Neurother. 2010 May;10(5):729-45. **Key Finding**: Oxidative stress has been strongly implicated in the pathophysiology of neurodegenerative disorders such as Alzheimer's. This article reviews the antioxidant potential of polyphenol compounds such as anthocyanin from berries, catechins and the flavins from tea, curcumin from turmeric and resveratrol from grapes.

Neuroprotective properties of resveratrol in different neurodegenerative disorders. Albani D, Polito L, Signorini A, Forioni G. Biofactors. 2010 Sep;36(5):370-6.**Key Finding**: "Resveratrol has neuroprotective features both in vitro and in vivo in models of **Alzheimer's disease**, but it has proved to be beneficial also in **ischemic stroke, Parkinson's disease, Huntington's disease, and epilepsy**. Here we summarize the invitro and in vivo experimental results highlighting the possible role of resveratrol as neuroprotective bio factor with a particular focus on Alzheimer's disease."

*Mitochondria-targeted antioxidants protect against amyloid-beta toxicity in **Alzheimer's disease** neurons.* Manczak M, Mao P, Calkins MJ, Et al. J Alzheimers Dis. 2010;20 Suppl 2:S609-31. **Key Finding**: "The purpose of our study was to investigate the effects of the mitochondria-targeted antioxidants MitoQ and SS31, and the anti-aging agent **resveratrol** on neurons from a mouse model of Alzheimer's disease. These findings suggest that MitoQ and SS31 prevent Abeta toxicity, which would warrant the study of MitoQ and SS31 as potential drugs to treat patients with Alzheimer's disease."

Resveratrol as a therapeutic agent for neurodegenerative diseases. Sun AY, Wang Q, Simonyi A, Sun GY. Mol Neurobiol. 2010 Jun;41(2-3):375-83. **Key Finding**: "Excess production of reactive oxygen species in the brain has been implicated as a common underlying risk factor for the pathogenesis of a number of neurodegenerative disorders, including **Alzheimer's disease, Parkinson's disease, and stroke**. In this review we place emphasis on recent studies implicating the neuroprotective effects of resveratrol. These studies show that the beneficial effects of resveratrol are not only limited to its antioxidant and anti-inflammatory action but also include activation of sirtuin 1 and vitagenes, which can prevent the deleterious effects triggered by oxidative stress."

Piceatannol attenuates 4-hydroxynonenal-induced apoptosis of PC12 cells by blocking activation of c-Jun N-terminal kinase. Jang YJ, Kim JE, Kang NJ, Lee KW, Lee HJ. Ann N Y Acad Sci. 2009 Aug;1171:176-82. **Key Finding:** "These results indicate that piceatannol, an analogue of resveratrol, has therapeutic potential in the prevention of **Alzheimer's disease**."

*A review of antioxidants and **Alzheimer's disease**.* Frank B, Gupta S. Ann Clin Psychiatry. 2005 Oct-Dec;17(4):269-86. **Key Finding:** Over 300 articles were reviewed of antioxidants helpful in the prevention of Alzheimer's disease and 187 articles were selected for inclusion. Agents that show promise helping prevent AD include: 1) aged garlic extract, 2) curcumin, 3) melatonin, 4) resveratrol, 5) Ginkgo biloba extract, 6) green tea, 7) vitamin C and 8) vitamin E.

Amyotrophic lateral sclerosis

An in vitro screening cascade to identify neuroprotective antioxidants in ALS. Barber SC, Higginbottom A, Mead RJ, Barber S, Shaw PJ. Free Radic Biol Med. 2009 Apr 15;46(8):1127-38. **Key Finding:** "**Amyotrophic lateral sclerosis (ALS)** is a neurodegenerative disease characterized by progressive dysfunction and death of motor neurons. We have developed an in vitro screening cascade to identify antioxidant molecules capable of rescuing NSC34 motor neuron cells expressing an ALS-associated mutation of superoxide dismutase 1. The top-performing molecules identified include caffeic acid phenethyl ester, esculetin, and resveratrol."

Antioxidation

*Activation of the erythrocyte plasma membrane redox system by resveratrol: a possible mechanism for **antioxidant** properties.* Rizvi SI, Pandey KB. Pharmacol Rep. 2010;62(4):726-32. **Key Finding**: "The role of resveratrol in activating the erythrocyte PMRS and AFR reductase may assume significant in all disease conditions in which there is a decrease in plasma antioxidant potential."

Antioxidant activities of curcumin and combinations of this curcuminoid with other phyto-chemicals. Aftab N, Vieira A. Phytother Res. 2009 Nov 19. (Epub ahead of print). **Key Finding:** "The main goal of the present study was to compare antioxidant activities of curcumin with those of **resveratrol**. Combination of the two were examined for potential synergism in a heme-enhanced oxidation reaction. Curcumin and resveratrol together (5 muM each) resulted in a synergistic antioxidant effect: 15.5 +/- 1.7% greater than an average of individual activities. This synergy was significantly greater than that of curcumin together with the flavonol quercetin."

*Resveratrol protects against irradiation-induced hepatic and ileal damage via its **anti-oxidative** activity.* Velioglu-Ogunc A, Sehirli O, Toklu HZ, Ozyurt H, Mayadagli A, Eksioglu-Demiralp E, Erzik C, Cetinel S, Yegen BC, Sener G. Free Radic Res. 2009 Aug 25:1-12. **Key Finding:** "The present study was undertaken to determine whether resveratrol could ameliorate ionizing radiation-induced oxidative injury. Resveratrol treatment reversed all biochemical indices, as well as histopathological alterations induced by irradiation. In conclusion, supplementing cancer patients with adjuvant therapy of resveratrol may have some benefit for a more successful radiotherapy."

Antiviral

*Resveratrol exhibits a strong cytotoxic activity in cultured cells and has an **antiviral** action against polyomavirus: potential clinical use.* Berardi V, Ricci F, Castelli M, Galati G, Risuleo G. J Exp Clin Cancer Res. 2009 Jul 1;28:96. **Key Finding:** "Resveratrol is cytotoxic and inhibits, in a dose dependent fashion, the synthesis of polyomavirus DNA in the infected cell. The cytotoxic and antiviral properties of resveratrol make it a potential candidate for the clinical control of proliferative as well as viral pathologies."

Atherosclerosis

Inhibition of proliferation and migration by piceatannol in vascular smooth muscle cells. Lee B, Lee EJ, Kim DI, Park SK, Kim WJ, Moon SK. Toxicol In Vitro. 2009 Oct;23(7):1284-91. **Key Finding:** "Piceatannol may be an effective therapeutic approach to treat **atherosclerosis**. The present study investigated for the first time the card protective effects of piceatannol on vascular smooth muscle cells."

Resveratrol blocks interleukin-18-EMMPRIN cross-regulation and smooth muscle cell migration. Venkatesan B, Valente AJ, Reddy VS, Siwik DA, Chandrasekar B. Am J

Physiol Heart Circ Physiol. 2009 Aug;297(2):H874-86. **Key Finding:** "Resveratrol, via its antioxidant and anti-inflammatory properties, has the potential to inhibit the progression of **atherosclerosis** by blocking IL-18 and EMMPRIN cross-regulation and SMC migration."

Cancer (bladder; breast; colon; esophageal; liver; leukemia; lung; ovarian; pancreatic; prostate)

Resveratrol in the chemoprevention and treatment of **hepatocellular Carcinoma**. Bishayee A, Politis T, Darvesh AS. Cancer Treat Rev. 2010 Feb;36(1):43-53. **Key Finding**: "Using naturally occurring phytochemicals and dietary compounds endowed with potent antioxidant and anti-inflammatory properties is a novel approach to prevent and control hepatocellular carcinoma, the most common type of **liver cancer**. One such compound, resveratrol, present in grapes, berries, peanuts, has emerged as a promising molecule that inhibits carcinogenesis with a pleiotropic mode of action."

Evaluation of anti-invasion effect of resveratrol and related methoxy analogues on human hepatocarcinoma cells. Weng CJ, Wu CF, Huang HW, Et al. J Agric Food Chem. 2010 Mar 10;58(5):2886-94. **Key Finding**: "These results suggest that resveratrol and its related methoxy analogue MR-3 might exert anti-invasive activity against hepatoma cells {**liver cancer**} through regulation of MMP-2, MMP-9, TIMP-1, and TIMP-2."

Resveratrol suppresses colitis and **colon cancer** *associated with* **colitis**. Cui X. Jin Y. Hofseth AB. Et al. Cancer Prev Res. 2010 Apr;3(4):549-59. **Key Finding**: "We used a dextran sulfate sodium mouse model of colitis. The current study indicates that resveratrol is a useful, nontoxic complementary and alternative strategy to abate colitis and potentially colon cancer associated with colitis."

Resveratrol suppresses IGF-1 induced human **colon cancer** *cell proliferation and elevates apoptosis via suppression of IGF-1R/Wnt and activation of p53 signaling pathways.* Vanamala J, Reddivari L, Radhakrishran S, Tarver C. BMC Cancer. 2010 May 26;10:238. **Key Finding**: "For the first time, we report that resveratrol suppresses colon cancer cell proliferation and elevates apoptosis even in the presence of IGF-1 via suppression of IGF-1R/Akt/Wnt signaling pathways and activation of p53, suggesting its potential role as a chemotherapeutic agent."

Pterostilbene inhibits colorectal aberrant crypt foci (ACF) and **colon carcinogenesis** *via suppression of multiple signal transduction pathways in azoxymethane-treated mice.* Chiou YS, Tsai ML, Wang YJ, Et al. J Agric Food Chem. 2010 Aug 11;58(15):8833-41. **Key Finding**: "All of these results revealed that pterostilbene, a natural dimethylated analogue of resveratrol, is an effective antitumor agent capable of preventing inflammation-associated colon tumorigenesis."

Resveratrol induces growth arrest and apoptosis through activation of FOXO transcription factors in **prostate cancer** *cells.* Chen Q, Ganapathy S, Singh KP, Et al. PLoS One. 2010 Dec 14;5(12):15288. **Key Finding**: "These data suggest that FOXO transcription factors mediate anti-proliferative and pro-apoptotic effects of resveratrol in part due to activation of extrinsic apoptosis pathway."

Resveratrol enhances antitumor activity of TRAIL in **prostate cancer** *xenografts through activation of FOXO transcription factor.* Ganapthay S, Chen Q, Singh KP, Et al. PLoS One. 2010 Dec 28;5(12):e15627. **Key Finding**: "These data suggest that resveratrol can enhance the apoptosis-inducing potential of TRAIL by activating FKHRL1 and its target genes. The ability of resveratrol to inhibit tumor growth, metastasis and angiogenesis, and enhance the therapeutic potential of TRAIL suggests that resveratrol alone or in combination with TRAIL can be used for the management of prostate cancer."

Resveratrol regulated the PTEN/AKT pathway through androgen receptor-dependent and – independent mechanisms in **prostate cancer** *cell lines.* Wang Y, Romigh T, He X, Et al. Hum Mol Genet. 2010 Nov 15;19(22):4319-29. **Key Finding**: "Resveratrol may act as potential adjunctive treatment for late-stage hormone refractory prostate cancer. For the first time, out study demonstrates the mechanism by which the androgen receptor regulates PTEN expression at the transcription level."

Resveratrol prevents epigenetic silencing of BRCA-1 by the aromatic hydrocarbon receptor in human **breast cancer** *cells.* Papoutsis AJ, Lamore SD, Wondrak GT, Et al. J Nutr. 2010 Sep;140(9):1607-14. **Key Finding**: "These results support the hypothesis that epigenetic silencing of the BRCA-1 gene by the aromatic hydrocarbon receptor is preventable with resveratrol and provide the molecular basis for the development of dietary strategies."

Resveratrol induces apoptosis and cell cycle arrest of human T24 **bladder cancer** *cells in vitro and inhibits tumor grown in vivo.* Bai Y, Mao QO, Qin J, Et al. Cancer Sci. 2010 Feb;101(2):488-93. **Key Finding**: "These findings suggest that resveratrol could be an important chemoprevention agent for bladder cancer."

Anticancer activity and molecular mechanism of resveratrol-bovine serum albumin nanoparticles on subcutaneously implanted human primary **ovarian carcinoma** *cells in nude mice.* Guo I, Peng Y, Yap J, Et al. Cancer Biother Radiopharm. 2010 Aug;25(4):471-7. **Key Finding:** "This study investigates the antitumor effects and functional mechanism of resveratrol-bovine serum albumin nanoparticles on human primary ovarian carcinoma cells in nude mice."

2,3', 4, 4',5'-Pentamethoxy-trans-stilbene, a resveratrol derivative, inhibits colitis-associated colorectal carcinogenesis in mice. Li H, Wu WK, Li ZJ, Et al. Br J Pharmacol. 2010 Jul;160(5);1352-61. **Key Finding**: The resveratrol methoxylated derivative "effectively suppressed colon carcinogenesis in an ACM/DSS animal model and may merit further clinical investigation as a chemo prophylactic agent against colitis-associated **colon cancer** in humans."

Antiproliferative effect of resveratrol in **pancreatic cancer** *cells.* Cui J, Sun R., Yu Y, Et al. Phytother Res. 2010 Nov;24(11):1637-44. **Key Finding**: "Resveratrol inhibited the proliferation of pancreatic cancer cells by inducing apoptotic cell death. There was different sensitivity to resveratrol in different pancreatic cancer cell lines."

Resveratrol modulates angiogenesis through the GSK3B/B-catenin/TGF-dependent pathway in human endothelial cells. Wang H, Zhou H, Zou Y, Et al. Biochem Parmacol. 2010 Nov 1;80(9):1386-95. **Key Finding**: "We observed that resveratrol was able to modulate the expression of VEGF and the formation of vascular network in a biphasic pattern. Our findings may have implications in the management of **cardiovascular disease** and other conditions such as **cancer** by the use of resveratrol"

Clinical pharmacology of resveratrol and its metabolites in **colorectal cancer** *patients.* Patel KR, Brown VA, Jones DJ, Et al. Cancer Res. 2010 Oct 1;70(19):7392-9. **Key Finding**: "The results suggest that daily p.o. doses of resveratrol at 0.5 or 1.0 g. produce levels in the human gastrointestinal tract of an order of magnitude sufficient to elicit anticarcinogenic effects. Resveratrol merits further clinical evaluation as a potential colorectal cancer chemo preventive agent."

Resveratrol promotes autophagic cell death in chronic myelogenous **leukemia** *cells via JNK-mediated p62/SQSTM1 expression and AMPK activation.* Puissant A, Robert G, Fenouille N, Et al. Cancer Res. 2010 Feb 1;70(3):1042-52. **Key Finding**: "Autophagy that is induced by starvation or cellular stress can enable cancer cell survival by sustaining energy homeostasis and eliminating damaged organelles and proteins.

We concluded that resveratrol triggered autophagic cell death in leukemia (CML) cells via both JNK-mediated p62 overexpression and AMPK activation."

*Arachidin-1, a **Peanut** Stilbenoid, Induces Programmed Cell Death in Human **Leukemia** HL-60 Cells.* Huang CP, Au LC, Chiou RY, Et al J Agric Food Chem. 2010 Nov 10 {Epub ahead of print}. **Key Finding**: "**Resveratrol**, a stilbenoid isolated from germinating peanut kernels, possesses anticancer activity and studies have indicated that it induces programmed cell death in human leukemia HL-60 cells. In this study, the anticancer activity of these stilbenoid was determined in HL-60 cells."

*Resveratrol, a red wine polyphenol, suppresses **pancreatic cancer** by inhibiting leukotriene A hydrolase.* Oi N, Jeong CH, Nadas J, Et al. Cancer Res. 2010 Dec 1;70(23):9755-64. **Key Finding**: "Resveratrol is a well-known polyphenolic compound of red wine {and grapes} with cancer chemo preventive activity. However, the basis for this activity is unclear. Our findings identify LTA(4)H as a functionally important target {in pancreatic cancer} for mediating the anticancer properties of resveratrol.

*Resveratrol and quercetin cooperate to induce senescence-like growth arrest in C6 rat **glioma cells**.* Zamin LL, Filippi-Chiela EC, Dillenburg-Pilla P, Horn F, Salbego C, Lenz G. Cancer Sci. 2009 Sep;100(9):1655-62. **Key Finding:** "Resveratrol and quercetin chronically administered presented a strong synergism in inducing senescence-like growth arrest. These results suggest that the combination of polyphenols can potentialize their antitumoral activity, thereby reducing the therapeutic concentration needed for glioma treatment."

*Genistein and resveratrol, alone and in combination, suppress prostate **cancer** in SV-40 tag rats.* Harper CE, Cook LM, Patel BB, Wang J, Eltoum IA, Arabshahi A, Shirai T, Lamartiniere CA. Prostate. 2009 Nov 1;69(15):1668-82. **Key Finding:** "Genistein and resveratrol, alone and in combination, suppress prostate cancer development in the SV-40 Tag (rat) model. Regulation of SRC-3 and growth factor signaling proteins are consistent with these nutritional polyphenols reducing cell proliferation and increasing apoptosis in the prostate."

*Natural compounds in chemoprevention of **esophageal squamous cell tumors**— experimental studies.* Szumilo J. Pol Merkur Lekarski. 2009 Feb;26(152):156-61. **Key Finding:** "In esophageal squamous cell carcinoma—this belongs to the group of the most aggressive tumors of digestive system with poor prognosis. Chemo preventive properties of many complex diets and pure natural compounds were evaluated. Most studies were performed on rats exposed to chemical carcinogens. The best effects were achieved after administration of diallyl sulfide and phenethyl isothiocyanate. Lyophilized black raspberries, blackberries and straw-berries, as well as products obtained from leaves and buds of tea plant, ellagic acid and resveratrol were also very effective."

*Evaluation of anti-**leukemia** effect of resveratrol by modulating SATA3 signaling.* Li T, Wang W, Chen H, Li T, Ye L. Int Immunopharmacol. 2009 Sep 29. (Epub ahead of print). **Key Finding:** "Resveratrol is a natural occurring phytoalexin present in grapes and berries that has been shown to have chemo preventive/ therapeutic activity. In this study, we examine its anti-leukemia effect both in vitro and in vivo. Our data indicate that resveratrol contributes to inhibiting growth, inducing apoptosis and cell cycle arrest in the three leukemia cell lines (Jurkat, SUP-B15, and Kasumi-1) and reducing the phosphorylation of STAT3, mean-while modulating the expression of Bcl-2 and Bax."

*Resveratrol in the chemoprevention and treatment of **hepatocellular carcinoma**.* Bishayee A, Politis T, Darvesh AS. Cancer Treat Rev. 2009 Nov 10. (Epub ahead of print). **Key Finding:** "Hepatocellular carcinoma commonly develops in patients with chronic liver disease. Resveratrol, present in grapes, berries and peanuts, has emerged as a promising molecule that inhibits carcinogenesis with a pleiotropic mode of action. This review examines the current knowledge on mechanism-based in vitro and in vivo studies on the chemo preventive and chemotherapeutic potential of resveratrol in **liver cancer**."

*Resveratrol Induces Apoptosis in Human SK-HEP-1 **Hepatic Cancer** Cells.* Choi HY, Chong SA, Nam MJ. Cancer Genomics Proteomics. 2009 Sep-Oct;6(5):263-8. **Key Finding:** "Resveratrol causes hepatic cancer cell death by suppressing the expression of antioxidant proteins. Resveratrol inhibited cell proliferation, gener-ated reactive oxygen species, and caused DNA single-strand breaks."

*Pterostilbene Inhibits **Breast Cancer** In Vitro Through Mitochondrial Depolarization and Induction of Caspase-Dependent Apoptosis.* Alosi JA, McDonald DE, Schneider JS, Privette AR, McFadden DW. J Surg Res. 2009 Aug 18. (Epub ahead of print). **Key Finding:** "Pterostilbene, an analogue of resveratrol found in blueberries, has both antioxidant and antiproliferative properties. Pterostilbene treatment inhibits the growth of breast cancer in vitro through caspase-dependent apop-tosis. Further in vitro mechanistic studies and in vivo experiments are warranted to determine its potential for the treatment of breast cancer."

*Pterostilbene Inhibits **Lung Cancer** Through Induction of Apoptosis.* Schnieder JG, Alosi JA, McDonald DE, McFadden DW. J Surg Res. 2009 Jul 21. (Epub ahead of print). **Key Finding:** "We investigated the effects of pterostilbene, an analog of resveratrol found in blueberries, on lung cancer, in vitro. Pterostilbene significantly decreased cell viability in lung cancer cells in a concentration and time-dependent manner. Further in vitro mechanistic studies and in vivo experiments are warranted to determine the potential role for pterostilbene in lung cancer treatment or prevention."

Curcumin synergizes with resveratrol to inhibit **colon cancer.** Majumdar AP, Banerjee S, Nautiyal J, Patel BB, Patel V, Du J, Yu Y, Elliott AA, Levi E, Sarkar FH. Nutr Cancer. 2009;61(4):544-53. **Key Finding:** "Our current data suggest that the combination of curcumin and resveratrol could be an effective preventive/therapeutic strategy for colon cancer. The combination of curcumin and resveratrol was found to be more effective in inhibiting growth of p53-positive (wt) and p53-negative colon cancer HCT-116 cells in vitro and in vivo in SCID xenografts of colon cancer HCT-116 (wt) cells than either agent alone."

Apoptosis induced by capsaicin and resveratrol in **colon carcinoma** *cells requires nitric oxide production and caspase activation.* Kim MY, Trudel LJ, Wogan GN. Anticancer Res. 2009 Oct;29(10):3733-40. **Key Finding:** "We examined the role of nitric oxide and influence of p53 status during apoptosis induced by these agents in two isogenic HCT116 human colon carcinomas, wild-type p53 and complete knockout of p53 cells. Capsaicin and resveratrol, alone or in combination, inhibited cell growth and promoted apoptosis by the elevation of nitric oxide; combined treatment in p53-WT cells was most effective. These findings offer exciting opportunities to improve the effectiveness of colon cancer treatment."

Resveratrol induces apoptosis and cell cycle arrest of human T24 **bladder cancer** *cells in vitro and inhibits tumor growth in vivo.* Bai Y, Mao QQ, Qin J, Zheng XY, Wang YB, Yang K, Shen HF, Xie LP. Cancer Sci. 2009 Oct 27 (Epub ahead of print). **Key Finding:** "Treatment of bladder cancer cells with resveratrol resulted in a significant decrease in cell viability. These findings suggest that resveratrol could be an important chemoprevention agent for bladder cancer."

Resveratrol suppresses growth of human **ovarian cancer** *cells in culture and in a murine xenograft model: eukaryotic elongation factor 1A2 as a potential target.* Lee MH, Choi BY, Kundu JK, Shin YK, Na HK, Surh YJ. Cancer Res. 2009 Sep 15;69(18):7449-58. **Key Finding:** "Pretreatment with resveratrol attenuated proliferation of serum-starved PA-1 cells stimulated with insulin or serum. Resveratrol also activated caspase-9, -7, and -3 and induced apoptosis in PA-1 cells in the presence of insulin or serum."

*Resveratrol, a multi-targeted agent, can enhance antitumor activity of gemcitabine in vitro and in orthotropic mouse model of human **pancreatic cancer**.* Harikumar KB, Kunnunmakkara AB, Sthei G, Diagaradjane P, Anand P, Pandey MK, Gelovani J, Krishnan S, Guha S, Aggarwal BB. Int J Cancer. 2009 Nov 11 (Epub ahead of print). **Key Finding:** "Our results demonstrate that resveratrol can synergize the effects of gemcitabine, a standard treatment for pancreatic cancer, through suppression of markers of proliferation, invasion, angiogenesis and metastasis."

*Effects of diverse dietary phytoestrogens on cell growth, cell cycle and apoptosis in estrogen-receptor-positive **breast cancer** cells.* Sakamoto T, Horiguchi H, Oguma E, Kayama F. J Nutr Biochem. 2009 Oct 2 (Epub ahead of print). **Key Finding:** "Resveratrol might be the most promising candidate for hormone replacement therapy and chemoprevention of breast cancer due to its estrogenic activity and high antitumor activity."

*Resveratrol enhances p53 acetylation and apoptosis in **prostate cancer** by inhibiting MTA1/NuRD complex.* Kai L, Samuel SK, Levenson AS. Int J Cancer. 2009 Oct 6. (Epub ahead of print). **Key Finding:** "Our study identifies MTA1 as a new molecular target of resveratrol that may have important clinical applications for prostate cancer chemoprevention and therapy, and points to the combination of resveratrol with HDAC inhibitors as an innovative therapeutic strategy for the treatment of prostate cancer."

*Influence of dietary resveratrol on early and late molecular markers of 1,2-dimethylhydrazine-induced **colon carcinogenesis**.* Sengottuvelan M, Deeptha K, Nalini N. Nutrition. 2009 Nov-Dec;25(11-12):1169-76. **Key Finding:** "Our study demonstrates that the chemo preventive efficacy of resveratrol could be attributed to its action on multiple direct targets of carcinogenesis. The results clearly indicate that chronic resveratrol supplementation inhibited the colon cancer development through modulating the early and late events of carcinogenesis and helped to maintain the colonic mucosal integrity."

*Mechanisms of apoptotic effects induced by resveratrol, dibenzoylmethane, and their analogues on human **lung carcinoma** cells.* Weng CJ, Yang YT, Ho CT, Yen GC. J Agric Food Chem. 2009 Jun 24;57(12):5235-43. **Key Finding:** "We have demonstrated that resveratrol, DBM, and their analogues could be effective candidates for chemoprevention of lung cancer."

*Suppression of Heregulin-{beta}1/HER2-Modulated Invasive and Aggressive Phenotype of **Breast Carcinoma** by Pterostilbene via Inhibition of Matrix Metalloproteinase-9, p38 Kinase Cascade and Akt Activation.* Pan MH, Lin YT, Lin CL, Wei CS, Ho CT, Chen

WJ. Evid Based Complement Alternat Med. 2009 Jul 16 (Epub ahead of print). **Key Finding:** "Pterostilbene, a natural analog of resveratrol, exerts its cancer chemo preventive activity similar to resveratrol by inhibiting cancer cell proliferation and inducing apoptosis. We found that pterostilbene was able to suppress HRG-beta1-mediated cell invasion, motility and cell transformation of MCF-7 human breast carcinoma."

2, 3', 4, 4', 5'-Pentamethoxy-trans-stilbene, a resveratrol derivative, is a potent inducer of apoptosis in **colon cancer** *cells via targeting microtubules.* Li H, Wu WK, Zheng Z, Che CT, Yu L, Li ZJ, Wu YC, Cheng KW, Yu J, Cho CH, Wang M. Biochem Pharmacol. 2009 Nov 1;78(9):1224-32. **Key Finding:** "These data suggest that the resveratrol derivative is a potent inducer of apoptosis via targeting microtubules and may merit investigation as a potential chemo prophylactic and therapeutic agent for colon cancer."

Induction of a reversible, non-cytotoxic S-phase delay by resveratrol: implications for a mechanism of **lifespan** *prolongation and* **cancer** *protection.* Zhou R, Fukui M, CHoi HJ, Zhu BT. Br J Pharmacol. 2009 Sep;158(2):462-74. **Key Finding:** "Resveratrol has been shown to prolong lifespan and prevent cancer formation. At present, the precise cellular mechanisms of resveratrol's action are still not clearly understood, and this is the focus of this study. It is hypothesized that the induction of a non-cytotoxic S-phase delay may represent a useful mechanistic strategy for lifespan prolongation and cancer prevention."

*Involvement of mitochondria and recruitment of Fas/CD95 signaling in lipid rafts in resveratrol-mediated anti***myeloma** *and anti***leukemia** *actions.* Reis-Sobreiro M, Gajate C, Mollinedo F. Oncogene. 2009 Sep 10;28(36):3221-34. **Key Finding:** "We have found that resveratrol induced apoptosis in multiple myeloma and T-cell leukemia cells through co-clustering of Fas/CD95 death receptor and lipid rafts, whereas normal lymphocytes were spared."

Anti-inflammatory action of pterostilbene is mediated through the p38 mitogen-activated protein kinase pathway in **colon cancer** *cells.* Paul S, Rimando AM, Lee HJ, Ji Y, Reddy BS. Suh N. Cancer Prev Res. 2009 Jul;2(7):650-7. **Key Finding:** "Our data suggest that the p38 mitogen-activated protein kinase cascade is a key signal transduction pathway for eliciting the anti-inflammatory action of pterostilbene in cultured HT-29 colon cancer cells."

Inhibitory effect of resveratrol on the growth of human **colon cancer** *1s174t cells and its subcutaneously transplanted tumor in nude mice and the mechanism of action.* Chen J, Dong XS, Guo XG. Zhonghua Zhong Liu Za Zhi (Chinese). 2009 Jan;31(1):15-9. **Key**

Finding: "Resveratrol can inhibit the growth of 1s174t cells through apoptosis induction. The mechanism is probably related to inhibition of anti-apoptotic factor bcl-2 and enhancement of expression of apoptotic factor bax."

Resveratrol: cellular actions of a potent natural chemical that confers a diversity of health benefits. Marques FZ, Markus MA, Morris BJ. Int J Biochem Cell Biol. 2009 Nov;41(11):2125-8. **Key Finding:** "Resveratrol has health benefits in common age-related diseases such as **cancer, type 2 diabetes, cardiovascular disease, and neurological conditions.** Resveratrol has positive effects on metabolism and can increase the lifespan of various organisms. Its effects arise from its capacity to interact with multiple molecular targets involved in diverse intracellular pathways."

*Growth inhibition of human **colon cancer** cells by plant compounds.* Duessel S, Heuertz RM, Ezekiel UR. Clin Lab Sci. 2008 Summer;21(3):151-7. **Key Finding**: "The purpose of this study was to determine if resveratrol from red grapes, cinnamaldehyde from cinnamon, and piperine from black pepper has anti-proliferative effects on colon cancer. All phytochemicals displayed anti-proliferative effects on DLD-1 colon cancer cells in culture. These results taken together with everyday dietary availability of concentrations used in this study strongly suggest that regular intake of low doses of these phytochemicals offer preventive effects against colon cancer."

Chemo preventive anti-inflammatory activities of curcumin and other phytochemicals mediated by MAP kinase phosphatase-5 in prostate cells. Nonn L, Duong D, Peehl DM. Carcinogenesis. 2007 Jun;28(6):1188-96. **Key Finding:** The mediating anti-inflammatory activities of curcumin, **resveratrol** and gingerol were examined. "Our findings show direct anti-inflammatory activity of MKP5 in prostate cells and suggest that up-regulation of MKP5 by phytochemicals may contribute to their chemo preventive actions by decreasing **prostatic inflammation**."

*Resveratrol-caused apoptosis of human **prostate carcinoma** LNCaP cells is mediated via modulation of phosphatidylinositol 3'-kinase/Akt pathway and Bcl-2 family proteins.* Aziz MH, Nihal M, Fu VX, Jarrard DF, Ahmad N. Mol Cancer Ther. 2006 May;5(5):1335-41. **Key Finding:** "This study was conducted to evaluate the chemo preventive/antiproliferative potential of resveratrol against prostate cancer and its mechanism of action. We suggest that resveratrol could be developed as an agent for the management of prostate cancer."

*Polyphenolic phytochemicals versus non-steroidal **anti-inflammatory** drugs: which are better cancer chemo preventive agents?* Gescher A. J Chemother. 2004 Nov;16

Suppl 4:3-6. **Key Finding:** "As non-steroidal anti-inflammatory drugs possess unwanted side effects, polyphenol phytochemicals such as curcumin and **resveratrol** are promising alternatives. They suppress **carcinogenesis** in the ApcMin+ mouse model. Clinical pilot studies of curcumin show that it is safe at doses of up to 3.6g daily, and that the levels of curcumin which can be achieved in the gastrointestinal tract exert pharmacological activity."

*Role of chemo preventive agents in **cancer** therapy.* Dorai T, Aggarwal BB. Cancer Lett. 2004 Nov 25;215(2):129-40. **Key Finding:** "Chemo preventive agents include genistein, **resveratrol**, diallyl sulfide, S-allyl cysteine, allicin, lycopene, capsaicin, curcumin, 6-gingerol, ellagic acid, ursolic acid, silymarin, anethol, catechins and eugenol. Because these agents have been shown to suppress cancer cell proliferation, inhibit growth factor signaling pathways, induce apoptosis, inhibit NF-kappaB, AP-1 and JAK-STAT activation pathways, inhibit angiogenesis, suppress the expression of anti-apoptotic proteins, inhibit cyclooxygenase-2, they may have untapped therapeutic value. These chemo preventive agents also have very recently been found to reverse chemo resistance and radio resistance in patients undergoing cancer treatment."

Resveratrol in raw and baked blueberries and bilberries. Lyons MM, Yu C, Toma RB, Cho SY, Reiboldt W, Lee J, Van Breemen RB. J Agric Food Chem. 2003 Sep 24;51(20):5867-70. **Key Finding:** "Although blueberries and bilberries were found to contain resveratrol, the level of this **chemo protective** compound in these fruits was <10% that reported for grapes. Furthermore, cooking or heat processing of these berries will contribute to the degradation of resveratrol."

Cardiovascular disease

*Resveratrol and **cardiovascular health**.* Das M, Das DK. Mol Aspects Med. 2010 Dec;31(6):503-12. **Key Finding:** "Overall observation indicates that resveratrol has a high therapeutic potential for the treatment of cardiovascular diseases."

Resveratrol modulates angiogenesis through the GSK3B/B-catenin/TGF-dependent pathway in human endothelial cells. Wang H, Zhou H, Zou Y, et al. Biochem Parmacol. 2010 Nov 1;80(9):1386-95. **Key Finding**: "We observed that resveratrol was able to modulate the expression of VEGF and the formation of vascular network in a biphasic pattern. Our findings may have implications in the management of **cardiovascular disease** and other conditions such as **cancer** by the use of resveratrol"

Effects of Longevinex (modified resveratrol) on **cardio protection** *and its mechanisms of action.* Mukherjee S, Ray D, Lekli I, et al. Can J Physiol Pharmacol. 2010 Nov;88(11):1017-25. **Key Finding**: "We designed a study with a resveratrol formulation that contained resveratrol supplemented with 5% quercetin and 5% rice bran phytate (commercially known as Longevinex.) Sprague-Dawley rats were gavaged with either Longevinext or vehicle and sacrificed after 1 or 3 months. The results appear to suggest that Longevinext induces longevity after prolonged feedings via induction of autophagy, while it converts death signals into survival signals and provides cardio protection within a relatively short period of time."

Antiatherogenic properties of flavonoids: implications for **cardiovascular health.** Mulvihill EE, Huff MW. Can J Cardiol. 2010 Mar;26 Suppl A:17A-21A. **Key Finding**: "The present review summarizes data suggesting that flavonoids improve endothelial function, inhibit low-density lipoprotein oxidation, decrease blood pressure and improve dyslipidemia. A large number of studies have reported the impact of consuming flavonoid-rich foods on biomarkers of cardio-vascular disease risk in healthy volunteers or at-risk individuals."

Dietary polyphenols: focus on resveratrol, a promising agent in the prevention of **cardiovascular diseases** *and control of glucose homeostasis.* Borriello A, Cucciolla V, Della Ragione F, Galletti P. Nutr Metab Cardiovasc Dis. 2010 Oct;20(8):618-25. **Key Finding**: "This article reports the actions of resveratrol on cardiovascular diseases and the molecular bases of its activity."

Co-ordinated autophagy with resveratrol and gamma-tocotrienol confers a synergetic **cardio protection.** Lekli I, Ray D, Mukherjee S, Gurusamy N, Ahsan MK, Juhasz B, Bak I, Tosaki A, Gherghiceanu M, Popescu IM, Das DK. J Cell Mol Med. 2009 Oct 3 (Epub ahead of print). **Key Finding:** "Palm-oil derived gamma-tocotri-enol and resveratrol from grapes acted synergistically providing greater degree of cardio protection simultaneously generating greater amount of survival signal through the activation of Akt-Bcl-2 survival pathway. It is tempting to speculate that during ischemia and reperfusion autophagy along with enhanced survival signals helps to recover the (rat heart) cells from injury."

Cellular mechanisms of **cardio protection** *by calorie restriction: state of the science and future perspectives.* Marzetti E, Wohlgemuth SE, Anton SD, Bernabei R, Carter CS, Leeuwenburgh C. Clin Geriatr Med. 2009 Nov;25(4):715-32. **Key Finding:** "Preclinical studies indicate that specific compounds, such as **resveratrol,** may mimic many of the effects of calorie restriction, thus potentially obviating the need for drastic food intake reductions. Results from ongoing clinical trials will reveal whether the intriguing alternative of calorie restriction represents a safe and effective strategy to promote cardiovascular health and delay cardiac **aging** in humans."

Cardio protection by resveratrol: A novel mechanism via autophagy involving the mTORC2 pathway. Gurusamy N, Lekli I, Mukherjee S, Ray D, Ahsan MK, Gherghiceanu M, Popescu LM, Das DK. Cardiovasc Res. 2009 Dec 3. (Epub ahead of print). **Key Finding:** "Based on our previous reports that cardio protection induced by ischemic preconditioning induces autophagy and that resveratrol induces preconditioning-like effects, we sought to determine if resveratrol could induce autophagy. Our results indicate that at lower dose, resveratrol-mediated cell survival is, in part, mediated through the induction of autophagy involving mTOR-Rictor survival pathway."

Physiological concentrations of dietary polyphenols regulate vascular endothelial cell expression of genes important in **cardiovascular** *health.* Nicholson SK, Tucker GA, Brameld JM. Br J Nutr. 2009 Dec 21:1-6. **Key Finding:** "Previous cell culture-based studies have shown potential health beneficial effects on gene expression of dietary polyphenols. The present study investigated effects of physiological concentrations of different classes of dietary polyphenol on the expression of genes important in cardiovascular health. Only three of the eleven polyphenols tested –resveratrol, quercetin and epigallocatechin gallate—had biological activity with observed effects on gene expression that would be expected to result in vasodilation and reduced **blood pressure**."

A new insight into resveratrol as an **atheroprotective** *compound: inhibition of lipid peroxidation and enhancement of cholesterol efflux.* Berrougui H, Grenier G, Loued S, Drouin G, Khalil A. Atherosclerosis. 2009 Dec;207(2):420-7. **Key Finding:** "Resveratrol is known for its anti-atherogenic properties and is thought to be beneficial in reducing the incidence of cardiovascular diseases. However, the mechanism of action by which it exerts its anti-atherogenic effect remains unclear. We investigated the relationship between the antioxidant effects of resveratrol and its ability to promote cholesterol efflux. We found that resveratrol appears to be a natural antioxidant and enhances cholesterol efflux and means it could be used to prevent and treat **cardiovascular disease**."

Resveratrol Supplementation Gender Independently Improves Endothelial Reactivity and Suppresses Superoxide Production in Healthy Rats. Soylemez S, Sepici A, Akar F. Cardiovasc Drugs

Ther. 2009 Oct 7. (Epub ahead of print). **Key Finding:** "Our results suggest that resveratrol supplementation could improve the capacity of endothelial function and suppression of oxidative stress under physiological conditions. Resveratrol ingestion indicates a potential for **cardiovascular** health promotion."

Resveratrol: cellular actions of a potent natural chemical that confers a diversity of health benefits. Marques FZ, Markus MA, Morris BJ. Int J Biochem Cell Biol. 2009 Nov;41(11):2125-8. **Key Finding:** "Resveratrol has health benefits in common age-related diseases such as **cancer, type 2 diabetes, cardiovascular disease, and neurological conditions.** Resveratrol has positive effects on metabolism and can increase the lifespan of various organisms. Its effects arise from its capacity to interact with multiple molecular targets involved in diverse intracellular pathways."

Colitis

*Resveratrol suppresses colitis and **colon cancer** associated with **colitis.*** Cui X, Jin Y, Hofseth AB, Et al. Cancer Prev Res. 2010 Apr;3(4):549-59. **Key Finding:** "We used a dextran sulfate sodium mouse model of colitis. The current study indicates that resveratrol is a useful, nontoxic complementary and alternative strategy to abate colitis and potentially colon cancer associated with colitis."

*Resveratrol (trans-3,5,4'-trihydroxystilbene) induces SIRT1 and down-regulates NF-{kapp} B activation to abrogate DSS-induced **colitis**.* Singh UP, Singh N, Singh B, Hofseth LJ, Price BL, Nagarkatti M, Nagarkatti P. J Pharmacol Exp Ther. 2009 Nov 30 (Epub ahead of print). **Key Finding:** "This study demonstrates for the first time that SIRT1 is involved in colitis, functioning as an inverse regulator of NF-kappaB activation and inflammation. Furthermore, our results indicate that resveratrol may protect against colitis through up-regulation of SIRT1 in immune cells in the colon."

Diabetes

*Resveratrol, **obesity and diabetes**.* Szkudelska K, Szkudelski T. Eur J Pharmacol. 2010 Jun 10;635(1-3):1-8. **Key Finding:** "The broad spectrum of effects of resveratrol has been enlarged by new data demonstrating a great potency of this compound in relation to obesity and diabetes. Data point to the potential possibility of use of resveratrol in preventing and/or treating obesity and diabetes."

Resveratrol improves left ventricular diastolic relaxation in **type 2 diabetes** *by inhibiting oxidative/nitrative stress: in vivo demonstration with magnetic resonance imaging.* Zhang H, Morgan B, Potter BJ, Et al. Am J Physiol Circ Physiol. 2010 Oct;299(4):H985-94. **Key Finding**: "This study was designed to elucidate the mechanisms by which resveratrol protects against diabetes-induced cardiac dysfunction. Resveratrol protects against cardiac dysfunction by inhibiting oxidative/nitrative stress and improving nitric oxide availability."

Insulin and resveratrol act **synergistically**, *preventing cardiac dysfunction in diabetes, but the advantage of resveratrol in diabetics with acute* **heart attack** *is antagonized by insulin.* Huang JP, Huang SS, Deng JY, Et al. Free Radic Biol Med. 2010 Dec 1;49(11):1710-21. **Key Finding**: "These results indicate that insulin and resveratrol synergistically prevented cardiac dysfunction in diabetes and this may be in parallel with activation of the insulin-mediated Akt/GLUT4 signaling pathway. Insulin counteracted the advantage of resveratrol in **diabetics** with acute heart attack."

Central administration of resveratrol improves diet-induced **diabetes**. Ramadori G, Gautron L, Fujikawa T, Vianna CR, Elmquist JK, Coppari R. Endocrinology. 2009 Dec;150(12):5326-33. **Key Finding:** "Our results unveiled a previously unrecognized key role for the central nervous system in mediating the antidiabetic actions of resveratrol. Central nervous system resveratrol delivery improves hypothalamic nuclear factor-kappaB inflammatory signaling."

Resveratrol: cellular actions of a potent natural chemical that confers a diversity of health benefits. Marques FZ, Markus MA, Morris BJ. Int J Biochem Cell Biol. 2009 Nov;41(11):2125-8. **Key Finding:** "Resveratrol has health benefits in common age-related diseases such as **cancer, type 2 diabetes, cardiovascular disease, and neurological conditions.** Resveratrol has positive effects on metabolism and can increase the lifespan of various organisms. Its effects arise from its capacity to interact with multiple molecular targets involved in diverse intracellular pathways."

Metabolic effects of resveratrol in mammals—a link between improved insulin action and **aging**. Frojdo S, Durand C, Pirola L. Curr Aging Sci. 2008 Dec;1(3):145-51. **Key Finding:** "Resveratrol, a polyphenol, has been shown to possess lifespan-promoting properties in yeast and metazoans, including small mammals. The action of resveratrol has been linked to its capability to i) prolong lifespan following chronic administration to mice and ii) protect from the development of diet-induced obesity and obesity-dependent metabolic disorders. Here we summarize the current understanding on how resveratrol displays its remarkable properties by acting on the control of insulin secretion and by modulation of insulin action in peripheral insulin-responsive tissues. Resveratrol has the potential to prevent the establishment of insulin-resistance and thus postpone or even prevent the onset of **type 2 diabetes**."

Epilepsy

Neuroprotective properties of resveratrol in different neurodegenerative disorders. Albani D, Polito L, Signorini A, Forioni G. Biofactors. 2010 Sep;36(5):370-6.**Key Finding**: "Resveratrol has neuroprotective features both in vitro and in vivo in models of **Alzheimer's disease**, but it has proved to be beneficial also in **ischemic stroke, Parkinson's disease, Huntington's disease, and epilepsy**. Here we summarize the in vitro and in vivo experimental results highlighting the possible role of resveratrol as neuroprotective bio factor with a particular focus on Alzheimer's disease."

Huntington's disease

Neuroprotective properties of resveratrol in different neurodegenerative disorders. Albani D, Polito L, Signorini A, Forioni G. Biofactors. 2010 Sep;36(5):370-6.**Key Finding**: "Resveratrol has neuroprotective features both in vitro and in vivo in models of **Alzheimer's disease**, but it has proved to be beneficial also in **ischemic stroke, Parkinson's disease, Huntington's disease, and epilepsy**. Here we summarize the in vitro and in vivo experimental results highlighting the possible role of resveratrol as neuroprotective bio factor with a particular focus on Alzheimer's disease."

Hypertension

*Resveratrol and small artery compliance and remodeling in the spontaneously **hypertensive** rat.* Behbathari J, Thandapily SJ, Louis XL, Et al. Am J Hypertens. 2010 Dec;23(12):1273-8. **Key Finding**: "Small arteries from the spontaneously hypertensive rat exhibit abnormal stiffness and geometry. This study investigated the effects of resveratrol on small arteries. The ability of resveratrol to limit the increase in compliance of spontaneously hypertensive rat arteries is likely related to inhibitory effects on remodeling and pro-growth ERK signaling."

Resveratrol Prevents the Development of Pathological Cardiac Hypertrophy and Contractile Dysfunction in the SHR Without Lowering Blood Pressure. Thandapilly SJ, Wojciechowski P, Behbahani J, Louis XL, Yu L, Juric D, Kopilas MA, Anderson HD, Netticadan T. Am J Hypertens. 2009 Nov 26. (Epub ahead of print). **Key Finding:** "Resveratrol treatment was beneficial in preventing the development of concentric hypertrophy and **cardiac dysfunction** in spontaneously hypertensive rats. The cardio protective effect of resveratrol may be partially mediated by a reduction in oxidative stress. Thus, resveratrol may have potential in preventing cardiac impairment in patients with essential **hypertension.**"

*Physiological concentrations of dietary polyphenols regulate vascular endothelial cell expression of genes important in **cardiovascular** health.* Nicholson SK, Tucker GA, Brameld JM. Br J Nutr. 2009 Dec 21:1-6. **Key Finding:** "Previous cell culture-based studies have shown potential health beneficial effects on gene expression of dietary polyphenols. The present study investigated effects of physiological concentrations of different classes of dietary polyphenol on the expression of genes important in cardiovascular health. Only three of the eleven polyphenols tested −resveratrol, quercetin and epigallocatechin gallate—had biological activity with observed effects on gene expression that would be expected to result in vasodilation and reduced **blood pressure.**"

*Resveratrol prevents monocrotaline-induced pulmonary **hypertension** in rats.* Csiszar A, Labinskyy N, Olson S, Pinto JT, Gupte S, Wu JM, Hu F, Ballabh P, Podlutsky A, Losonczy G, de Cabo R, Mathew R, Wolin MS, Ungvari Z. Hypertension. 2009 Sep;54(3):668-75. **Key Finding:** "Our studies show that resveratrol exerts anti-inflammatory, antioxidant, and antiproliferative effects in the pulmonary arteries, which may contribute to the prevention of pulmonary hypertension."

Neurodegenerative diseases (in general)

*Heme oxygenase1: another possible target to explain the **neuroprotective** action of resveratrol, a multifaceted nutrient-based molecule.* Bastianetto S, Quirion R. Exp Neurol. 2010 Oct;225(2):237-9. **Key Finding**: "Numerous animal and in vitro studies have shown that this polyphenol is neuroprotective and can reverse various types of cognitive deficits."

Neuroprotective properties of resveratrol in different neurodegenerative disorders. Albani D, Polito L, Signorini A, Forioni G. Biofactors. 2010 Sep;36(5):370-6.**Key Finding**: "Resveratrol has neuroprotective features both in vitro and in vivo in models of **Alzheimer's disease**, but it has proved to be beneficial also in **ischemic stroke, Parkinson's disease, Huntington's disease, and epilepsy**. Here we summarize the invitro and in vivo experimental results highlighting the possible role of resveratrol as neuroprotective bio factor with a particular focus on Alzheimer's disease."

Resveratrol as a therapeutic agent for neurodegenerative diseases. Sun AY, Wang Q, Simonyi A, Sun GY. Mol Neurobiol. 2010 Jun;41(2-3):375-83. **Key Finding**: "Excess production of reactive oxygen species in the brain has been implicated as a common underlying risk factor for the pathogenesis of a number of neurodegenerative disorders, including **Alzheimer's disease, Parkinson's disease, and stroke**. In this review we place emphasis on recent studies implicating the neuroprotective effects of resveratrol. These studies show that the beneficial effects of resveratrol are not only limited to its antioxidant and anti-inflammatory action but also include activation of sirtuin 1 and vitagenes, which can prevent the deleterious effects triggered by oxidative stress."

Neuroprotective *effects of resveratrol on ischemic injury mediated by modulating the release of neurotransmitter and neuromodulator in rats.* Li C, Yan Z, Yang J, Chen H, Li H, Jiang Y, Zhang Z. Neurochem Int. 2009 Dec 21 (Epub ahead of print). **Key Finding:** "This study provides the first in vivo evidence that resveratrol could exert neuroprotective effect against **ischemia injury** by modulating the release of multiple neurotransmitters and neuromodulators during ischemia/reperfusion."

*Protective effect of resveratrol in severe **acute pancreatitis**-induced **brain injury**.* Jha RK, Ma Q, Sha H, Palikhe M. Pancreas. 2009 Nov;38(8):947-53. **Key Finding:** "The protective effect of resveratrol might be associated with the up-regulation of Bcl-2 and down-regulation of Bax and caspase-3."

Resveratrol: cellular actions of a potent natural chemical that confers a diversity of health benefits. Marques FZ, Markus MA, Morris BJ. Int J Biochem Cell Biol. 2009 Nov;41(11):2125-8. **Key Finding:** "Resveratrol has health benefits in common age-related diseases such as **cancer, type 2 diabetes, cardiovascular disease, and neurological conditions.** Resveratrol has positive effects on metabolism and can increase the lifespan of various organisms. Its effects arise from its capacity to interact with multiple molecular targets involved in diverse intracellular pathways."

Protective effects of resveratrol and quercetin against MPP+ -induced oxidative stress act by modulating markers of apoptotic death in dopaminergic neurons. Bournival J, Quessy P, Martinoli MG. Cell Mol Neurobiol. 2009 Dec;29(8):1169-80. **Key Finding:** "These findings support the role of these natural polyphenols in preventive and/or complementary therapies for several human **neurodegenerative diseases** caused by oxidative stress and apoptosis."

Obesity

Resveratrol, ***obesity and diabetes****.* Szkudelska K, Szkudelski T. Eur J Pharmacol. 2010 Jun 10;635(1-3):1-8. **Key Finding**: "The broad spectrum of effects of resveratrol has been enlarged by new data demonstrating a great potency of this compound in relation to obesity and diabetes. Data point to the potential possibility of use of resveratrol in preventing and/or treating obesity and diabetes."

Osteoarthritis

Chondroprotective effects and mechanisms of resveratrol in advanced glycation end products-stimulated chondrocytes. Liu FC, Hung LF, Wu WL. Arthritis Res Ther. 2010;12(5):R167. **Key Finding**: "Accumulation of advanced glycation end products (AGEs) in joints contributes to the pathogenesis of cartilage damage in osteoarthritis. The present study reveals not only the effects and mechanisms regarding how resveratrol may protect cartilage from AGEs-mediated damage but also the potential therapeutic benefit of resveratrol in the treatment of **osteoarthritis**."

Synergistic chondroprotective effects of curcumin and resveratrol in human articular chondrocytes: inhibition of IL-1beta-induced NF-kappaB-mediated inflammation and apoptosis. Csaki C, Mobasheri A, Shakibaei M. Arthritis Res Ther. 2009 Nov 4;11(6):R165. **Key Finding:** "Currently available treatments for **osteoarthritis** are restricted to non-steroidal anti-inflammatory drugs, which exhibit numerous side effects and are only temporarily effective. Naturally occurring polyphenol compounds, such as curcumin and resveratrol, are potent agents for modulating inflammation. The aim of this study was to investigate the potential synergistic effects of curcumin and resveratrol on IL-1beta-stimulated human chondrocytes in vitro. Treatment with curcumin and resveratrol suppressed NF-kappaB-regulated gene products involved in inflammation. We propose that combining these natural compounds may be a useful strategy in osteoarthritis therapy as compared with separate treatment with each individual compound."

Parkinson's disease

Resveratrol as a therapeutic agent for neurodegenerative diseases. Sun AY, Wang Q, Simonyi A, Sun GY. Mol Neurobiol. 2010 Jun;41(2-3):375-83. **Key Finding**: "Excess production of reactive oxygen species in the brain has been implicated as a common underlying risk factor for the pathogenesis of a number of neurode-generative disorders, including **Alzheimer's disease, Parkinson's disease, and stroke**. In this review we place emphasis on recent studies implicating the neuroprotective effects of resveratrol. These studies show that the beneficial effects of resveratrol are not only limited to its antioxidant and anti-inflammatory action but also include activation of sirtuin 1 and vitagenes, which can prevent the deleterious effects triggered by oxidative stress."

Neuroprotective properties of resveratrol in different neurodegenerative disorders. Albani D, Polito L, Signorini A, Forioni G. Biofactors. 2010 Sep;36(5):370-6.**Key Finding**: "Resveratrol has neuroprotective features both in vitro and in vivo in models of **Alzheimer's disease**, but it has proved to be beneficial also in **ischemic stroke, Parkinson's disease, Huntington's disease, and epilepsy**. Here we summarize the in vitro and in vivo experimental results highlighting the possible role of resveratrol as neuroprotective bio factor with a particular focus on Alzheimer's disease."

Resveratrol protects dopamine neurons against lipopolysaccharide-induced neurotoxicity through its anti-inflammatory actions. Zhang F, Shi JS, Zhou H, Et al. Mol Pharmacol. 2010 Sep;78(3):466-77. **Key Finding**: "**Parkinson's disease** is the second most common neurodegenerative disease characterized by a progressive loss of dopamine neurons in the substantia nigra. Accumulating evidence indicates that inhibition of microglia-mediated neuroinflammation may become a reliable protective strategy for Parkinson's disease. The results of this study clearly demonstrated that resveratrol protected dopamine neurons."

Periodontal disease

*Protective effect of resveratrol on apoptosis of human **periodontal** ligament cells in vitro.* Lu HX, Lin SS, Liu SS, Niu ZY. Zhonghua Kou Qiang Yi Xue Za Zhi (Chinese). 2009 Aug;44(8):469-73. **Key Finding:** "Resveratrol reduced oxidative stress and apoptosis in an experimental human periodontal ligament cell injury model induced by H2O2. Resveratrol plays a key role in the human periodontal ligament cell protection against oxidative injury."

Resveratrol inhibits Porphyromonas gingivalis lipopolysaccharide-induced endothelial adhesion molecule expression by suppressing NF-kappaB activation. Park HJ, Jeong SK, Kim SR, Bae SK, Kim WS, Jin SD, Koo TH, Jang HO, Yun I, Kim KW, Bae MK. Arch Pharm Res. 2009 Apr;32(4):583-91. **Key Finding:** "These findings suggest that resveratrol significantly attenuates the P. gingivalis LPS-induced monocyte adhesion to the endothelium by suppressing the expression of the NF-kappaB-dependent cell adhesion molecules, suggesting its therapeutic role in **periodontal** pathogen-induced vascular inflammation."

Prostate inflammation

Chemo preventive anti-inflammatory activities of curcumin and other phytochemicals mediated by MAP kinase phosphatase-5 in prostate cells. Nonn L, Duong D, Peehl DM. Carcinogenesis. 2007 Jun;28(6):1188-96. **Key Finding:** The mediating anti-inflammatory activities of curcumin, **resveratrol** and gingerol were examined. "Our findings show direct anti-inflammatory activity of MKP5 in prostate cells and suggest that up-regulation of MKP5 by phytochemicals may contribute to their chemo preventive actions by decreasing **prostatic inflammation**."

Respiratory diseases (asthma, chronic obstructive pulmonary disease)

Antioxidant and anti-inflammatory effects of resveratrol on airway disease. Wood LG, Wark PA, Garg ML. Antioxid Redox Signal. 2010 Nov 15;13(10):1535-48. **Key Finding**: "Respiratory diseases such as **asthma and chronic obstructive pulmonary disease** are characterized by airway inflammation, which develops in response to various stimuli. Resveratrol demonstrates both antioxidative and anti-inflammatory functions and may have a protective role in respiratory diseases."

Stroke

Resveratrol as a therapeutic agent for neurodegenerative diseases. Sun AY, Wang Q, Simonyi A, Sun GY. Mol Neurobiol. 2010 Jun;41(2-3):375-83. **Key Finding**: "Excess production of reactive oxygen species in the brain has been implicated as a common underlying risk factor for the pathogenesis of a number of neurodegenerative disorders, including **Alzheimer's disease, Parkinson's disease, and stroke**. In this review we place emphasis on recent studies implicating the neuroprotective effects of resveratrol. These studies show that the beneficial effects of resveratrol are not only limited to its antioxidant and anti-inflammatory action but also include activation of sirtuin 1 and vitagenes, which can prevent the deleterious effects triggered by oxidative stress."

Resveratrol protects against experimental **stroke:** *putative neuroprotective role of heme oxygenase 1.* Sakata Y, Zhuang H, Kwansa H, Et al. Exp Neurol. 2010 Jul'224(1):325-9. **Key Finding**: "This study revealed that resveratrol selectively induces heme oxygenase 1 in a dose- and time-dependent manner in cultured mouse cortical neuronal cells and provides neuroprotection from free-radical or excitotoxicity damage."

Neuroprotective properties of resveratrol in different neurodegenerative disorders. Albani D, Polito L, Signorini A, Forioni G. Biofactors. 2010 Sep;36(5):370-6.**Key Finding**: "Resveratrol has neuroprotective features both in vitro and in vivo in models of **Alzheimer's disease**, but it has proved to be beneficial also in **ischemic stroke, Parkinson's disease, Huntington's disease, and epilepsy**. Here we summarize the in vitro and in vivo experimental results highlighting the possible role of resveratrol as neuroprotective bio factor with a particular focus on Alzheimer's disease."

Ulcer (gastric)

Protective and therapeutic effects of resveratrol on acetic acid-induced **gastric ulcer**. Solmaz A, Sener G, Cetinel S, Yuksel M, Yegen C, Yegen BC. Free Radic Res. 2009 Jun;43(6):594-603. **Key Finding:** "Results demonstrate that resveratrol has both protective and therapeutic effects on oxidative gastric damage by suppressing pro-inflammatory cascades, including the activation of pro-inflammatory cyto-kines, accumulation of neutrophils and release of oxygen-derived free radicals."

Wound healing

The effects of resveratrol on the healing of left colonic anastomosis. Cakmak GK, Irkorucu O, Ucan BH, Tascilar O, Emre AU, Karakaya K, Bahadir B, Acikgoz S, Pasoglu H, Ankarali H, Ugurbas E, Demirtas C, Comert M. J Invest Surg. 2009 Sep-Oct;22(5):353-61. **Key Finding:** "The study results suggest that exogenous resveratrol administration exerts a positive effect on experimental colonic wound healing in the rat. Although the precise cellular mechanisms by which resveratrol enhance anastomotic **wound healing** is not clear, stimulation of neovascular-ization, generation of collagen synthesis, inhibition of over inflammation, and restriction of oxidative injury seems to be of paramount importance."

Sea Vegetables (see also Algae)

"SEA VEGETABLES" IS A GENERAL TERM for various types of multicellular algae, such as brown, red, and green algae, that exist in brackish water or seawater. In Asia, they have been used medicinally and as a food source for thousands of years.

A popular use of sea vegetables is to dry them and form it into sheets, which in Japan is called nori and is most often used to wrap sushi. Sea vegetables are high in iodine, which is essential for human thyroid function, and also contain high concentrations of magnesium and calcium. Much of the medical science research on the benefits of sea vegetables has focused on cancer, particularly breast, lung, and skin cancer.

Cancer (Breast; Leukemia; Lung; Skin)

The mechanism of fucoidan-induced apoptosis in leukemic cells: involvement of ERK1/2, JNK, glutathione, and nitric oxide. Jin JO, Song MG, Kim YN, Et al. Mol Carcinog. 2010 Aug;49(8):771-82. **Key Finding**: "Fucoidan, a sulfated polysaccharide in brown seaweed, has various biological activities including anti-tumor activity. We investigated the effects of fucoidan on the apoptosis of human promyleoid **leukemic cells** and fucoidan-mediated signaling pathways. Our results suggest that activation of MEKK1, MEK1, ERK1/2, and JNK, depletion of gluta-thione, and production of NO are important mediators in fucoidan-induced apoptosis of human leukemic cells."

A case-control study on seaweed consumption and the risk of breast cancer. Yang YJ, Nam SJ, Kong G, Kim MK. Br J Nutr. 2010 May;103(9):1345-53. **Key Finding**: "Gim (Porphyra sp.) and miyeck (Udaria pinnatifida) are seaweeds most consumed by Koreans. We investigated the association between the intake of gim and miyeck and the risk of **breast cancer** in a case-control study of 362 women aged 30-65 years old who were histologically confirmed to have breast cancer. Controls visiting the same hospital were matched to cases according to their age and menopausal status. The daily intake of gim was inversely associated with the risk of breast cancer, whereas miyeck consumption did not have any significant associations. These results suggest that high intake of gim may decrease the risk of breast cancer."

Evaluating the possible genotoxic, mutagenic and tumor cell proliferation-inhibition effects of a non-anticoagulant, but antithrombotic algal heterofucan. Almedia-Lima J, Costa LS, Silva NB, Et al. J Appl Toxicol. 2010 Oct;30(7):708-15. **Key Finding**: "Fucan is a term used to denominate a family of sulfated polysaccharides extracted mainly from brown seaweeds. Our research group purified a non-anticoagulant hetero-fucan (fucan A) which displays antithrombotic activity in vivo. Tumor-cell (HeLa, PC3, PANC, HL60) proliferation was inhibited. Non-tumor cell lines prolifera-tion were not affected by this molecule."

*Seaweed Prevents **Breast Cancer**?* Funahashi H, Imai T, Mase T, Sekiya M, Yokoi K, Hayashi Y, Shibata A, Hayashi T, Nishikawa M, Suda N, Hibi Y, Mizuno Y, Tsukamura K, Hayakawa A, Tamuma S. Jpn J Cancer Res. 2001 May;92:483-487. **Key Finding:** "We found earlier that the seaweed, *wakame*, showed a suppressive effect on the proliferation of DMBA-induced rat mammary tumors, possibly via apoptosis induction. In the present study, powdered *mekabu* was used in solution. It showed an extremely strong suppressive effect on rat mammary carcinogenesis when used in daily drinking water, without toxicity. In vitro, *mekabu* solution strongly induced apoptosis in 3 kinds of human breast cancer cells. These effects were stronger than those of a chemotherapeutic agent widely used to treat human breast cancer. Furthermore, no apoptosis induction was observed in normal human mammary cells."

*Potent suppressive effect of Japanese edible seaweed, Enteromorpha prolifera (Sujiao-nori) on initiation and promotion phases of chemically induced mouse **skin tumorigenesis**.* Hiqashi-Okaj K, Otani S, Okai Y. Cancer Lett. 1999;140(1-2):21-25. **Key Finding:** "These results suggest that E. prolifera has a potent suppressive activity against chemically induced mouse skin tumorigenesis through the suppression at the initiation and promotion phases, and that pheophytin-a might be partially associated with the in vivo anticarcinogenic activity."

*Anticancer Activity of a Natural Product, Viva-Natural, Extracted from Undaria pinnatifida on Intraperitoneally Implanted Lewis **Lung Carcinoma**.* Furusawa E, Furusawa S. Oncology. 1985;42:364-369. **Key Finding:** "A natural product, named Viva-Natural, extracted from dietary seaweed Undaria pinnatifida has been found to be therapeutically active against Lewis lung carcinoma. Viva-Natural also demonstrated moderate prophylactic activity against LLC in allogeneic mice. A combination therapy of Viva-Natural and standard anticancer drugs was addi-tively or synergistically effective."

Antitumor effect of seaweeds. II. Fractionation and partial characterization of the poly-saccharide with antitumor activity from Sargassum fulvellum. Yamamoto I, Nagumo T, Fujihara M, Takahashi M, Ando Y. Jpn J Exp Med. 1977 Jun;47(3):133-40. **Key Finding:** "An almost purified antitumor polysaccharide fraction was obtained by fractional precipitation and ethanol from hot-water extract of Sargassum fulvellum. The fraction showed remarkable tumor-inhibiting effect against sarcoma-180 implanted subcutaneously in mice. The results of chemical and physical analyses suggested that the active substance may be either a sulphated peptidoglycuronoglycan or a sulphated glycuronoglycan."

Detoxification

Seaweed accelerates the excretion of dioxin stored in rats. Morita K, Nakano T. J Agric Food Chem. 2002 Feb 13;50(4):910-7. **Key Finding:** "These findings suggest that the administration of seaweed such as wakame is efficient in preventing the absorption and reabsorption of dioxin from the gastrointestinal tract and might be useful in treatment of humans exposed to dioxin."

Diabetes

Algae consumption and risk of type 2 diabetes: Korean National Health and Nutrition Exami-nation Survey in 2005. Lee HJ, Kim HC, Vitek L, Nam CM. J Nutr Sci Vitaminol (Tokyo). 2010;56(1):13-8. **Key Finding**: "Our results suggest that dietary algae consumption may decrease the risk of diabetes mellitus in Korean men."

Spinach

SPINACH WAS APPARENTLY FIRST CULTIVATED in ancient Persia and then spread along trading routes to India and China. Not until the ninth century was it introduced to southern Europe, and several hundred years later, to England.

It is one of the most nutritious of all vegetables, with high levels of antioxidants and vitamins A, C, E, and K, along with zinc, iron, selenium, folic acid, omega-3 fatty acids, and numerous other nutrients. Studies indicate that spinach consumption can help reduce the risk of at least nine types of cancer.

Aging

Dietary supplementation with blueberries, spinach, or spirulina reduces ischemic brain damage. Wang Y, Chang CF, Chou J, Chen HL, Deng X, Harvey BK, Cadet JL, Bickford PC. Exp Neurol. 2005 May;193(1):75-84. **Key Finding:** "Free radicals are involved in neurodegenerative disorders, such as **ischemia** and **aging**. We have previously demonstrated that treatment with diets enriched with blueberry, spinach, or spirulina have been shown to reduce neurodegenerative changes in aged animals. The purpose of this study was to determine if these diets have neuroprotective effects in focal ischemic brain in Sprague-Dawley rats. Animals treated with blueberry, spinach, or spirulina had significantly lower caspase-3 activity in the ischemic hemisphere. In conclusion, our data suggest that chronic treatment with blueberry, spinach, or spirulina reduces ischemia/reperfusion-induced apoptosis and cerebral infarction."

*Oxidative stress protection and vulnerability in **aging:** putative nutritional implications for intervention.* Joseph JA, Denisova NA, Bielinski D, Fisher DR, Shukitt-Hale B. Mech Ageing Dev. 2000 Jul 31;116(2-3):141-53. **Key Finding:** "Among the most effective agents that antagonized cellular oxidative stress were the combination of polyphenols found in fruits (e.g. blueberry extract) with high antioxidant activity. Subsequent experiments using dietary supplementation with fruit (strawberry) or vegetable (spinach) extracts have shown that such extracts are also effective in forestalling and reversing the deleterious effects of behavioral aging in F344 rats."

*Reversals of age-related declines in neuronal signal transduction, **cognitive,** and **motor behavioral deficits** with blueberry, spinach, or strawberry dietary supplementation.*

Joseph JA, Shukitt-Hale B, Denisvoa NA, Bielinski D, Martin A, McEwen JJ, Bickford PC. J Neurosci. 1999 Sep 15;19(18):8114-21. **Key Finding:** "Our previous study had shown that rats given dietary supplements of fruits and vegetable extracts with high antioxidant activity for 8 months beginning at 6 months of age retarded age-related declines in neuronal and cognitive function. The present study showed that such supplements (strawberry, spinach or blueberry) fed for 8 weeks to 19-month-old Fischer 344 rats were also effective in reversing age-related deficits in several neuronal and behavioral parameters. These findings suggest that, in addition to their known beneficial effects on **cancer** and **heart disease,** phytochemicals present in antioxidant-rich foods may be beneficial in reversing the course of neuronal and behavioral **aging.**"

Membrane and receptor modifications of oxidative stress vulnerability in **aging.** *Nutritional considerations.* Joseph JA, Denisova N, Fisher D, Shukitt-Hale B, Bickford P, Prior R, Cao G. Ann N Y Acad Sci. 1998 Nov 20;854:268-76. **Key Finding:** "Evidence suggests that oxidative stress may contribute to the pathogenesis of age-related decrements in **neuronal function** and that OS vulnerability increases as a function of age. In studies attempts have been made to determine whether increased OS protection via nutritional increases in antioxidant levels in rats (strawberry extracts, dried aqueous extract, spinach, or blueberry extracts) would protect against exposure to 100% O2 (a model of accelerated neuronal aging.) Results indicated that these diets were effective in preventing OS-induced decrements in several parameters, suggesting that although there maybe increases in OS vulnerability in aging, phytochemicals present in antioxidant-rich foods may be beneficial in reducing or retarding the functional central nervous system deficits seen in aging or oxidative insult."

Antioxidation

Antioxidant *and antiproliferative activities of common vegetables.* Chu YF, Sun J, Wu X, Liu RH. J Agric Food Chem. 2002 Nov 6;50(23):6910-6. **Key Finding:** "In this study, 10 common vegetables were selected on the basis of consumption per capita data in the U.S. Broccoli possessed the highest total phenolic content, followed by spinach, yellow onion, red pepper, carrot, cabbage, potato, lettuce, celery, and cucumber. Red pepper had the highest total antioxidant activity, followed by broccoli, carrot, spinach, cabbage, yellow onion, celery, potato, lettuce and cucumber. Antiproliferative activities were also studied in vitro using human **liver cancer** cells. Spinach showed the highest inhibitory effect, followed by cabbage, red pepper, onion, and broccoli."

Serum antioxidant *capacity is increased by consumption of strawberries, spinach, red wine or vitamin C in elderly women.* Cao G, Russell RM, Lischner N, Prior RL. J Nutr. 1998 Dec;128(12):2383-90. **Key Finding:** "In this study we investigated the responses in serum total antioxidant capacity following consumption of strawberries (240 g), spinach (294 g), red wine (300 ml) or vitamin C (1250 mg) in eight elderly women. The results showed that the total antioxidant capacity of serum determined as ORAC, TEAC and FRAP, using the area under the curve, increased significantly by 7-25% during the 4-h period following consumption. The total antioxidant capacity of urine determined by ORAC increased (P<0.05) by 9.6, 27.5 and 44.9% for strawberries, spinach, and vitamin C respectively during the 24-h period following these treatments."

Atherosclerosis

Phytoestrogens and human health effects: weighing up the current evidence. Humfrey CD. Nat Toxins. 1998;6(2):51-9. **Key Finding:** "Phytoestrogens are present in beans, sprouts, cabbage, spinach, soybean, grains and hops. Epidemiological studies suggest that foodstuffs containing phytoestrogens may have a beneficial role in protecting against a number of chronic diseases and conditions. For **cancer of the prostate, colon, rectum, stomach and lung**, the evidence is most consistent for a protective effect. Soya and linseed may have beneficial effects on the risk of **breast cancer** and may help to alleviate **postmenopausal symptoms**. Soya also appears to have beneficial effects on blood lipids which may help to reduce the risk of **cardiovascular disease and atherosclerosis.**"

Cancer (breast; cervical; colon; gallbladder; gastric; liver; prostate; rectum; stomach)

*Phytochemicals that counteract the cardio toxic side effects of **cancer chemotherapy**.* Piasek A, Bartoszek A, Namiesnik J. Postepy Hig Med Dosw (Polish). 2009 Apr 17;63:142-58. **Key Finding**: "Dietary intervention with antioxidants (such as in tomato, garlic, spinach) may be a safe and effective way of alleviating the toxicity of anticancer chemotherapy and preventing **heart failure.**"

*Identifying efficacious approaches to chemoprevention with chlorophyllin purified chlorophylls and freeze-dried spinach in a mouse model of transplacental **carcinogenesis**.* Castro DJ, Lohr CV, Fischer KA, Waters KM, Webb-Robertson BJ, Dashwood RH, Bailey GS, Williams DE. Carcinogenesis. 2009 Feb;30(2):315-20. **Key Finding**: "Coadministration of chlorophyllin provided significant protection against DBP-initiated carcinogenesis. Coadministration of CHL also reduced lung tumor multiplicity in mice by approximately 50%."

Anti-tumor effect of orally administered spinach glycolipid fraction on implanted cancer cells, colon-26, in mice. Maeda N, Kokai Y, Ohtani S, Sahara H, Et al. Lipids. 2008 Aug;43(8):741-8. **Key Finding**: "These results suggest that the orally administered glycolipid fraction from spinach could suppress **colon tumor** growth in mice by inhibiting the activities of neovascularization and cancer cellular proliferation in tumor tissue."

Inhibitory effect on replicative DNA polymerases, human cancer cell proliferation, and in vivo **anti-tumor** *activity by glycolipids from spinach.* Maeda N, Hada T, Yoshida H, Mizushina Y. Curr Med Chem. 2007;14(9):955-67. **Key Finding**: "The spinach Fraction-II containing SQDG might be a potent anti-tumor compound and may be a healthy food substance with anti-tumor activity."

Prospective study of fruit and vegetable intake and risk of **prostate cancer**. Kirsh VA, Peters U, Mayne ST, Subar AF, Et al. J Natl Cancer Inst. 2007 Aug 1;99(15):1200-9. **Key Finding**: "High intake of broccoli, cauliflower, may be associated with reduced risk of aggressive prostate cancer. We found some evidence that risk of aggressive prostate cancer decreased with increasing spinach consumption."

Differential attenuation of oxidative/nitrosative injuries in early prostatic neoplastic lesions in TRAMP mice by dietary antioxidants. Tam NN, Nyska A, Maronpot RR, Kissling G, Lomnitski L, Et al. Prostate. 2006 Jan 1;66(1):57-69. **Key Finding**: "Our data indicate that in TRAMP mice, OS/NS injuries are likely involved in early **prostatic tumorigenesis** and can be modulated by various antioxidants such as from spinach extracts."

Correlates between vegetable consumption and **gallbladder cancer**. Rai A, Mohapatra SC, Shukla HS. Eur J Cancer Prev. 2006 Apr;15(2):134-7. **Key Finding**: "A significant inverse trend was observed for green leafy vegetables and gallbladder cancer. An inverse association was observed for spinach, cabbage and fenugreek leaves."

Green vegetables, red meat and **colon cancer**: *chlorophyll prevents the cytotoxic and hyper proliferative effects of haem in rat colon.* De Vogel J, Jonker-Termont DS, Van Lieshout EM, Katan MB, Van der Meer R. Carcinogenesis. 2005 Feb;26(2):387-93. **Key Finding**: "We studied whether green vegetables inhibit the unfavorable colonic effects of haem from red meat. Spinach or an equimolar amount of chlorophyll supplement in the haem diet in rats inhibited the haem effect completely. Haem clearly inhibited exfoliation of colonocytes, an effect counteracted by spinach and chlorophyll."

Inhibitory effect of glycolipids from spinach on in vitro and ex vivo angiogenesis. Matsubara K, Matsumoto H, Mizushina Y, Mori M, Naksjima N, Et al. Oncol Rep. 2005 Jul;14(1):157-60. **Key Finding**: "These results demonstrate that glycolipids from spinach would suppress **tumor** growth by suppressing angiogenesis and might be candidates for anti-**cancer** or anti-angiogenic materials."

Effects of DNA polymerase inhibitory and antitumor activities of lipase-hydrolyzed glycolipid fractions from spinach. Maeda N, Hada T, Murakami-Nakai C, Kuriyama I, Ichikawa H, Fukumori Y, Et al. J Nutr Biochem. 2005 Feb;16(2):121-8. **Key Finding**: "Spinach glycolipid fraction might be a potent antitumor compound. This glycolipid fraction was an inhibitor of DNA polymerases and a growth inhibitor of NUGC-3 human **gastric cancer** cells."

Inhibitory effects of glycolipids fraction from spinach on mammalian DNA polymerase activity and human cancer cell proliferation. Kuriyama I, Musumi K, Yonezawa Y, Takemura M, Maeda N, Et al. J Nutr Biochem. 2005 Oct;16(10):594-601. **Key Finding**: "Of the six subspecies of spinach tested, "Anna" had the largest amount of SQDG, strongest inhibitory activity toward DNA polymerase and greatest effect on human **cancer** cell proliferation. Based on these results, the glycolipids fraction from spinach is potentially a source of food material for a novel anticancer activity."

*Retinoic acid and retinoid receptors: potential chemo preventive and therapeutic role in **cervical cancer***. Abu J, Batuwangala M, Herbert K, Symonds P. Lancet Oncol. 2005 Sep;6(9):712-20. **Key Finding**: "Retinoids are derivatives of vitamin A which can be obtained from spinach, carrots, sweet potatoes, mangos and others. Retinoids regulate various important cellular functions in the body through specific nuclear retinoic-acid receptors and retinoid-X receptors, which are encoded by separate genes. Several experimental and epidemiological studies have shown the antiproliferative activity of retinoids and their potential use in **cancer** treatment and chemoprevention. Emerging clinical trials have shown the chemotherapeutic and chemo preventive potential of retinoids in cancerous and precancerous conditions of the **uterine cervix**."

*Unique natural antioxidants (NAOs) and derived purified components inhibit cell cycle progression by down regulation of ppRb and E2F in human PC3 **prostate cancer** cells.* Bakshi S, Bergman M, Dovrat S, Grossman S. FEBS Lett. 2004 Aug 27;573(1-3):31-7. **Key Finding**: "In the present study, we explored the signaling mechanism through which unique natural antioxidant derived from spinach extract exerts their beneficial effects in the chemoprevention of prostate cancer using human PC3 cells."

Potential anticancer effect of red spinach (Amaranthus gangeticus) extract. Sani HA, Rahmat A, Ismail M, Rosli R, Endrini S. Asia Pac J Clin Nutr. 2004;13(4):396-400. **Key Finding**: "A. gangeticus inhibited the proliferation of **liver cancer** cell line HepG2 and **breast cancer** cell line MCF-7 and **colon cancer** cell line Caco-2."

*Slowing tumorigenic progression in TRAMP mice and **prostatic carcinoma** cell lines using natural antioxidant from spinach, NAO-a comparative study of three antioxidants.* Nyska A, Suttie A, Bakshi S, Et al. Toxicol Pathol. 2003 Jan-Feb;31(1):39-51. **Key Finding**: "The anti-oxidative and antiproliferative properties of NAO from spinach leaves may explain its efficacy in slowing the spontaneous prostatic carcinogenic progress in the TRAMP model and its effects in the cell lines."

***Antioxidant** and antiproliferative activities of common vegetables.* Chu YF, Sun J, Wu X, Liu RH. J Agric Food Chem. 2002 Nov 6;50(23):6910-6. **Key Finding:** "In this study, 10 common vegetables were selected on the basis of consumption per capita data in the U.S. Broccoli possessed the highest total phenolic content, followed by spinach, yellow onion, red pepper, carrot, cabbage, potato, lettuce, celery, and cucumber. Red pepper had the highest total antioxidant activity, followed by broccoli, carrot, spinach, cabbage, yellow onion, celery, potato, lettuce and cucumber. Antiproliferative activities were also studied in vitro using human **liver cancer** cells. Spinach showed the highest inhibitory effect, followed by cabbage, red pepper, onion, and broccoli."

*Carotenoids affect proliferation of human **prostate cancer** cells.* Kotake-Nara E, Kushiro M, Zhang H, Sugawara T, Miyashita K, Nagao A. Nutrition. 2001 Dec;131(12):3303-6. **Key Finding**: "When the prostate cancer cells were cultured in a carotenoid-supplemented medium for 72 h at 20 micromol/L,5,6-monoepoxy carotenoids, namely, neoxanthin from spinach and fucoxanthin from brown algae, significantly reduced cell viability."

*Carotenoids and **colon cancer**.* Slattery ML, Benson J, Curtin K, Ma KN, Schaeffer D, Potter JD. Am J Clin Nutr. 2000 Feb;71(2):575-82. **Key Finding:** "Lutein was inversely associated with colon cancer in both men and women studied. The major dietary sources of lutein in subjects with colon cancer and in control subjects were spinach, broccoli, lettuce, tomatoes, oranges and orange juice, carrots, celery, and greens. These data suggest that incorporating these foods into the diet may help reduce the risk of developing colon cancer."

*Effects of spinach powder fat-soluble extract on proliferation of human **gastric adenocarcinoma** cells.* He T, Huang CY, Chen H, Hou YH. Biomed Environ Scit. 1999

Dec;12(4):247-52. Key Finding: "The results indicated that extract of spinach powder inhibited the proliferation and colony forming ability of SGC-7901 cells. And in MTT assay, it inhibited the viability of SGC-7901 cells, but no inhibitory effect was observed on the viability of lymphocytes in peripheral blood of healthy people."

Phytoestrogens and human health effects: weighing up the current evidence. Humfrey CD. Nat Toxins. 1998;6(2):51-9. **Key Finding:** "Phytoestrogens are present in beans, sprouts, cabbage, spinach, soybean, grains and hops. Epidemiological studies suggest that foodstuffs containing phytoestrogens may have a beneficial role in protecting against a number of chronic diseases and conditions. For **cancer of the prostate, colon, rectum, stomach and lung**, the evidence is most consistent for a protective effect. Soya and linseed may have beneficial effects on the risk of **breast cancer** and may help to alleviate **postmenopausal symptoms**. Soya also appears to have beneficial effects on blood lipids which may help to reduce the risk of **cardiovascular disease and atherosclerosis.**"

Cardiovascular disease

Phytoestrogens and human health effects: weighing up the current evidence. Humfrey CD. Nat Toxins. 1998;6(2):51-9. **Key Finding:** "Phytoestrogens are present in beans, sprouts, cabbage, spinach, soybean, grains and hops. Epidemiological studies suggest that foodstuffs containing phytoestrogens may have a beneficial role in protecting against a number of chronic diseases and conditions. For **cancer of the prostate, colon, rectum, stomach and lung**, the evidence is most consistent for a protective effect. Soya and linseed may have beneficial effects on the risk of **breast cancer** and may help to alleviate **postmenopausal symptoms**. Soya also appears to have beneficial effects on blood lipids which may help to reduce the risk of **cardiovascular disease and atherosclerosis.**"

Cognition

Effect of fruits, vegetables, or vitamin E-rich diet on vitamins E and C distribution in peripheral and brain tissues: implications for brain function. Martin A, Prior R, Shukitt-Hale B, Cao G, Joseph JA. J Gerontol A Biol Sci Med Sci. 2000 Mar;55(3):B144-51. **Key Finding**: "Compared to the control group, rats supplemented with strawberry, spinach or vitamin E showed a significant enhancement in striatal dopamine release. These findings suggest that other nutrients present in fruits and vegetables, in addition to the well-known antioxidants, may be important for **brain function**."

Reversals of age-related declines in neuronal signal transduction, **cognitive,** *and* **motor behavioral deficits** *with blueberry, spinach, or strawberry dietary supplementation.* Joseph JA, Shukitt-Hale B, Denisvoa NA, Bielinski D, Martin A, McEwen JJ, Bickford PC. J Neurosci. 1999 Sep 15;19(18):8114-21. **Key Finding:** "Our previous study had shown that rats given dietary supplements of fruits and vegetable extracts with high antioxidant activity for 8 months beginning at 6 months of age retarded age-related declines in neuronal and cognitive function. The present study showed that such supplements (strawberry, spinach or blueberry) fed for 8 weeks to 19-month-old Fischer 344 rats were also effective in reversing age-related deficits in several neuronal and behavioral parameters. These findings suggest that, in addition to their known beneficial effects on **cancer** and **heart disease,** phytochemicals present in antioxidant-rich foods may be beneficial in reversing the course of neuronal and behavioral **aging.**"

Long-term dietary strawberry, spinach, or vitamin E supplementation retards the onset of age-related neuronal signal-transduction and cognitive behavioral deficits. Joseph JA, Shukitt-Hale B, Denisova NA, Prior RL, Cao G, Martin A, Taglialatela G, Bickford PC. J Neurosci. 1998 Oct 1;18(19):8047-55. **Key Finding:** "Phytochemicals present in antioxidant-rich foods such as spinach may be beneficial in retarding functional age-related CNS and **cognitive behavioral deficits** and, perhaps, may have some benefit in **neurodegenerative disease.**"

Membrane and receptor modifications of oxidative stress vulnerability in **aging.** *Nutritional considerations.* Joseph JA, Denisova N, Fisher D, Shukitt-Hale B, Bickford P, Prior R, Cao G. Ann N Y Acad Sci. 1998 Nov 20;854:268-76. **Key Finding:** "Evidence suggests that oxidative stress may contribute to the pathogenesis of age-related decrements in **neuronal function** and that OS vulnerability increases as a function of age. In studies attempts have been made to determine whether increased OS protection via nutritional increases in antioxidant levels in rats (strawberry extracts, dried aqueous extract, spinach, or blueberry extracts) would protect against exposure to 100% O2 (a model of accelerated neuronal aging.) Results indicated that these diets were effective in preventing OS-induced decrements in several parameters, suggesting that although there maybe increases in OS vulnerability in aging, phytochemicals present in antioxidant-rich foods may be beneficial in reducing or retarding the functional central nervous system deficits seen in aging or oxidative insult."

Diabetes

*Dietary sources of aldose reductase inhibitors: prospects for alleviating **diabetic** complications.* Sarawat M, Muthenna P, Suryanarayana P, Petrash JM, Reddy GB. Asia Pac J Clin Nutr. 2008;17(4):558-65. **Key Finding**: "Among 22 dietary sources tested for aldose reductase inhibitory potential to treat secondary complications of diabetes, 10 showed considerable inhibitory potential. These include spinach, black pepper, cumin, and lemon."

Menopausal symptoms (post)

Phytoestrogens and human health effects: weighing up the current evidence. Humfrey CD. Nat Toxins. 1998;6(2):51-9. **Key Finding:** "Phytoestrogens are present in beans, sprouts, cabbage, spinach, soybean, grains and hops. Epidemiological studies suggest that foodstuffs containing phytoestrogens may have a beneficial role in protecting against a number of chronic diseases and conditions. For **cancer of the prostate, colon, rectum, stomach and lung**, the evidence is most consistent for a protective effect. Soya and linseed may have beneficial effects on the risk of **breast cancer** and may help to alleviate **postmenopausal symptoms**. Soya also appears to have beneficial effects on blood lipids which may help to reduce the risk of **cardiovascular disease and atherosclerosis.**"

Strawberries

CULTIVATED STRAWBERRIES, OFTEN CALLED GARDEN STRAWBERRIES, are relatively new in the diet of humans, having been bred for the first time in eighteenth-century France using two wild varieties found in North and South America. The strawberry quickly became associated with love and lovers in poetry and verse because of its shape and lush flavor and texture.

Research has shown that garden strawberries contain a variety of flavo-noids that benefit human health. They have been proven beneficial for fifteen health conditions, ranging from cancer (six types) to gout and obesity. Some of the more recent research has focused on the role of phytochemicals in strawberry to help retard the aging process and protect cognitive function.

Aging

*Grape juice, berries, and walnuts affect **brain aging** and behavior.* Joseph JA, Shukitt-Hale B, Willis LM. J Nutr. 2009 Sep;139(9):1813S-7S. **Key Finding:** "Research from our laboratory has suggested that dietary supplementation with fruit or vegetable extracts high in antioxidants (e.g. blueberries, strawberries, walnuts and Concord grape juice) can decrease the enhanced vulnerability to oxidative stress that occurs in aging and these reductions are expressed as improvements in behavior. Collaborative findings indicate that blueberry or Concord grape juice supplementation in humans with mild **cognitive impairment** increased verbal memory performance, thus translating our animal findings to humans."

*Beneficial effects of fruit extracts on neuronal function and behavior in a rodent model of accelerated **aging**.* Shukitt-Hale B, Carey AN, Jenkins D, Rabin BM, Joseph JA. Neurobiol Aging. 2007 Aug;28(8):1187-94. **Key Finding:** "Previous research has shown that diets supplemented with 2% blueberry or strawberry extracts have the ability to retard and even reverse age-related deficits in behavior and signal transduction in rats. This study evaluated the efficacy of these diets on irradiation-induced deficits in these parameters by maintaining rats on these diets or a control diet from 8 weeks prior to being exposed to whole-body irradiation. The strawberry diet offered better protection against spatial deficits in the maze because strawberry-fed animals were better able to retain place information compared to controls. The blueberry diet, on the other hand, seemed to improve reversal learning, a behavior more dependent on intact striatal function."

Potential impact of strawberries on human health: a review of the science. Hannum SM. Crit Rev Food Sci Nutr. 2004;44(1):1-17. **Key Finding:** "Individual compounds in strawberries have demonstrated anti**cancer** activity in several different experimental systems, blocking initiation of carcinogenesis, and suppressing progression and proliferation of tumors. Preliminary animal studies have indicated that diets rich in strawberries may also have the potential to provide benefits to the **aging brain**."

Oxidative stress protection and vulnerability in **aging***: putative nutritional implications for intervention.* Joseph JA, Denisova NA, Bielinski D, Fisher DR, Shukitt-Hale B. Mech Ageing Dev. 2000 Jul 31;116(2-3):141-53. **Key Finding:** "Among the most effective agents that antagonized cellular oxidative stress were the combination of polyphenols found in fruits (e.g. blueberry extract) with high antioxidant activity. Subsequent experiments using dietary supplementation with fruit (strawberry) or vegetable (spinach) extracts have shown that such extracts are also effective in forestalling and reversing the deleterious effects of behavioral aging in F344 rats. Thus, it appears that the beneficial effects of the polyphenols found in fruits and vegetables in **neuronal aging** and behavior may be similar to those seen with respect to carcinogenesis and cardiovascular disease."

Reversals of age-related declines in neuronal signal transduction, **cognitive,** *and* **motor behavioral deficits** *with blueberry, spinach, or strawberry dietary supplementation.* Joseph JA, Shukitt-Hale B, Denisvoa NA, Bielinski D, Martin A, McEwen JJ, Bickford PC. J Neurosci. 1999 Sep 15;19(18):8114-21. **Key Finding:** "Our previous study had shown that rats given dietary supplements of fruits and vegetable extracts with high antioxidant activity for 8 months beginning at 6 months of age retarded age-related declines in neuronal and cognitive function. The present study showed that such supplements (strawberry, spinach or blueberry) fed for 8 weeks to 19-month-old Fischer 344 rats were also effective in reversing age-related deficits in several neuronal and behavioral parameters. These findings suggest that, in addition to their known beneficial effects on **cancer** and **heart disease,** phytochemicals present in antioxidant-rich foods may be beneficial in reversing the course of neuronal and behavioral **aging.**"

Dietary antioxidants modulation of **aging** *and immune-endothelial cell interaction.* Meydani M. Mech Ageing Dev. 1999 Nov;111(2-3):123-32. **Key Finding:** "In this brief review, the importance of dietary antioxidant intervention on longevity and age-associated changes in bodily functions and diseases are discussed. Vitamin E supplementation improves cell-mediated immunity in mice and in humans. In addition to modulating the oxidation of low-density lipoproteins, vitamin E can modulate immune/endothelial cells interactions, thus reducing the risk of **cardiovascular disease**. Antioxidants such as vitamin E from food sources or supplements appear to be promising for successful aging by improving immune function."

Membrane and receptor modifications of oxidative stress vulnerability in **aging**. *Nutritional considerations.* Joseph JA, Denisova N, Fisher D, Shukitt-Hale B, Bickford P, Prior R, Cao G. Ann N Y Acad Sci. 1998 Nov 20;854:268-76. **Key Finding:** "Evidence suggests that oxidative stress may contribute to the pathogenesis of age-related decrements in **neuronal function** and that OS vulnerability increases as a function of age. Results indicated that rat diets supplemented with vitamin E, strawberry extracts, or blueberry extracts were effective in preventing OS-induced decrements in several parameters (e.g., nerve growth factor decreases) suggesting that although there may be increases in OS vulnerability in aging, phytochemicals present in antioxidant-rich foods may be beneficial in reducing or retarding the functional central nervous system deficits seen in aging or oxidative insult."

Antioxidation

Strawberry *consumption is associated with increased* **antioxidant** *capacity in serum.* Henning SM, Seeram NP, Zhang Y, Et al. J Med Food. 2010 Feb;13(1):116-22. **Key Finding**: "Daily consumption of strawberries resulted in a modest but significant increase in antioxidant capacity in a healthy population."

Prevention of **oxidative DNA damage** *by bioactive berry components.* Aiyer HS, Kichambare S, Gupta RC. Nutr Cancer. 2008;60 Suppl 1:36-42. **Key Finding:** "The hormone 17ss-estradiol (E(2)) causes oxidative DNA damage via redox cycling of its metabolites. In this study, ACI rats were fed either AIN-93M diet or diets supplemented with 0.5% each of mixed berries (strawberry, blueberry, blackberry, and red and black raspberry), blueberry along or ellagic acid. Ellagic acid (EA) diet significantly reduced E(2)-induced levels of 8-oxodG. Blueberry alone also significantly reduced the levels. Mixed berries were ineffective. In addition, aqueous extracts of berries (2%) and EA (100 microM) were tested for their efficacy in diminishing oxidative DNA adducts induced by redox cycling of 4E(2) catalyzed by copper chloride in vitro. EA was the most efficacious (90%) followed by extracts of red raspberry (70%), blueberry and strawberry (50% each; P<0.001)."

Prevention of **oxidative DNA damage** *by bioactive berry components.* Aiyer HS, Kichambare S, Gupta RC. Nutr Cancer. 2008;60 Suppl 1:36-42. **Key Finding:** "In this study, ACI rats (8 wk. old) were fed either AIN-93M diet or diets supplemented with 0.5% each of mixed berries (strawberry, blueberry, blackberry, and red and black raspberry), blueberry alone, or ellagic acid. Ellagic acid diet significantly reduced E(2)-induced levels of 8-oxodG, P-1, P-2, and PL-1 by 79, 63, 44, and 67% respectively. Blueberry diet also significantly reduced the levels of P-1, P-2, and PL-1 subgroups by 77, 43, and 68% respectively. Mixed berries were, however, ineffective. In addition, aqueous extracts of berries and EA were tested for their efficacy in diminishing oxidative DNA adducts induced by redox cycling of 4E(2) catalyzed by copper chloride in vitro. Ellagic acid was the most efficacious (90%) followed by extracts of red raspberry (70%), blueberry, and strawberry (50% each)."

Efficiency of apples, strawberries, and tomatoes for reduction of **oxidative stress** *in pigs as a model for humans.* Pajk T, Rezar V, Levart A, Salobir J. Nutrition. 2006 Apr;22(4):376-84. **Key Finding:** "Our findings support the hypothesis that supplementation with apples, strawberries, or tomatoes effectively decreases oxidative stress by decreasing MDA formation in the body and by protecting mononuclear blood cells against increased DNA damage. This effect was particularly pronounced in the group supplemented with a fruit mixture; among the single fruit supplements, the most beneficial effect was obtained with apples."

Strawberry and its anthocyanin reduce **oxidative stress**-*induced apoptosis in PC12 cells.* Heo HJ, Lee CY. J Agric Food Chem. 2005 Mar 23;53(6):1984-9. **Key Finding:** "Strawberry showed the highest cell protective effects among the fresh fruit samples. The overall relative **neuronal cell protective** activity of three fruits (strawberry, banana and orange) by three tests followed the decreasing order strawberry>banana>orange. The protective effects appeared to be due to the higher phenolic contents including anthocyanin, and anthocyanin in strawberries seemed to be the major contributors."

Antioxidant *and antiproliferative activities of common fruits.* Sun J, Chu YF, Wu X, Liu RH. J Agric Food Chem. 2002 Dec 4;50(25):7449-54. **Key Finding:** "Phytochemicals, especially phenolic, in fruits and vegetables are suggested to be the major bioactive compound for the health benefits associated with reduced risk of chronic diseases such as **cardiovascular disease** and **cancer**. Cranberry had the highest total phenolic content, followed by apple, red grape, strawberry, pineapple, banana, peach, lemon, orange, pear, and grapefruit. Cranberry had the highest total antioxidant activity followed by apple, red grape, strawberry, peach, lemon, pear, banana, orange, grapefruit and pineapple. Antiproliferation activities were also studied in vitro using HepG(2) human liver-cancer cells, and cranberry showed the highest inhibitory effect followed by lemon, apple, straw-berry, red grape, banana, grapefruit and peach."

Antioxidant activity in fruits and leaves of blackberry, raspberry, and strawberry varies with cultivar and developmental stage. Wang SY, Lin HS. J Agric Food Chem. 2000 Feb;48(2):140-6. **Key Finding:** "Of the ripe fruits tested, on the basis of wet weight of fruit, cv. Jewel black raspberry and blackberries may be the richest source for antioxidants. On the basis of the dry weight of fruit, strawberries had the highest ORAC activity followed by black raspberries (cv. Jewel), blackberries, and red raspberries."

Scavenging capacity of berry crops on superoxide radicals, hydrogen peroxide, hydroxyl radicals, and singlet oxygen. Wang SY, Jiao H. J Agric Food Chem. 2000 Nov;48(11):5677-84. **Key Finding:** "The antioxidant activities against superoxide radicals, hydrogen peroxide, hydroxyl radicals and singlet oxygen was evaluated in fruit juice from different cultivars of thorn less blackberries, blueberries, cranberries, raspberries, and strawberries. Among the different cultivars, juice of Hull Thorn less blackberry, Earliglow strawberry, Early Black cranberry, Jewel raspberry, and Elliot blueberry had the highest antioxidant capacity against superoxide radicals, hydrogen peroxide, hydroxyl radicals and singlet oxygen. In general, blackber-ries had the highest antioxidant capacity inhibition. Strawberry was second best. With regard to O(2) scavenging activity, strawberry had the highest value, while blackberry was second. Cranberries had the lowest inhibition activity."

The effects of dietary **antioxidants** *on* **psychomotor performance** *in aged mice.* Shukitt-Hale B, Smith DE, Meydani M, Joseph JA. Exp Gerontol. 1999 Sep;34(6):797-808. **Key Finding:** "Male C57BL/6NIA mice were provided one of six different antioxidant diets: vitamin E, glutathione, vitamin E plus gluta-thione, melatonin, strawberry extract, or control, beginning at 18 months of age. A battery of motor tests —rod walk, wire hang, plank walk, and inclined screen— was administered before and after dietary treatment. Psychomotor performance was lower in 18-month-old mice compared with 4-month old mice; however, no further decline was seen from 18 to 24 months on any measure. Chronic dietary antioxidant treatments were not effective in reversing age-related defi-cits in psychomotor behavior, except for the glutathione diet on inclined screen performance. It seems that motor deficits may be difficult to reverse even with antioxidant treatment."

Serum antioxidant *capacity is increased by consumption of strawberries, spinach, red wine or vitamin C in elderly women.* Cao G, Russell RM, Lischner N, Prior RL. J

Nutr. 1998 Dec;128(12):2383-90. **Key Finding:** "In this study we investigated the responses in serum total antioxidant capacity following consumption of strawberries (240 g), spinach (294 g), red wine (300 ml) or vitamin C (1250 mg) in eight elderly women. The results showed that the total antioxidant capacity of serum determined as ORAC, TEAC and FRAP, using the area under the curve, increased significantly by 7-25% during the 4-h period following consumption. The total antioxidant capacity of urine determined by ORAC increased (P<0.05) by 9.6, 27.5 and 44.9% for strawberries, spinach, and vitamin C respectively during the 24-h period following these treatments."

Cancer (breast; cervical; colon; leukemia; oral; prostate)

*Inhibitory effects of flavonoids isolated from Fragaria ananassa Duch on IgE-mediated degranulation in rat basophilic **leukemia** RBL-2H3.* Itoh T, Ninomiya M, Yasuda M, Koshikawa K, Deyashiki Y, Nozawa Y, Akao Y, Koketsu M. Bioorg Med Chem. 2009 Aug 1;17(15):5374-9. **Key Finding:** "We isolated four kinds of flavonoids from strawberry and examined the effect of these flavonoids on the degranulation in RBL-2H3 cells. The flavonoids were found to suppress the degranulation from Ag-stimulated RBL-2H3 cells to different extents."

*Strawberry polyphenols are equally cytotoxic to tumorigenic and normal human **breast and prostate** cell lines.* Weaver J, Briscoe T, Hou M, Goodman C, Kata S, Ross H, McDougall G, Stewart D, Riches A. Int J Oncol. 2009 Mar;34(3):777-86. **Key Finding:** "The cytotoxic effects of strawberry polyphenols were investigated on normal cells and tumor cells derived from the same patient. The strawberry extract was cytotoxic with doses of approximately 5 microg/ml causing a 50% reduction in cell survival in both the normal and the tumor lines. After fractionation of the strawberry sample, the cytotoxicity was retained in the tannin-rich fraction and this fraction was considerably more toxic to all cells (normal or turmoil cell lines or lymphocytes) than the anthocyanin-rich fraction. From these findings we conclude that there is little evidence to assume that polyphenols from strawberry have a differential cytotoxic effect on tumor cells relative to comparable normal cells from the same tissue derived from the same patient."

*Lupeol, a novel anti-**inflammatory** and anti-**cancer** dietary triterpene.* Saleem M. Cancer Lett. 2009 Nov 28;285(2):109-15. **Key Finding:** "Lupeol, a triterpene (also known as Fagarsterol) found in white cabbage, green pepper, strawberry, olive, mangoes and grapes was reported to possess beneficial effects as a therapeutic and preventive agent for a range of disorders. This mini review provides detailed account of preclinical studies conducted to determine the utility of Lupeol as a therapeutic and chemo preventive agent for the treatment of inflammation and cancer."

Differential effects of black raspberry and strawberry extracts on BaPDE-induced activation of transcription factors and their target genes. Li J, Zhang D, Stoner GD, Huang C. Mol Carcinog. 2008 Apr;47(4):286-94. **Key Finding:** "These results suggest that black raspberry and strawberry components may target different signaling pathways in exerting their **anti-carcinogenic** effects." For example, tumor necrosis factor-alpha (TNF-alpha) induction by BaPDE was blocked by extract fractions of both black raspberries and strawberries, whereas vascular endothelial growth factor (VEGF) expression, which depends on AP-1 activation, was suppressed by black raspberry fractions but not strawberry fractions.

*Berry extracts exert different antiproliferative effects against **cervical** and **colon cancer** cells grown in vitro.* McDougall GJ, Ross HA, Ikeji M, Stewart D. J Agric Food Chem. 2008 May 14;56(9):3016-23. **Key Finding:** "Polyphenol-rich berry extracts were screened for their antiproliferative effectiveness using human cervical cancer (HeLa) cells grown in microtiter plates. Rowan berry, raspberry, lingonberry, cloudberry, arctic bramble, and strawberry extracts were effective, but blueberry, sea buckthorn and pomegranate extracts were considerably less effective. The most effective extracts (strawberry>arctic bramble>cloudberry>lingonberry) gave EC 50 values in the range of 25-40 microg/(mL of phenols). These extracts were also effective against human colon cancer (CaCo-2) cells, which were generally more sensitive at low concentrations but conversely less sensitive at higher concentrations. The strawberry, cloudberry, arctic bramble and the raspberry extracts share common polyphenol constituents, especially the ellagitannins, which have been shown to be effective antiproliferative agents."

*Isolation and identification of strawberry phenolic with antioxidant and human **cancer** cell antiproliferative properties.* Zhang Y, Seeram NP, Lee R, Feng L, Heber D. J Agric Food Chem. 2008 Feb 13;56(3):670-5. **Key Finding:** "The current study reports the isolation and structural characterization of 10 phenolic compounds from strawberry extracts. The 10 were evaluated for antioxidant and human cancer cell antiproliferative activities. Among the pure compounds, the anthocyanin was the most potent antioxidants. Crude extracts inhibited the growth of human **oral, colon**, and **prostate cancer** cells."

*Blackberry, black raspberry, blueberry, cranberry, red raspberry, and strawberry extracts inhibit growth and stimulate apoptosis of human **cancer** cells in vitro.* Seeram NP, Adams LS, Zhang Y, Lee R, Sand D, Scheuller HS, Heber D. J Agric Food Chem. 2006 Dec 13;54(25):9329-39. **Key Finding:** "The berry extracts were evaluated for their ability to inhibit the growth of human **oral, breast, colon and prostate tumor cell** lines at concentrations ranging from 25 to 200 micro g/ml. With increasing concentration of berry extract, increasing inhibition of cell proliferation in all of the cancer cell lines was observed, with different degrees of potency between cell lines. The berry extracts were also evaluated for their ability to stimulate apoptosis of the COX-2 expressing **colon cancer** cell line, HT-29. Black raspberry and strawberry extracts showed the most significant pro-apoptotic effects against this cell line."

*In vitro **antileukemic** activity of extracts from berry plant leaves against sensitive and multidrug resistant HL60 cells.* Skupien K, Oszmianski J, Kostrzewa-Kowak D, Tarasiuk J. Cancer Lett. 2006 May 18;236(2):282-91. **Key Finding:** "It was found that the blueberry extract was the most efficient against sensitive HL60 cell line (about 2-fold more active than strawberry and raspberry extracts) but presented much lower activity towards resistant cells. In contrast, strawberry and raspberry extracts exhibited the high cytotoxic activity against sensitive leukemia HL60 cell line as well as its MDR sublines."

*Protection against **esophageal cancer** in rodents with lyophilized berries: potential mechanisms.* Stoner GD, Chen T, Kresty LA, Aziz RM, Reinemann T, Nines R. Nutr Cancer. 2006;54(1):33-46. **Key Finding:** "Our laboratory has been evaluating the ability of lyophilized (freeze-dried) black raspberries, blackberries and strawberries to inhibit carcinogen-induced cancer in the rodent esophagus. At 25 wks. of the bioassay, all three berry types were found to inhibit the number of esophageal tumors in NMBA-treated animals by 24-56% relative to NMBA controls. Black raspberries and strawberries were also tested in a post initiation scheme and were found to inhibit NMBA-induced esophageal tumorigenesis by 31-64% when administered in the diet following treatment of the animals with NMBA. Berries, therefore, inhibit tumor promotion and progression events as well as tumor initiation."

*Antioxidant levels and inhibition of **cancer cell proliferation** in vitro by extracts from organically and conventionally cultivated strawberries.* Olsson ME, Andersson CS, Oredsson S, Berglund RH, Gustavsson KE. J Agric Food Chem. 2006 Feb 22;54(4):1248-55. **Key Finding:** "The ratio of ascorbate to dehydroascorbate was significantly higher in the organically cultivated strawberries. The strawberry extracts decreased the proliferation of both HT29 **colon cancer** cells and MCF-7 **breast cancer** cells in a dose-dependent way. The inhibitory effect for the highest concentration of the extracts was in the range of 41-63% inhibition compared to controls for the HT29 cells and 26-56% for MCF-7 cells. The extracts from organically grown strawberries had a higher antiproliferative activity for both cell types at the highest concentration than the conventionally grown, and this might indicate a higher content of secondary metabolites with anticarcinogenic properties in the organically grown strawberries."

Extracts From Organically and Conventionally Cultivated Strawberries Inhibit **Cancer** *Cell Proliferation In Vitro.* Olsson ME, Andersson SC, Berglund RH, Gustavsson KE, Oredsson S. ISHS Acta Horticulturae 744: International Symposium on Human Health Effects of Fruits and Vegetables. 2005. **Key Finding:** "The strawberry extracts inhibited cell proliferation in colon cancer cells HT29 and breast cancer cells MCF-7 in a concentration dependent way. Extracts from organically grown strawberries inhibited cell proliferation to a higher extent than conventionally grown at the two highest concentrations. The content of ascorbate was 36% higher and the ratio of ascorbate to dehydroascorbate was eight-fold higher in the organically grown strawberries than in the conventionally grown. Ascorbate is suggested to act synergistically with other substances in the extracts."

Comparative effects of food-derived polyphenols on the viability and apoptosis of a human hepatoma cell line (HepG2). Ramos S, Alia M, Bravo L, Goya L. J Agric Food Chem. 2005 Feb 23;53(4):1271-80. **Key Finding:** "Dietary polyphenols have antioxidant and antiproliferative properties that might explain their beneficial effect on **cancer** prevention. The aim of this study was to investigate the effects of different pure polyphenols (quercetin, chlorogenic acid and (-)-epicatechin) and natural fruit extracts (strawberry and plum) on viability or apoptosis of human hepatoma HepG2 cells. The treatment of cells for 18 h with quercetin and fruit extracts reduced cell viability in a dose-dependent manner; however, chlorogenic acid and (1)-epicatechin had no prominent effects on the cell death rate. Similarly, quercetin and strawberry and plum extract, rather than chlorogenic acid and (1)-epicatechin, induced apoptosis in HepG2 cells. Moreover, quercetin and fruit extracts arrested the G1 phase in the cell cycle progression prior to apoptosis."

The relationship between intake of vegetables and fruits and **colorectal adenoma-carcinoma** *sequence.* Lee SY, Choi KY, Kim MK, Kim KM, Lee JH, Meng KH, Lee WC. Korean J Gastroenterol (from Korean). 2005 Jan;45(1):23-33. **Key Finding:** "These findings suggest that the intake of vegetables and fruits may act differently in developmental steps of colorectal adenoma-carcinoma sequence.

For this study, 539 cases with histopathologically confirmed incidental colorectal adenoma, 162 cases with colorectal cancer and 2,576 controls were collected. In female, the high intake of raw green and yellow vegetables was found to be negatively associated with the risk of adenoma with mild dysplasia. In male, the high intake of banana, pear, apple and watermelon among fruits were negatively associated with the risk of colorectal cancer."

Inhibitory effect on activator protein-1, nuclear factor-kappaB, and cell transformation by extracts of strawberries (Fragaria x ananassa Duch.). Wang SY, Feng R, Lu Y, Bowman L, Ding M. J Agric Food Chem. 2005 May 18;53(10):4187-93. **Key Finding:** "Strawberry extracts inhibited the proliferation of human **lung epithelial cancer** cell line A549 and decreased TPA-induced neoplastic transformation of JB6 P+ mouse epidermal cells."

Potential impact of strawberries on human health: a review of the science. Hannum SM. Crit Rev Food Sci Nutr. 2004;44(1):1-17. **Key Finding:** "Individual compounds in strawberries have demonstrated anti**cancer** activity in several different experimental systems, blocking initiation of carcinogenesis, and suppressing progression and proliferation of tumors. Preliminary animal studies have indicated that diets rich in strawberries may also have the potential to provide benefits to the **aging brain**."

Antimutagenic activity of berry extracts. Hope Smith S, Tate PL, Huang G, Magee JB, Meepagala KM, Wedge DE, Larcom LL. J Med Food. 2004 Winter;7(4):450-5. **Key Finding:** "Identification of phytochemicals useful in dietary prevention and intervention of **cancer** is of paramount importance. Juice from strawberry, blueberry, and raspberry fruit significantly inhibited **mutagenesis** caused by both carcinogens tested (methyl methanesulfonate and benzo{a}pyrene). Ethanol extracts from freeze-dried fruits of strawberry cultivars (Sweet Charlie and Carlsbad) and blueberry cultivars (Tifblue and Premier) were also tested. Of these, the hydrolysable tannin-containing fraction from Sweet Charlie strawberries was most effective at inhibiting mutations."

Antioxidant and antiproliferative activities of strawberries. Meyers KJ, Watkins CB, Pritts MP, Liu RH. Agric Food Chem. 2003 Nov 5;51(23):6887-92. **Key Finding:** "Strawberries contain high levels of antioxidants, which have been correlated with a decreased risk of chronic disease. To more fully characterize the antioxidant profiles and possible associated health benefits of this fruit, the total free and bound phenolic, total flavonoid, and total anthocyanin contents of eight strawberry cultivars (Earliglow, Annapolis, Evangeline, Allstar, Sable, Sparkle, Jewel, and Mesabi) were measured. Free phenolic contents differed by 65% between the highest (Earliglow) and the lowest (Allstar) ranked cultivars. The total flavonoid content of Annapolis was 2-fold higher than that of Allstar, which had the lowest content. The anthocyanin content of the highest ranked cultivar, Evangeline, was more than double that of the lowest ranked cultivar, Allstar. The proliferation of HepG(2) human **liver cancer** cells was significantly inhibited in a dose-dependent manner after exposure to all strawberry cultivar extracts, with Earliglow exhibiting the highest antiproliferative activity and Annapolis exhibiting the lowest."

*Anticarcinogenic Activity of Strawberry, Blueberry, and Raspberry Extracts to **Breast and Cervical Cancer** Cells.* Wedge DE, Meepagala KM, Magee JB, Smith SH, Huang G, Larcom LL. J Med Food. 2001 Spring;4(1):49-51. **Key Finding:** "Freeze-dried fruits of two strawberry cultivators, Sweet Charlie and Carlsbad, and two blueberry cultivars, Tifblue and Premier, were sequentially extracted and tested separately for in vitro anticancer activity on cervical and breast cancer cell lines. Ethanol extracts from all four fruits strongly inhibited CaSki and SiHa cervical cancer cell lines and MCF-7 and T47-D breast cancer cell lines. An unfractionated aqueous extract of raspberry and the ethanol extract of Premier blueberry significantly inhibited mutagenesis by both direct-acting and metabolically active carcinogens."

*Failure of dietary lyophilized strawberries to inhibit 4-(methylnitrosamino)-1-(3-pyridyl)-1-butanone-and benzo{a}pyrene-induced **lung tumorigenesis** in strain A/J mice.* Carlton PS, Kresty LA, Stoner GD. Cancer Lett. 2000 Oct 31;159(2):113-7. **Key Finding:** "At 24 weeks, there were no differences in tumorigenesis between the strawberry group and the control group. Therefore, lyophilized strawberries at 10% in the diet failed to inhibit NNK- and B{a}P-induced mouse lung tumorigenesis."

*Isothiocyanates and freeze-dried strawberries as inhibitors of **esophageal cancer**.* Stoner GD, Kresty LA, Carlton PS, Siglin JC, Morse MA. Toxicol Sci. 1999 Dec;52(2 Suppl):95-100. **Key Finding:** "A group of aryl alkyl isothiocyanates were tested for their abilities to inhibit tumorigenicity and DNA methylation induced by the esophageal-specific carcinogen, N-nitrosomethylbenzylamine (NMBA) in the F344 rat esophagus. Phenylpropyl isothiocyanate (PPITC) was more potent (inhibiting esophageal cancer) than either phenylethyl isothiocyanate (PEITC) or benzyl isothiocyanate (BITC). A freeze-dried strawberry preparation was also evaluated for its ability to inhibit NMBA-esophageal tumorigenesis. It proved to be an effective inhibitor, although not as potent as either PEITC or PPITC. The inhibitory effect of the berries could not be attributed solely to the content of the chemo preventive agent, ellagic acid, in the berries."

Cardiovascular disease

Strawberries decrease **atherosclerotic** markers in subjects with metabolic syndrome. Basu A, Fu DX, Wilkinson M, Et al. Nutr Res. 2010 Jul;30(7):462-9. **Key Finding**: "Short-term freeze-dried strawberry supplementation improved selected atherosclerotic risk factors, including dyslipidemia and circulating adhesion molecules in subjects with metabolic syndrome."

Cardiovascular effects in vitro of aqueous extract of wild strawberry (Fragaria vesca, L.) leaves. Mudnic I, Modun D, Brizic I, Vukovic J, Generalic I, Katalinic V, Bilusic T, Ljubenkov I, Boban M. Phytomedicine. 2009 May;16(5):462-9. **Key Finding:** "The extract did not significantly affect heart rate and contractibility, main parameters of the cardiac action that determine oxygen demands, while coronary flow increased up to 45% over control value with a simultaneous decrease of oxygen extraction by 34%. The results indicate that the aqueous extract of wild strawberry leaves is a direct, endothelium-dependent vasodilator, action of which is mediated by NO and cyclooxygenase products and which potency is similar to that of the hawthorn aqueous extract."

Strawberry extract caused endothelium-dependent relaxation through the activation of PI3 kinase/akt. Edirisinghe I, Burton-Freeman B, Varelis P, Kappagoda T. J Agric Food Chem. 2008 Oct 22;56(20):9383-90. **Key Finding:** "Polyphenol compounds are vasodilators and help to lower the risk of **cardiovascular diseases**. We hypothesized that a freeze-dried strawberry powder that is rich in polyphenol compounds would cause an endothelium-dependent relaxation (EDR) through the activation of phosphatidylinositol-3 (PI3)-kinase/protein kinase B (akt) in rabbit aorta. Our novel findings suggest that the EDR induced by strawberry extract was mediated by activation of the PI3 kinase/akt signaling pathway, resulting in phosphorylation of eNOS."

Strawberry intake, lipids, C-reactive protein, and the risk of **cardiovascular disease** *in women.* Sesso HD, Gaziano JM, Jenkins DJ, Buring JE. J Am Coll Nutr. 2007 Aug;26(4):303-10. **Key Finding:** "Strawberry intake was unassociated with the risk of incident cardiovascular disease, lipids, or C-reactive protein in middle-aged and older women, though higher strawberry intake may slightly reduce the likelihood of having elevated CRP levels. Additional epidemiologic data are needed to clarify any role of strawberries in CVD prevention."

Anti-angiogenic property of edible berries. Roy S, Khanna S, Alessio HM, Vider J, Bagchi D, Bagchi M, Sen CK. Free Radic Res. 2002 Sep;36(9):1023-31. **Key Finding:** "The ORAC values of strawberry powder and grape seed proanthocyanidin extract were higher than cranberry, elderberry or raspberry seed. Wild bilberry and blueberry extracts possessed the highest ORAC values. Each of the berry samples studied significantly inhibited both H2O2 as well as TNF alpha induced vascular endothelial growth factor expression by the human keratinocytes. Matrigel assay using human dermal micro vascular endothelial cells showed that edible berries impair **angiogenesis.**"

***Antioxidant** and antiproliferative activities of common fruits.* Sun J, Chu YF, Wu X, Liu RH. J Agric Food Chem. 2002 Dec 4;50(25):7449-54. **Key Finding:** "Phytochemicals, especially phenolic, in fruits and vegetables are suggested to be the major bioactive compound for the health benefits associated with reduced risk of chronic diseases such as **cardiovascular disease** and **cancer**. Cranberry had the highest total phenolic content, followed by apple, red grape, strawberry, pineapple, banana, peach, lemon, orange, pear, and grapefruit. Cranberry had the highest total antioxidant activity followed by apple, red grape, strawberry, peach, lemon, pear, banana, orange, grapefruit and pineapple. Antiproliferation activities were also studied in vitro using HepG(2) human liver-cancer cells, and cranberry showed the highest inhibitory effect followed by lemon, apple, strawberry, red grape, banana, grapefruit and peach."

Effects of tomato extract on human platelet aggregation in vitro. Dutta-Roy AK, Crosbie L, Gordon MJ. Platelets. 2001 Jun;12(4):218-27. **Key Finding:** "Among all fruits tested in vitro for their anti-platelet property, tomato had the highest activity followed by grapefruit, melon, and strawberry, whereas pear and apple had little or no activity. All these data indicate that tomato contains very potent anti-platelet components, and consuming tomatoes might be beneficial both as a preventive and therapeutic regime for **cardiovascular disease.**"

*Dietary antioxidants modulation of **aging** and immune-endothelial cell interaction.* Meydani M. Mech Ageing Dev. 1999 Nov;111(2-3):123-32. **Key Finding:** "In this brief review, the importance of dietary antioxidant intervention on longevity and age-associated changes in bodily functions and diseases are discussed. Vitamin E supplementation improves cell-mediated immunity in mice and in humans. In addition to modulating the oxidation of low-density lipoproteins, vitamin E can modulate immune/endothelial cells interactions, thus reducing the risk of **cardiovascular disease**. Antioxidants such as vitamin E from food sources or supplements appear to be promising for successful aging by improving immune function."

Cholesterol

*Freeze-dried strawberry powder improves **lipid profile** and lipid peroxidation in women with metabolic syndrome: baseline and post intervention effects.* Basu A, Wilkinson M, Penugonda K, Simmons B, Betts NM, Lyons TJ. Nutr J. 2009 Sep 28;8:43. **Key Finding:** "We tested the hypothesis that freeze-dried strawberry powder will lower fasting lipids and biomarkers of oxidative stress and inflammation at four weeks compared to baseline. Short-term supplementation of freeze-dried strawberries appeared to exert **hypocholesterolemic** effects and decrease lipid peroxidation in women with **metabolic syndrome**."

*The effect of strawberries in a **cholesterol**-lowering dietary portfolio.* Jenkins DJ, Nguyen TH, Kendall CW, Faulkner DA, Bashyam B, Kim IJ, Ireland C, Patel D, Vidgen E, Josse AR, Sesso HD, Burton-Freeman B, Josee RG, Leiter LA, Singer W. Metabolism. 2008 Dec;57(12):1636-44. **Key Finding:** "We conclude that strawberry supplementation reduced oxidative damage to LDL while maintaining reductions in blood lipids and enhancing diet palatability. Added fruit may improve the overall utility of diets designed to lower **coronary heart disease** risk."

Cognition

*Grape juice, berries, and walnuts affect **brain aging** and behavior.* Joseph JA, Shukitt-Hale B, Willism LM. J Nutr. 2009 Sep;139(9):1813S-7S. **Key Finding:** "Research from our laboratory has suggested that dietary supplementation with fruit or vegetable extracts high in antioxidants (e.g. blueberries, strawberries, walnuts and Concord grape juice) can decrease the enhanced vulnerability to oxidative stress that occurs in aging and these reductions are expressed as improvements in behavior. Collaborative findings indicate that blueberry or Concord grape juice supplementation in humans with mild **cognitive impairment** increased verbal memory performance, thus translating our animal findings to humans."

Potential impact of strawberries on human health: a review of the science. Hannum SM. Crit Rev Food Sci Nutr. 2004;44(1):1-17. **Key Finding:** "Individual compounds in strawberries have demonstrated anti**cancer** activity in several different experimental systems, blocking initiation of carcinogenesis, and suppressing progression and proliferation of tumors. Preliminary animal studies have indicated that diets rich in strawberries may also have the potential to provide benefits to the **aging brain**."

Effect of fruits, vegetables, or vitamin E-rich diet on vitamins E and C distribution in peripheral and brain tissues: implications for **brain function**. Martin A, Prior R, Shukitt-Hale B, Cao G, Joseph JA. J Gerontol A Biol Sci Med Sci. 2000 Mar;55(3):B144-51. **Key Finding:** "It is concluded that supplementation or depletion of alpha-tocopherol for 8 months results in marked changes in vitamin E levels in brain tissue and peripheral tissues, and varied distribution of alpha-tocopherol throughout the different brain regions examined. In addition, compared to control group, rats supplemented with strawberry, spinach or vitamin E showed a significant enhancement in striatal ·dopamine release. These findings suggest that other nutrients present in fruits and vegetables, in addition to the well-known antioxidants, may be important for brain function."

Reversals of age-related declines in neuronal signal transduction, **cognitive,** *and* **motor behavioral deficits** *with blueberry, spinach, or strawberry dietary supplementation.* Joseph JA, Shukitt-Hale B, Denisvoa NA, Bielinski D, Martin A, McEwen JJ, Bickford PC. J Neurosci. 1999 Sep 15;19(18):8114-21. **Key Finding:** "Our previous study had shown that rats given dietary supplements of fruits and vegetable extracts with high antioxidant activity for 8 months beginning at 6 months of age retarded age-related declines in neuronal and cognitive function. The present study showed that such supplements (strawberry, spinach or blueberry) fed for 8 weeks to 19-month-old Fischer 344 rats were also effective in reversing age-related deficits in several neuronal and behavioral parameters. These findings suggest that, in addition to their known beneficial effects on **cancer** and **heart disease,** phytochemicals present in antioxidant-rich foods may be beneficial in reversing the course of neuronal and behavioral **aging.**"

Membrane and receptor modifications of oxidative stress vulnerability in **aging**. *Nutritional considerations.* Joseph JA, Denisova N, Fisher D, Shukitt-Hale B, Bickford P, Prior R, Cao G. Ann N Y Acad Sci. 1998 Nov 20;854:268-76. **Key Finding:** "Evidence suggests that oxidative stress may contribute to the pathogenesis of age-related decrements in **neuronal function** and that OS vulnerability increases as a function of age. Results indicated that rat diets supplemented with vitamin E, strawberry extracts, or blueberry extracts were effective in preventing OS-induced decrements in several parameters (e.g., nerve growth factor decreases) suggesting that although there may be increases in OS vulnerability in aging, phytochemicals present in antioxidant-rich foods may be beneficial in reducing or retarding the functional central nervous system deficits seen in aging or oxidative insult."

Coronary artery disease

*The effect of strawberries in a **cholesterol**-lowering dietary portfolio.* Jenkins DJ, Nguyen TH, Kendall CW, Faulkner DA, Bashyam B, Kim IJ, Ireland C, Patel D, Vidgen E, Josse AR, Sesso HD, Burton-Freeman B, Josee RG, Leiter LA, Singer W. Metabolism. 2008 Dec;57(12):1636-44. **Key Finding:** "We conclude that strawberry supplementation reduced oxidative damage to LDL while maintaining reductions in blood lipids and enhancing diet palatability. Added fruit may improve the overall utility of diets designed to lower **coronary heart disease** risk."

Diabetes

*Phenolic-linked variation in strawberry cultivars for potential dietary management of **hyperglycemia** and related complications of **hypertension**.* Cheplick S, Kwon YI, Bhowmik P, Shetty K. Bioresourc Technol. (EPub 2009) 2010 Jan;101(1):404-13. **Key Finding:** "Strawberry cultivars with combined inhibitory potential against alpha-glucosidase and angiotensin-1-converting enzyme activity and with moderate or low alpha-amylase inhibitory potential could be targeted for potential management of hyperglycemia-linked **type 2 diabetes** and related complications of hypertension."

Gout

Impact of strawberries on human health: insight into marginally discussed bioactive compounds for the Mediterranean diet. Tulipani S, Mezzetti B, Battino M. Public Health Nutr. 2009 Sep;12(9A):1656-62. **Key Finding:** "The mechanisms responsible for the potential health-promoting effects of strawberry may not be necessarily searched in the activity of phytochemicals. Particularly, a greater interest should be addressed to show whether a prolonged strawberry consumption may effectively improve the folate status and reduce the incidence of folate-related pathological conditions. Furthermore, the hypouricaemic effects of cherries need to be evaluated also in respect to strawberry intake, and the mechanisms of actions and **anti-gout** potentialities need to be studied in detail."

Hypercholesteremia

*Efficiency of pharmacologically-active antioxidant phytomedicine Radical Fruits in treatment **hypercholesteremia** in men.* Abidov M, Jimenez Del Rio M, Ramazanov A,

Kalyuzhin O, Chkhikvishvili I. Georgian Med News. 2006 Nov;(140):78-83. **Key Finding:** "Radical Fruits is a dietary supplement that contains standardized extracts and concentrates of prune, pomegranate, apple, grape, raspberry, blueberry, white cherry and strawberry. Forty-four non-obese, non-smoking, non-diabetic hypercholesteremic male volunteers took part in a 4 week double-blind, randomized, placebo-controlled clinical trial. Administration of pharmacologically active antioxidant supplement Radical Fruit in hypercholesteremic men significantly increased plasma HDL and reduced total cholesterol and LDL, and urinary oxidative and inflammatory isoprostanes and thromboxane."

*Determination of malondialdehyde (MDA) by high-performance liquid chromatography in serum and liver as a biomarker for oxidative stress. Application to a rat model for **hypercholesterolemia** and evaluation of the effect of diets rich in phenolic antioxidants from fruits.* Mateos R, Lecumberri E, Ramos S, Goya L, Bravo L. J Chromatogr B Analyt Technol Biomed Life Sci. 2005 Nov 15;827(1):76-82. **Key Finding:** "A significant decrease of serum and liver MDA concentrations in animals fed diets containing 0.3% of polyphenols from strawberry, cocoa or plum was observed in the normocholesterolemic groups. This reduction was especially noteworthy in the hypercholesterolemic animals, with increased MDA levels indicating enhanced lipid peroxidation in the controls, yet with values parallel to the normocholesterolemic groups in animals fed the polyphenol-rich diets. These results point out the beneficial effects of phenolic antioxidants from fruits in preventing oxidative damage in vivo.

Hypertension

*Phenolic-linked variation in strawberry cultivars for potential dietary management of **hyperglycemia** and related complications of **hypertension**.* Cheplick S, Kwon YI, Bhowmik P, Shetty K. Bioresourc Technol. 2010 Jan;101(1):404-13. **Key Finding:** "Strawberry cultivars with combined inhibitory potential against alpha-glucosidase and angiotensin-1-converting enzyme activity and with moderate or low alpha-amylase inhibitory potential could be targeted for potential management of hyperglycemia-linked **type 2 diabetes** and related complications of hypertension."

Influenza

*Effect of long-term dietary antioxidant supplementation on **influenza virus** infection.* Han SN, Meydani M, Wu D, Bender BS, Smith DE, Vina J, Cao G, Prior RL,

Meydani SN. J Gerontol A Biol Sci Med Sci. 2000 Oct;55(10):B496-503. **Key Finding:** "This study compared the effect of vitamin E on the course of influenza infection with that of other antioxidants—glutathione, melatonin, strawberry extract. Among the antioxidants tested, only vitamin E was effective in reducing pulmonary viral titers and preventing an influenza-mediated decrease in food intake and weight loss. In addition to its antioxidant activity, other mechanisms might be involved in vitamin E's beneficial effect on lowering viral titer and preventing weight loss."

Neurodegenerative diseases

*Strawberry and its anthocyanin reduce **oxidative stress**-induced apoptosis in PC12 cells.* Heo HJ, Lee CY. J Agric Food Chem. 2005 Mar 23;53(6):1984-9. **Key Finding:** "Strawberry showed the highest cell protective effects among the fresh fruit samples. The overall relative **neuronal cell protective** activity of three fruits (strawberry, banana and orange) by three tests followed the decreasing order strawberry>banana>orange. The protective effects appeared to be due to the higher phenolic contents including anthocyanin, and anthocyanin in strawberries seemed to be the major contributors."

Long-term dietary strawberry, spinach, or vitamin E supplementation retards the onset of age-related neuronal signal-transduction and cognitive behavioral deficits. Joseph JA, Shukitt-Hale B, Denisova NA, Prior RL, Cao G, Martin A, Taglialatela G, Bickford PC. J Neurosci. 1998 Oct 1;18(19):8047-55. **Key Finding:** "Phytochemicals present in antioxidant-rich foods such as spinach may be beneficial in retarding functional age-related CNS and **cognitive behavioral deficits** and, perhaps, may have some benefit in **neurodegenerative disease**."

Obesity

Purified berry anthocyanin but not whole berries normalize lipid parameters in mice fed an obesogenic high fat diet. Prior RL, Wu X, Gu L, Hager T, Hager A, Wilkes S, Howard L. Mol Nutre Food Res. 2009 Nov;53(11):1406-18. **Key Finding:** "Administering purified anthocyanin from blueberry and strawberry via drinking water prevented the development of **dyslipidemia** and obesity in mice, but feeding diets containing whole berries or purple corn ACNs did not alter the development of **obesity**."

Whole berries versus berry anthocyanin: interactions with dietary fat levels in the C57BL/6J mouse model of **obesity**. Prior RL, Wu X, Gu L, Hager TJ, Hager A, Howard LR. J Agric Food Chem. 2008 Feb 13;56(3):647-53. **Key Finding:** "Male mice were given freeze-dried powders from whole blueberries or strawberries, or purified anthocyanin extracts from the two berries. After 8 weeks, mice fed the 60% calories from fat diet plus purified anthocyanin from blueberry in the drinking water had lower body weight gains and body fat than the controls. Anthocyanin's fed as the whole blueberry did not prevent and may have actually increased obesity. However, feeding purified anthocyanin from blueberries or strawberries reduced obesity."

Thrombosis (blood clots)

An experimentally **antithrombotic** *strawberry variety is also effective in humans*. Naemura A, Ohira H, Ikeda M, Koshikawa K, Ishii H, Yamamoto J. Pathophysiol Haemost Thromb. 2006;35(5):398-404. **Key Finding:** "The strawberry variety (KYSt-4; Nohime) which earlier inhibited experimental thrombosis **arterial thrombotic disease)** showed antithrombotic effects in humans, while the experimentally inactive variety as well as the relevant control was ineffective."

Anti-thrombotic effect of strawberries. Naemura A, Mitani T, Ijiri Y, Tamura Y, Yamashita T, Okimura M, Yamamoto J. Blood Coagul Fibrinolysis. 2005 Oct;16(7):501-9. **Key Finding:** "Because of the high mortality, prevention of **arterial thrombotic disease** has top priority in developed countries. Strawberry varieties were tested in this study for their anti-thrombotic effect. Of the tested strawberry varieties, KYSt-4, KYSt-11 and KYSt-17 showed significant anti-thrombotic effect. The dual mechanism of the effect may involve a direct inhibition of both platelet function and antioxidant activities."

Tomatoes

SOMETIMES CALLED THE "LOVE APPLE," the tomato is a member of the nightshade family and is native to South America. The Aztecs domesticated it and consumed it in large quantities, even giving it the name tomato, which means "swelling fruit." Many historians believe that early European explorers, such as Hernán Cortés, brought the tomato back to the European continent, where it was soon adopted into Spanish, and eventually Italian, cuisine.

Strangely, tomatoes were considered unfit for human consumption in Britain and North America well into the eighteenth century. However, they are rich in lycopene and other phytochemicals and have been shown to have health benefits that include reducing the risk for various cancers, particularly colon and prostate cancer.

Antioxidation

Administration of tomato and paprika beverages modifies hepatic glucose and lipid metabolism in mice: a DNA microarray analysis. Aizawa K, Matsumoto T, Inakuma T, Ishijima T, Nakai Y, Abe K, Amano F. J Agric Food Chem. 2009 Nov 25;57(22):10964-71. **Key Finding**: "To examine whether the expression of hepatic genes, including biomarkers, is affected by the ingestion of tomato or paprika, mice were given tomato beverage, paprika beverage, or water control for 6 weeks. The ingestion of tomato or paprika un-regulated the expression of 687 and 1045 genes and down-regulated the expression of 841 and 653 genes respectively. These changes in gene expression suggest that tomato ingestion promotes flycogen accumulation and stimulates some specific steps in fatty acid oxidation. Paprika ingestion promoted the entire glucose and fatty acid metabolic pathways to improve lipid profiles."

Efficiency of apples, strawberries, and tomatoes for reduction of **oxidative stress** *in pigs as a model for humans.* Pajk T, Rezar V, Levart A, Salobir J. Nutrition. 2006 Apr;22(4):376-84. **Key Finding:** "Our findings support the hypothesis that supplementation with apples, strawberries, or tomatoes effectively decreases oxidative stress by decreasing MDA formation in the body and by protecting mononuclear blood cells against increased DNA damage. This effect was particularly pronounced in the group supplemented with a fruit mixture; among the single fruit supplements, the most beneficial effect was obtained with apples."

Atherosclerosis

Protective activity of tomato products on in vivo markers of lipid oxidation. Visioli F, Riso P, Grande S, Galli C, Porrini M. Eur J Nutr. 2003 Aug;42(4):201-6. **Key Finding**: "These results further support a role for tomato products in the prevention of lipid peroxidation, a risk factor of **atherosclerosis** and **cardiovascular disease**."

Cancer (breast; cervical; colon; liver; lung; pancreatic; prostate; renal; stomach)

Antimutagenic effects of lycopene and tomato puree. Polivkova Z, Et al. J Med Food. 2010 Dec;13(6):1443-50. **Key Finding**: "Results indicate that lycopene, a tomato carotenoid, has antimutagenic effects, although the effects are lower than that of tomato puree, which contains a complex mixture of bioactive phytochemicals. The antimutagenic effect is connected with the chemo preventive role of lycopene, tomatoes, and tomato products in the prevention of **carcinogenesis**."

*Changes in free amino acid, phenolic, chlorophyll, carotenoid and glycoalkaloid contents in tomatoes during 11 stages of growth and inhibition of **cervical and lung human cancer cells** by **green tomato extracts**.* Choi SH, Lee SH, Kim HJ, Et al. J Agric Food Chem. 2010 Jul 14;58(13):7547-56. **Key Finding**: "Widely consumed Korean tomatoes of the variety Doturakworld were analyzed. Hel299 lung cells, A549 lung cancer cells, and HeLa cervical carcinoma cells were highly susceptible to inactivation by glycoalkaloid-rich green tomato extracts."

Differential effects of lycopene consumed in tomato paste and lycopene in the form of a purified extract on target genes of cancer prostatic cells. Talvas J, Caris-Veyrat C, Guy L, Et al. Am J Clin Nutr. 2010 Jun;91(6):1716-24. **Key Finding**: "Studies indicate that tomato consumers are protected against **prostate cancer**. Dietary lycopene can affect gene expression."

*Dietary lycopene and tomato extract supplementation inhibit nonalcoholic steatohepatitis-promoted **hepatocarcinogenesis** in rats.* Wang Y, Ausman LM, Greenberg AS, Et al. Int J Cancer. 2010 Apr 15;126(8):1788-96. **Key Finding**: "These data indicate that lycopene and tomato extract can inhibit NASH-promoted hepatocarcinogenesis mainly as a result of reduced oxidative stress, which could be fulfilled through different mechanisms."

*Induction of apoptosis by tomato using space mutation breeding in human **colon cancer** SW480 and HT-29 cells.* Shi J, Yang B, Feng P, Et al. J Sci Food Agric. 2010

Mar 15;90(4):615-21. **Key Finding**: "These data suggest that consumption of tomato using space mutation breeding may provide benefits to inhibit growth of colon cancer cells."

Foods groups and **renal cell carcinoma**: *results from a case-control study.* Grieb SM, Theis RP, Burr D, Benardot D, Siddiqui T, Asal NR. J Am Diet Assoc. 2009 Apr;109(4):656-67. **Key Finding**: "Incident cases were identified from hospital records and the Florida cancer registry, and population controls frequency matched by age, sex, and race were identified. Eating habits were assessed through the use of the 70-item Block food frequency questionnaire. Findings include the decreased risk of renal cell carcinoma with tomato consumption."

Prostate cancer *and vegetable consumption.* Chan R, Lok K, Woo J. Mol Nutr Food Res. 2009 Feb;53(2):201-16. **Key Finding**: "There is accumulating evidence to support the consumption of lycopene, in particular tomato and tomato-based products, as protective factors against prostate cancer. Evidence on the protective role of beta-carotene was inconsistent from cohort and case-control studies."

Effect of beta-carotene-rich tomato lycopene beta-cyclase (tlcy-b) on cell growth inhibition in HT-29 **colon adenocarcinoma** *cells.* Palozza P, Bellovino D, Simone R, Boningsegna A, Cellini F, Monastra G, Gaetani S. Br J Nutr. 2009 Jul;102(2):207-14. **Key Finding**: "Inhibition of cell growth by tomato digestate was dose-dependent and resulted from an arrest of cell cycle progression at the GO/G1 and G2/M phase and by apoptosis induction."

Tomatoes and lycopene in prevention and therapy—is there an evidence for prostate diseases? Ellinger S, Ellinger J, Muller SC, Stehle P. Aktuelle Urol. (German) 2009 Jan;40(1):37-43. **Key Finding**: "The consumption of tomatoes and tomato products may probably protect from **prostate cancer**—at least when considering low-grade prostate cancer. Thus, regular consumption of these foods can be recommended for the prevention of prostate cancer."

Phytochemicals that counteract the cardio toxic side effects of **cancer chemotherapy**. Piasek A, Bartoszek A, Namiesnik J. Postepy Hig Med Dosw (Polish). 2009 Apr 17;63:142-58. **Key Finding**: "Dietary intervention with antioxidants (such as in tomato, garlic, spinach) may be a safe and effective way of alleviating the toxicity of anticancer chemotherapy and preventing **heart failure**."

Tomatine-containing green tomato extracts inhibit growth of **human breast, colon, liver and stomach cancer** *cells.* Friedman M, Levin CE, Lee SU, Kim HJ, Lee IS, Byun JO, Kozukue N. J Agric Food Chem. 2009 Jul 8;57(13):5727-33.

Key Finding: "Tomato plants synthesize the glycoalkaloids dehydrotomatine and alpha-tomatine, possibly as a defense against bacteria, fungi, viruses, and insects. Six green and three red tomato extracts were investigated for their ability to induce cell death in human cancer and normal cells using a micro culture tetrazolium (MTT) assay. Compared to the untreated controls, the high-tomatine green tomato extracts strongly inhibited the following human cancer cell lines: breast (MCF-7), colon (HT-29), gastric (AGS), and hepatoma liver (HepG2), as well as normal human liver cells. There was little inhibition of the cells by the three low-tomatine red tomato extracts."

Concomitant supplementation of lycopene and eicosapentaenoic acid inhibits the proliferation of human **colon cancer** *cells.* Tang FY, Cho HJ, Pai MH, Chen YH. Nutr Biochem. 2009 Jun;20(6):426-34. **Key Finding**: "Our novel findings suggest that lycopene and EPA synergistically inhibited the growth of human colon cancer HT-29 cells even at low concentrations."

A combination of tomato and soy products for men with recurring **prostate cancer** *and rising prostate specific antigen.* Grainger EM, Schwartz SJ, Wang S, Unlu NZ, Boileau TW, Ferketich AK, Monk JP, Gong MC, Bahnson RR, DeGroff VL, Clinton SK. Nutr Cancer. 2008;60(2):145-54. **Key Finding:** "Forty-one men with recurrent asymptomatic prostate cancer were randomized among 2 groups. Group A consumed tomato products but no soy. Group B consumed soy but no tomatoes. Serum prostate-specific antigen decreased for 14 men, 34% of the total. Mean serum vascular endothelial growth factor for the entire group was reduced from 87 to 51 ng/ml. Further studies combining tomato and soy foods to determine efficacy for prostate cancer prevention or management are encouraged."

Effects of carrot and tomato juice consumption on faecal markers relevant to **colon carcinogenesis** *in humans.* Schnabele K, Briviba K, Bub A, Roser S, Pool-Zobel BL, Rechkemmer G. Br J Nutr. 2008 Mar;99(3):606-13. **Key Finding**: "In the present study, 2-week interventions with carotenoid-rich juices led only to minor changes in investigated luminal biomarkers relevant to colon carcinogenesis."

Lycopene has limited effect on cell proliferation in only two of seven human cell lines (both cancerous and noncancerous) in an in vitro system with doses across the physiological range. Burgess LC, Rice E, Fischer T, Seekins JR, Burgess TP, Sticka SJ, Klatt K. Toxicol In Vitro. 2008 Aug;22(5):1297-300. **Key Finding**: "Seven cell types, cancerous and noncancerous, were treated with lycopene from 0.0001 to 10 microM for 24, 48 and 72 hours. The Hep-G2 **liver adenocarcinoma** cell line showed a reduction at the high doses after 24 h and the IMR-90, noncancerous lung cell line, showed a reduction at the highest dose after 72 h. The A431 **skin carcinoma**, DU-145 **prostate carcinoma**, HS-68 noncancerous skin, A549 **lung carcinoma**, and HS-578T **breast carcinoma**, all showed no reduction in proliferation."

*A combination of tomato and soy products for men with recurring **prostate cancer** and rising prostate specific antigen.* Grainger EM, Schwartz SJ, Wang S, Unlu NZ, Boileau TW, Ferketich AK, Monk JP, Gong MC, Bahnson RR, DeGroff VL, Clinton SK. Nutr Cancer. 2008;60(2):145-54. **Key Finding**: "Prostate cancer patients will consume diets rich in tomato products and soy with excellent compliance and bioavailability of phytochemicals. Further studies combining tomato and soy foods to determine efficacy for prostate cancer prevention or management are encouraged."

*Effects of lycopene on the insulin-like growth factor (IGF) system in premenopausal **breast cancer** survivors and women at high familial breast cancer risk.* Voskuil DW, Vrieling A, Korse CM, Et al. Nutr Cancer. 2008;60(3):342-53. **Key Finding**: "This randomized controlled trial shows that 2 mo of lycopene supplementation has no effect on serum total IGF-I in the overall study population. However, lycopene effects were discordant between the 2 study populations showing beneficial effects in high-risk healthy women but not in breast cancer survivors."

Contribution of tomato phenolic to suppression of COX-2 expression in KB cells. Shen YC, Chen SL, Zhuang SR, Wang CK. J Food Sci. 2008 Jan;73(1):C1-10. **Key Finding:** "These results suggest that tomato phenolic may play an important role in the chemoprevention of **cancer**."

*Interaction of tomato lycopene and ketosamine against rat **prostate tumorigenesis**.* Mossine VV, Chopra P, Mawhinney TP. Cancer Res. 2008 Jun 1;68(11):4384-91. **Key Finding**: "We investigated whether ketosamines, a group of carbohydrate derivatives present in dehydrated tomato products, may interact with lycopene against prostate tumorigenesis. One ketosamine, FruHis, strongly synergized with lycopene against proliferation of the highly metastatic rat prostate adenocarcinoma MAT-LyLu cell line in vitro. The FruHis/lycopene combination significantly inhibited in vivo tumor formation by MAT-LyLu cells in syngeneic Copenhagen rats. FruHis, therefore, may exert tumor preventive effect through its antioxidant activity and interaction with lycopene."

*Lycopene inhibits growth of human **colon cancer** cells via suppression of the Akt signaling pathway.* Tang FY, Shih CJ, Cheng LH, Ho HJ, Chen HJ. Mol Nutr Food Res.

2008 Jun;52(6):646-54. **Key Finding**: "Lycopene inhibited cell proliferation of human colon cancer cells via suppression of the Akt signaling pathway and downstream targeted molecules."

*Combinations of tomato and broccoli enhance **antitumor** activity in dunning r3327-h prostate adenocarcinomas.* Canene-Adams K, Lindshield BL, Wang S, Jeffery EH, Clinton SK, Erdman JW Jr. Cancer Res. 2007 Jan 15;67(2):836-43. Epub 2007 Jan 9. **Key Finding:** "The combination of tomato and broccoli was more effective at slowing tumor growth than either tomato or broccoli alone and supports the public health recommendations to increase the intake of a variety of plant components."

*Serum lycopene, other carotenoids, and **prostate cancer** risk: a nested case-control study in the prostate, lung, colorectal and ovarian cancer screening trial.* Peters U, Leitzmann MF, Chatterjee N, Wang Y, Albanes D, Gelmann EP, Friesen MD, Riboli E, Hayes RB. Cancer Epidemiol Biomarkers Prev. 2007 May;16(5):962-8. **Key Finding**: "In this large prospective study, high serum beta-carotene concentrations were associated with increased risk for aggressive, clinically relevant prostate cancer. Lycopene and other carotenoids were unrelated to prostate cancer. Consistent with other recent publications, these results suggest that lycopene or tomato-based regimens will not be effective for prostate cancer prevention."

*Tomato lycopene extract supplementation decreases insulin-like growth factor-I levels in **colon cancer** patients.* Walfisch S, Walfisch Y, Kirilov E, Linde N, Mnitentag H, Agbaria R, Sharoni Y, Levy J. Eur J Cancer Prev. 2007 Aug;16(4):298-303. **Key Finding**: "The results support our suggestion that tomato lycopene extract has a role in the prevention of colon and possibly other types of cancer."

*Fruits, vegetables, soy foods and **breast cancer** in pre- and postmenopausal Korean women: a case-control study.* Do MH, Lee SS, Kim JY, Jung PJ, Lee MH. Int J Vitam Nutr Res. 2007 Mar;77(2):130-41. **Key Finding**: "High tomato intake was associated with reduced breast cancer risk in premenopausal women. In postmenopausal women, green pepper intake showed an inverse association of breast cancer risk."

*Lycopene and soy isoflavones in the treatment of **prostate cancer**.* Vaishampayan U, Hussain M, Banerjee M, Seren S, Sarkar FH, Fontana J, Forman JD. Cher ML. Powell I. Pontes JE. Kucuk O. Nutr Cancer. 2007;59(1):1-7. **Key Finding**: "The data suggest that lycopene and soy isoflavones have activity in prostate cancer patients with PSA relapses disease and may delay progression of both hormone-refractory and hormone-sensitive prostate cancer. However, there may not be an additive effect between the 2 compounds when taken together."

Lycopene inhibits PDGF-BB-induced signaling and migration in human dermal fibroblasts through interaction with PDGF-BB. Chiang HS, Wu WB, Fang JY, Chen DF, Chen BH, Huang CC, Chen YT, Hung CF. Life Sci. 2007 Nov 10;81(21-22):1509-17. **Key Finding**: "Our results provide the first evidence showing that lycopene is an effective inhibitor of migration of stromal fibroblasts (**melanoma**) and this effect may contribute to its antitumor activity."

Lycopene supplementation elevates circulating insulin-like growth factor binding protein-1 and -2 concentrations in persons at greater risk of ***colorectal cancer***. Vrieling A, Voskuil DW, Bonfrer JM, Korse CM, van Doorn J, Cats A, Depla AC, Timmer R, Witteman BJ, Van Leeuwen FE, Van't Veer LJ, Rookus MA, Kampman E. Am J Clin Nutr. 2007 Nov;86(5):1456-62. **Key Finding**: "This is the first study known to show that lycopene supplementation may increase circulating IGFBP-1 and IGFBP-2 concentrations. Higher circulating insulin-like growth factor IGF-I concentrations have been related to a greater risk of cancer."

Gene signature of ***breast cancer*** *cell lines treated with lycopene.* Chalabi N, Delort L, Le Corre L, Satih S, Bignon YJ, Bernard-Gallon D. Pharmacogenomics. 2006 Jul;7(5):663-72. **Key Finding**: "Based on the observed results, lycopene seems to exert regulation on apoptosis, cell cycle and DNA repair mechanisms according to estrogen and retinoic acid receptor status."

Dietary intake of ***lycopene*** *is associated with reduced* ***pancreatic cancer*** *risk.* Nkondjock A, Ghadirian P, Johnson KC, Krewski D. Canadian Cancer Registries Epidemiology Research Group. J Nutr. 2005 Mar;135(3):592-7. **Key Finding:** "In this study, we investigated the possible association between dietary carotenoids and pancreatic cancer risk. A case-control study of 462 histologically confirmed pancreatic cancer cases and 4721 population-based controls in 8 Canadian provinces took place. The results of this study suggest that a diet rich in tomatoes and tomato-based products with high lycopene content may help reduce pancreatic cancer risk."

Role of lycopene and tomato products in ***prostate*** *health.* Stacewicz-Sapuntzakis M, Bowen PE. Biochem Biophys Acta. 2005 May 30;1740(2):202-5. **Key Finding:** "We conducted a small intervention trial among patients diagnosed with prostate adenocarcinoma. Tomato sauce pasta was consumed daily for 3 weeks. Oxidative DNA damage in leukocytes and prostate tissues was significantly diminished the latter mainly in the tumor cell nuclei, possibly due to the antioxidant properties of lycopene. Quite surprising was the decrease in blood prostate-specific antigen, which was explained by the increase in apoptotic death of prostate cells, especially in carcinoma regions. Other phytochemicals in tomato may act in synergy with lycopene to potentiate protective effects and to help in the maintenance of prostate health."

Relationship between plasma carotenoids and **prostate cancer**. Chang S, Erdman JW, Clinton SK, Vadiveloo M, Strom SS, Yamamura Y, Duphorne CM, Spitz MR, Amos CI, Contois JH, Gu X, Babaian RJ, Scardino PT, Hursting SD. Nutr Cancer. 2005;53(2):127-34. **Key Finding:** "These findings suggest that, in these 118 men with nonmetastatic prostate cancer and 52 healthy men from the same area, higher circulating levels of alpha-cryptoxanthin, alpha-carotene, trans-beta-carotene, and lutein and zeaxanthin may contribute to lower prostate cancer risk but not to disease progression."

Tomato *phytochemicals and* **prostate cancer** *risk*. Campbell JK, Canene-Adams K, Lindshield BL, Boileau TW, Clinton SK, Erdman JW Jr. J Nutr. 2004 Dec;134(12 Suppl):3486S-3492S. **Key Finding:** "This paper reviews the epidemiological evidence, evaluating the relationship between prostate cancer risk and tomato consumption, and presents experimental data from this and other laboratories that support the hypothesis that whole tomato and its phytochemical components reduce the risk of prostate cancer."

The role of tomato products and lycopene in the prevention of **prostate cancer**: *a meta-analysis of observational studies*. Etminan M, Takkouche B, Caamano-Isorna F. Cancer Epidemiol Biomarkers Prev. 2004 Mar;13(3):340-5. **Key Finding**: "Our results show that tomato products may play a role in the prevention of prostate cancer. However, this effect is modest and restricted to high amounts of tomato intake. Further research is needed to determine the type and quantity of tomato products with respect to their role in preventing prostate cancer."

Prostate carcinogenesis in N-methyl-N-nitrosourea (NMU)-testosterone-treated rats fed tomato powder, lycopene, or energy-restricted diets. Boileau TW, Liao Z, Kim S, Lemeshow S, Erdman JW Jr, Clinton SK. J Natal Cancer Inst. 2003 Nov 5;95(21):1578-86. **Key Finding:** "Consumption of tomato powder but not lycopene inhibited prostate carcinogenesis, suggesting that tomato products contain compounds in addition to lycopene that modify **prostate carcinogenesis**. Diet restriction also reduced the risk of prostate cancer. Tomato phytochemicals and diet restriction may act by independent mechanisms."

Botanicals in **cancer** *chemoprevention*. Park EJ, Pezzuto JM. Cancer Metastasis Rev. 2002;21(3-4):231-55. **Key Finding:** "In this review, we discuss the cancer chemo preventive activity of cruciferous vegetables such as cabbage and broccoli, Allium vegetables such as garlic and onion, green tea, citrus fruits, tomatoes, berries, ginger and ginseng. Phytochemicals of these types have great potential in the fight against human cancer, and a variety of delivery methods are available as a result of their occurrence in nature."

*Tomatoes, lycopene, and **prostate cancer**: progress and promise.* Hadley CW, Miller EC, Schwartz SJ, Clinton SK. Exp Biol Med. 2002 Nov;227(10):869-80. **Key Finding:** "In contrast to the pharmacologic approach with pure lycopene, many nutritional scientists direct their attention upon the diverse array of tomato products as a complex mixture of biologically active phytochemicals that together may have anti-prostate cancer benefits beyond those of any single constituent."

*Tomato products, lycopene, and **prostate cancer** risk.* Miller EC, Giovannucci E, Erdman JW Jr, Bahnson R, Schwarz SJ, Clinton SK. Urol Clin North Am. 2002 Feb;29(1):83-93. **Key Finding:** "It is reasonable to recommend to the general population the consumption of tomato products at approximately one serving per day or five servings per week as part of an overall healthy dietary pattern that may reduce the risks of prostate cancer, other malignancies, or other chronic diseases."

*Tomatoes, lycopene, and **prostate cancer**: progress and promise.* Hadley CW, Miller EC, Schwartz SJ, Clinton SK. Exp Biol Med. 2002 Nov;227(10):869-80. **Key Finding:** "In contrast to the pharmacologic approach with pure lycopene, many nutritional scientists direct their attention upon the diverse array of tomato products as a complex mixture of biologically active phytochemicals that together may have anti-prostate cancer benefits beyond those of any single constituent."

Oral Consumption of Bitter Gourd and Tomato Prevents Lipid Peroxidation in Liver Associated with DMBA Induced Skin Carcinogenesis in Mice. De S, Chakraborty J, Das S. Asian Pac J Cancer Prev. 2000;1(3):203-206. **Key Finding:** "The protective role of two commonly consumed natural dietary items – bitter gourd and tomato— against endogenous as well as 7,12-dimethylbenz(a)anthracene (DMBA) include lipid peroxidation in the livers of mice was investigated. The rationale for such an approach is that lipid peroxidation has been suggested to play a key role in human cancer development. Our observations support the hypothesis that natural combinations of phytochemicals present in the fruit juices exert **cancer**-protective effects via a decrease in lipid peroxidation."

Tomatoes, tomato-rich foods, lycopene and cancer of the upper aero digestive tract: a case-control in Uruguay. De Stefani E, Oreggia F, Boffetta P, Deneo-Pellegrini H, Ronco A,

Mendilaharsu M. Oral Oncol. 2000 Jan;36(1):47-53. **Key Finding:** "In order to study the relationship between tomatoes, tomato products, lycopene and **cancers** of the upper aero digestive tract; **oral cavity, pharynx, larynx, esophagus;** a case-control study was carried out in Uruguay involving 238 cases and 491 hospitalized controls. We found that the joint effect of lycopene and total phytosterols was associated with a significant reduction in risk for these cancers."

Carotenoids and **colon cancer**. Slattery ML, Benson J, Curtin K, Ma KN, Schaeffer D, Potter JD. Am J Clin Nutr. 2000 Feb;71(2):575-82. **Key Finding:** "Lutein was inversely associated with colon cancer in both men and women studied. The major dietary sources of lutein in subjects with colon cancer and in control subjects were spinach, broccoli, lettuce, tomatoes, oranges and orange juice, carrots, celery, and greens. These data suggest that incorporating these foods into the diet may help reduce the risk of developing colon cancer."

Tomato lycopene and its role in human health and chronic diseases. Agarwal S, Rao AV. CMAJ. 2000 Sep 19;163(6):739-44. **Key Finding:** "In this article we outline the possible mechanisms of action of lycopene and review the current understanding of its role in human health and disease prevention."

Role of diet modification in **cancer** *prevention.* Abdulla M, Gruber P. Biofactors. 2000;12(1-4):45-51. **Key Finding:** "A number of epidemiological and experimental studies have shown that vitamin C and E, Beta-carotene and the essential trace element selenium can reduce the risk of cancer. Consistent observations during the last few decades that cancer risk is reduced by a diet rich in vegetables, fruits, legumes, grains and green tea have encouraged research to identify several plant components especially phytochemicals that protects against DNA damage. This paper reviews current knowledge."

Retinol, beta-carotene and **cancer**. Wald N. Cancer Surv. 1987;6(4):635-51. **Key Finding**: "A low serum beta-carotene level is associated with a high risk of cancer, but here the association persists for many years before the diagnosis of cancer, indicating that it probably also precedes its development. The dietary and serum studies are therefore consistent in showing a long-term inverse association between beta-carotene and the risk of cancer."

Cardiovascular disease

Effect of lycopene from cooked tomatoes on serum antioxidant enzymes, lipid peroxidation rate and lipid profile in **coronary heart disease**. Bose KS, Agrawal BK. Singapore

Med J. 2007 May;48(5):415-20. **Key Finding**: "These findings suggest that tomato lycopene may have considerable therapeutic potential as an antioxidant but may not be used as a hypolipidemic agent in coronary heart disease."

Are the health attributes of lycopene related to its antioxidant function? Erdman JW Jr, Ford NA, Lindshield BL. Arch Biochem Biophys. 2009 Mar 15;483(2):229-35. **Key Finding**: "We conclude that there is an overall shortage of supportive evidence for the 'antioxidant hypotheses as lycopene's major in vivo mechanism of action in decreasing **cardiovascular disease** and **prostate cancer** risk. Our laboratory has postulated that metabolic products of lycopene, the lycopenoids, may be responsible for some of lycopene's reported bioactivity."

Protective activity of tomato products on in vivo markers of lipid oxidation. Visioli F, Riso P, Grande S, Galli C, Porrini M. Eur J Nutr. 2003 Aug;42(4):201-6. **Key Finding**: "These results further support a role for tomato products in the prevention of lipid peroxidation, a risk factor of **atherosclerosis** and **cardiovascular disease**."

Effects of tomato extract on human platelet aggregation in vitro. Dutta-Roy AK, Crosbie L, Gordon MJ. Platelets. 2001 Jun;12(4):218-27. **Key Finding:** "Among all fruits tested in vitro for their anti-platelet property, tomato had the highest activity followed by grapefruit, melon, and strawberry, whereas pear and apple had little or no activity. All these data indicate that tomato contains very potent anti-platelet components, and consuming tomatoes might be beneficial both as a preventive and therapeutic regime for **cardiovascular disease**."

Cholesterol

*Tomato powder is more protective than lycopene supplement against **lipid peroxidation** in rats.* Alshatwi AA, Al Obaaid MA, Al Sedairy SA, Al-Assaf AH, Zhang LL, Lei KY. Nutr Res. 2010 Jan;30(1):66-73. **Key Finding**: "Liver total cholesterol was markedly lowered by tomato powder or lycopene-beadlet treatment, but liver triglycerides were lowered to one fourth by only tomato powder treatment. Tomato powder appeared to be more protective because of its additional ability to prevent the H(2)O(2)-induced rise in serum MDA and seemed to lower liver triglycerides more than lycopene treatment."

Contribution of tomato phenolic to antioxidation and down-regulation of blood lipids. Shen YC, Chen SL, Wang CK. J Agric Food Chem. 2007 Aug 8;55(16):6475-81. **Key Finding**: "A human clinical trial was conducted to examine plasma antioxidation, status of blood lipids, and phenolic responses after ingestion of fresh tomato,

tomato juice, and a lycopene drink. Tomato phenolic showed fair antioxidant activity (57-71%) and also synergistically promoted the antioxidation (81-100%) of tomato carotenoids. In the human clinical study, total antioxidant capacity and phenolic contents of plasma were increased after administration of fresh tomato and tomato juice, but no significant difference was found for lycopene drink consumption. **Triglyceride levels** and low-density lipoprotein **cholesterol** were decreased after administration of fresh tomato and tomato juice, and high-density lipoprotein cholesterol was increased."

Colitis

5-ASA and lycopene decreases the oxidative stress and inflammation induced by iron in rats with **colitis**. Reifen R, Nissenkorn A, Matas Z, Bujanover Y. J Gastroenterol. 2004 Jun;39(6):514-9. **Key Finding:** "Significantly more severe colitis, including necrosis, ulceration, and hemorrhage, was seen in colonic biopsies of rats with colitis when iron was supplemented. This pathology was attenuated when iron was given in combination with 5-aminosalicylic acid and/or lycopene."

Lycopene supplementation attenuates the inflammatory status of **colitis** *in a rat model.* Reifen R, Nur T, Matas Z, Halpern Z. Int J Vitam Nutr Res. 2001 Nov;71(6):347-51. **Key Finding:** "We propose that the dietary supplementation of lycopene may be an effective approach for reducing the level of oxidative stress and improving the inflammatory status of colitis."

Dementia

Vascular action of polyphenols. Ghosh D, Scheepens A. Mol Nutr Food Res. 2009 Mar;53(3):322-31. **Key Finding**: "Several epidemiological studies suggest that the regular consumption of foods and beverages rich in flavonoids is associated with a reduction in the risk of several pathological conditions ranging from **hypertension to coronary heart disease, stroke and dementia**. The major polyphenols shown to have some of these effects in humans are primarily from tomatoes (polyphenols and nonpolyphenolics), soy, pomegranate, grape seed and berries."

Eye disease

Chemistry, distribution, and metabolism of tomato carotenoids and their impact on human health. Khachik F, Carvalho L, Bernstein PS, Muir GJ, Zhao DY, Katz NB. Exp

Biol Med. 2002 Nov;227(10):845-51. **Key Finding:** "In this review we identified and quantified the complete spectrum of carotenoids from pooled human retinal pigment epithelium, ciliary body, iris, lens, and the uveal tract and in other tissues of the human eye to gain a better insight into the metabolic pathways of ocular carotenoids. Lycopene and a wide range of dietary carotenoids have been detected in high concentrations in ciliary body and retinal pigment epithelium. The possible role of lycopene and other dietary carotenoids in the prevention of age-related macular degeneration and other **eye diseases** is discussed."

Hypertension

Vascular action of polyphenols. Ghosh D, Scheepens A. Mol Nutr Food Res. 2009 Mar;53(3):322-31. **Key Finding**: "Several epidemiological studies suggest that the regular consumption of foods and beverages rich in flavonoids is associated with a reduction in the risk of several pathological conditions ranging from **hypertension to coronary heart disease, stroke and dementia**. The major polyphenols shown to have some of these effects in humans are primarily from tomatoes (polyphenols and nonpolyphenol), soy, pomegranate, grape seed and berries."

*The effects of natural antioxidants from tomato extract in treated but uncontrolled **hypertensive** patients.* Paran E, Novack V, Engelhard YN, Hazan-Halevy I. Cardiovasc Drugs Ther. 2009 Apr;23(2):145-51. **Key Finding**: "Tomato extract when added to patients treated with low doses of ACE inhibition, calcium channel blockers or their combination with lose dose diuretics, had a clinically significant effect reduction of blood pressure by more than 10 mmHg systolic and more than 5 mmHg diastolic pressure."

*Dark chocolate or tomato extract for **prehypertension**: a randomized controlled trial.* Ried K, Frank OR, Stocks NP. BMC Complement Altern Med. 2009 Jul 8;9:22. **Key Finding**: "Our study did not find a blood pressure lowering effect of dark chocolate or tomato extract in a prehypertensive population of 36 prehypertensive healthy adult volunteers."

*Effect of lycopene from tomatoes (cooked) on plasma antioxidant enzymes, lipid peroxidation rate and lipid profile in grade-I **hypertension.*** Bose KS, Agrawal BK. Ann Nutr Metab. 2007;51(5):477-81. **Key Finding**: "These findings suggest that tomato lycopene may have considerable natural therapeutic potential as an antioxidant but may not be used as a hypolipidemic agent in hypertension."

Inflammatory bowel diseases

*Dietary Factors in the Modulation of **Inflammatory Bowel Disease** Activity.* Shah S. MedGenMed. 2007;9(1):60. **Key Finding:** "Two studies have indicated that lycopene, an antioxidant, found in high quantities in foods that have a natural red color (e.g. tomato, watermelon, pink grapefruit) may play a role in attenuating the inflammatory process. Studies done using indoacetamide rat model of colitis showed that lycopene attenuated the inflammatory response."

Stroke

Vascular action of polyphenols. Ghosh D, Scheepens A. Mol Nutr Food Res. 2009 Mar;53(3):322-31. **Key Finding**: "Several epidemiological studies suggest that the regular consumption of foods and beverages rich in flavonoids is associated with a reduction in the risk of several pathological conditions ranging from **hypertension to coronary heart disease, stroke and dementia**. The major polyphenols shown to have some of these effects in humans are primarily from tomatoes (polyphenols and nonpolyphenol), soy, pomegranate, grape seed and berries."

Walnuts (see Nuts)

Wheatgrass (chlorophyll)

DURING THE 1930S AN AMERICAN AGRICULTURAL CHEMIST, Charles F. Schnabel, initiated a series of experiments in which he found that wheatgrass (sprouts of the common wheat plant grown in Kansas) not only returned dying hens to good health, but stimulated them to produce eggs at double their previous rate. Schnabel began marketing wheatgrass to humans in powdered form, touting its health benefits.

We now know that wheatgrass is the best source of life-giving chlorophyll of any plant. It is also rich in protein, vitamin E, vitamin B_{12}, and phosphorus. Over the past few decades, studies have found wheatgrass consumption to be particularly beneficial to people suffering from anemia, colitis, and other inflammatory bowel disorders.

Anemia (and blood transfusions)

The role of iron chelation activity of wheat grass juice in patients with mylodysplastic syndrome. Mukhopadhyay S, Basak J, Kar M, Mandal S, Mukhopadhyay A. J Clin Oncol. 2009 May 20;27(155):7012. **Key Finding:** "The mean serum Ferritin level of the patients was 2,250 (range 650-4,800) before wheat grass treatment. The mean reduced to 950 (range 68-1680). The mean interval between transfusions was found increased. Wheat grass juice is an effective iron chelator and its use in reducing serum ferritin should be encouraged in **myelodysplastic syndrome** and other diseases where repeated blood transfusion is required."

Wheat Grass Juice Reduces Transfusion Requirement in Patients with Thalassemia Major: A Pilot Study. Marwaha RK, Bansal D, Kaur S, Trehan A. Ind Pediatrics. 2004 July 17;41:716-720. **Key Finding:** "Several of our patients in the thalassemia unit began consuming wheat grass juice after anecdotal accounts of beneficial effects on **blood transfusion** requirements. These encouraging experiences prompted us to evaluate the effect of wheat grass juice on transfusion requirements in patients with transfusion dependent beta thalassemia. A beneficial effect of wheat grass juice was defined as decrease in the requirement of packed red cells by 25% or more. Sixteen cases were analyzed. Blood transfusion requirement fell by 25% or more in 50% of patients with a decrease of 40% or more in three patients. No perceptible adverse effects were recognized."

Antioxidation

Evaluation of antioxidant profile and activity of amalaki (Emblica officinalis), spirulina and wheat grass. Shukla V, Vashistha M, Singh SN. Ind J Clin Biochem. 2009 Jan;24(1):70-75. **Key Finding:** "Total antioxidant activity of aqueous extract of amalki, spirulina and wheatgrass at 1mg/ml concentration were 7.78, 1.33 and 0.278 mmol/l respectively. Alcoholic extract of wheat grass showed 50% inhibition in FeCI2- ascorbic acid induced lipid peroxidation of rat liver homogenates in vitro. Both aqueous and alcoholic extracts of amalaki inhibited activity of rat liver glutathione S-transferase in vitro in dose dependent manner. The aqueous extracts of both amalki and spirulina also showed protection against t-BOOH induced cytotoxicity and production of ROS in cultured C6 glial cells."

Cancer (breast; colon)

*Administering wheatgrass juice in supportive care of terminally ill **cancer** patients.* Basak J, Bhattacharjee C, Dey S, Adhikari S, Mukhopadhyay S, Mukhopadhyay A. Annals of Oncology. 2008 July;19(Suppl 5). **Key Finding:** "Wheatgrass juice was used for anemic patients to increase hemoglobin levels. We concluded that wheatgrass is an effective alternative to blood transfusion. Its use in terminally ill cancer patients should be encouraged."

*Wheatgrass Juice May Improve Hematological Toxicity Related to Chemotherapy in **Breast Cancer** Patients: A Pilot Study.* Bar-Sela G, Tsalic M, Fried G, Goldberg H. Nutrition and Cancer. 2007 Jun;58(1):43-48. **Key Finding:** "It was found that wheatgrass juice taken during FAC chemotherapy may reduce myelotoxicity, dose reductions, and need for GCSF support, without diminishing efficacy of chemotherapy."

*Heme and chlorophyll intake and risk of **colorectal cancer** in the Netherlands cohort study.* Balder HF, Vogel J, Jansen MC, Weijenberg MP, Van den Brandt PA, Westenbrink S, van der Meer R, Godlbohm RA. Cancer Epidemiol Biomarkers Prev. 2006 Apr;15(4):717-25. **Key Finding:** "Our data suggest an elevated risk of colon cancer in men with increasing intake of heme iron and decreasing intake of chlorophyll. Further research is needed to confirm these results."

Tumors from rats given 1,2-dimethylhydrazine plus chlorophyllin or indole-3-carbinol contain transcriptional changes in beta-catenin that are independent of beat-catenin mutation status. Wang R, Dashwood WM, Bailey GS, Williams DE, Dashwood RH. Mutat Res.

2006 Oct 10;601(1-2):11-8. **Key Finding:** "Tumors induced in the rat by 1, 2-dimethylhydrazine contains mutations in beta-catenin, but the spectrum of such mutations can be influenced by phytochemicals such as chlorophyllin and indole-3-carbinol. In the present study, we determined the mutation status of beta-catenin in more than 50 DMH-induced **colon tumors** and small intestine tumors. Similar findings have been reported in primary human colon cancers and their liver metastases."

Chlorophyll, chlorophyllin, and related tetrapyrroles are significant inducers of mammalian phase 2 cytoprotective genes. Fahey JW, Stephenson KK, Dinkova-Kostova AT, Egner PA, Kensler TW, Talalay P. Carcinogenesis. 2005 Jul;26(7):1247-55. **Key Finding:** Plant chlorophylls and carotenoids, which play central roles in photosynthesis, have the ability to induce mammalian phase 2 proteins that protect cells against oxidants and electrophiles. "One of the most potent inducers was isolated from chlorophyllin, a semisynthetic water-soluble chlorophyll derivative. Although chlorophyll itself is low in inducer potency, it may nevertheless account for some of the disease-protective effects attributed to diets rich in green vegetables because it occurs in much higher concentrations in those plants than the widely studied phytochemicals."

Green vegetables, red meat and **colon cancer**: *chlorophyll prevents the cytotoxic and hyper proliferative effects of haem in rat colon.* De Vogel J, Jonker-Termon DS, Van Lieshout EM, Katan MB, Van der Meer R. Carcinogenesis. 2005 Feb;26(2):387-93. **Key Finding:** "We studied whether green vegetables inhibit the unfavorable colonic effects of haem (from red meat) in rat colons. We conclude that green vegetables may decrease colon cancer risk because chlorophyll prevents the detrimental, cytotoxic and hyperproliferative colonic effects of dietary haem."

Promotion versus suppression of rat **colon carcinogenesis** *by chlorophyllin and chlorophyll: modulation of apoptosis, cell proliferation, and beta-carenin/Tcf signaling.* Blum CA, Xu M, Orner GA, Dario Diaz G, Li Q, Dashwood WM, Bailey GS, Dashwood RH. Mutat Res. 2003 Feb-Mar;523-524:217-23. **Key Finding:** "The results suggest that further investigation of the dose-response for suppression versus promotion by chlorophyll and chlorophyllin is warranted, including studies of the beta-catenin/Tcf signaling pathway and its influence on cell proliferation and apoptosis in the colonic crypt."

Inhibitory effects of chlorophyllin, hemin, and tetrakis (4-benzoic acid)porphyrin on oxidative DNA damage and mouse skin inflammation induced by 12-0-tetradecanoylphorbol-13-acetate as a possible **anti-tumor** *promoting mechanism.* Park KK, Park JH, Jung YJ, Chung

WY. Mutat Res. 2003 Dec 9;542(1-2):89-97. **Key Finding:** "These results demonstrate that the antioxidative properties of porphyrins such as chlorophyllin are important for inhibiting TPA-induced tumor promotion."

Beta-Catenin mutation in rat **colon tumors** *initiated by 1, 2-dimethylhydrazine and 2-amino-3-methylimidazo (4, 5-fquinoline, and the effect of post-initiation treatment with chlorophyllin and indole-3-carbinol.* Blum CA, Xu M, Orner GA, Fong AT, Bailey GS, Stoner GD, Horio DT, Dashwood RH. Carcinogenesis. 2001 Feb;22(2):315-20. **Key Finding:** "Two dietary phytochemicals, chlorophyllin and indole-3-carbinol, given post-initiation, shifted the pattern of beta-catenin mutations in rat colon tumors. The results indicate that the mechanism might involve the altered expression of beat-catenin/Tcf/Lef target genes."

Chlorophyllin intervention reduces aflatoxin-DNA adducts in individuals at high risk for **liver cancer.** Egner PA, Wang JB, Zhu YR, Zhang BC, Wu Y, Zhang QN, Qian GS, Kuang SY, Gange SJ, Jacobson LP, Helzlsouer KJ, Bailey GS, Groopman JD, Kensler TW. Proc Natl Acad Sci. 2001 Dec 4;98(25):14601-6. **Key Finding:** "Chlorophyllin consumption at each meal led to an overall 55% reduction in median urinary levels of aflatoxin biomarker compared with those taking placebo. Thus, prophylactic interventions with chlorophyllin or supplementation of diets with foods rich in chlorophylls may represent practical means to prevent the development of hepatocellular carcinoma or other environmentally induced cancers."

Effect of dietary phytochemicals on **cancer** *development (review).* Waladkhani AR, Clemens MR. Int J Mol Med. 1998 Apr;1(4):747-53. **Key Finding:** "Phytochemicals can inhibit carcinogenesis by inhibiting phase I enzymes, and induction of phase II enzymes, scavenge DNA reactive agents. Suppress the abnormal proliferation of early lesions, and inhibit certain properties of the cancer cell. There are many biologically plausible reasons why consumption of plant foods might slow or prevent the appearance of cancer. These include the presence in plant foods of such potentially anticarcinogenic substances as carotenoids, chlorophyll, flavonoids, indole, isothiocyanate, polyphenolic compounds, protease inhibitors, sulfides, and terpens. The specific mechanisms of action of most phytochemicals in cancer prevention are not yet clear but appear to be varied."

Non-specific inhibition of cytochrome P450 activities by chlorophyllin in human and rat liver microsomes. Yun CH, Jeong HG, Jhoun JW, Guengerich FP. Carcinogenesis. 1995 Jun;16(6):1437-40. **Key Finding:** "These results suggest that the antigenotoxic effect of chlorophyllin might be due to inhibition of P450 enzymes involving bio activation of carcinogens in addition to molecular complex formation between carcinogens and chlorophyllin."

Chemo preventive properties of chlorophyllin: inhibition of aflatoxin B1 (AFB1)-DNA binding in vivo and **anti-mutagenic** *activity against AFB1 and two heterocyclic amines in the Salmonella mutagenicity assay.* Dashwood RH, Breinholt V, Bailey GS. Carcinogenesis. 1991 May;12(5):939-42. **Key Finding:** "These studies support a chlorophyllin inhibitory mechanism involving complex formation with the carcinogen in the gut coupled with electrophile scavenging or further complexion in the target organ."

Colitis

Wheatgrass juice in the treatment of active distal **ulcerative colitis**: *a randomized double-blind placebo-controlled trial.* Ben-Ayre E, Goldin E, Wengrower D, Stamper A, Kohn R, Berry E. Scand J Gastroenterol. 2002 Apr;37(4):444-9. **Key Finding:** "Twenty-one patients completed the study. Treatment with wheatgrass was associated with significant reductions in the overall disease activity index and in the severity of rectal bleeding. Wheatgrass juice appeared effective and safe as a single or adjuvant treatment of active distal ulcerative colitis."

Inflammatory bowel diseases

Dietary Factors in the Modulation of **Inflammatory Bowel Disease** *Activity.* Shah S. MedGenMed. 2007;9(1):60. **Key Finding:** "The components of wheatgrass juice include chlorophyll, vitamins A, C, and E, and various amino acids. It has been demonstrated that wheatgrass juice is anti-mutagenic. One constituent of wheatgrass is apigenin, which is believed to possess both anti-inflammatory and antioxidant properties. Some believe that this constituent may be beneficial in ulcerative colitis. A randomized controlled trial of wheatgrass juice in the management of ulcerative colitis has demonstrated some efficacy."

Index

Medical conditions, diseases, and major topics appear in *italicized* typeface; additionally, major topics also appear in **bold** typeface.

oxygen radical absorbance capacity (ORAC)
and, 97–98, 102, 103, 104, 108,
124, 417, 477
phenolics in, 95, 98, 101, 107, 118, 422, 426
phytochemicals in, 95, 99, 100, 101, 104,
105, 344, 351, 353
polyphenols in, 95, 96, 100, 105, 106, 108,
407, 409, 411, 419, 471, 495, 496,
497
prostate cancer and, 421
resveratrol in, 432, 436
stomach cancer and, 421
stroke and, 407, 409, 411, 495, 497
tumor necrosis factor (TNF) and, 477
tumors and, 99, 100, 101, 103
ulcers and, **108**
UV-B and, 95
vascular disease and, **108–9**
vascular endothelial growth factor (VEGF)
and, 97–98, 103–4, 124
beta-carotene (b-carotene), 18, 397, 486, 489,
493
beta-cryptoxanthin, *bladder cancer/oranges* and,
385
beta-glucans, in *mushrooms,* 332, 338
bilberries
anthocyanins and, 98, 118
as antimicrobial, 426
as *antioxidant,* 97–98, 103, 104, 417
atherosclerosis and, 98
cancer and, 104, 125, 181, 441
colon cancer and, 101, 422
Helicobacter pylori (H. pylori) and, 107–8
intestinal pathogens and, 107
oxygen radical absorbance capacity (ORAC)
and, 124, 477
resveratrol and, 441
tumor necrosis factor (TNF) and, 477
vascular disease and, 108–9
bitter gourd, *skin cancer* and, 492
blackberries/blackberry juice
anthocyanins in, 98, 243, 418
as *antibacterial,* 415
as *anti-inflammatory,* 97
as *antioxidant,* 97, 100, 102, 116, 121, 416,
420, 469
apoptosis and, 178, 422
breast cancer and, 101, 102, 122, 178, 422,
472
cancer and, 95, 97, 102, 121, 122, 422
cardiovascular (coronary artery/heart) disease
and, 95
cholesterol (hypercholesterolemia) and, 95
cognition and, 105
colon cancer and, 102, 122, 178, 422, 472
cultivated, 95
esophageal cancer and, 99, 102–3, 423, 436,
472

intestinal cancer and, 101, 178
memory and, 105
oral cancer and, 102, 122, 178, 422, 472
oxidative damage/stress and, 97, 115–16
oxygen radical absorbance capacity (ORAC)
and, 469
polyphenols in, 95
prostate cancer and, 101, 102, 122, 178, 422,
472
stomach cancer and, 101, 178
as wild, 95
black cabbage, isothiocyanate in, 159
black cherry juice, as *antioxidant,* 97
black chokeberry, *intestinal pathogens* and, 107
black cumin, 164–65, 265, 297
black currants/black currant juice
as *antibacterial,* 415
as *antioxidant,* 401
breast cancer and, 101, 178, 421
cancer and, 56, 121, 386–87
colon cancer and, 101, 422
inflammation and, 251
intestinal cancer and, 101, 178, 421
lipids and, 386–87
peripheral arterial disease and, 251
polyphenols in, 401
prostate cancer and, 101, 178, 421
stomach cancer and, 101, 178, 421
black garlic, *diabetes* and, 285
black grapes, 255, 311, 417
black pepper, 164, 170, 230, 300, 321, 391,
393, 398, 440, 464
black raspberries
about, 415
angiogenesis and, 424–25
anthocyanin in, 421–22
apoptosis and, 178, 421, 422, 424, 472
breast/mammary cancer and, 102, 120, 122,
178, 418, 420, 422, 472
cancer and, 415, 419
colon cancer and, 102, 122, 178, 422, 423,
425, 472
colorectal cancer and, 418
esophageal cancer and, 99, 102–3, 419, 423,
425, 436, 472
inflammation and, 419
NFkappa-B and, 421–22, 424, 425
oral cancer and, 102, 122, 178, 421, 422, 424,
472
oxidative damage/stress and, 97, 115–16
oxygen radical absorbance capacity (ORAC)
and, 469
prostate cancer and, 102, 122, 178, 422, 472
skin cancer and, 419, 421–22
tumor necrosis factor (TNF) and, 419, 471
tumors and, 423–24, 425
vascular endothelial growth factor (VEGF)
and, 419, 423, 424, 471

black soybeans, 79, 80

black tea, 97, 165, 266

bladder *cancer/ischemia*
   blueberry juice and, 384
   broccoli and, 142–43, 144, 147
   capsaicin and, 395
   cranberry juice and, 176, 384
   diallyl trisulfide and, 259, 260
   garlic and, 259, 260, 268
   mushrooms and, 324, 325, 327, 331–32
   oranges/orange juice and, **384,** 385
   resveratrol and, 433, 437
   soy and, 77, 78

blood cancer, garlic and, 264

blood clots. *See* **thrombosis (blood clots)**

blood oranges, *obesity* and, 389

blood pressure
   blueberries and, 110, 132
   chlorella and, 42
   cinnamon and, 165–66, 167, 169, 170
   cranberries/cranberry juice and, 182, 183, 188
   epigallocatechin gallate and, 443, 447
   flavonoids and, 442
   garlic and, 275, 276, 278, 279, 280, 282, 286–87
   mushrooms and, 334, 335
   nuts and, 344, 347–48, 351, 353, 364
   olive oil and, 356, 364
   onions and, 368, 380
   phytoestrogens and, 81
   pomegranate juice and, 402, 409–10
   quercetin and, 380, 443, 447
   resveratrol and, 443, 447
   soy and, 81, 88
   spirulina to reduce, 19, 20, 26, 30
   tomatoes and, 496
   walnuts and, 347–48

blood transfusions. *See* **anemia (and blood transfusions)/sickle cell anemia**

blueberries *(Vaccinium)/blueberry juice*
   about, **110**
   aging (ageing) and, **110–14,** 128, 310, 339, 348
     cognition and, 129, 456–57, 463, 466, 479
     flavonoids and, 101, 111, 119, 121, 138, 183, 188
     neurodegeneration and, 4, 37, 135, 456
     polyphenols and, 113, 118, 456, 466
   Alzheimer's disease and, **114–15,** 128, 134
   anthocyanins in, 98, 119, 123, 127, 128, 135, 136–37, 482, 483
   as *anti-inflammatory,* 6, 130, 134, 135, 136
   as antimutagenic, 425, 426
   as *antioxidant,* **115–18**
     aging (ageing) and, 111, 114, 310, 339, 348, 456, 457, 465, 466, 478
     atherosclerosis and, 118
     bladder ischemia and, 384

cancer and, 97–98, 100, 103, 104, 121, 404, 417, 420, 463
cardiovascular (coronary artery/heart) disease and, 125, 463
cataracts and, 126
cervical cancer and, 100
cognition and, 126, 127, 128, 129, 463
cranberries vs., 173
DNA damage and, 416
ischemia and, 172
neurodegeneration and, 40–41, 133, 134, 135
oxidative damage/stress and, 46–47, 310, 456
polyphenols and, 97
stroke and, 125, 138
apoptosis and, 5, 113, 122, 123, 126, 133, 135, 178, 422
atherosclerosis and, 98, 101, 111, **118–19,** 121, 138, 183, 188
blood pressure and, 110, 132
Blueberin, 131
breast/mammary cancer and, 101, 102, 104, 119, 120, 122, 178, 420, 421, 422, 425, 436, 472, 475
cancer and, 110, **119–25**
   DNA damage and, 116–17
   flavonoids and, 101, 111, 119, 121, 138, 183, 188
   OptiBerry and, 97–98, 103
   oxygen radical absorbancy capacity (ORAC) and, 103–4, 124, 477
   phytochemicals and, 113–14, 129, 456–57, 463, 466, 474, 479
   resveratrol and, 441
cardiovascular (coronary artery/heart) disease and, 114, **125,** 129, **131,** 138, 457, 463
cataracts and, **126**
cerebral infarction and, 5, 37, 113, 135, 138, 456
cervical cancer and, 100, 104, 425, 471, 475
chlorogenic acid (CLA) in, 98
cholesterol and, 110
cognition/cognitive impairment and, 105, 110, 111, **126–29,** 133, 310, 348, 463, 465, 478, 479
colitis and, **130**
colon cancer and, 100, 102, 119, 121–22, 123, 178, 422, 472
cytotoxicity and, 115
diabetes and, 110, **130–31,** 136
DNA damage and, 46–47, 97, 105, 115–16, 116–17
dyslipidemia and, 136, 482
flavonoids in, 101, 111, 115, 121, 123, 127, 138, 183, 188
flavonols in, 118, 123, 127
gastric cancer and, 122

myocardial infarction and, 227, 286
  osteoporosis and, 231, 289
  prostate cancer and, 394
  psoriasis and, 232
  septic shock and, 233, 290
N-nitrosoimethylamine (NDMA) and, 271
prostate cancer and, 392, 394
reactive oxygen species (ROS) and, 393, 394
tongue cancer and, 391
tumors and, 271, 298, 393–94, 397
Capsicum. See **peppers (Capsicum)**
carcinoma, C-phycocyanin (C-PC) and, 13–14
cardamom, *cancer/immune system* and, 391
cardiac hypertrophy, curcumin and, 228
cardiomyopathy, garlic and, 284
cardiovascular (coronary artery/heart)
    disease. *See also* specific types of
  Allium vegetables and, 262
  almonds and, 344, 348, 349, 350, 351, 353
  apples and, 44, **58–60,** 59, 173, 181, 184
  avocados and, 67, 68
  bananas and, 173, 181, 184
  beans (legumes) and, 72, 78, 79–80, **80–82,**
      85, 89, 91
  berries and, 99, **104–5,** 344, 353, 407, 409,
      411, 495, 497
  blackberries and, 95
  blueberries and, 114, **125,** 129, **131,** 138,
      457, 463
  broccoli and, 58, 139, **151–52**
  Brussels sprouts and, **156**
  caloric/dietary restriction and, 428, 442–43
  cherries and, 249
  cinnamon and, 162, 163, **165,** 166, 169
  C-phycocyanin (C-PC) to protect against, 10
  cranberries and, 173, 175, 179, 181, **182–84,**
      185
  curcumin and, 200, 203, 214, **223,** 225, **227,**
      231, 232
  epicatechin and, 375
  flavonoids and, 58, 59, 152, 375, 376, 378,
      407, 409, 411, 442, 495, 496, 497
  flavonols and, 378
  *fruits/*vegetables and, 48, 57, 76, 80, 86, 152,
      156, 173, **247,** 276, 306
  gamma-tocotrienol and, 442
  garlic/garlic extract and, 252, 253, 254, 255,
      262, 270, **274–77,** 279, 281, 284,
      291, 314–15, 458, 486
  grapefruit and, 173, 181, 184, **305–6,** 307,
      388, 494
  grapes/grape juice/grape seeds and, 254, 274–75,
      310, **314–16,** 407, 409, 411, 495,
      497
  green tea and, 408
  hazelnut and, 254, 274–75, 314
  isoflavones and, 378

lemons and, 173, 181, 184
Longevinex (rice bran phytate) and, 442
low-density lipoprotein (LDL) and, 156,
    182, 183
lycopene and, 152, 276, 493–94
macadamia nuts and, 343, 345
melons and, 306, 494
mushrooms and, 324
nuts and, **342–43,** 347, **348–51,** 352, 353,
    362, 364
olives/olive oil and, 356, 357, 360, **361–62,**
    362–63, 364, 365
omega-3 fatty acids and, 200, 343, 345
onions and, 59, **374–76, 378–79**
oranges and, 173, 181, 184, 306, **388**
oxidative stress and, 182
peaches and, 173, 181, 184
peanuts and, 342, 344, 349
pears and, 173, 181, 184
phenolics and, 311, 314, 315, 468, 477
phytochemicals and, 48, 156, 184, 311, 314,
    315, 463, 466, 468, 477, 479
phytoestrogens and, 72, 78, 80, 81, 82, 93,
    152, 156, 276
pineapples/pineapple juice and, 173, 181,
    184, 306, 388
pistachio nuts (pistachios) and, 342–43, 344,
    345, 350
polyphenols and, 476
pomegranates/pomegranate juice and, 402, 406,
    406, 407, **407,** 408, 409, **409,** 410,
    411, **411,** 495, **495,** 497, **497**
prostate health and, 266
pulses and, 88
quercetin and, 375, 376, 442
red grapes and, 173, 181, 184
resveratrol and, 428, 434, 440, **441–44,** 445,
    447, 448
soy/soya and
  cholesterol and, 80
  diabetes and, 86
  isoflavones and, 81
  lipids and, 72, 79, 80, 81, 82, 91, 458,
      462, 464
  menopausal symptoms and, 77, 90
  phytoestrogens and, 78, 462, 464
  polyphenols and, 407, 409, 411, 495, 497
spinach and, 114, 129, 262, 457, 458, **462,**
    463, 486
strawberries and, 114, 129, 173, 181, 184,
    457, 463, **476–77, 480,** 494
sucrose and, 104–5, 106, 108
tea and, 59
tofu and, 378
tomatoes and, 262, 306, 407, 409, 411, 458,
    477, 485, 486, **493–95,** 497
vitamin C (ascorbic acid) and, 408

diabetes and, 162, 163, **165–69**
flavonoids in, 169
glucose and, 165, 166, 167–68, 169
glycemia and, 166
human immunodeficiency virus (HIV) and, **169**
hyperglycemia/hypoglycemia and, 167, 170
hypertension and, 162, **169–70**
immune system health and, 162, **170**
inflammation and, 170
insulin resistance and, 162, 165, 167, 169, 170,
    230, 300, 398
leukemia and, 163–64
lipids and, 167–68, 169
low-density lipoprotein (LDL) and, 169
lymphoma and, 163
melanoma and, 163, 164
metabolic syndrome and, 165, 167, 168–69
obesity and, 165, 166, **170,** 230, 300, 398
polycystic ovary syndrome and, 167
polyphenols in, 167, 170
tumors and, 163, 164
Cinnulin, 165
cirrhosis, chlorella/spirulina and, 9, 14
citrus fruit(s). *See also* specific types of
cancer and, 150, 160, 246, 267, 298, 303,
    321, 373, 492
colon cancer and, 304
colorectal cancer and, 244
esophageal cancer and, 244
flavonoids in, 305
forestomach cancer and, 305
hesperidin in, 243, 305
immune system and, 321
laryngeal cancer and, 244
liminoids and, 303
limonene in, 244–45, 320
limonin in, 304
lung cancer and, 305
monoterpene in, 245
naringenin in, 305
naringin in, 178
oral cancer and, 244
pharyngeal cancer and, 244
skin cancer and, 304
stomach cancer and, 244
stroke and, 94
citrus limonoids, *cytotoxicity* and, 319
citrus pectin, *hypocholesterolemia* and, 321
CLA (chlorogenic acid), in *berries,* 98
cloudberries, 100, 107, 118, 419–20, 422, 426,
    471
cloves
    as antimicrobial, 164–65, 265
    cancer and, 164–65, 265, 297
    insulin resistance and, 170, 230, 300, 398
    NF-kappaB and
        Alzheimer's disease and, 294

arthritis and, 203, 256, 410
asthma and, 204
atherosclerosis and, 204, 257, 295
cancer and, 216, 266, 298
Crohn's disease and, 284, 300
diabetes and, 285
human immunodeficiency virus (HIV) and, 228
inflammatory diseases and, 410
multiple sclerosis and, 230, 288
myocardial infarction and, 227, 286
osteoporosis and, 231, 289
psoriasis and, 232
septic shock and, 233, 290
obesity and, 170, 230, 300, 398
cocoa, polyphenols in, 481
cognition/*cognitive impairment/brain function. See
    also memory/**memory impairment**
algae and, **21–22**
apples and, 44
beans (legumes) and, 79–80, **84–85,** 91
berries and, **105**
blueberries and, 105, 110, 111, **126–29,** 133,
    310, 339, 348, 463, 465, 478, 479
chlorella and, 23
Concord grape juice and, 111, 310, 339,
    348, 465, 478
cranberries and, 171
curcmin and, **224**
nuts and, **348**
olive oil and, 356, 362
phytochemicals and, 463
phytoestrogens and, 82, 93
reactive oxygen species (ROS) and, 111
soy and, 84–85
spinach and, **462–63,** 479
strawberries and, 462, 463, 465, **478–79**
vitamin E and, 462, 479
walnuts and, 126, 348, 465
colitis
algae and, **22**
blueberries and, 130
cranberries and, **185**
curcumin and, 225, 228
garlic and, 283
ginger and, **299–300**
grapes and, **317**
iron and, 495
lycopene and, 309, 495, 497
olive oil and, 357
proanthocyanidin and, 317
probiotics and, 130
resveratrol and, 432, 434, **444**
selenium and, 37
tomatoes and, **495**
wheatgrass (chlorophyll/chlorophyllin) and, 498,
    502

colon cancer
   2,3', 4, 4',5'-Pentamethoxy-trans-stilbene
     and, 434, 439
   allyl sulfur compounds and, 264
   almonds and, 341
   apples/apple juice and, 50, 51, 52, 53, 55–56,
     387
   arctic brambles and, 419–20, 471
   berries and, 100, 101, 102, 122, 419–20,
     422–23
   bilberries and, 422
   blackberries and, 122, 178, 422, 472
   black currants and, 422
   black pepper and, 164, 393, 440
   black raspberries and, 122, 178, 422, 425,
     472
   blueberries and, 100, 102, 119, 121–22, 123,
     178, 422, 472
   Brassica vegetables and, 145, 155
   broccoli and, 145–46, 149, 151, 387
   Brussels sprouts and, 155
   cabbage and, 159–60, 412
   capsaicin and, 391, 392, 395, 437
   carotenoids and, 247, 387, 461, 487, 493
   carrots and, 151, 387, 487
   celery and, 151, 387
   chlorella and, 13
   chlorophyll/chlorophyllin and, 459, 499–
     500, 501
   cinnamaldehyde and, 393, 440
   cinnamon and, 164, 393
   cloudberries and, 419–20, 422, 471
   cranberries and, 122, 177, 178, 179–80, 422,
     472
   cruciferous vegetables and, 149
   cucurbitacins and, 412
   curcumin and, 206, 209, 213, 214, 218, 219,
     220–21, 222, 437
   diallyl sulfide/diallylsulfides and, 259, 264
   diosgenin and, 236
   ellagitannins and, 403, 405
   fenugreek and, 235, 236
   fiber (dietary) and, 51
   fruits/vegetables and, 159–60, 412
   fucoxanthin and, 219
   garlic and, 252, 259, 260, 261, 264, 266, 270
   gingerols and, 297
   grapefruit and, 303–4
   grape seeds and, 312, 313
   greens and, 151, 387
   green vegetables and, 459, 500
   indole-3-carbinol (I3C) and, 501
   iron and, 499
   lemons/limes and, 319
   lettuce and, 151, 159–60, 387, 412
   liminoids and, 319, 384
   limonene and, 304

   lingonberries and, 419–20, 422, 471
   lutein and, 150–51, 219, 387, 461, 493
   lycopene and, 219, 486, 487, 488–89
   mushrooms and, 325, 326, 330
   nobiletin and, 246
   nuts and, 341
   olives/olive oil and, 356, 357, 359, 360
   onions and, 371
   oranges/orange juice and, 151, 247, 384, 387
   phytochemicals and, 164, 393
   phytoestrogens and, 72, 79, 82, 91, 458,
     462, 464
   phytosterols and, 384
   piperine and, 393, 440
   polyphenols and, 51, 55
   pomegranates/pomegranate juice and, 100, 403,
     404, 405
   prickly pear fruit and, 244
   procyanidins and, 50
   pterostilbene and, 433, 439
   pulses and, 79
   pumpkins and, 159–60, 412
   quercetin and, 214, 221
   raspberries and, 419–20, 422
   red grapes and, 164, 393
   red meat and, 459
   red raspberries and, 122, 178, 418, 422, 472
   resveratrol and, 391, 393, 432, 433, 434, 437,
     438, 439–40, 444
   Rowan berries and, 419–20
   shogaols and, 297
   soy and, 73, 74–75, 79
   spinach and, 151, 387, 459, 461
   spirulina and, 18
   strawberries and, 122, 178, 419–20, 422, 471,
     472, 473
   sulforaphane and, 149
   tangeretin and, 246
   tetrahydrocurcumin (THC) and, 219
   thiacremonone and, 261
   tomatoes and, 151, 387, 484, 485–86, 486–87
   urolothins and, 403
   walnuts and, 341
   wheatgrass (chlorophyll/chlorophyllin) and,
     499–500
colorectal adenoma/colorectal adenomatous polyps/
     colorectal cancer
   algae and, **43**
   apples and, 50, 54, 474
   bananas and, 247, 474
   beans (legumes) and, 72
   Brussels sprouts juice and, 154, 155
   cherries and, 386
   cinnamon and, 163
   citrus fruit and, 244
   colorectal adenoma as precursor to *colorectal*
     cancer, 371

glucose and, 172, 186
glycosides in, 177, 180, 181
Helicobacter pylori and, 107–8, 175, 182, 190, 191
hyperglycemia and, 186
hypertension (high blood pressure) and, 186–87, **187–88**
inflammation and, 173, 174, 182, 183, 189, 369
influenza and, 188
intestinal cancer and, 101, 178, 421
intestinal pathogens and, 107
ischemia/ischemic stroke and, 101, 115, 119, 121, 138, 172, 183, 188
kidney stones and, 188
lipids and, 179, 186
liver cancer and, 48, 57, 58, 173, 181, 184, 311, 314, 315, 468–69, 477
low-density lipoprotein (LDL)/high-density lipoprotein (HDL) and, 182, 183–84, 185, 186
lung cancer and, 177, 180
lymphoma and, 177
myricetin in, 181
neurodegeneration and, 101, 119, 121, 138, 183, **188–89**
oral cancer and, 102, 122, 177, 178, 179–80, 422, 472
oral streptococii and, 190
ovarian cancer and, 175
oxidative damage/stress and, 172, 179, 184, 189, 192
oxygen radical absorbance capacity (ORAC) and, 124
P. gingivalis and, 189, 190
periodontis and, **189–90**
phenolic content in
cancer and, 48, 57, 58, 173, 175, 180–81, 182, 184, 301, 311, 314, 315, 477
cardiovascular (coronary artery/heart) disease and, 48, 57, 58, 173, 175, 180–81, 182, 184, 301, 311, 314, 315, 468–69, 477
diabetes and, 186–87
Helicobacter pylori (H. pylori) and, 190
hypertension and, 186–87
infections and, 175, 182, 192
phytochemicals in, 171, 175, 177, 178–80, 182, 184, 185, 187–88
polyphenols in, 182, 183, 185, 188–89, 191
proanthocyanidin in, 124, 125, 175, 176, 177, 179, 180, 181, 182, 186, 189, 191, 194
prostate cancer and, 101, 102, 122, 175, 176, 177, 178, 179–80, 421, 422, 472
pyelonephritis and, 173
pyuria and, 196

quercetin in, 98, 181
rutin in, 178
salicylic acid and, 193
skin cancer and, 180
spigallocatechin in, 181
squamous cell carcinoma and, 313
stomach cancer and, 101, 178, 421
triglycerides and, 172, 184
triterpenoids in, 177
tumors and, 179, 180
ulcers/peptic ulcers and, 175, 182, 190
urinary tract infections and, 171, 174, 175, 182, **191–96**
urostomies and, 196
V. harveyi and, 191
vascular diseases and, 101, 119, 121, 138, 183, 189
vasico-ureteric reflux and, 173
vitamin C (ascorbate/ascorbic acid) and, 172, 173

Crohn's disease
curcumin and, 200, 203, 214, 223, **225,** 231, 232
ginger and, **299–300**
inflammation and, 299
NF-kappaB and
curcumin and, 203, 204, 216, 227, 229, 231, 232, 233, 410
garlic and, 255, 257, 266, **284,** 285, 286, 288, 289, 290
ginger and, 294, 295, 298, 300
pomegranates and, 410
cruciferous vegetables
apoptosis and, 149, 160
cancer and, 143, 148, 150, 160, 267, 298, 373, 491–92
carotenoids in, 270
colon cancer and, 149
colorectal cancer and, 148
indole-3-carbinol in, 155, 160
isothiocyanates and, 149, 158
lung cancer and, 148, 155, 158
pancreatic cancer and, 149
prostate cancer and, 160
stroke and, 94
sulforaphane in, 159
cucumbers, 5, 45, 47, 139, 160, 390, 396, 457, 461
Cucumis trigonus Roxb., diabetes and, 248
cumin
diabetes and, 321, 464
NF-kappaB and
Alzheimer's disease and, 294
arthritis and, 203, 256, 410
asthma and, 204
atherosclerosis and, 204, 257, 295
cancer and, 216, 266, 298

dithiines, *cholesterol* and, 282
diuretic, prickly pear fruit as, 242
DMBA (7,12-dimethylbenzanthracene). *See*
7,12-dimethylbenz{a}anthracene
(DMBA)
DNA damage
apples/apple juice and, 46–47, 51, 116–17
berries and, 97, 100, 115–16, 116–17
blueberries (Vaccinium)/blueberry juice and,
46–47, 97, 105, 115–16, 116–17
cranberry juice and, 179
onions and, 367
quercetin and, 46, 116–17
red raspberry and, 97, 115–16
strawberries and, 46, 97, 115–16
sulforaphane and, 142–43
tomatoes and, 46
duodenal cancer, curcumin and, 220, 222
duodenal ulcers. See **ulcers**/*duodenal ulcers/peptic*
ulcers/ulcerative colitis
dyslipidemia, 10, 37, 136, 442, 476, 482
dyspepsia, cranberries/Pongamia pinnata and, 190,
251

E

E. coli, 191, 192–93, 194, 195, 232, 233, 415
EF24, *cancer* and, 211
EGCG (epigallocatechin (-3-) gallate), *oral cancer*
and, 218–19
elderberries, 97–98, 103, 104, 107–8, 108–9,
124, 169
ellagic acid
angiogenesis and, 441
apoptosis and, 297, 441
in *berries,* 95, 97, 115–16, 400, 411, 420
breast/mammary cancer and, 120
cancer and, 297, 441
DNA damage and, 97
esophageal cancer and, 99, 436, 476
inflammation and, 400
NF-kappaB and, 297, 441
Alzheimer's disease and, 294
arthritis and, 203, 256, 410
asthma and, 204
atherosclerosis and, 204, 257, 295
cancer and, 216, 266, 298
Crohn's disease and, 284, 300
diabetes and, 285
human immunodeficiency virus (HIV) and,
228
inflammatory diseases and, 410
multiple sclerosis and, 230, 288
myocardial infarction and, 227, 286
osteoporosis and, 231, 289
psoriasis and, 232

septic shock and, 233, 290
oxidative damage and, 416, 467, 468
in *pomegranates,* 400, 411
prostate cancer and, 403
in *raspberry juice,* 417
skin damage/wrinkles and, 95, 400, 411
ellagitannins, 100, 107, 118, 403, 405, 417,
420, 422, 471
endometrial cancer, 205, 260, 261, 370
endothelial dysfunction/function, 71–72, 81, 87, 88,
89, 316, 375, 442, 444
endotoxemia, chlorella and, 38
enoki/enokitake mushrooms, 326, 332–33
Enteromorpha prolifera, *skin cancer* and, 454
EOMA cell, *berries* and, 99, 102, 108
epicatechin, 44, 59, 181, 375, 473
epigallocatechin gallate (ECGC), 218–19, 443,
447
epilepsy, 308, 429, **446,** 448, 450, 452
erectile dysfunction, *antioxidants* and, **106**
ergothioneine, *atherosclerosis/mushrooms* and, 324
esophageal adenocarcinoma/esophageal cancer/
esophageal squamous cell carcinoma
Allium vegetables and, 373
berries and, 99, 102
blackberries and, 99, 102–3, 423, 436, 472
black raspberries and, 99, 102–3, 419, 420,
423, 425, 436, 472
broccoli and, 140
capsaicin and, 394
citrus fruit and, 244
cranberries and, 176
diallyl sulfide and, 272, 435–36
ellagic acid and, 99, 436, 476
fruits and, 261, 370
garlic and, 260, 261, 269, 370
lycopene and, 492–93
mushrooms and, 331
olive oil and, 358
onions and, 261, 370
phenethyl isothiocyanate and, 435–36
phytosterols and, 492–93
raw vegetables and, 373
resveratrol and, 99, 435–36
soy and, 78
strawberries and, 423, 436, 472, 475–76
tea and, 99, 436
tomatoes and, 492–93
vegetables and, 370
estrogen, 71, 73, 219, 220
eugenol
angiogenesis and, 297, 441
apoptosis and, 297, 441
cancer and, 297, 441
NF-kappaB and, 297, 441
Alzheimer's disease and, 294
arthritis and, 203, 256, 410

leukemia and, 470
low-density lipoprotein (LDL) and, 442
lung cancer and, 57, 58, 304, 371, 373
in *nuts,* 340
in *olives,* 358, 359
in *onions,* 57, 58, 59, 304, 369
in *oranges,* 387–88
in prickly pear fruit, 244
in purple grapes, 311
in *raspberries/raspberry juice,* 417–18
in *strawberries,* 465, 474–75
stroke and, 407, 409, 411, 495, 496, 497
in sweetie fruit, 308
in tea, 58, 59
in white grapefruit, 57
flavonols, 47, 48, 61, 71, 118, 123, 127, 175,
    177, 182, 371, 378
flaxseed, 76, 165, 266, 343, 353–54, 413
folate/folic acid, 4, 256, 342, 345, 354, 456
forestomach cancer, 220, 222, 305
formononetin, *colorectal adenoma* and, 371
fruit(s). *See also* specific types of
about, **241**
alimentary cancer and, 58
Alzheimer's disease and, **241**
as *antifungal,* **242**
as *antioxidant,* 48, 57, 58, 116, 120–21, 172,
    173, 180–81, 184, **242–43,** 339,
    404, 416, 420
arthritis and, **243**
atherosclerosis and, **243**
breast cancer and, 56, 159–60
cancer and, 241, **244–47**
    antioxidant activity and, 100, 116, 120–21,
        404, 416, 420
    cellular differentiation and, 220
    death risk and, 76, 80, 86
    phenolics and, 48, 57, 58, 173, 180–81,
        184, 301, 311, 314, 315, 468–69,
        477
    phytochemicals and, 493
    prostate cancer, 66
cardiovascular (coronary artery/heart) disease and,
    57, 58, 76, 80, 86, 152, 156, 173,
    247, 276, 306
cerebrovascular disease and, **247**
cholesterol and, 106
colon cancer and, 159–60
colorectal cancer and, 55, 246–47, 270, 474–75
death risk and, 86
dementia and, 241, **248**
diabetes and, **248–49**
esophageal cancer and, 261, 370
flavonoids in, 58
gastric cancer and, 159–60, 244
hyperlipidemia and, **250**
immune function and, **250**

inflammation and, **251**
lung cancer and, 159–60, 245
minerals in, 241
oxidative stress and, 116, 121, 416, 420
oxygen radical absorbance capacity (ORAC)
    and, 120–21
peripheral arterial disease and, **251**
phenolics in, 48, 58, 100, 120, 173, 180–81,
    184, 314, 315, 468, 477
phytochemicals in, 57, 58, 173, 180–81,
    241, 311, 314, 315, 468, 477
polyphenols in, 113, 118
Radical Fruits, 106
respiratory tract cancer and, 58
squamous cell carcinoma and, 261
stroke and, 94
ulcers and, 251
vitamins in, 241
weight loss and, 64
fucan, 11, 42–43, 454
fucoidan, *leukemia* and, 11, 453
fucoxanthin, 219, 461

G

galangin, *breast cancer* and, 305, 387
gallbladder cancer, 393, 459
gallocatechins, 181, 400
gallstone diseases/gallstones, 236–37, 277, 278,
    349, 377–78, 379, **379,** 393
gambogic acid, *cancer* and, 297
gamma-tocotrienol, *cardiovascular (coronary artery/
    heart) disease* and, 442
Ganoderma (mushroom), 246, 335, 336
garlic/garlic extract/garlic juice/garlic oil/garlic
    powder
    7,12-dimethylbenz{a}anthracene (DMBA)
        and, 269–70, 272
    about, 252
    acute myeloid leukemia and, 267
    aging and, **252,** 253, 255, 276, 291
    AIDS and, 255, 257, 266, 284, 285, 286,
        288, 289, 290
    Alistate, 290
    alk(en)yl thiosulfates in, 372
    allergies and, 255, 257, 266, 284, 285, 286,
        288, 289, 290
    allicin and, 269, 272–73, 274, 275, 280, 284
    alliin and, 269
    allylic compounds and, 374
    Alzheimer's disease and, 200, 252, 253, 255,
        257, 275, 276, 277, 291, **294,** 430
    angiogenesis and, 264–65, 293
    as *antibacterial,* 253
    as *anti-inflammatory,* 255
    as antimicrobial, 164–65, 262, 265, 280, 287

I

carteonoids in, 412
colon cancer and, 159–60, 412
cucurbitacins in, 412–13
diabetes and, 88, 89, 412, **413**
gastric cancer and, 159–60, 412
glucose and, 413
hyperglycemia and, 88, 89, **413,** 414
hypertension (high blood pressure) and, 88, 89,
    413, **414**
iron in, 412
lung cancer and, 159–60, 412
melanoma and, 413
Moschatin in, 413
nicotinic acid in, 413
phenolic compounds in, 88, 89, 413, 414
phytochemicals in, 88, 89, 413, 414
phytosterols in, 412
potassium in, 412
prostate cancer/hyperplasia and, 412, **414**
riboflavin in, 412
trigonelline in, 413
vitamins in, 412
punicalagins, 400, 405
purple cabbage, isothiocyanate in, 159
purple grapes/purple grape juice, 49, 311, 313,
    316, 318
purple raspberries, 415
pyelonephritis, cranberries and, 173
pyridoxine, in spirulina, 4
pyuria, cranberry juice and, 196

Q

quercetin
    as antimicrobial, 381
    as *antioxidant,* 60, 200, 295, 375
    apoptosis and, 473
    in *apples/apple juice,* 44, 46–47, 48–49, 50–51,
        56, 57, 116–17, 304, 373
    arthritis and, 174, 203, 369
    atherosclerosis and, 375
    blood pressure and, 380, 443, 447
    in *blueberries,* 46
    bone formation/loss and, 369
    breast cancer and, 305, 387
    broccoli and, 142
    cancer and, 370, 387
    cardiovascular (coronary/heart) disease and, 375,
        376, 442
    cerebral ischemia and, 376–77
    cerebrovascular disease and, 59–60
    colon cancer and, 214, 221
    in *cranberries,* 98, 181
    curcumin and, 200, 201, 431
    diabetes and, 238
    DNA damage and, 46, 116–17

glioma and, 435
hepatomas and, 473
hypertension and, 380
inflammation and, 174, 369
leukemia and, 370
in lingonberries, 98
lung cancer and, 304, 371
in *onions,* 48–49, 304, 367, 368, 369, 370,
    371, 373, 375, 376, 380, 381
oxidative stress and, 375
resveratrol and, 442
thrombosis (blood clots) and, 376

R

rabies virus, spirulina and, 28
Radical Fruits, *hypercholesterolemia* and, 106, 426,
    480–81
raisins, *oral health* and, 318
**raspberries/raspberry juice/raspberry
    seeds.** *See also* specific types of
    about, **415**
    anthocyanins in, 98, 242–43, 415, 417, 418
    as *antibacterial,* 107, **415,** 426
    as antimicrobial, 415, 426
    as antimutagenic, 425, 426
    as *antioxidant,* 97–98, 100, 103, 104, 116,
        121, 404, 415, **416–18,** 420, 469
    atherosclerosis and, 98
    breast cancer and, 101, 178, 421, 475
    cancer and, 103, 104, 121, 124, **418–26,** 474
    cervical cancer and, 100, 419, 422, 471, 475
    colon cancer and, 100, 101, 419–20, 422
    cytokines and, 417
    E. coli and, 415
    ellagic acid in, 417
    ellagitannins in, 100, 107, 417, 420, 422,
        471
    flavonoids in, 417–18
    gastroenteritis and, 415
    Helicobacter pylori and, 107–8
    hypercholesterolemia and, 106, **426,** 481
    intestinal cancer/pathogens and, 101, 107, 178,
        421, 426
    leukemia and, 122–23, 423, 472
    mutagenesis and, 426, 474
    oxidative damage/stress and, 416, 417
    oxygen radical absorbance capacity (ORAC)
        and, 124
    phenolic content in, 415, 416–17, 417–18
    phytochemicals in, 422
    polyphenols in, 100, 420, 422, 471
    proanthocyanidin in, 124, 417
    prostate cancer and, 101, 178, 421
    reactive oxygen species (ROS) and, 416
    stomach cancer and, 101, 178, 421

S

saffron, 165, 266
salicylic acid, *cranberry juice* and, 193
S-allyl cysteine/S-allylcysteine/S-allyl-L-
    cysteine/S-allylmercaptocysteine/S-
    allylmercapto-L-cysteine (SAMC)
  angiogenesis and, 297, 441
  apoptosis and, 262, 297, 441
  cancer and, 297, 441
  garlic and, 262, 270, 289
  gastric cancer and, 262
  neurodegeneration and, 289
  NF-kappaB and, 297, 441
    Alzheimer's disease and, 294
    arthritis and, 203, 256, 410
    asthma and, 204
    atherosclerosis and, 204, 257, 295
    cancer and, 216, 266, 298
    Crohn's disease and, 284, 300
    diabetes and, 285
    human immunodeficiency virus (HIV) and,
        228
    inflammatory diseases and, 410
    multiple sclerosis and, 230, 288
    myocardial infarction and, 227, 286
    osteoporosis and, 231, 289
    psoriasis and, 232
    septic shock and, 233, 290
  prostate cancer and, 263
Salmonella, 107, 223, 232, 415, 426
SAMC (S-allylmercapto-L-cysteine). *See* S-allyl
    cysteine/S-allylcysteine/S-allyl-L-
    cysteine/S-allylmercaptocysteine/S-
    allylmercapto-L-cysteine (SAMC)
saponins, in *beans (legumes),* 71
sarcoma, 211, 268
Sargassum fulvellum, *tumors* and, 455
sauerkraut, *chronic disease* and, 158
saw palmetto oil, *prostate hyperplasia* and, 414
Schisandra sphenathera, NF-kappaB and, 245
Schisantherin A., as *anti-inflammatory,* 245
schizandra, as *antioxidant,* 295
schleroderma, *avocados* and, **70**
sea buckthorn/sea buckthorn juice, 100, 101,
    121, 130, 178, 421, **455,** 471
sea vegetables, 2, 453, **453–55.** *See also*
    specific types of
seaweed, 10–11
selenium, 12, 13, 22, 37, 38, 41, 149, 456, 493
septic shock
  curcumin and, **232–33**
  NF-kappaB and
    curcumin and, 203, 204, 216, 227, 230,
        231, 232, 233, 410
    garlic and, 255, 257, 266, 284, 285, 286,
        288, 289, **290**

ginger and, 294, 295, 298, 300
pomegranates and, 410
serviceberries/serviceberry juice, 101, 121, 178
SFN (sulphoraphane). *See* sulforaphane (SFN)
shiitake *(Lentinula edodes)* mushrooms, 323, 325,
    326, 327–28, 328–29, 330, 331, 332,
    336, 337, 338
shogaols, *cancer* and, 296–97
**sickle cell anemia (and blood
    transfusions),** 29, 38, **290–91, 498,**
    499
silymarin, 174, 203, 288, 297, 369, 441
simvastatin, Hawthorn fruit and, 243, 250
skeletal muscle damage, 42, 137
skin health/problems. See also melanoma
  skin aging/damage, 233, 400, 411, 427
  skin cancer
    6-gingerol and, 296
    7,12-dimethylbenz{a}anthracene
        (DMBA) and, 272, 374
    apples and, 52
    bitter gourd and, 492
    black raspberries and, 419, 421–22
    broccoli and, 140, 141, 144–45, 147, 370
    citrus fruits and, 304
    coumarins and, 222–23
    cranberries and, 180
    curcumin and, 220, 222, 223
    diallyl sulfide and, 264
    Enteromorpha prolifera and, 454
    garlic and, 264, 272
    ginger and, 294
    limonene and, 304, 320
    luteolin and, 370
    lycopene and, 488
    mushrooms and, 328
    olive oil and, 360, 363
    onions and, 140, 370
    pomegranates and, 404
    resveratrol and, 427
    sea vegetables and, 453
    tomatoes and, 488, 492
  skin condition, in *urostomy* patients, *cranberry juice*
      and, 196
  skin papillo magenesis, chlorella and, 16
  skin photoprotection, red orange and, 385
smokers/smoking, chlorella as *antioxidant* to, 8
smoothies, spirulina in, 7
sodium spirulan, *atherosclerosis* and, 9–10
soy/soy products. *See also under* isoflavones/
    isoflavonoids; phytoestrogens
  aging/age-related diseases/diseases of old age and,
      77, 90
  atherosclerosis and, 79, 82, 91, 462, 464
  bladder cancer and, 77, 78
  blood pressure and, 81, 88
  body fat and, 84

watermelon(s)/watermelon juice, 55, 56, 122,
247, 308, 474, 497
weight loss, 29, **64,** 86, 92, **309, 338,** 366,
482
Welsh onion, 377, 380
wheatgrass (chlorophyll/chlorophyllin)/
wheatgrass juice
about, **498**
amino acids in, 502
anemia and, 498, 499
as anti-inflammatory, 502
as antimutagenic, 502
as antioxidant, 8, **499,** 501, 502
apigenin in, 502
breast cancer and, 499
cancer and, 458–59, **499–502**
colitis and, 498, **502**
colon cancer and, 459, 499–500, 501
colorectal cancer and, 499
dioxin and, 24
inflammatory bowel diseases and, 498, **502**
iron and, 498
lipids and, 499
liver cancer and, 501
myelodysplastic syndrome and, 498
myelotoxicity and, 499
phosphorous in, 498
protein in, 498
thalassemia and, 498
tumors and, 500–501
vitamins in, 498, 502
white button mushrooms, breast cancer/
phytochemicals and, 329
white cabbage, 157–58, 359, 392, 470
white cherries, hypercholesterolemia and, 106, 426,
481
white currants, 101, 121, 178, 421
white grapefruit, 57, 304, 373
white-green foods, cancer and, 152, 156, 266,
276
white kidney beans, diabetes and, 87
white onions, atherosclerosis and, 256
white tea, as antioxidant, 97
withanamides, Alzheimer's disease and, 96
wolfberry, Alzheimer's disease and, 241
wound healing/wounds, 70, 293, **293, 452**

X

xanthophyll, in green peppers, 397

Y

yellow onions, 139, 160, 369, 390, 396, 457,
461
yellow soybean, oxidative stress and, 80
yellow vegetables, 55, 247, 371, 474. See also
specific types of

Z

zerumbone, 297, 299
zhuling (Grifola umbellate pilat), bladder cancer and,
331–32
zinc, 26, 367, 456

About the Author

DR. BRIAN R. CLEMENT has directed the renowned Hippocrates Health Institute for more than three decades. He is internationally recognized for his relentless pursuit of complimentary health methods that support recovery and prevention of disease. For more than four decades, Dr. Clement has been personally involved in clinical research on a daily basis with the hundreds of thousands of people who have been through the program he developed and maintains. Research partners have included universities, physicians, and co-workers at the Institute itself. Many whole food supplement companies partner with Dr. Clement and Hippocrates in their pursuit to research the benefits of the products they offer. On several occasions, pioneering efforts have grown out of Clement's passionate pursuit for excellence.

Dr. Clement employs his mission statement, to unify the vast world of health professions, to set a round table and encourage discussion among his peers and adversaries. He believes it is time to put the person/patient first and stop perpetuating narrow perceptions and condemnation of what we do not understand as professionals. As the incidence of disease increases, Clement's determination equals it. His observation that catastrophic disorders are now affecting the youngest among us has him acutely concerned. When recently addressing a medical conference, he stated, "Disease is surmountable once we are willing to reengage sincere observation and utilization of the biological world that surrounds us." Dr. Clement hopes this three-volume series, *Food IS Medicine*, will make both patients and practitioners aware of the large quantity of scientific data that documents how the food we eat can either be our best friend or our worst foe.